BRONCHIAL ASTHMA

WITHDRAWN

BRONCHIAL ASTHMA

Principles
of Diagnosis
and Treatment

Second Edition

Edited by

M. ERIC GERSHWIN, M.D.

Section of Rheumatology/Allergy and Clinical Immunology
Department of Medicine
University of California
Davis, California

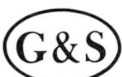

Grune & Stratton, Inc.

Harcourt Brace Jovanovich, Publishers

Orlando   New York   San Diego   Boston   London
San Francisco   Tokyo   Sydney   Toronto

Library of Congress Cataloging-in Publication Data

Bronchial asthma.

Includes bibliographies and index.
1. Asthma.   I. Gershwin, M. Eric, 1946–
[DNLM: 1. Asthma—diagnosis.   2. Asthma—therapy.
WF 553 B8693]
RC591.B753   1986   616.2′38   86-4721
ISBN 0-8089-1814-1

Grune & Stratton, Inc.
Orlando, Florida 32887

Distributed in the United Kingdom by
Grune & Stratton, Ltd.
24/28 Oval Road, London NW 1

Library of Congress Catalog Number 86-4721
International Standard Book Number 0-8089-1814-1
Printed in the United States of America
86 87 88 89   10 9 8 7 6 5 4 3 2 1

From M.E.G. with love to Tracy, who started it all.

"They asked if the sneezles
came after the wheezles,
Or if the first sneezle came first."

A.A. Milne from "Sneezles" in *Now We are Six,* Dutton and Co.,
New York, 1927

Contents

PART II: SPECIAL PROBLEMS

PART III: PATIENT MANAGEMENT

Preface to the First Edition

Asthma is the most common chronic disease of childhood and among the most frequent complaints of adults. When a national study was undertaken in 1975, asthma was found to account for nearly 2 million outpatient clinic visits and was the most frequent cause of absence from school and work. Moreover, more than 90 percent of patients with asthma required some form of intermittent drug therapy. These overwhelming statistics, as well as the chronic physically restrictive nature of asthma, result in significant stress to patients and families. Nonetheless, despite the widespread nature of asthma and the fact that it has been well characterized throughout recorded medical history, the basic disease process remains difficult to define. Indeed, asthma is clearly a syndrome of multiple etiologies interacting in the common pathway of reversible obstructive airway disease.

Because of the ubiquitous nature of asthma, a variety of physicians in many disciplines are called upon to treat patients. Although the majority of research of this disease occurs at large university medical centers, the bulk of medical care is delivered throughout the community. Indeed, asthma is a lifelong disease process that requires considerable education on the part of both the physician and the patient. At the University of California we have emphasized the need for continued feedback in postgraduate medical education. Toward this end we have sponsored a number of courses in the diagnosis and management of asthma and have often been requested to provide a textbook appropriate for the clinical practitioner. As an academician, this presents a formidable task because the patient population served by the university is often considerably more severe and/or acute than patients served in other facilities. Nonetheless, we strongly feel that a text that emphasizes the diagnosis and clinical management of patients with bronchial asthma would be well received and would serve as an important supplement to more detailed treatises. Moreover, the number of significant advances in the pharmacotherapy, immunotherapy, and biochemistry of bronchial asthma continue to necessitate up-to-date approaches.

With few exceptions, the approach to the treatment of asthma, as well as the general avenue of problem solving, has changed little over the past 25 years. There will never be a substitute for a thorough history and physical examination conducted by a skilled and concerned physician. Nonetheless, the discovery and study of IgE and its mediators, the significant improvement in the recognition of contributions of the major histocompatability loci and regulatory influences on lymphocyte subpopulations, and the refinements in pulmonary physiology, pharmacotherapeutics, and diagnostic technology have significantly influenced our concepts of etiology and intervention of disease. Patients with asthma may now look forward to a normal life span, uncomplicated by severe morbidity. Indeed, the care of patients with asthma can be a rewarding experience for both physicians and patients.

Newer technology must also ultimately be transferred from research ventures to training programs and then to community physicians. This volume has been aimed at just such a goal. It is with eager anticipation that its contributors look forward to the realization of these vistas, similar presentations in the future, and, most importantly, to the improved care and quality of life of patients who suffer from asthma.

Preface to the Second Edition

Asthma affects nearly 2 percent of the population, is especially troublesome in childhood, and accounts for more than 2 million outpatient clinic visits per year. In some studies, it is the most frequent cause of absence from school and work; 10 million Americans suffer from asthma. For many patients, asthma is merely a minor nuisance and requires only occasional use of medications. For others it is a chronic, unrelenting struggle. The care of asthmatics crosses many medical disciplines, including family practice, pediatrics, internal medicine as well as the subspecialties of allergy and chest medicine. Because of the ubiquitous problems encountered in the management of asthma, there are many textbooks available for physicians, nurses, chest physiotherapists, and of course, medical student education. These include impressive encyclopedic treatises and several smaller specialty books.

The principal objective of the first edition of this text, published six years ago, was to provide a shorter but very readable volume that would have utility to the practicing physician, but still would be sophisticated enough for university medical school libraries and, of course, subspecialists. This was a formidable task but the positive feedback and reviews of the first edition were very satisfactory. We have attempted to uphold the standard of the first edition in this second edition. The contributors to this volume are experts in their fields. Their tasks were to write material that is patient-oriented with abundant use of tables and figures. We prefer listing suggested reading at the end of a chapter, rather than a long annotated list of references. One of the major goals at the University of California at Davis is to further physician education in the diagnosis and management of asthma. It is from this experience that this book originally grew. The editor of the volume, myself, became an allergist, and became interested in asthma after one of my children developed and became especially bothered by asthma. This second edition, spurred by the extraordinarily good reviews of the first edition, attempts to further these goals of physician education towards a useful book that will be helpful to patients.

There are three major objectives of the text. First, we present data on definitions of asthma, study of epidemiology, pulmonary physiology and description of type I hypersensitivity reactions. We do not an attempt to explain the extraordinarily important basic science or the frontiers in immunology that have developed and continue to contribute to an understanding of asthma. Rather we present data that has clinical applications. Second, there is a section on special problems and considerations involved in any patient with asthma. These include the perennial issues of infections, the role of aspirin, metabisulfite and preservatives, the contribution of air pollution, and the special circumstances of allergic bronchopulmonary aspergillosis, occupational asthma, and of course, exercise and asthma. All of these are covered in individual chapters. Third, and most important is the detailed analysis of patient management. These include not only separate chapters on asthma in childhood versus asthma and adults, but also the pregnant asthmatic, asthma and anesthesia, and the problems of status asthmaticus in children and adults. Finally, because of the continued emphasis on aerosol treatment, we have a new chapter on the clinical considerations and decision-making using aerosol delivery systems. The majority of the second edition has been completely rewritten and approximately one third of the contributors are new to this edition. Indeed, we conclude with a new chapter on preventive medicine and patient education, describing many of the things that patients can obtain and find available through local support groups and respiratory societies.

As with any book there are going to be errors, including omissions. We have attempted to reduce these as much as possible. This is likewise true in the new self-assessment exam at the end, where the contributors have done their best to review all of our data. Ultimately such problems are my responsibility and (hopefully), are few in number. With the printing of a second edition comes the disturbing statistical feature that death from asthma has not changed, and perhaps, may even be increasing. Moreover, the incidence of asthma may be slightly increasing. These features are alarming and raise issues of the widespread influences of technology and urbanization. These are likewise discussed but clearly must await new data and the third edition.

Many people were extremely helpful in putting this volume together. To Steve Nagy goes my thanks for running our clinics, giving me the time to write and edit. Judy and Mark Van der Water, with their usual steadfast diligence, checked the accuracy of references. Finally a very special note of appreciation to Nikki Rojo, who organized and typed this whole book.

Contributors

JOANN BLESSING-MOORE, M.D.
Allergy/Pediatric Pulmonary Department
Palo Alto Medical Clinic
Clinical Faculty Department of Pediatrics
Stanford University/Children's Hospital at Stanford
Palo Alto, California

CARROLL E. CROSS, M.D.
Professor of Medicine and Physiology
Division of Pulmonary and Critical Care Medicine
University of California School of Medicine
Davis, California

HILLARY DON, M.D.
Associate Professor
Department of Anesthesia
School of Medicine
University of California;
Veterans Administration Medical Center
San Francisco, California

ROGER W. FOX, M.D.
Assistant Professor of Medicine
Department of Internal Medicine
Division of Allergy and Immunology
University of South Florida;
College of Medicine
James A. Haley V.A. Hospital
Tampa, Florida

DENNIS L. FUNG, M.D.
Associate Clinical Professor of Anesthesiology
Department of Anesthesiology
University of California School of Medicine
Davis, California

M. ERIC GERSHWIN, M.D.
Professor of Medicine
Chief, Division of Rheumatology/Allergy and Clinical Immunology
Department of Internal Medicine
University of California at Davis
Davis, California

SIMON GODFREY, M.D., Ph.D., F.R.C.P.
Professor of Pediatrics
Chairman, Department of Pediatrics
Haddassah University Hospital
Mount Scopus, P.O.B. 24035
Jerusalem, Israel

THEODORE A. GOODMAN, M.D.
Assistant Professor of Psychiatry
Department of Psychiatry
University of California at Davis
Davis, California

GEORGES M. HALPERN, M.D.
Visiting Scholar
Division of Rheumatology/Allergy and Clinical Immunology
Department of Internal Medicine
University of California School of Medicine
Davis, California

FREDERICK W. HANSON, M.D.
Professor of Obstetrics and Gynecology
Division of Reproductive Biology and Medicine
Department of Obstetrics and Gynecology
University of California School of Medicine
Davis, California

ROBERT S. HOWARD, J.D., Ph.D., M.D.
Pulmonary Medicine Fellow
Division of Pulmonary Medicine
University of California, Davis, Medical Center
Davis, California

GARY INCAUDO, M.D.
Assistant Clinical Professor
Departments of Medicine and Pediatrics
University of California at Davis
Davis, California

RICHARD E. KANNER, M.D., F.A.C.P., F.C.C.P.
Associate Professor of Medicine
Division of Respiratory, Critical Care, and Occupational Medicine
Department of Internal Medicine
University of Utah School of Medicine
Salt Lake City, Utah

EDWIN L. KLINGELHOFER, Ph.D.
Professor Emeritus of Psychology
Department of Psychology
California State University
Sacramento, California

GEOFFREY KURLAND, M.D.
Assistant Professor of Pediatrics
Chief, Pediatric Pulmonary Diseases
Department of Pediatrics
University of California at Davis Medical Center
Sacramento, California

ALBIN B. LEONG, M.D.
Assistant Clinical Professor of Pediatrics
Department of Pediatrics
University of California at Davis Medical Center
Sacramento, California

GLEN A. LILLINGTON, M.D., M.S. (Med), F.R.C.P.(C), F.A.C.P.
Professor of Medicine
Chief, Division of Pulmonary-Critical Care Medicine
Department of Medicine
University of California (Davis) School of Medicine
Davis, California

RICHARD F. LOCKEY, M.D.
Professor of Medicine and Pediatrics
Chief, Division of Allergy and Immunology
University of South Florida;
College of Medicine
James A. Haley V.A. Hospital
Tampa, Florida

MANUEL LOPEZ, M.D.
Associate Professor of Medicine
Head, Clinical Immunology Laboratories
Section of Clinical Immunology
Department of Medicine
Tulane University School of Medicine
New Orleans, Louisiana

JOHN MILLS, M.D., F.A.C.P.
Professor of Medicine, Microbiology, and Pharmacy
University of California, San Francisco
Chief, Division of Infectious Diseases
San Francisco General Hospital
San Francisco, California

STEPHEN M. NAGY, JR., M.D.
Clinical Professor of Medicine
Codirector, Allergy Clinic
Department of Medicine
University of California School of Medicine
Davis, California

HAROLD S. NOVEY, M.D., F.A.C.P.
Clinical Professor of Medicine
Division of Basic and Clinical Immunology
Department of Medicine
University of California, Irvine Medical Center
Orange, California

GEORGE T. O'CONNOR, M.D.
Research Fellow in Clinical Epidemiology of Lung Disease
Department of Medicine
Channing Laboratory, Brigham and Women's Hospital
Harvard Medical School
Boston, Massachusetts

PHILIP E.S. PALMER, M.D., F.R.C.P. (Ed), F.R.C.R.
Professor of Diagnostic Radiology
Department of Radiology
University of California School of Medicine
Davis, California

GIBBE H. PARSONS, M.D.
Associate Professor of Medicine
Division of Pulmonary Medicine and Critical Care
University of California, Davis, School of Medicine
Davis, California

OTTO G. RAABE, Ph.D.
Professor of Civil Engineering and of Veterinary Pharmacology and
Toxicology
University of California at Davis
Davis, California

JOHN SALVAGGIO, M.D.
Henderson Professor of Medicine
Chairman, Department of Internal Medicine
Tulane University School of Medicine
New Orleans, Louisiana

MARC SCHENKER, M.D.
Assistant Professor of Medicine
Director, Occupational and Environmental Health Unit
Department of Internal Medicine
University of California, Davis
Davis, California

ARIF SEYAL, M.D.
Clinical Instructor in Medicine
Division of Allergy
Department of Internal Medicine
University of California at Davis
Davis, California

R. MICHAEL SLY, M.D.
Director of Allergy and Immunology
Children's Hospital National Medical Center;
Professor of Child Health and Development
George Washington University School of Medicine and Health Sciences
Washington, D.C.

N. TY SMITH, M.D.
Professor of Anesthesiology
Department of Anesthesiology
University of California School of Medicine
San Diego, California

FRANK E. SPEIZER, M.D.
Associate Professor in Medicine
Channing Laboratory, Brigham and Women's Hospital
Harvard Medical School
Boston, Massachusetts

JOE P. TUPIN, M.D.
Professor of Psychiatry
Department of Psychiatry
University of California at Davis
Davis, California

SVERRE VEDAL, M.D.
Assistant Professor of Medicine
Department of Medicine
University of British Columbia
Vancouver General Hospital
Vancouver, British Columbia, Canada

ADAM WANNER, M.D.
Professor of Medicine
Chief, Division of Pulmonary Medicine
Department of Internal Medicine
University of Miami School of Medicine
Miami, Florida

STEPHEN I. WASSERMAN, M.D.
Professor of Medicine
Chief, Division of Allergy
University of California School of Medicine
San Diego, California

SUETARO WATANABE, M.D.
Research Associate Professor of Medicine
Division of Respiratory, Critical Care, and Occupational Medicine
Department of Internal Medicine
University of Utah School of Medicine
Salt Lake City, Utah

SCOTT T. WEISS, M.D., M.S.
Associate Professor of Medicine
Channing Laboratory, Brigham and Women's Hospital
Harvard Medical School
Boston, Massachusetts

PART I

Definitions and Host Responses to Bronchospasm

George T. O'Connor
Scott T. Weiss
Frank E. Speizer

1

The Epidemiology of Asthma

Population-based studies of asthma provide information on disease occurrence, natural history, and etiologic risk factors. These data may give the practitioner insights of clinical importance and may offer the investigator clues regarding the etiology and pathophysiology of the disease. In addition, quantitative information on asthma occurrence, morbidity, and mortality is of value to health care planners. This chapter will focus on the definition of asthma, an epidemiologic view of bronchial reactivity, incidence and prevalence, risk factors, and natural history of the disease.

DEFINITION OF ASTHMA

A critical first step in the study of any disease is the creation of a precise definition. This has been a major problem with studies of asthma. While there is no universally accepted definition of asthma, most investigators and clinicians would agree with a conceptual definition of asthma focusing on bronchial hyperreactivity, episodic or variable airflow limitation, and the presence of symptoms related to these physiologic abnormalities. An often-quoted conceptual definition is that proposed by the American Thoracic Society in 1962:

Asthma is a disease characterized by an increased responsiveness of the trachea and bronchi to various stimuli and manifested by a widespread narrowing of the airways that changes in severity either spontaneously or as a result of therapy.

BRONCHIAL ASTHMA, Second Edition
ISBN 0-8089-1814-1

The term "asthma" is not appropriate for the bronchial narrowing which results solely from widespread bronchial infection . . .; from destructive disease of the lung e.g., pulmonary emphysema; or from cardiovascular disorders.

Even if such a conceptual definition is accepted, a number of difficulties remain. There is no agreement on what number or severity of symptoms must be present to constitute a diagnosis of asthma. It is not certain whether individuals with bronchial hyperreactivity and symptomatic episodes of increased airflow limitation in the setting of chronic bronchitis and/or fixed airflow limitation should be considered to have asthma. There is evidence that such hyperreactivity may differ from that found in "pure" or atopic asthma. It is unclear whether "wheezy bronchitis" in children is distinct from asthma by virtue of an infectious etiology or whether the former is in fact indistinguishable from the latter.

As difficult as it is to agree upon a conceptual definition, the choice of an operational definition of asthma for use in epidemiologic study may be even more problematic. An operational definition must be precise and concrete, consisting of criteria which may be met by objective data feasible to collect.

A number of different operational definitions have been used for the study of asthma. Some of these definitions have been based solely on subjective criteria, while others have relied on more objective data. For example, a case of asthma may be defined as an affirmative response when a subject is asked whether he or she has or has had asthma or has been diagnosed by a physician as having asthma. Such an operational definition is susceptible to bias due to the tendency for physicians to diagnose young, atopic, and non-smoking subjects as "asthmatic" while labeling older, nonatopic, and smoking persons with similar symptoms as having "chronic obstructive pulmonary disease." Access to medical care obviously may influence the likelihood of being labeled as asthmatic in such a definition of disease. Alternatively, an operational definition of asthma may be based on the presence of specific symptoms, such as attacks of wheezing and dyspnea. Nonspecificity of symptoms is the major problem with such a definition. Symptoms in combination with the results of physician examination, pulmonary function testing, and/or bronchial challenge testing could be used in an operational definition of asthma; however, cost would be increased, number of subjects reduced, and criteria difficult to agree upon. Finally, hospital or practitioner records indicating a diagnosis of asthma may be used, but selection bias and observer bias limit the value of such an operational definition of asthma.

PREVALENCE AND INCIDENCE

Asthma is a common disease which is responsible for a large number of hospital admissions and outpatient visits. The overall point prevalence of asthma—i.e., the prevalence of recently active asthma—in the United States is approximately 3–4 percent according to several population-based surveys (see Table 1-1). Slightly higher prevalence has been found in the south and west of the U.S. than in other regions. A population-based study in Tucson, Arizona found an overall prevalence of 6.6 percent. This high prevalence in Tucson may reflect the effects of migration or of environmental factors such as allergen exposure. The cumulative prevalence of asthma—i.e., the prevalence of having ever had asthma—was found to be similar in Michigan and in Connecticut in studies of population-based samples: 7 percent among males and 5–6 percent among females.

Asthma prevalence has been reported to be slightly higher among males than females. Male predominance is most striking among children, in whom male:female ratios of up to 2:1 have been found in some population-based samples. Different asthma prevalences in boys and girls may result from differing patterns of lung growth, differences in environmental exposures, or differential biases in disease reporting or detection. During most of adulthood, there appears to be little difference in prevalence between men and women. Male predominance among those 65 years old and over was found in the 1970 National Health Survey but has not been observed in other investigations.

The prevalence of asthma varies with age (Fig. 1-1). Prevalence is relatively high in childhood, declining in adolescence and young adulthood, and then rising during middle age and later years. High remission rates among childhood asthmatics and the occurrence of bronchial hyperreactivity associated with chronic obstructive pulmonary disease in older individuals are probably important determinants of this relationship of asthma prevalence to age.

The incidence of *new* cases of asthma also varies with age. The Tucson group has studied asthma incidence using a prospective design, following 3432 subjects who initially denied asthma for an average of 3.5 years (Table 1-2). Forty-nine new diagnoses of asthma were made, an overall incidence of .0041 cases per person-year. The highest incidence of new cases of asthma occurred among children, but new cases occurred throughout adulthood as well. About half of the new diagnoses of asthma in subjects 40 years old and older were made in individuals already carrying a diagnosis of chronic bronchitis or emphysema. In a population survey in Tecumseh, Michigan, almost 50 percent of asthmatic respondents dated the onset of asthma to before age ten, while 25 percent had experienced the onset of asthma after age 40.

The prevalence of asthma has been investigated throughout the world, but many of these studies suffer from imprecise or unstated operational definitions of asthma. These data indicate a wide range of point prevalence, from less than 1 percent among Tokyo school children to a remarkable 35 percent among similar-aged children in the Western Caroline Islands. Among industrialized western nations, reported point prevalence has varied from 1 to

Table 1-1
Asthma Prevalence, U.S. Studies

Location (Authors)	Year Reported	Point Prevalence	Cumulative Prevalence	Comments
Berlin, New Hampshire (Ferris and Anderson)	1962	0.4%M 0.7%F		Age ≥25. Definition: Bronchial asthma diagnosed and still present. "Still present" may have reduced reporting of asthma.
Iowa (Smith and Knowler)	1965	3.2–3.8%		Narrow definition requiring attacks precipitated by specific exposures or worse in early-morning hours.
National Health Survey	1970	3%		Survey of national sample of households. Definition: Saw physician for asthma within past 12 months. South and West greater than Northeast.
Tecumseh, Michigan (Broder et al.)	1974	4.2%M 3.5%F	7.2%M 6.0%F	Probable asthma diagnosed when asthma or wheezing reported by subject along with 2 out of 3 other criteria (associated with attacks of shortness of breath, attributed to allergens, or diagnosis by examining physician).
Tucson, Arizona (Dodge and Burrows)	1980	6.9%M 6.3%F		Definition: Ever had asthma *and* has seen physician about asthma *and* attack or therapy within past year.
Lebanon, Connecticut (Schachter et al.)	1984		7%M 5%F	Age ≥7. Definition: Ever had bronchial asthma.

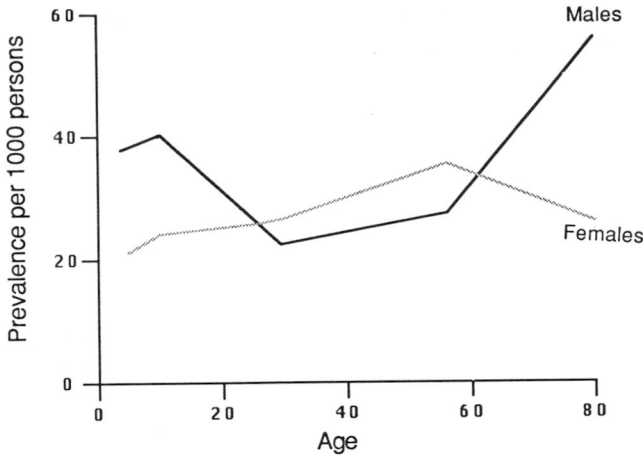

Fig. 1-1. Prevalence of asthma in the United States, 1970, by age and sex, based on data from the Health Interview Survey of the U.S. National Center for Health Statistics. (From Speizer FE: "Epidemiological Aspects of Asthma," Triangle 17:117–123, 1978. Used with permission.)

Table 1-2

Observed and Expected Asthma Incidence by Age and Sex[a]

Age	Asthma Incidence		Expected* Asthma Incidence	
	Men	Women	Men	Women
0–4	1.4†	0.9	1.4	1.0
5–9	1.0	0.7	0.4	0.6
10–14	0.2	0.3	0.3	0.3
15–19	—	—	0.2	0.2
20–29	0.2	0.4	0.1	0.3
30–39	—	0.4	0.2	0.2
40–49	—	0.4	0.1	0.2
50–59	—	0.5	0.3	0.2
60–69	0.3	0.8	0.2	0.2
>70	0.2	0.6	††	††

[a] Adapted from Dodge R, Burrows B: The prevalence and incidence of asthma and asthma-like symptoms in a general population sample. Am Rev Respir Dis 122:567–575, 1980
* Estimates made retrospectively from cross-sectional data on age of disease onset.
† Incidence expressed as cases per 100 person-years at risk.
†† Number of subjects in this group is too small to determine retrospective estimates of incidence.

7

6 percent. While results of different studies cannot be compared with certainty, the magnitude of variation suggests important genetic and environmental determinants of asthma which have yet to be elucidated.

Although it is difficult to compare the results of prevalence studies from different time periods because of methodologic differences, there is evidence to suggest that the prevalence of asthma may be increasing. A 1928–1931 U.S. Public Health Service survey found asthma prevalence to be less than 1 percent for all age groups, substantially less than the prevalence found by more recent reports. A similar trend is suggested by reports from other countries such as Japan, where it has been estimated that the prevalence of asthma doubled between 1955 and 1971. Whether a real increase in asthma prevalence with time is occurring will remain uncertain until a large population can be followed longitudinally using standard methodology.

BRONCHIAL REACTIVITY

Increased bronchial reactivity to nonspecific bronchoconstricting stimuli is a characteristic shared by all asthmatics and is a fundamental property of the disease. Bronchial hyperreactivity per se, however, does not constitute asthma and is found in some individuals with no history or symptoms of asthma. Thus, bronchial hyperreactivity is necessary but may not be sufficient for asthma to occur, and other physiologic and immunologic factors also must play important roles.

In population-based samples, bronchial reactivity has been found to occur in a unimodal distribution skewed toward hyperresponsiveness (Fig. 1-2). Asthmatics fall at the most responsive end of the curve, and most nonasthmatics fall in the middle or least responsive portions of the curve, but there

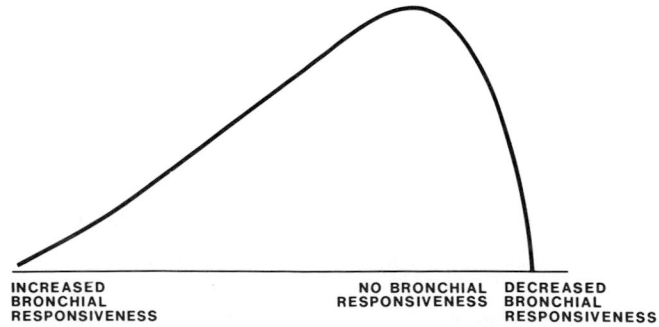

INCREASED   NO BRONCHIAL   DECREASED
BRONCHIAL   RESPONSIVENESS   BRONCHIAL
RESPONSIVENESS   RESPONSIVENESS

Fig. 1-2. Idealized distribution of bronchial reactivity in a population-based sample.

is overlap between the responsiveness of asthmatics and normals. The bronchial reactivity of a particular individual or group is determined by a variety of factors. (Heredity is an important determinant of bronchial reactivity as indicated by the greater intrapair correlation for methacholine responsiveness in monozygotic twins than in dizygotic twins. Environmental factors also appear to be important determinants of bronchial reactivity. There is evidence that respiratory infection, exposure to specific antigens, exposure to air pollutants, and cigarette smoking may all affect bronchial reactivity. Bronchial reactivity may change over time, but at present no data are available on longitudinal tracking of bronchial reactivity in population-based samples.

Preliminary evidence from several sources indicates that bronchial reactivity may vary with age in a pattern similar to that of asthma prevalence. Relatively high reactivity is found in childhood, declining to a low point in young adulthood, then increasing throughout middle age and later years (Fig. 1-3). In a population-based sample of subjects aged 6–58, Weiss et al. found that 22 percent of subjects less than 24 years old, but only 7 percent of subjects over 24 years old, experienced a drop in FEV_1 of 9 percent or greater in response to eucapneic hyperpnea with cold air. Relatively high bronchial reactivity in childhood may relate to the high incidence of respiratory infection in this group or to intrinsic properties of growing lungs. The high level of reactivity among the elderly may result from the effects of long-term environmental exposures or from the aging process itself. This relationship of bronchial reactivity to age may play a major role in the relationship between asthma prevalence and age.

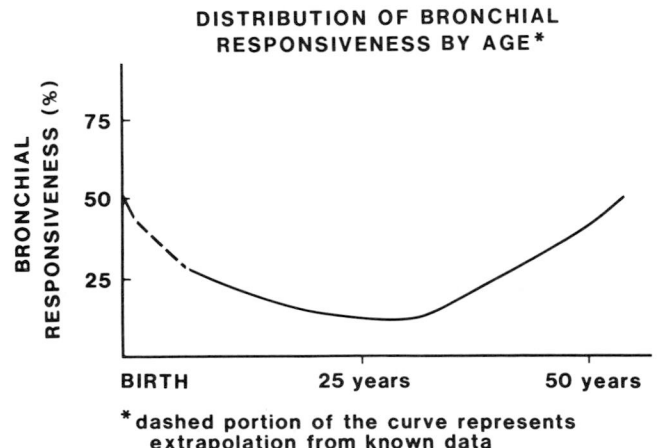

DISTRIBUTION OF BRONCHIAL RESPONSIVENESS BY AGE*

*dashed portion of the curve represents extrapolation from known data

Fig. 1-3. Relationship between bronchial reactivity and age. (Based on unpublished data from East Boston, Tucson, and the Netherlands.)

Nonspecific bronchial challenge testing is a very valuable tool for investigating the pathophysiology of asthma, but its role in clinical practice is limited. The majority of cases of asthma can be diagnosed on the basis of history, physical exam, and routine spirometry with bronchodilator testing, and only a minority of problematic cases (e.g., the occasional asthmatic who presents with unexplained cough as the only symptom) requires nonspecific challenge testing to establish a diagnosis. Bronchial challenge testing may be used to monitor the long-term effects of asthma therapy, but most pulmonary physicians do not find this necessary. Nonspecific bronchial challenge testing may be useful in the occupational setting, both to screen for hyperreactive individuals who might require protection from certain workplace exposures and to document adverse effects among exposed workers. Challenge testing with specific agents encountered in the workplace may be useful in some situations to document individual susceptibility to particular exposures. Finally, in population-based studies, nonspecific challenge testing may provide a marker for identifying people who may subsequently be at risk of developing asthma or other chronic obstructive lung disease upon exposure to other risk factors.

RISK FACTORS FOR ASTHMA

Possible risk factors for the development of asthma are listed in Table 1-3, along with important findings which link each factor to asthma. Asthma appears to be a multifactorial disease which may be caused by genetic or environmental factors or by the interaction of both in some individuals.

Heredity

Heredity is an important risk factor for the development of asthma, but little is known about the mode of inheritance. Familial aggregation of asthma has been well documented, but this finding alone does not determine whether common genetic makeup or common environmental exposures, or both, are responsible. A large study of twins in Sweden found a 19-percent concordance for asthma among monozygotic twins, compared to 4.8-percent concordance among dizygotic twins. This finding suggests a genetic contribution to the development of asthma, although common environmental exposures cannot be entirely excluded as a cause of such concordance, since monozygotic twins share more common environmental exposure than do dizygotic twins. Since asthma is a common, multifactorial disease which may involve incomplete penetrance, a precise mode of inheritance is not likely to be

Table 1-3

Selected Possible Risk Factors for Asthma

Risk Factors	Evidence
Heredity	Familial aggregation
	Twin concordance studies
	Twin intrapair correlation of bronchial reactivity
Atopy	Clinical importance of allergic ("extrinsic") asthma
	Association of asthma prevalence with serum IgE level, blood eosinophil count
Respiratory infection	Increased bronchial reactivity with URI
	Wheezing, increased bronchial reactivity following severe childhood lower respiratory infection
Cigarette smoking	
Active	Increase in airway resistance after acute smoking
	Increased bronchial reactivity among chronic smokers
	Wheeze among smokers
Passive	Associations between childhood asthma and persistent wheeze and maternal smoking
Air pollution	Increased morbidity among asthmatics during acute air pollution episodes
	SO_2 and O_3 cause bronchoconstriction in asthmatics
	O_3 increases bronchial reactivity in normal subjects
Occupational exposures	Clinical importance
	In vitro effects of TDI on bronchial smooth muscle
	Cotton bract extract increases bronchial reactivity in normal, previously unexposed subjects
Chemicals in food and drugs	ASA, tartarizine dye, and sodium metabisulfite precipitate asthma in sensitive individuals

established. The inherited trait may be the genetic predisposition to bronchial hyperreactivity, and asthma may only occur when there is interaction with other risk factors.

Atopy

Allergy plays a major role in many cases of asthma by precipitating or aggravating symptoms. Such patients ("extrinsic" asthma), as well as some patients whose symptoms cannot be related to allergen exposure ("intrinsic" asthma), frequently display evidence of an atopic disposition: increased immediate hypersensitivity to skin testing with common allergens, elevated serum IgE level, and blood eosinophilia. A positive association between asthma prevalence and both skin test reactivity and serum IgE level has been observed in population-based samples. Many asthmatics, however, do not have allergic symptoms or findings of atopy. Furthermore, many individuals with allergic symptoms and laboratory manifestations of atopy do not have asthma.

Whether there is a direct relationship between atopy and nonspecific bronchial reactivity is not known. Numerous investigators have found that subjects with hay fever have bronchial reactivity which is greater than that of subjects without hay fever, although less than that of asthmatics. Population-based studies of atopy, as assessed by skin testing, and nonspecific bronchial reactivity have yielded conflicting results. Welty et al. studied 171 adults in East Boston, Massachusetts, by means of eucapneic hyperventilation with subfreezing air (cold air challenge test) and skin tests using 4 common environmental antigens. There was no significant association between skin test reactivity and bronchial reactivity. Cockroft et al. studied 400 randomly selected college students by means of histamine challenge tests and allergy skin tests. The prevalence of bronchial hyperreactivity increased with increasing atopic grade. There was a small correlation between the concentration of histamine provoking a 20-percent reduction in FEV_1 (PC_{20}) and atopy grade among the subgroup with bronchial hyperreactivity, but no correlation was found for the overall sample. These studies differ not only in the populations sampled but also in the tests of airway responsiveness and in the definitions of atopy used. The potential for atopy and the potential for bronchial hyperreactivity may be independently inherited traits. Allergens may act as modifiers of bronchial responsiveness in atopic individuals by provoking the release of substances such as histamine, prostaglandins, and leukotrienes. Such a mechanism could account for the increased airway responsiveness found in hay fever sufferers. Genetic independence of bronchial reactivity and atopy has not been confirmed.

Respiratory Infection

Respiratory infection can precipitate exacerbations in asthmatic individuals, but its role in causing the development of asthma is not certain. A number of studies have found evidence of a relationship between respiratory infection and bronchial reactivity. Some investigators have found increased bronchial reactivity in association with viral upper respiratory infection in otherwise healthy subjects. This effect of a respiratory infection may be due to vagally mediated reflexes, decreased beta-adrenergic sensitivity, increased mucosal permeability, or alterations of immunologic status.

Long-term effects of respiratory infection on asthma symptoms and bronchial reactivity are more difficult to study. Several studies have found increased respiratory symptoms and airway responsiveness in subjects with histories of severe childhood respiratory infections requiring hospitalization. The follow-up of only approximately one-third of the patients identified from hospital records in these studies is a source of possible selection bias. A recent study by Pullan and Hey identified 180 infants hospitalized for proven respiratory syncytial virus (RSV) lower respiratory infections and evaluated 130 of these children 10 years later. Compared to a group of control children, the RSV-infected children were more likely to have experienced wheezing and had greater bronchial reactivity. Fewer of the RSV-infected children had positive allergy skin tests than did the controls. Parental cigarette smoking was more common among the RSV-infected children than among the controls and must be considered a potential confounder in this study.

Weiss et al. examined bronchial reactivity to hyperpnea with cold air 5 years after a 2-year prospective assessment of respiratory illness in children aged 5–9. Children with a prior history of croup or bronchiolitis or more than 2 acute lower respiratory illnesses in the 2 years of prospective study had greater bronchial reactivity to cold air than did children without such infections.

These findings may reflect damage to the growing lungs caused by respiratory infection. Alternatively, certain children may be more susceptible to severe respiratory infections because of an existing predisposition to bronchial hyperreactivity. Only longitudinal studies of respiratory symptoms and bronchial reactivity starting in childhood will be able to resolve this issue. The long-term impact of respiratory infection in adults on bronchial reactivity and respiratory symptoms has not been studied.

Cigarette Smoke

A link between exposure to cigarette smoke and the development of asthma has been found in a number of physiologic studies. An acute increase in airway resistance has been observed immediately after cigarette smoking, although an acute change in bronchial reactivity after smoking has not been demonstrated. Longtime cigarette smokers were found to have greater bronchial reactivity than nonsmokers in one investigation of healthy volunteers. Cigarette smoking has been found to increase airway mucosal permeability, which could increase penetration of bronchoconstricting agents or allergens. Cigarette smoking is associated with elevation of serum IgE and blood eosinophilia, suggesting alteration of immune status as another possible mechanism by which smoking may be related to asthma.

Epidemiologic data on active cigarette smoking and asthma are not conclusive. Although the prevalence of asthma has been found not to differ between current smokers and never smokers, this does not exclude the possibility of an etiologic association of smoking and asthma. If smokers tend to develop asthma but asthmatics tend to either stop smoking or not take up smoking in the first place, then an increased prevalence of asthma among current smokers might not occur. If this is the case, one would expect an increased prevalence of asthma among ex-smokers. Population-based studies in Tucson, Arizona and Tecumseh, Michigan have reported slightly greater asthma prevalence among ex-smokers than among other groups, but the differences were not statistically significant. In the Tucson study, subjects who developed new onset of asthma during prospective follow-up were more likely to be smokers than were those not developing asthma, although this difference was significant only for subjects less than 40 years of age and the number of new cases of asthma was small.

Studies of passive cigarette smoke exposure and asthma have yielded suggestive but inconclusive results. The symptoms of many asthmatic children are exacerbated by parental smoking and often improve when parents stop smoking, but this does not establish a causal relationship. Gortmaker et al. analyzed data from 2 random household-health surveys and found a significant association between maternal smoking and childhood asthma. They calculated that from 18 to 34 percent of asthma in their sample could be attributed to maternal smoking. The possibility of recall bias cannot be excluded, however, so these data must be interpreted with caution. Weiss et al. studied 650 children aged 5–9 and found a significant association between persistent wheeze and parental cigarette smoking. Bronchial reactivity to cold air, however, was not significantly correlated with parental smoking in 173 children aged 12–16 studied by the same group. The relationship between passive smoking and bronchial reactivity is currently being investigated in several population-based studies.

Air Pollution

Air pollution is another environmental exposure which may play a role in the development of asthma. Asthmatics have experienced increased mortality and morbidity during severe air pollution episodes and also have been found to experience increased morbidity and hospital admissions in association with more typical levels of specific pollutants. Laboratory investigations have documented bronchoconstriction following controlled exposure to sulfur dioxide. Temporary increases in bronchial reactivity have been observed in normal subjects following brief exposure to high concentrations of ozone. Recent exposure-chamber studies have observed increased bronchial reactivity in normal subjects exercising while exposed to ozone levels similar to those currently encountered in parts of the U.S. The current evidence from population-based data on the relation between the prevalence of wheeze or asthma and air pollution suggests that exacerbation of disease is increased with increasing pollution levels, but there is no conclusive evidence that current U.S. levels of pollution are causing an increased incidence of disease.

Occupational Exposures

Asthma may be aggravated or occur for the first time in relation to exposure to substances encountered in the workplace, but it is not known whether certain occupational exposures are capable of causing bronchial hyperreactivity and asthma de novo or whether they are providing the stimulus needed for a latent asthmatic predisposition to become clinically manifest. For example, exposure to Toluene Diisocyanate (TDI), a recognized cause of occupational asthma in about 5 percent of exposed workers, may result in hypersensitivity associated with tolyl-specific IgE, but there is also evidence of a direct effect of TDI on bronchial smooth muscle. Investigations utilizing measurements of bronchial reactivity prior to employment and after a period of workplace exposure may help resolve the question of causation and further define factors which determine individual susceptibility.

Byssinosis provides another important model of how an environmental exposure can actually cause symptomatic bronchial hyperreactivity. Byssinosis is an occupational disorder in which wheezing, dyspnea, cough, and bronchial hyperreactivity appear to be caused by exposure to high levels of cotton dust encountered in the textile industry. No evidence of any allergic mechanism has been found, and inhalation of cotton bract extract has been shown to increase bronchial reactivity in normal subjects exposed for the first time. Some component of cotton bract extract appears to exert a pharmacological effect causing increased bronchial reactivity. Symptomatic byssinosis is much more common among smokers than among nonsmokers, suggesting an important interaction between cigarette smoke and cotton dust exposure.

Drugs and Food Additives

The many medications and food additives to which present-day populations are exposed include a variety of substances which may precipitate asthma attacks in sensitive individuals. A few examples include aspirin, tartarazine food dye, bisulfites (the use of which has recently been restricted in the U.S.), and a number of antibiotics. These agents may exacerbate asthma by a variety of mechanisms. Antibiotics, for example, may lead to IgE-mediated hypersensitivity reactions. Aspirin leads to asthma attacks in sensitive individuals by inhibiting cyclooxygenase and thereby altering the distribution of arachidonic acid metabolites. There is no evidence that these substances represent an important cause of the development of asthma or bronchial hyperreactivity in population-based samples; however, for the individual patient it is critical to identify these specific sensitivities, and important insights into the pathophysiology of asthma may result from the study of these phenomena.

Interrelationship Between Risk Factors

Important interrelationships exist between the possible risk factors which have been discussed separately. Cigarette smoking is associated with elevations of serum IgE and blood eosinophil counts. Both active and passive smoking are associated with an increased frequency of respiratory infection. There is some evidence that infection may predispose to the development of atopy, but this remains controversial. Investigation of the role of any of these factors in the pathogenesis of asthma must account for potential confounding by the other factors as well as real biologic interaction between them.

NATURAL HISTORY

Course and Severity

The course of asthma is quite variable, some asthmatics remaining subject to symptoms indefinitely while others experience complete remission. A number of studies have indicated that 30–70 percent of childhood asthmatics greatly improve or become asymptomatic by adulthood. Asthma during adulthood is less likely to remit than is childhood disease, although some adult asthmatics do improve or remit. The importance of asthma therapy, avoidance of allergens, and elimination of other environmental exposures in causing remission, rather than merely controlling symptoms temporarily, is not known, but there is evidence that bronchodilators and avoidance of allergens may lead to substantial long-term reductions in nonspecific bronchial reactivity. Frequency of asthma attacks has been found to correlate negatively with likelihood of remission.

The severity of asthma varies greatly, from individuals only rarely symptomatic enough to require even minimal therapy to asthmatics who are repeatedly hospitalized and require continuous intensive medical regimens, including systemic corticosteroids. Childhood asthma associated with atopy is more severe than is that without associated atopy. Among childhood asthmatics, earlier age of onset is associated with increased severity. Other factors which determine the severity of asthma have yet to be identified.

Mortality

Mortality due to asthma is difficult to assess with certainty since physicians may list other causes of death (e.g., respiratory failure, bronchitis, chronic obstructive pulmonary disease) when asthma is the true cause. Furthermore, deaths due to complications of asthma therapy may not be diagnosed or reported as such. Despite these limitations, it would appear that death due to asthma is quite rare. Recent U.S. mortality data indicate approximately 3000 asthma deaths each year in the U.S., an overall rate of approximately 1.5 deaths/100,000 person-years. In the 5–34 year-old age group, in which there occur few other diseases to confuse the diagnosis, there have been 300–400 annual asthma deaths recently. Mortality due to asthma may actually be greater than these figures reflect, however, if in some cases asthma leads to irreversible decline in lung function which is subsequently labeled chronic obstructive pulmonary disease. Long-term follow-up studies of cohorts of asthma patients have reported 10- to 20-year case fatality rates from 0–2 percent. The parallel increase in asthma mortality and the use of over-the-counter beta-agonist inhaler in Great Britain in the 1960s suggested that overuse of these inhalers was associated with an increased risk of death, particularly among young asthmatics. The epidemic was controlled by better patient and physician education and by making the inhaler a prescription item only. This led to a substantial reduction in sales of these agents, and presumably reduced abuse, which was associated with reduced mortality.

Development of Chronic Airway Obstruction

Asthma may cause or contribute to the development of irreversible fixed airflow limitation in some patients. Asthmatics have been shown to experience a more rapid decline in FEV_1 over time than do nonasthmatics in population-based samples. In a study of 34 smokers with chronic bronchitis, Barter and Campbell found that subjects with bronchial hyperreactivity experienced a more rapid decline of FEV_1 over time than did normally reactive subjects. Because of the selected nature of these patients and inadequate control for initial level of pulmonary function and quantity of cigarettes smoked, these data cannot be considered conclusive. These findings are consistent, however, with the so-called Dutch hypothesis of the pathogenesis of chronic obstructive pulmonary disease, originally proposed in the 1960s by Orie and Van der Lende. These investigators suggested that intrinsic host characteristics such as bronchial responsiveness and atopy are important determinants of how individuals will respond to subsequent exposures. Some cigarette smokers develop wheezing and dyspnea, while others develop cough and mucous hypersecretion, and still others remain asymptomatic. Some of these individuals may experience episodic reversible airflow limitation as a result of smoking, while others develop fixed airway obstruction. Combinations of these abnormalities also might occur, making it difficult to sort out which are primary effects and which are secondary. Whether asthma is part of the complex interplay of host and environmental risk factors for the development of chronic obstructive pulmonary disease is unknown at present. The effect of bronchial reactivity on the rate of decline of pulmonary function and the modification of this effect by bronchodilator therapy are subjects of current investigation.

REFERENCES

Broder I, Higgins MW, Matthews KP, et al: Epidemiology of asthma and allergic rhinitis in a total community, Tecumseh, Michigan. III. Second survey of the community. J Allergy Clin Immunol 53:127, 1974

Cockroft DW, Berscheid BA, Murdock KY: Unimodal distribution of bronchial responsiveness to inhaled histamine in a random human population. Chest 83:751–754, 1983

Dodge RR, Burrows B: The prevalence and incidence of asthma and asthma-like symptoms in a general population sample. Am Rev Respir Dis 122:567–575, 1980

Gortmaker SL, Walker DK, Jacobs FH, et al: Parental smoking and the risk of childhood asthma. Am J Public Health 72:574–579, 1982

Gregg I: Epidemiological aspects, in Clark TJH, Godfrey S (eds): Asthma, 2nd ed. London, Chapman and Hall, 1983

Pullan CR, Hey EN: Wheezing, asthma, and pulmonary dysfunction 10 years after infection with respiratory syncgtial virus in infancy. Br Med J 284:1665–1669, 1982

Schachter EN, Doyle CA, Beck GJ: A prospective study of asthma in a rural population. Chest 85:623, 1984

Weiss ST, Speizer FE: The epidemiology of asthma: Risk factors and natural history, in Weiss EB, Segal MS, Stein M (eds): Bronchial Asthma: Risk Factors and Natural History, 2nd ed. Boston, Little, Brown and Co., 1985, pp. 14–23

Weiss ST, Tager IB, Munoz A, et al: The relationship of respiratory infections in early childhood to the occurrence of increased levels of bronchial responsiveness and atopy. Am Rev Respir Dis 131:573–578, 1985

Weiss ST, Tager IB, Speizer FE, et al: Persistent wheeze: Its relation to respiratory illness, cigarette smoking, and level of pulmonary function in a population sample of children. Am Rev Respir Dis 122:697–707, 1980

Weiss ST, Tager IB, Weiss JW, et al: Airways responsiveness in a population sample of adults & children. Am Rev Respir Dis 129:898–902, 1984

Welty C, Weiss ST, Tager IB, et al: The relationship of airways responsiveness to cold air, cigarette smoking, & atopy to respiratory symptoms and pulmonary function in adults. Am Rev Respir Dis 130:198–203, 1984

Stephen I. Wasserman

2

The Pathophysiology of Mediators in Asthma

The term asthma denotes a symptom complex characterized by wheezing and dyspnea caused by bronchial obstruction. Consequent to bronchospasm, excessive mucoid sputum production, mucosal edema, basement membrane thickening, and muscular hypertrophy are alveolar hypoventilation, regional ventilation-perfusion imbalances, hyperinflation of the lungs, and atelectasis. Pathologic examination of the lungs in cases of fatal status asthmaticus reveals atelectasis and extensive plugging of small airways by mucus, eosinophils, Charcot-Leyden crystals, and desquamated pulmonary epithelium. Although the precise genesis of the pathophysiologic alterations characteristic of asthma has not been defined, a body of information regarding the generation and physiologic effects of biochemical mediators and the regulatory role of the adrenergic and cholinergic nervous systems in human and animal asthma is now available. This information provides insight into the mechanism by which bronchospasm and inflammatory alterations of the airways may be generated. In addition, an understanding of the interrelationships of mediator generation and release, smooth muscle activation, mucus production, and airway inflammation should provide clues as to the recurrent, yet chronic, nature of asthma.

BRONCHIAL ASTHMA, Second Edition
ISBN 0-8089-1814-1

MAST CELLS

Mast cells are present in human lung in the bronchial lumen, in the bronchial mucosa in intra-epithelial locations, in deeper perivenular collections, and in the intra-alveolar septa at concentrations of $1-7 \times 10^6$ cells/g of lung tissue. Each mast cell possesses several hundred metachromatically staining granules, each surrounded by a bilayer membrane. Lung mast-cell granules possess a subgranular architecture of repeating electron-dense units in a scroll or lattice pattern of unknown functional significance. The mast cell membrane is ruffled and possesses 50–300,000 receptors for the Fc portion of IgE. IgE molecules belong to an immunoglobulin class defined by its activity in mediating immediate hypersensitivity reactions and by its characteristic physicochemical properties. It is comprised of two heavy and light chains linked by disulfide bridges with a total molecular weight (m.w.) of 190,000. It is heat labile, but does not form precipitates with specific antigen, and it does not fix complement. The serum concentration of IgE is under genetic control, being higher in atopic than in normal individuals. Papain digests IgE into three fragments, two of which (Fab) bind specific antigen and one of which (Fc) binds to the specific receptors on the mast cell surface. Receptors for the anaphylatoxins, C3a and C5a, fragments of the third and fifth components of complement, respectively, have been attributed to the mast cell upon functional criteria. In addition, mast cells may be degranulated by nonimmunologic stimuli. Thus, enzymes, ionophores, polycationic amines and proteins, biologically active peptides such as substance P, radiocontrast media, cytokines, and opiates may all effect mast-cell degranulation. While it is generally assumed that atopic individuals exhibit their antigen-induced symptoms as a result of IgE-dependent mast cell activation, the demonstration of non-IgE-mediated mechanisms for mast cell mediator release does not diminish the role of IgE in allergy, but rather, yields additional information on how mediators could be generated.

Recent work in rodents has demonstrated the existence of two different types of mast cells: connective tissue and mucosal. These cells differ in type and amount of specific granular constituents, in type of molecules generated upon activation, in their responsiveness to activators and regulatory drugs, and in their staining properties. In the human, similar heterogeneity has been postulated based upon the presence of two types of mast cells in the gut as identified by metachroniasia under various fixation techniques and by a variance of size, density, mediator content, and mediator release in human lung mast cells. In the rodent, both mast cells have their origin in a bone marrow precursor; the mucosal type differentiates in response to a T-lymphocyte product, interleukin 3, while the signal for connective tissue mast cell development is unknown. Factors relevant to human mast cell growth and differentiation remain unknown.

ACTIVATION AND DEGRANULATION OF MAST CELLS

The IgE-dependent degranulation of mast cells is initiated by the bridging of pairs of cell-bound IgE by specific antigen. Activation begins immediately upon bridging and secretion is complete within minutes. Bridging of IgE molecules pari passu induces bridging of mast cell IgE receptors which, in turn, in some unknown manner, initiates a sequence of membrane events. The earliest events appear to be increases in phospholipase C-induced generation of diacylglycerol from membrane phospholipids, and inositol triphosphate liberation. Associated with these membrane events is energy-dependent calcium-ion entry into the cell. Consequent to these steps are: an elevation of intracellular cyclic AMP, utilization of both cAMP-dependent and calcium-phospholipid-dependent protein kinases with phosphorylation of proteins, fusion of perigranular membranes with each other and with plasmalemma, pore formation, changes in cell-surface charge, and release of preformed mediators and generation of unstored mediators. Mediator release and generation is energy-dependent and noncytolytic, but does not require actual degranulation. Granules may be exposed to the external environment by formation of small pores which form in the fused penta-laminar plasmalemma-granule membrane and solubilization of mediators may then ensue (Fig. 2-1).

Degranulation may be modulated at several steps in its sequence by endogenous or exogenous agents. Some of these agents act on specific mast cell receptors, while others are thought to affect various enzymes important in mast cell activation or in the generation of specific mediators. Thus, beta-adrenergic agonists inhibit mast cell degranulation and augment intracellular

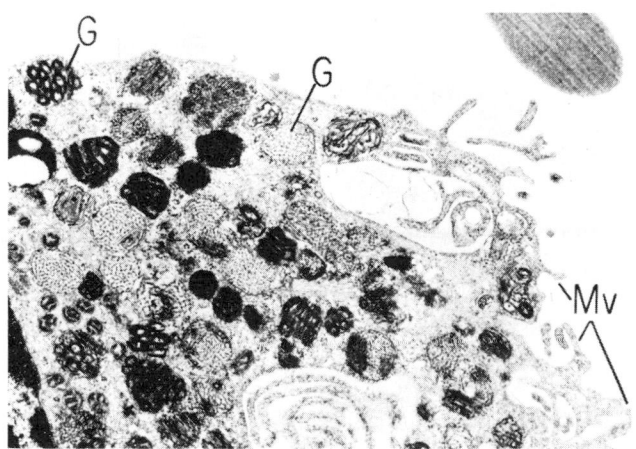

Fig. 2-1. Activation and degranulation of mast cells.

cyclic AMP concentration via their interaction with a beta$_2$-adrenergic receptor linked to adenylcyclase. Adenosine by its interaction with an A$_2$ receptor also causes increases in cyclic AMP but augments mediator release. Examples of enzyme inhibitors which block mast cell mediator release include DFP which inhibits serine protease action, and S-adenosyl homocystein plus 3-deazoadenosine which inhibit phospholipid methylation.

MAST-CELL-DEPENDENT MEDIATORS

Mast cells possess within their granules a variety of amines, peptides, and proteins, and complex polysaccharides with vasoactive, bronchospastic, and chemotactic properties as well as a variety of active enzymes and structural proteoglycans. Mast cell activation leads to the release of these preformed granular elements as well as to the generation of potent bronchospastic, vasoactive, and chemotactic substances. Some unstored mediators are generated directly by activated mast cells, whereas others are dependent upon the effect of mast cell products on other cells or constituents of the local microenvironment.

The mast-cell-derived preformed and newly generated mediators are biologically available during inflammatory events. The relevance of these mediators to asthma has been derived from studies of the pathophysiologic alterations induced by the individual mediators, identification of the mediators in tissue or biologic fluids of patients experiencing asthma, and the known pathophysiology of asthma.

Mediators not only possess the ability to induce immediate tissue responses such as rapid-onset, brief-duration alterations in pulmonary function, but may also mediate a prolonged inflammatory response. The fact that IgE and mast cells are relevant to prolonged inflammatory events has been documented by passive transfer with isolated IgE of delayed inflammatory responses in skin, and by the dependence upon IgE antibody for similar delayed alterations in pulmonary mechanics following inhalation of antigen. In lung, these delayed responses are prevented by pretreatment with disodium cromoglycate, which supports the central role of the mast cell. Histopathologic assessment of delayed cutaneous responses reveals an influx of neutrophils, eosinophils, basophils, lymphocytes, and mononuclear leukocytes, the deposition of fibrin, and vascular abnormalities which may progress to vasculitis. In the lung, IgE-dependent mast cell activation leads to rapid edema, hyperemia, and mucus release followed by neutrophil and then eosinophil exudation. Although some of the mediators responsible for the early and later phases of the IgE-mast-cell reaction can be surmised from the kinetics of their in vitro effects, their absolute identification and means of participation in disease require further definition.

The postulated role of the mast cell and its mediators in inflammation may provide insight into the clinical evolution of some disorders, such as the progression of seasonal to perennial asthma and may also provide insight into the local homeostatic regulation of the lung environment and thereby the defense of the lung. Although much remains to be clarified, the rapidly expanding understanding of target cell activation, together with the identification of mast-cell-derived mediators, provides a framework for the definition of the complex processes that eventuate in asthma.

Bronchospastic and Vasoactive Mediators (Table 2-1)

HISTAMINE

Histamine, the product of decarboxylation of the amino acid histidine, is ionically bound to proteoglycan-protein backbones of mast cell granules and is displaced by sodium exchange in the extracellular fluid. Histamine is catabolized by either oxidative deamination (histaminase) or by combined methylation and oxidative deamination (histaminase plus histamine N-methyl transferase). The former enzyme is located in eosinophils and neutrophils, whereas the latter is found in mononuclear leukocytes. The pulmonary effects of histamine are expressed as both direct and reflex constriction of both large- and small-airways smooth muscle, causing increased airway resistance and decreased compliance. Histamine also dilates small radicles of the pulmonary vasculature and increases the distance between endothelial cells of the venules, thereby increasing the potential for transudation of plasma and for extravasation of leukocytes.

The biologic activities of histamine are expressed by its interaction with either of two specific classes of receptors on target cells. Those receptors designated H_1 predominate in skin and smooth muscle and are blocked by classic antihistamines, while H_2 receptors predominate in the stomach and are selectively inhibited by ranitidine and cimetidine. Bronchoconstriction, vasodilation, and increased cGMP are H_1 effects, while H_2 effects include inhibition of both human-lymphocyte-mediated cytotoxicity and IgE-mediated histamine release from basophils due to elevation in cAMP content. Histamine inhibits chemotaxis through H_2 receptors, presumably by stimulating adenylate cyclase and increasing cAMP, whereas it augments chemotaxis via an H_1 effect thought to be a consequence of cGMP elevation. The combined effects of histamine upon H_1 and H_2 receptors are required for the full expression of wheal and flare responses, flushing, headache, and cardiac rhythm disturbances.

Histamine has been detected in the circulation of asthmatics after experimental induction of bronchospasm by antigen or exercise.

Table 2-1
Mast-cell-dependent Mediators—Bronchospasmic and Vasoactive

Mediator	Structural Characteristics	Functions	Identification in Asthma	Inactivation
Histamine (preformed)	β-imidazolyl-ethylamine mol wt 111	Contraction of smooth muscle, increase of vascular permeability, stimulation of suppressor T lymphocytes, generation of prostaglandins, stimulation of mucus release, elevation of cAMP (H2) and cGMP (H1)	+ human	Histaminase (diamine oxidase) or Histamine N-methyl transferase
Leukotrienes C4, D4, E4 (newly generated)	C-6 sulfido peptide adduct of leukotriene A_4 (arachidionic acid metabolite)	Contraction of smooth muscle, increase of vascular permeability, synergistic with histamine generation of prostaglandins, enhancement of mucus release, cause cardiac dysfunction	+ guinea pig	Lipoxygenase, hypochlorous acid, H_2O_2, O^-, OH^-
PAF (newly generated)	mol wt ~ 400 1-0-alkyl-2-acetyl sn-glyceryl-3-phosphorylcholine	Release of platelet amines, cause of leukocyte and platelet aggregation, sequestration of platelets, cause of hypotension and cardiac dysfunction	+ rabbit	Phospholipases, acetyl hydrolase
PGD$_2$ (newly generated)	C_{20} Fatty acid (archidonic acid metabolite)	Contraction of smooth muscle, cause of wheal and flare, enhancement of leukocyte motility	+ human	Prostaglandin dehydrogenase
Adenosine (newly generated)	Purine nucleoside	Vasodilation, bronchospasm, enhancement of mast cell secretion	+ human	Adenosine deaminase

PRODUCTS OF ARACHIDONIC ACID OXIDATION

In the human, products of arachidonic acid metabolism comprise the prostaglandins and thromboxanes, the hydroxyeicosatetraenoic acids, and the family of leukotrienes (Fig. 2-2). Arachidonic acid, a 20-carbon fatty acid with four double bonds, is present as one of the fatty acids in the majority of mammalian cell membrane phospholipids. When it is mobilized from cell membrane phospholipids by the action of phospholipase C and diacylglycerol lipase or by phospholipase A_2, it is then either converted to prostaglandins and thromboxanes via a cyclo-oxygenase-dependent pathway or to hydroperoxyeicosatetraenoic acid (HPETE) and then to monohydroxy fatty acids or to leukotrienes.

Prostaglandin D_2 is the cyclooxygenase product generated directly by human mast cells upon immunologic activation, and $PGF_2\alpha$ and PGE_2 are

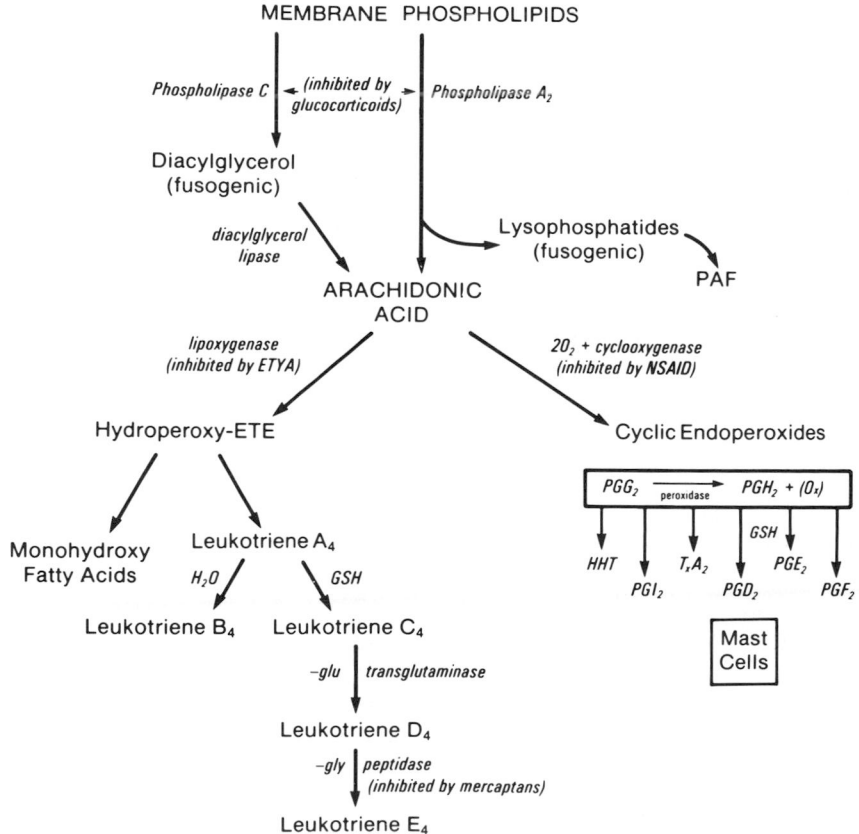

Fig. 2-2. Metabolic pathway of prostanoid generation.

also present after IgE-dependent activation of human lung fragments. The latter are thought to be generated from other lung cells by the action of mast cell mediators including histamine and a peptide termed prostaglandin-generating factor. PGD_2 is a potent bronchoconstrictor; it can induce wheal and flare responses and is capable of potentiating leukocyte infiltration induced by various chemotactic factors. It has been identified in lavage fluids from antigen-challenged allergic asthmatics.

Action of a mast cell 5-lipoxygenase enzyme followed by the action of a specific glutathione transfer enzyme termed leukotriene C_4 synthetase leads to the generation of the family of leukotrienes once termed "slow-reacting substance of anaphylaxis" (SRS-A). The three peptido-leukotrienes LTC_4, D_4, and E_4 possess intact glutathione, cysteinylglycine, and cysteine respectively. These molecules are potent bronchoconstrictors 100–1000-fold more active than histamine on a molar basis. They induce wheal and flare cutaneous responses, augment respiratory mucus secretion, impair cardiac performance, and contract gastrointestinal smooth muscle. They each interact with a specific receptor to induce their effects, and in general LTD_4 is most and LTE_4 least potent. The presence of the hydrophobic portion and the sulfidopeptide chain are required for full biologic activity. Degradation of leukotrienes proceeds via oxidative processes including those mediated by peroxides and hypochlorous acid. Sulfidopeptide leukotrienes have not yet been identified in human asthma, but they are known to be generated by human lung mast cells and inhibition of their action by the semiselective inhibitor FPL-55712 can inhibit some forms of experimental bronchospasm.

PLATELET ACTIVATING FACTOR (PAF)

PAF is generated subsequent to IgE processes in rodent mucosal-type mast cells and may also be a product of human lung mast cells, as well as human neutrophils, eosinophils and monocyte-macrophages. It is phospholipid of the structure 1-0 alkyl, 2-acetyl-sn-glycerol-3-phosphocholine. Maximal activity is achieved with C16-18 alkyl substituents and progressive loss of activity occurs with shorter or longer alkyl moieties. Loss of the acetyl or choline portions is associated with complete functional inactivity. In humans, PAF is rapidly degraded by an acid labile plasma acetyl hydrolase. PAF has been identified in the blood of patients with physical urticaria, but has yet to be identified in those with asthma, although the finding of elevated Platelet Factor IV levels in asthma may reflect the action of PAF. This mediator can induce bronchoconstriction, wheal and flare responses, platelet and neutrophil aggregation, hypotension, and even death upon its intravenous administration. The majority of the effects are fully expressed in platelet-depleted animals, suggesting that PAF is a direct agonist on a variety of cells and tissues.

ADENOSINE

The nucleoside adenosine is generated and released by mast cells upon their activation probably as a consequence of ATP hydrolysis. Adenosine levels increase in the blood of patients experiencing allergen-induced bronchospasm. Adenosine is a potent bronchoconstrictor in asthmatic humans, is a coronary vasodilator, an inhibitor of platelet activation, and an augmentor of secretagogue-mediated mast cell activation. Adenosine effects are inhibited by xanthines such as aminophylline and adenosine is degraded by adenosine deaminase or removed by its uptake into cells via a specific transport system.

Chemotactic Mediators (Table 2-2)

EOSINOPHIL CHEMOTACTIC FACTOR OF
ANAPHYLAXIS (ECF-A)

The first mast-cell-associated chemotactic factor described, ECF-A, was identified in the anaphylactic supernatant of challenged guinea pig lung fragments and subsequently in the analogous human tissue and in isolated mast cells. This factor is preferentially chemotactic for eosinophils. It also deactivates this cell type to further migration. A small molecule of about 400 daltons, ECF-A has also been identified preformed in human lung and isolated mast cells. This mediator from human lung has been structurally characterized as two acidic tetrapeptides with the amino acid sequence Val/Ala-Gly-Ser-Glu. ECF-A-like small molecules have been identified in the serum of patients with IgE-mediated mast cell activation in cold urticaria and asthma.

INTERMEDIATE-MOLECULAR-WEIGHT EOSINOPHIL
CHEMOTACTIC PEPTIDES

In addition to low-molecular-weight ECF-A tetrapeptides, human lung contains chemotactic factors of molecular weight 1200–2500 with specificity for eosinophil polymorphonuclear leukocytes. These factors are preformed, immunologically releasable, and capable of deactivating eosinophils. Molecules with similar molecular weights have been identified in the sera of patients undergoing cold-induced IgE-mediated mast cell degranulation and allergen-induced asthma.

HIGH-MOLECULAR-WEIGHT NEUTROPHIL
CHEMOTACTIC FACTORS (HMW-NCF)

HMW-NCF has been described in rat mast cells, human lung fragments, and the serum of patients with physical urticaria and exercise-induced or antigen-inhalation asthma. HMW-NCF has been characterized as a 660,000-

Table 2-2
Mast-cell-dependent Mediators—Chemotactic

Mediator	Structural Characteristics	Functions	Identification in Asthma	Inactivation
ECF-A (preformed)	Val/Ala-Gly-Ser-Glu mol wt 360–390	Chemotactic attraction and deactivation of eosinophils	unknown	Aminopeptidase Carboxypeptidase A
ECF-oligopeptides (preformed)	Peptides mol wt 1300–2500	Chemotactic attraction and deactivation of eosinophils	unknown	unknown
NCF (preformed)	Neutral protein mol wt ~660,000	Chemotactic attraction and deactivation of neutrophils	+ human	unknown
Lipid chemotactic factors (newly generated)	PAF LTB$_4$ HETEs	Chemotactic attraction of neutrophils and eosinophils	unknown	unknown
Histamine (preformed)	β-imidazolyl-ethylamine mol wt = 111	Enhancement of eosinophil and neutrophil migration	+ human	Histaminase (diamine oxidase) or Histaminase N-methyl transferase
Monocyte, basophil, and lymphocyte chemotactic factors	Unknown	Chemotactic activation of lymphocytes, monocytes, and basophils	unknown	unknown

dalton neutral protein which attracts and deactivates neutrophils in vitro. HMW-NCF appears to be a sensitive marker for mast cell activation, since it is present in serum following the challenge of allergic asthmatics with doses of antigen insufficient to induce bronchospasm, but it is not generated during methacholine-induced bronchospasm.

OTHER CHEMOTACTIC FACTORS

Factors of molecular weights 10,000–12,000 and 300–500 which are chemotactic for lymphocytes are generated by immunologic activation of rat mast cells, and similar uncharacterized activities have been noted in the blister fluid of patients with bullous pemphigoid associated with mast cell degranulation. Such activities in human or animal asthma await description.

Similarly, monocyte- and basophil-directed chemotactic activities have been identified in models of mast cell activation, but their chemical identification and presence in asthma has yet to be accomplished.

Other mast-cell-dependent chemotactic activities include the neutrophil-directed inflammatory factor of anaphylaxis and leukotriene B4, monohydroxy fatty acids (HETEs), and platelet activating factor, which display broad cellular specificity. Histamine and PGD_2 are known to modulate leukocyte responses induced by a variety of chemoattractants. These factors all demonstrate a broad spectrum of activity for various leukocytes, and their role, if any, in asthma is unknown.

Granule-associated Enzymes (Table 2-3)

PROTEASES

The major protein constituent of human mast cell granules is a tryptic protease termed tryptase. This 144,000-molecular-weight tetrameric enzyme is tightly bound to granular heparin and is not inhibited by plasma antitrypsins. It is capable of cleaving C3 to generate C3a, and it also can degrade kininogen, prekallikrein, and fibrinogen. Tryptase is released from human mast cells by IgE-mediated stimuli.

A captopril-insensitive, cathepsin-G-like chymotryptic protease is also present in human mast cell granules. This enzyme is a potent angiotensin-converting enzyme. Neither tryptase nor the chymotryptic enzyme have yet been identified in human asthma.

OTHER ENZYMES

The lysosomal hydrolases hexosaminidase, arylsulfatase, glucuronidase, superoxide dismutase, peroxidase, and carboxypeptidase have been identi-

Table 2-3
Mast-cell-dependent Mediators—Enzymes and Structural Components

Mediator	Structural Characteristics	Functions	Identification in Asthma	Inactivation
Heparin (preformed)	Proteoglycan mol wt ~ 60,000	Anticoagulation. Antithrombin III interaction. Inhibition of complement activation. Tryptase stabilization.	? + dog	Heparinase oxidation
Proteases Chymase	Protein	Proteolysis with chymotryptic specificity, angiotension conversion.	unknown	unknown
Tryptase (lung) Kallikrein of anaphylaxis (preformed)	Protein mol wt ~ 144,000	Proteolysis with tryptic specificity. Cleavage of kininogen, fibrinogen, C_3, Hageman factor.	unknown	unknown
Other enzymes peroxidase (preformed)	Protein	Generation of superoxide, H_2O_2.	unknown	unknown
arylsulfatase (preformed)	Protein mol wt ~ 100,000 (A)	Hydrolysis of various sulfate esters.	unknown	unknown
N-acetyl-β-D-glucosaminidase (preformed) (hexosaminidase)	Protein mol wt ~ 158,000	Cleavage of glucosamine residues.	unknown	unknown
β-glucocoronicase	Protein mol wt ~ 300,000	Cleavage of glucronide conjugates.	unknown	unknown
Superoxide dismutase (preformed)	Protein	Inactivation of superoxide.	unknown	unknown

fied in mast cells from a variety of sources. Their role in human asthma is undefined.

STRUCTURAL PROTEOGLYCANS HEPARIN

The sulfated, metachromatic, mucopolysaccharide heparin has been identified in human lung and localized to the mast cells isolated from human lung tissue. Human lung heparin is a proteoglycan of approximately 60,000 molecular weight, comprised of a protein core to which are attached, by xylosyl-seryl linkages, glycosaminoglycan side chains of average molecular weight 20,000. Human heparin interacts with human antithrombin III to accelerate anticoagulation. Heparin from other sources has been shown to inhibit generation of the convertase enzyme (C3bBb) responsible for the amplification of cleavage of the third component of complement (C3), to inhibit binding of the C1q fragment of complement to immune complexes, to inhibit the action of the activated first component of complement (C1s) upon its substrates, and to prevent binding of C2 to C4b. In addition, heparin has been shown to bind to Platelet Factor IV and to liberate lipoprotein lipase. Heparin also binds to and stabilizes tryptase and thereby potentiates its proteolytic activity on selected substrates, and acts as a growth factor for endothelial cells.

Rodent mucosal mast cells (and presumably human mucosal mast cells) lack heparin and instead possess an oversulfated form of chondroitin sulfate. This explains their lesser metachromasia when contrasted to heparin-containing mast cells, although other functions of these proteoglycans are not clearly identified.

MEDIATOR INTERACTIONS

The mediators of immediate-type hypersensitivity have been identified and assessed for their effects as isolated factors, and understanding of their interactions is fragmentary. It is known, however, that the spasmogenic effects of histamine and leukotrienes are synergistic, and, in addition, that the presence of either directly induces prostaglandin generation. The interactions of ECF-A, histamine, and ECF-oligopeptides are not fully delineated, but it is known that histamine in high concentrations inhibits and in low concentrations enhances ECF-A-induced eosinophil chemotaxis. In addition, PGD_2 enhances neutrophil chemotaxis, while heparin augments tryptase action. Given the number and complexity of mast-cell-dependent mediators, however, other potentially critical biologic interactions await elucidation.

DETERMINANTS OF ACTIVITY OF MAST CELL MEDIATORS

Following activation of mast cells by IgE-dependent or other mechanisms, the mediators generated and released and the myriad of their potential interactions provide the substrate for induction of inflammatory events. The putative role for the mast cell and its mediators in both the homeostatic as well as pathophysiologic induction of inflammation in the lung, and its participation in asthma, is strengthened by the location of the mast cell at the respiratory surface. Thus, the interaction of surface and intraluminal mast cells with antigen or other degranulating agents could, by the action of locally released vasoactive factors, lead to alterations of the respiratory epithelial barrier and permit access of inhaled material to the large number of more deeply situated mast cells. In addition, the presence of large numbers of interalveolar mast cells suggests their importance in the lung periphery as well. Of great importance has been the demonstration that solely mast-cell-dependent events can indeed cause both immediate and more persistent inflammatory processes. The biphasic response of airways to inhaled antigen may be comparable to the biphasic cutaneous model in which a wheal-and-flare response occurs within minutes of mast cell activation and reflects altered vascular permeability at the site, to be followed 2–6 hours later by inflammatory changes of an intense cellular infiltration secondary to chemotactic factor generation. This latter may be followed by frank vasculitis, perhaps due to leukocytic and/or mast cell enzyme activity. Elicitation of both phases by purely IgE-dependent mechanisms indicates that mast cell activation can contribute to subacute and chronic, as well as to acute, pathobiologic processes. This fact is central to according the mast cell an important role in asthma, since this disease is characterized by acute exacerbations superimposed on chronic inflammation and hyperirritability of the airway. Whether continued alteration in the threshold of airway response is due to mast cell mediators directly or to cellular infiltration is not established, but mast-cell-derived mediators alone or in combination could be critical by either route.

The mechanism by which mast cell mediators might provoke such biphasic inflammatory responses is depicted in Figure 2-3. The mast-cell-dependent generation of bronchospastic and vasoactive mediators establishes a local vasodilatory or humoral phase of inflammation, while the release of chemotactic mediators provokes a cellular phase of inflammation. The humoral phase, apparent within minutes, would lead to egress from the circulation of immunoglobulin and complement as well as fibrinolytic, procoagulant, and kinin-generating proteins. This response could be expected to be rapidly beneficial to the host by aiding removal of invading microorganisms or inhaled materials, by localizing and removing noxious agents, and

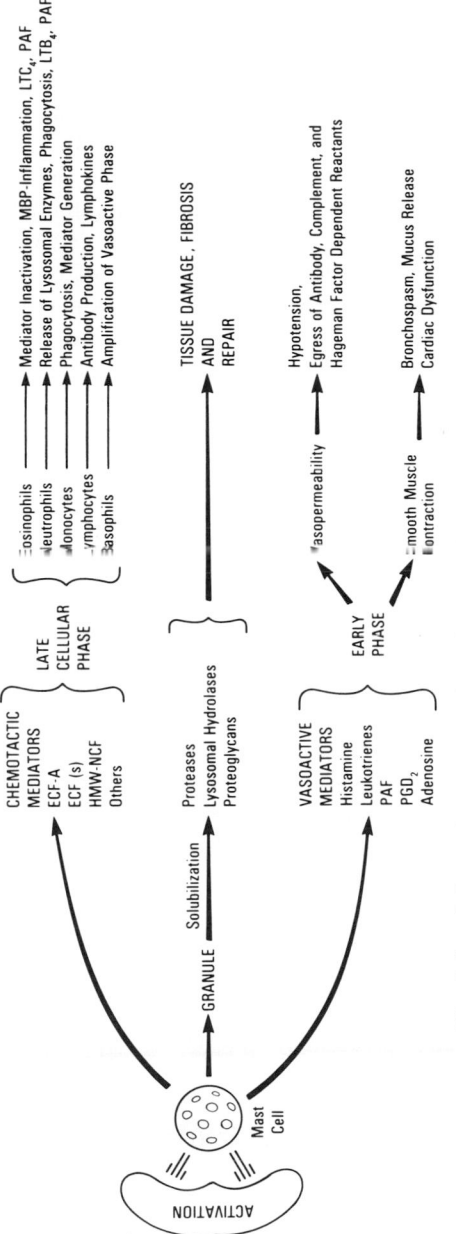

Fig. 2-3. Schematic representation of mast-cell-dependent inflammatory events.

33

by facilitating leukocyte migration through venular disconnections. On the other hand, an unregulated humoral phase might be expressed in disease as acute exacerbations of bronchospasm, alterations in tracheobronchial mucus flow or consistency, or as upper-airway obstruction due to edema. In fact, release of mucus by IgE-dependent mechanisms, perhaps through histamine, prostaglandins, and leukotrienes, has been demonstrated. The generation and release of chemotactic factors would, in a period of several hours, be expected to call to the local site a variety of inflammatory cells. These cells could prove beneficial not only by their phagocytic function but also by their ability to inactivate mediators. If accumulation of leukocytes were uncontrolled, however, the pathobiologic consequences of tissue infiltration with leukocytes would ensue. Clinically, such infiltration might be seen in the inflammatory bronchial epithelium of asthmatic patients or as vasculitis, or perhaps via the action of leukocytic lysosomal enzymes in the destruction of lung tissue and the induction of fibrosis. In addition, the eosinophil major basic protein can induce tracheobronchial epithelial cell desquamation in vitro, a finding reminiscent of the pathology of asthma known to occur in vivo. As chemotactic factors can activate leukocyte production of toxic oxygen species as well as induce secretion of granular contents, mast cell release of such materials may greatly augment local inflammation by action on resident as well as newly recruited leukocytes. However, by their capacities to deactivate leukocytes to further chemotactic response, mast cell chemotactic mediators might also inhibit localization of leukocytes. In cold urticaria, following mediator release by cold challenge, circulating neutrophils are rendered unresponsive to in vitro chemotactic stimulation. This effect is time-limited, but persists beyond the period in which measurable quantities of mediators are observed. Such an inhibitory action of chemotactic factors could prove beneficial by blunting exuberant inflammation or, if prolonged or ill-timed, might be harmful by preventing adequate host response to local insult. The release of mast cell proteases and lysosomal enzymes may itself lead to alterations in ground substances and to activation of such protein inflammatory cascades as complement, fibrinolysis, and coagulation. These processes would amplify inflammatory events and might prove beneficial to the elimination of microorganisms or toxic agents, but, if unregulated, might lead to tissue destruction, chronic inflammation, and fibrosis.

REGULATION OF MAST CELL MEDIATOR RELEASE AND ACTIVITY

The events which lead to the generation and release of mast cell mediators and thereby to the elicitation of mast-cell-dependent inflammatory events are regulated at several points. Thus, mast cell activation, the secretion of granules, the release of the preformed mediators and the generation of unstored mediators, the effect of mediators upon target cells, and, finally, the persistence in tissue of the mediators are all under biologic control.

The extent and effect of activation of the mast cell are determined by the availability of access of the eliciting agent to this cell, the amount of specific IgE antibody bound to the mast cell surface, and by the amount of eliciting agent. The mast cell itself might, by altering local permeability, allow increased antigen contact or, by the H_2 action of histamine, may suppress lymphocyte recognition of antigen and thereby prevent IgE immune response to antigen. Evidence also exists to suggest that mast cells from allergic patients are particularly sensitive to a variety of non-IgE-dependent stimuli and are thus able to release mediators after perturbations not associated with mediator release from non-atopic people.

Following secretion of the mast cell granule, the release of preformed mediators and thus the full expression of their activity is dependent upon the solubilities of each. Thus, B-glucuronidase, arylsulfatase A, histamine, ECF-A, and ECF-oligopeptides are fully soluble in physiologic buffers; hexosaminidase requires 0.5-M sodium chloride for full elution from the granule, and the protease-heparin complex requires 1.0-M sodium chloride for dissolution. While mechanism(s) by which the mast cell granule is solubilized in vivo remain unknown, this solubilization is clearly an important step in regulating the activity of mast cell inflammatory mediators. In vitro, oxidative processes can disrupt the intact granule.

Regulation of the action of mast cell mediators upon target cells may derive from alterations in cyclic nucleotide concentrations, or from the interaction of several mediators or their metabolites with the same target cell. Thus, histamine may be additive or inhibitory to ECF-A action upon eosinophils, depending upon the ratio of the two activities present. Mediators may also be synergistic on smooth muscle, as exemplified by leukotrienes and histamine action.

The regulation of the generation of unstored mediators has not been fully elucidated, but data suggest that the local microenvironment is critical to their generation. This is particularly important with regard to those mediators which can be generated by non-mast cells in response to mast cell mediators. Thus PAF, leukotrienes, HETEs, and prostaglandins can be generated from neutrophils, eosinophils, mononuclear leukocytes, or alveolar macrophages. The ratios of appropriate target cells thus may be crucial to the amount and type of mediator generated.

Finally, the persistence of the effect of mediators is also regulated. While this may reflect the amount of each mediator generated or released, mediator clearance by excretion, and probable tachyphylaxis to some, it is also affected by enzymatic inactivation of these biologic activities. Thus, eosinophils and neutrophils possess histaminase, while mononuclear leukocytes contain histamine methyl transferase, all capable of degrading histamine. Production of oxygen radicals by activated leukocytes can inactivate leukotrienes, while plasma exudation permits acetylhydrolase to inactivate PAF. Further regulatory interactions of course exist and their interrelationships to mediator generation, release, and persistence may be crucial to our understanding of the role of the mast cell in pulmonary pathophysiology.

REFERENCES

Atkins PC, Bedard PM, Zweiman B: Skin and systemic mediator release in antigen challenged allergic subjects. J Allergy Clin Immunol 69:94, 1982

Atkins PC, Zweiman B: Mediator release in local heat urticaria. J Allergy Clin Immunol 68:286–289, 1981

Ayars GH, Altman LC, Rosen H, et al: Phagocyte-mediated pneumocyte injury. Clin Res 30:426, 1982

Basran GS, Mareley J, Page C, et al: Platelet activating factors: A potential mediator of acute and chronic asthma. Clin Res 30:186, 1982

Bedard PM, Atkins PC, Zweiman B: Cellular inflammatory response and mediator release after antigen challenge. J Allergy Clin Immunol 69:146, 1982

Davis WB, Hunninghake G, Crystal R: Cytotoxicity of eosinophils for lung parenchymal cells. Clin Res 29:445, 1981

Flynn PG, Hammerschmidt DE, Redl H, et al: Platelet-granulocyte interactions in acute lung injury. Clin Res 30:429, 1982

Gleich GJ, Loegering DA, Frigas E, et al: The major basic protein of the eosinophil granule: Physiochemical properties, localization, and function, in Mahmoud AAF, Austen KF, Simon AS (eds): The Eosinophil in Health and Disease. New York, Grune & Stratton, 1980, pp. 79–97

Goetzl EJ: Mediators of immediate hypersensitivity derived from arachidonic acid. N Engl J Med 303:822–824, 1980

Goetzl EJ: Oxygenation products of arachidonic acid as mediators of hypersensitivity and inflammation. Med Clin North Am 65:809–828, 1981

Henderson WR, Jorg A, Klebanoff SJ: Eosinophil peroxidase-mediated inactivation of leukotrienes B_4, C_4, and D_4. J Immunol 128:2609–2613, 1982

Lee TH, Nagy L, Nagakura T, et al: Identification and partial characterization of an exercise-induced neutrophil chemotactic factor in bronchial asthma. J Clin Invest 69:889–899, 1982

Martin GL, Atkins PC, Dunsky EH, et al: Effects of theophylline, terbutaline, and prednisone on antigen-induced bronchospasm and mediator release. J Allergy Clin Immunol 66:204–212, 1980

Nagy L: The effect of disodium-cromoglycate on human serum neutrophil chemotactic activity in antigen-induced bronchospasm. Allerg Immunol 27:48–52, 1981

Nagy L: Serum neutrophil chemotactic activity and leukocyte count after house dust induced bronchospasm. Eur J Respir Dis 62:198–203, 1981

Nagy L, Lee TH, Kay AB: Neutrophil chemotactic activity in antigen-induced late asthmatic reactions. N Engl J Med 306:497–501, 1982

Oertel H, Kaliner M: The biologic activity of mast cell granules. III. Purification of inflammatory factors of anaphylaxis (IF-A) responsible for causing late-phase reactions. J Immunol 127:1398–1402, 1981

Oertel H, Kaliner M: The biologic activity of mast cell granules in rat skin: Effects of adrenocorticoids on late phase inflammatory responses induced by mast cell granules. J Allergy Clin Immunol 68:238–245, 1981

Orr TSC, Elliott ER, Altounyan REC, et al: Modulation of release of neutrophil chemotactic factor (NCF). Clin Allergy 10:491–496, 1980

Peters SP, Shulman ES, MacGlashen DW, et al: Pharmacologic and biochemical studies of human lung mast cells. J Allergy Clin Immunol 69:150, 1982

Schatz M, Wasserman SI, Patterson R: Eosinophil and immunologic lung disease. Med Clin North Am 65:1055–1071, 1981

Schenkel E, Atkins PC, Yost R, et al: Antigen-induced neutrophil chemotactic activity from sensitized lung. J Allergy Clin Immunol 70:321–325, 1982

Soter NA, Wasserman SI, Austen KF, et al: Release of mast cell mediators and alterations in lung function in patients with cholinergic urticaria. N Engl J Med 3302:604–609, 1980

Tennenbaum S, Oertel H, Henderson W, et al: The biologic activity of mast cell granules. I. Elicitation of inflammatory responses in rat skin. J Immunol 125:335, 1980

Virella G, Espinoza A, Patrick A, et al: Release of PAF by human PMN exposed to surface fixed immune complexes. Clin Res 30:360, 1982

Wasserman SI: Mast cell dependent chemotactic factors in human allergic disease in Kerr, Ganderton (eds): Proceedings of XIth International Congress of Allergology and Clinical Immunology. London, MacMillan Press Ltd., 1983, p 29

Wasserman SI, Austen KF, Soter NA: The functional and physiochemical characterization of three eosinophilotactic activities released into the circulation by cold challenge of patients with cold urticaria. Clin Exp Immunol 47:570–578, 1982

Wintroub B: Inflammation and mediators. Int J Dermatol 24:436–442, 1980

Carroll E. Cross

3

Pathogenic Mechanisms in Asthma

Asthma is a complex and heterogeneous disorder characterized by paroxysmal airway constriction, mucosal edema, inflammatory infiltrates in the airway walls, airway epithelial damage and desquamation, goblet cell hypertrophy, and mucus hypersecretion; it is precipitated by a multiplicity of stimuli. Although twin and family history studies suggest that genetic factors play a role in patient predisposition to allergies and asthma, there is no known definitive association between genetic factors (such as histocompatibility antigens) and asthma. Patients who exhibit this variable airway resistance are often arbitrarily subdivided into two groups: those with "allergic bronchial asthma," in whom immunologic mechanisms appear to play an important role, and those with "hyperreactive airways," in whom immunologic mechanisms may be difficult to document, but in whom a multitude of stimuli appear to be important in causing the asthmatic condition. Allergic asthma is almost certainly the result of release of mast-cell-derived mediators into the airway microenvironment. It is probable that mast cell mediator release is involved in other forms of asthma, such as exercise-induced bronchospasm.

Patients with allergic bronchial asthma almost always also exhibit hyperreactive airways. Excessive bronchomotor tone thus appears to play a pivotal role in all forms of asthma. Spasm of hyperreactive and hypertrophied bronchial smooth muscle in central, segmental, and subsegmental bronchi and/or in smaller peripheral bronchi and bronchioles causes the characteristic parox-

BRONCHIAL ASTHMA, Second Edition
ISBN 0-8089-1814-1

ysmal airway obstruction of asthmatic patients. The obstructive physiology is worsened by varying degrees of concomitant mucosal injury, edema, and inflammation and by overproduction and inspissation of respiratory tract secretions. These latter abnormalities dominate the clinically important sub-acute and chronic forms of asthma.

New knowledge related to respiratory tract morphology and neuroanatomy, biochemistry, immunology, and physiology has markedly enhanced understanding of the structure, function, and malfunction of the respiratory tract conducting airways. Over the past 10 years, there has been an explosion of new information about the basic nature of asthma, especially with respect to immune mechanisms and mediator-release phenomena, their interactions with airway afferent and efferent nervous system innervations, and airway hyperreactivity states. The most notable focus has perhaps been on the discovery of the lipoxygenase pathway of arachidonic acid (AA), a prominent constituent fatty acid of the phospholipid membrane component of both mast cells and phagocytes, and on nerve pathways modulating airway calibre. The clinical study of airway epithelial lining fluid obtained via bronchial lavage from asthmatics is beginning to provide further insights into disease processes which are not obtainable from physiological studies alone. It can be safely predicted that medical science is at the threshold of, in the next 10 years, taking therapeutic advantage of some of this new information. This chapter focuses upon selected aspects of airway cell biology as it potentially relates to two distinct pathogenic mechanisms that appear to be dominant in asthmatic patients: allergic bronchial asthma and airway hyperreactivity.

IMMUNOPATHOLOGIC CONSIDERATIONS: ALLERGIC BRONCHIAL ASTHMA

Current concepts of the pathophysiologic mechanisms operative in allergic bronchial asthma emphasize a rather clearly defined sequence of immunogenic and mast-cell-mediator-induced events and a less clearly defined series of airway responses to the various released mediators. The essential components for induction and completion of asthmagenic immune responses exist locally within the airways. As diagrammatically depicted in Figure 3-1, these include reaginic antibody immunoglobulin E (IgE)-producing mechanisms, respiratory tract mast cell "activation" phenomena, and various airway target cell responses to the released mast cell mediators.

It is currently believed that allergic asthma is mediated via macrophage-involved antigenic sensitization of T cell lymphocytes, which result in B cell lymphocyte stimulation with formation of IgE. The antigen-specific IgE subsequently attaches to specific receptors on airway mast cells and circulatory basophils. Following re-exposure to the antigen, the antigen bridges

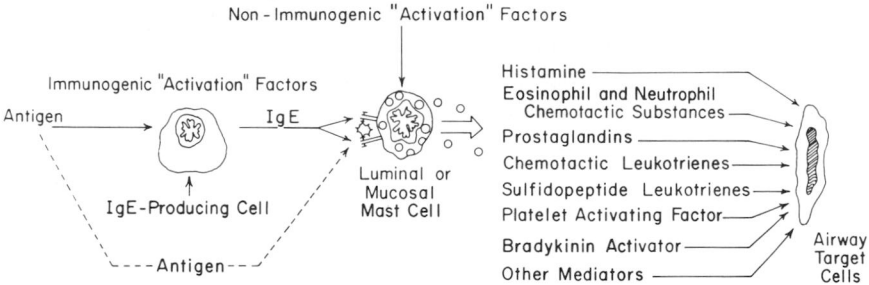

Fig. 3-1. Induction of the asthmagenic immune response in the lung.

between adjacent antigen-specific IgE molecules on the surface of respiratory tract mast cells. The aggregation of membrane antigen-specific IgE receptors triggers mast cell "activation," causing exocytosis of preformed mediator substances and de novo generation of other potential mediators of immune-inflammatory reactions.

The mediators are a diverse group of highly active biologic and pharmacologic agents which are capable of initiating both immediate and delayed local immune-inflammatory responses. The early (or immediate) phase causes bronchospasm, exudation of proteinaceous plasma into bronchial walls, and airway mucus glycoprotein secretion, whereas the late (or delayed) response is characterized by more intense specific phagocytic infiltrations into bronchial walls. The recruited phagocytes are capable of amplifying the mast-cell-initiated immune-inflammatory response. Both phases appear to be associated with a delayed and relatively inefficient mucociliary clearance, presumably secondary to released-mediator effects on the airway mucociliary apparatus.

A number of variables influence the specificity, severity, and temporal characteristics of airway responses to inhaled allergens. These include the intensity and persistence of the activation factors; the number, location, and type of the various airway mast cell populations; the contained quantity of membrane-associated IgE of the airway mast cell populations; mast cell membrane and intracellular controls regulating the generation and release of mediators; feedback mechanisms by which some released mediators influence subsequent mast cell responses; airway permeability to the various antigens and mediators; the reaction of mediators with target cells; the intrinsic responsiveness of the target cells; and the rates of removal of the released mediators from the airway via metabolism, airway microcirculatory flow, and, possibly, tracheobronchial clearance. For example, bronchoalveolar lavage studies have shown asthmatics to have increased numbers of recoverable mast cells when compared to nonasthmatics. These cells may have an increased tendency to release mediators. Both may contribute to the mechanism of bronchospasm seen in asthmatic patients.

Generation and release of airway mast cell mediators are modulated by agents specifically interacting with various mast cell membrane receptors and by substances acting on their cell surface membranes in nonspecific manners. The specific membrane receptors include adrenergic and cholinergic receptors, which in turn influence intracellular concentrations of cyclic adenosine (cAMP) and guanosine (cGMP) nucleotides, and receptors for selected mediators of inflammation such as receptors for histamine and certain metabolites of arachidonic acid. Nonspecific methods of pertubating mast cell membranes may indirectly modify the specific membrane receptor reactivities or modulate the membrane systems responsible for the transduction and translation of external receptor signals to the cell interior. For example, nonspecific mast cell surface membrane pertubations by osmotic, chemical, or toxic influences may be the underlying mechanism operative in exercise asthma and in such occupational asthmas as those related to platinum, nickel, and isocyanate (although for the occupational asthmas this is an unsettled matter at present; it seems likely that immunologic mechanisms play a role in subsets of some of these disorders).

The precise pathways by which aggregation of the receptors for antigen-specific IgE on mast cells (and basophils) triggers release of their metachromatic secretory granules and activates mediator release in these cells remain somewhat unsettled. Membrane molecular biology now emphasizes the role of the membrane G-proteins, which, are required in order to transduce the external cell membrane signals to the internal cell membrane. G-proteins can be either stimulatory or inhibitory towards signal transduction to two important inner membrane enzyme systems, the adenylate and guanylate cyclase system and the phospholipase C system. Adenylate and guanylate cyclase produces cAMP and cGMP from cell ATP and GTP, respectively, whereas phospholipase C cannibalizes phsphatidylinositol (PIP_2) from cell membrane phospholipid to generate inositol triphosphate (IP_3) and diacylglycerol (DG). The secondary messengers modulate such cell activities as: (1) calcium transport responsible for microtubular polymerization and preformed mediator secretion (cAMP, cGMP, and IP_3); (2) membrane phospholipase A_2 activation responsible for generation of AA from membrane phospholipid (DG); and (3) protein kinase C activation (DG). Oxidative AA pathways in turn lead to prostaglandin and leukotriene generation and their subsequent release from the mast cell. Protein kinase C activation triggers a wide range of biologic consequences, including the potentiation of stimuli initiating cell secretion. Although there is still a long way to go to obtain a complete picture of the complex interacting factors responsible for modulating mast cell mediator release, there is no doubt that a number of therapeutic agents effective in asthmatic states effect mast cell activation processes. The concept that airway mast cells play a key role in antigen-induced allergic asthma has been strengthened by morphological studies confirming that mast cell changes do indeed occur during allergen-induced hypersensitivity reactions and by direct measurements of mast-cell-derived mediator levels in airway lavage fluids after allergen inhalation.

In recent years, the list of immune-inflammatory mediators implicated in asthmatic airway reactions has increased considerably. Interpretations of the role that any one particular mediator plays in asthma are complicated by the fact that many of these mediators interact with each other (e.g., the prostanoid and histaminergic systems) and act at different locations (e.g., nerve cell, smooth muscle cell, proximal airways, peripheral airways). There is also the problem of considerable interspecies variation with respect to the types and amounts of mast cell mediators.

The primary or preformed mast cell mediators consist of vasoactive substances, chemotactic factors, enzymes, and proteoglycans. These include histamine, serotonin, eosinophilic chemotactic factor of anaphylaxis (ECF-A), neutrophilic chemotactic factor(s), and a variety of substances whose physiologic roles are yet to be fully determined. These latter substances include neutral proteases such as trypsin, other proteases with carboxypeptidase- and chymotrypsin-like activities, exoglycosidases such as arylsulfatase, and proteoglycans such as heparin. The secondary mediators include substances generated from cell membrane phospholipid and include platelet activating factor (PAF), the classical prostaglandins, thromboxanes, prostacyclins, and the chemotactic and sulfidopeptide leukotrienes. These mediators are believed to be important in immune-inflammatory reactions and are presumed to play an important role in asthma. A third group of mediators could include those formed outside of the mast cell, but as a result of in vivo mast cell release of "activators," such as the primary or preformed mediator proteases. Such externally generated substances include bradykinin and Hageman factor.

As diagrammatically depicted in Figure 3-2, these agents exert biologic influences on airway smooth muscle cells, epithelial and endothelial cells,

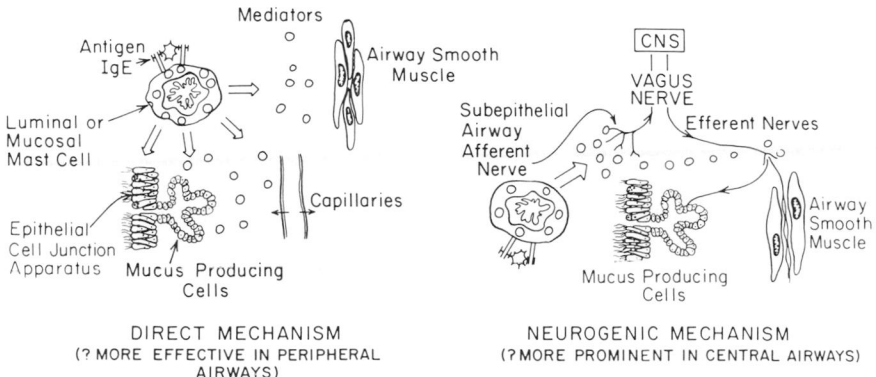

DIRECT MECHANISM
(? MORE EFFECTIVE IN PERIPHERAL AIRWAYS)

NEUROGENIC MECHANISM
(? MORE PROMINENT IN CENTRAL AIRWAYS)

Fig. 3-2. Direct and neurogenic mechanisms of airway immune response.

mucus-producing cells, subepithelial airway afferent nerve receptors, and probably on airway ganglion cells. The biologic effects of the released mediators can be direct and manifest regionally in the microenvironment of the activated mast cell, or these effects may be indirect and manifest throughout the airways via neurogenic reflexes. Stimulation of airway vagal afferent myelinated rapidly adapting stretch receptors results in both generalized airway bronchoconstriction and in mucus hypersecretion from airway mucus glands, both occurring via efferent cholinergic parasympathetic pathways. More recently, it has been suggested that airway afferent unmyelinated vagal C fibers may also be important, especially in histamine, serotonin, and bradykinin hyperresponsiveness. Awaiting full assessment are local axon constrictor fibers in afferent nerves, which respond to mucosal irritation and can cause local increases in mucosal blood flow and vascular permeability and cause local smooth muscle contraction by release of substance P. Nerve innervations appear to be most abundant in central airways, whereas respiratory mast cells are more plentiful in peripheral airways, suggesting that indirect neurogenic mechanisms may predominate in central airway constriction and that direct immune-inflammatory mediator effects may be more important in peripheral airway constriction.

Of the mediators released by respiratory tract mast cells, special focus has been placed upon histamine, the various chemotactic substances, the prostaglandins, the sulfidopeptide leukotrienes formerly known as SRS-A, and PAF. Histamine stimulates airway afferent vagal nerve endings, constricts bronchial smooth muscle, and increases endothelial permeability, particularly in bronchial venules; it possibly also affects epithelial cell intercellular junctions. The major cyclooxygenase product of mast cells, PGD_2, is a potent bronchoconstrictor. The sulfidopeptide leukotrienes constrict bronchial smooth muscle, increase endothelial permeability (possibly by potentiating the effects of histamine), cause mucus cell secretion, and retard mucociliary clearance mechanisms. The chemotactic substances selectively recruit eosinophils and neutrophils from the intravascular compartments in the airways. PAF, like the AA metabolites a mediator with potent biologic activity formed as a consequence endogenous phospholipid mobilization, has been implicated as a mediator of allergic and inflammatory processes. It is synthesized and released by a variety of cells, including phagocytes, basophils, mast cells, platelets and endothelial cells. This substance also contracts airway smooth muscle, even in the presence of cholinergic, histaminic, cyclooxygenase and lipoxygenase inhibitors. PAF also causes increases in microvascular permeability and potentiates release of lysosomal enzymes and AA metabolites from various cell types, thus potentially enhancing and/or perpetuating immune-inflammatory responses. Until a PAF assay and PAF antagonists are better developed, however, it will be difficult to assess its role in asthma.

It is important to consider the site of interaction of antigen, immune effector cells (including phagocytes), mast cells, their mediators, and the various target receptor cells. The permeability of the bronchial epithelial cells appears to be one important issue. Such a consideration calls attention to the availability of various antigenic proteins, mast cells and/or mast cell mediators to subepithelial target receptors. Although many uncertainties remain, it appears that immunologically produced IgE fixes to both luminal and submucosal mast cells. As schematically diagrammed in Figure 3-3, an inhaled antigen comes into contact with luminal surface mast cells (a small number of these have been shown to be present in human airways; this number appears to be increased in asthmatics), causing release of immune-inflammatory mediators from these cells. This mediator release presumably has profound effects on the adjacent airway mucosa.

The epithelial cells of the airways are bound together by tight intracellular bridges (tight junctions) that prevent movement of large molecules from

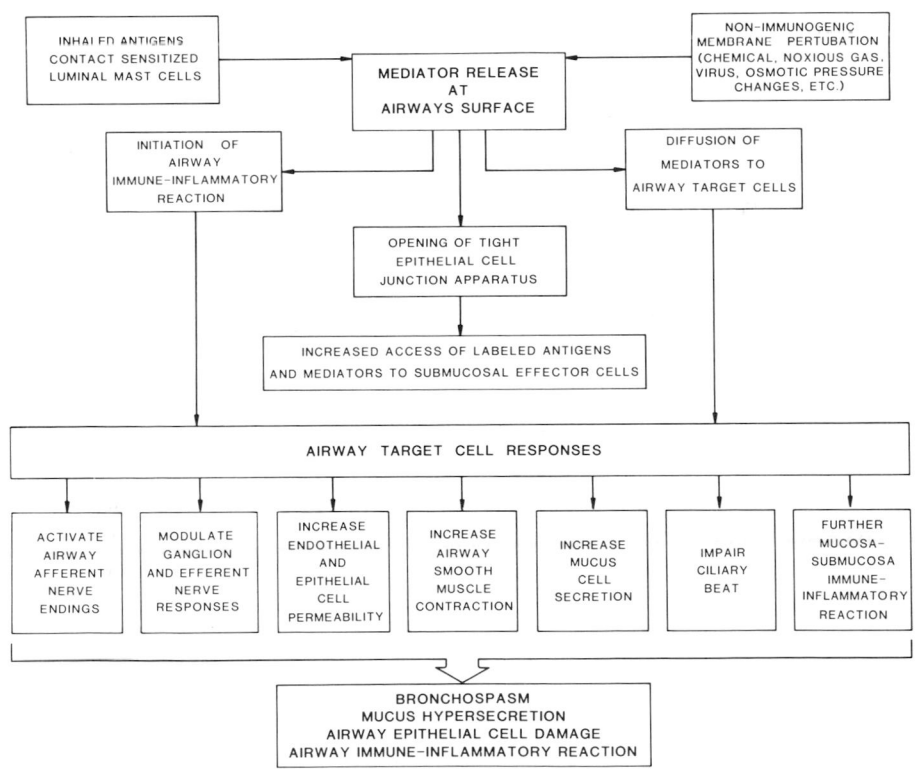

Fig. 3-3. Mast cell mediator responses.

the lumen into the submucosa, thus theoretically impeding the absorption of many noxious or immunologic substances from airway luminal surfaces. Airway responses initiated by mediator release and subsequent airway inflammatory reactions are associated with an opening of the tight intracellular bridges. The increase in mucosal permeability provides a direct access from airway lumen to airway mucosa-submucosa and smooth muscle. Thus, locally released mediators are capable of facilitating the influx of antigen to submucosal mast cells and thus locally amplifying the response. This increase in the access of mediators (and a variety of other stimuli or irritants) to the afferent neural plexis immediately below the junction apparatus also provides for a generalized neurogenic bronchoconstrictive response and augments intraluminal mediator availabilities to such other target cells as the submucosal smooth muscle cells and microvasculature endothelial cells. Thus, the tight junctions between the airway epithelial cells may play a critical role not only as a pathway for transepithelial ionic fluxes (as per other epithelial surfaces) but also as a "regulated" permeability barrier capable of modulating the transepithelial flux of both relatively small molecules ("mediators") and larger proteins (immunogenic substances). The fact that tight junctions can presumably be opened by mediators released by mast cells lying on or near the airway epithelial cells has implications for treatment, in that therapeutic agents given via inhalant routes could be expected to effectively reach these superficial mast cells in high concentrations. This fact also supports the concept that any respiratory tract injury mechanism which causes changes in airway epithelial plasma membranes also induces physiologically important changes in airway permeability.

Recent evidence has strongly suggested but not unequivocally proven that airway inflammation could represent the key ingredient in the development of airway hyperresponsiveness. The epithelial damage following an inflammatory reaction of the airways might induce airway hyperreactivity by several mechanisms. For example, it is probable that airway inflammatory reactions result in both increased airway permeability and increased airway responsiveness to bronchoconstrictive stimuli. This has two further implications.

First, airway epithelium damaged by acid, certain pollutants, or respiratory viruses appears to exhibit an increased absorption of inhaled antigenic proteins, suggesting a role for inflammation in augmenting the immune responsiveness of the airway. This could account for the high incidence of airway allergic phenomena in cystic fibrosis, a disease characterized by recurrent airways infection. Similarly, there appears to be a significant association between bronchiolitis in infancy and the development of asthma in childhood. It would explain the fact that acute bronchial infection or overwhelming exposure to agents causing noninfectious airway inflammation have been noted to herald the onset of asthma in adults. Finally, this would be compatible with the fact that classical allergic bronchial asthma has developed in some patients who had occupational and environmental asthmas that appear to be nonimmunogenic at the onset (and presumably secondary to chemical, pharmacologic, or toxic injury to airway epithelia).

Second, airways inflammation per se can induce allergic, asthma-like airway reactions. This is believed to occur via mechanisms of phagocyte and/ or mast cell activation, with various immune-inflammatory mediator releases playing the important contributory roles. This may account for the fact that respiratory tract infections (especially respiratory viruses) are among the stimuli most frequently evoking acute exacerbations of both allergic and nonallergic forms of asthma and may relate to the airway hyperreactivity states seen in some smokers and seen in bronchitis. It is probable that immune-inflammatory mediators released by phagocytes recruited into airway inflammatory foci provoke both direct and neurogenic bronchoconstrictive responses somewhat analogous to those elicited by the classical immunogenic mast cell release reactions (Fig. 3-2).

Although much literature has accumulated concerning the cytotoxicity of phagocyte-generated lysosomal enzyme substances and reactive oxygen species (such as O_2^-, H_2O_2, and $\cdot OH$), there is only fragmentary knowledge concerning the role of phagocytic mediators in inducing and sustaining bronchospastic conditions. Both lysosomal enzyme and oxidant-induced direct epithelial cell injury, and possibly concomitant nonimmunogenic mast cell mediator releases, appear to represent potential mechanisms whereby airway inflammatory responses could produce mediator inflammatory responses related bronchoconstriction. For example, it is interesting in a physiological sense that H_2O_2 and other reduced oxygen metabolites, released by phagocytes into their immediate microenvironment have been shown to cause mediator release from mast cells. However, whether or not mast cells themselves play a significant role in initiating and sustaining nonimmunologic inflammatory-related bronchoconstrictive processes in asthma remains to be fully documented. The recent concept of mast cell heterogeneity and the implications of the various mast cell subpopulations in asthma is another area in need of further investigation.

Much asthma research activity currently is focused upon detailed considerations of how acute transudative allergic airway responses lead to development of the chronic exudative inflammatory airway reactions which are characteristic of the more prolonged and severe human asthmatic episodes. Much of this focus upon the latter airway responses relates to studies of the pathogenesis of airway immune-inflammation processes which are characterized by the influx of polymorphonuclear phagocytes and varying amounts of eosinophils. The various chemotactic factors which attract phagocytes may be especially important in that the recruited and "activated" phagocytes serve to amplify the pre-existing, mast-cell-initiated immune-inflammatory responses and may be responsible for the epithelial damage seen in chronic forms of asthma. This phase also appears to be associated with a heightened airway hyperreactivity. Although eosinophils contain a number of substances that can inactivate immune-inflammatory mediators, their granular proteins, such as major basic protein and peroxidase, are potentially toxic to airway cells. It also appears that eosinophils are capable of releasing sulfidopeptide leukotrienes such as LTC_4 when appropriately activated. It seems likely that airway eosinophils contribute to pathophysiologic processes operative in asthma. This argument is strengthened by recent evidence suggesting that toxic eosinophilic cationic proteins may play a central part in the development of the visceral necrotizing granulomatous lesions seen in allergic granulomatosis and angiitis. The important therapeutic ramifications of agents designed to modulate or down-regulate phagocytic and eosinophilic recruitments to the airways in asthma is readily apparent!

Although the major cyclooxygenase products of AA generated by airway cells, including mast cells and phagocytes, have been shown to have potent effects on airway function for a number of years, their precise cumulative roles in allergic and nonallergic forms of bronchial asthma remain unclear. Prostaglandins such as PGD_2 and $PGF_2\alpha$, as well as thromboxanes, cause airway bronchoconstriction, whereas on the other hand PGE_2 and PGI_2 are generally recognized as having relaxant properties. Although several studies have implicated both PGD_2 and thromboxane to be important in the pathogenesis of airway hyperreactivity states, the precise relevance of their roles in the development of bronchospasm or airway hyperresponsiveness states remains to be further detailed. The recent demonstration that PGD_2 potentiates airway responsiveness to histamine and methacholine suggests that prostaglandins may exhibit important interactions with other transmitters known to be important in modulating airway smooth muscle tone. The discovery of the lipoxygenase pathway of biologically active AA oxidation products, termed leukotrienes, has yielded even further evidence that AA metabolites probably play an important role in the pathophysiology of bronchial asthma. Although the amount varies from cell to cell, most cells contain esterified AA as a constituent of their membrane phospholipid fraction and which can be released subsequent to membrane perturbation. AA metabolites are synthesized in various pathways by most cells in response to various stimuli and primarily act as tissue hormones. They are also likely to participate in the initiation and the regulation of immune-inflammatory reactions. They are found in inflamed tissue, their action is locally restricted, and they are capable of both up-regulating and down-regulating inflammatory responses. This has fostered the notion that they have a predominant function as intercellular or intracellular signals in the context of their putative role in cell and tissue immune-inflammatory processes.

The leukotrienes can operationally be divided into two groups: the dihydroxy acids, LTB_4 and its isomers and metabolites, potent chemotactic substances for polymorphonuclear leukocytes; and the sulfidopeptide leukotrienes LTC_4, LTD_4, and LTE_4 and LTF_4, bronchoconstrictive and vasoactive substances several orders of magnitude more potent than histamine. LCB_4 is one of the most potent known chemoattractant substances for polymorphonuclear leukocytes and also causes aggregation and degranulation of these cells. It has been shown to be present in effusions and exudates and has thus been implicated in the genesis of inflammatory responses in several tissues and diseases. Recently, aerosol administration of LCB_4 has been shown to induce airway hyperresponsiveness, perhaps via its effect to recruit phagocytes into the airway epithelium. The sulfidopeptide leukotrienes have been shown to be increased in respiratory tract inflammatory exudates, including those initiated by allergic reactions. LTC_4 and LTD_4 are about 3000 times as potent as histamine in provoking isolated human respiratory smooth muscle bronchoconstriction and are of much longer duration. LTC_4 appears to be important in the secretory function of mucus-producing airway cells and may even modulate alveolar macrophage "activation" and secretion processes. LTD_4 has been shown to impair airway tracheobronchial clearance mechanisms, although it is also a potent bronchoconstrictor. LTE_4, like histamine, is capable of increasing airway microvascular permeability (especially postcapillary permeability), but is far more potent. It has been reported to increase permeability by causing contraction of endothelial cells.

Although the lipoxygenase pathway of AA metabolism is capable of producing substances which could play a key role in the bronchospasm, inflammation, and mucus production which dominate the pathophysiology of severe forms of bronchial asthma, there is yet little information to suggest the physiologic functions that they may serve. As with the prostaglandins, some of the effects on airway cells of the spasmogenic sulfidopeptide leukotrienes appear to operate via receptor mechanisms. Reflex-mediated responses have also been described, based on the modulating effects that vagotomy and ganglionic blocker administrations have on some of their actions. In some systems, there appear to be separate pools of AA for the prostaglandins and the leukotrienes. This may not be the case for lung, since cyclooxygenase inhibitors which inhibit the generation of prostaglandins from human lung during antigen challenge have been found to greatly increase the output of leukotrienes.

Over the last few years, it has emerged that alveolar macrophages have important secretory functions. They represent the principal resident phagocytes in the lung and are known to possess an active AA metabolic pathway. Alveolar macrophages probably represent a potential major source of prostaglandin- and leukotriene-generation capability in the lung. (The membrane lipid of these cells contains high levels of esterified AA, up to 25 percent of its phospholipid fatty acid composition.) Alveolar macrophages release both prostaglandins and leukotrienes in response to a variety of both soluble and particulate stimuli (including pathogenic microorganisms). These macrophages have Fc membrane receptors which are able to bind to IgE in asthmatic patients and to be specifically activated by pneumoallergens. They thus seem capable, along with mast cells and polymorphonuclear leukocytes, of participating in mediator releases related to asthmatic airway responses. Recently, it has been shown that alveolar macrophages (as well as polymorphonuclear leukocytes) are capable of releasing factors that induce mediator release from mast cells and basophils. Alveolar macrophages also possess receptors for both prostaglandins and leukotrienes, suggesting a complicated role for these cells in immune-inflammatory reactions. However, the precise role of these cells in bronchial asthma remains poorly understood.

In spite of a wealth of information generated over the past two decades, there is as yet an incomplete understanding concerning the membrane events that signal both mast cell (or phagocyte) "activation" and secretion. The precise interrelationships between the various mast cell membrane receptors, the transducing and translating proteins, and the final second messengers such as cAMP, cGMP, and IP3, are complex and probably interdependent. As shown in Figure 3-4, it is probable that phosphatidylinositol (PIP_2) hydrolysis acts as a multifunctional transducer, the generated inositol triphosphate (IP_3) stimulating mediator release via increasing cytosolic calcium concentration whereas DG may activate AA metabolism through its activation of phospholipase A_2. Although it is not yet possible to obtain a complete picture of the various operative and interactive metabolic pathways, it is already apparent that physiologic, pathologic, and pharmacologic regulations can occur at almost all levels of this complex membrane activation sequence.

In some asthmatics (5–15 percent), cyclooxygenase inhibitors such as aspirin and indomethacin appear to induce asthmatic attacks via mast cell release mechanisms. Until discovery of the lipoxygenase pathway, it had been hypothesized that this nonsteroidal anti-inflammatory agent induction of bronchoconstriction in sensitive asthmatics could be explained by a decrease in the synthesis of bronchodilating prostaglandins. Since discovery of the lipoxygenase pathway, an alternative explanation has involved the overproduction of leukotrienes with strong bronchoconstrictor activities. Indeed, in some systems, including the lung, it has been demonstrated that cyclooxygenase inhibitors divert AA metabolism into lipoxygenase pathways. The degree to which this occurs in such cells, as the mast cell, depends upon whether or not the potential cell AA pool had equal access to enzymes subserving cyclooxygenase and lipoxygenase pathways of AA metabolism. Either explanation could serve if the susceptible asthmatics had an intrinsic sensitivity to bronchoconstrictor stimuli due to underactivity of counterbalancing bronchodilator pathways.

In certain situations, cyclooxygenase metabolites themselves may play an important role as regulators of airway cell function, much as we now

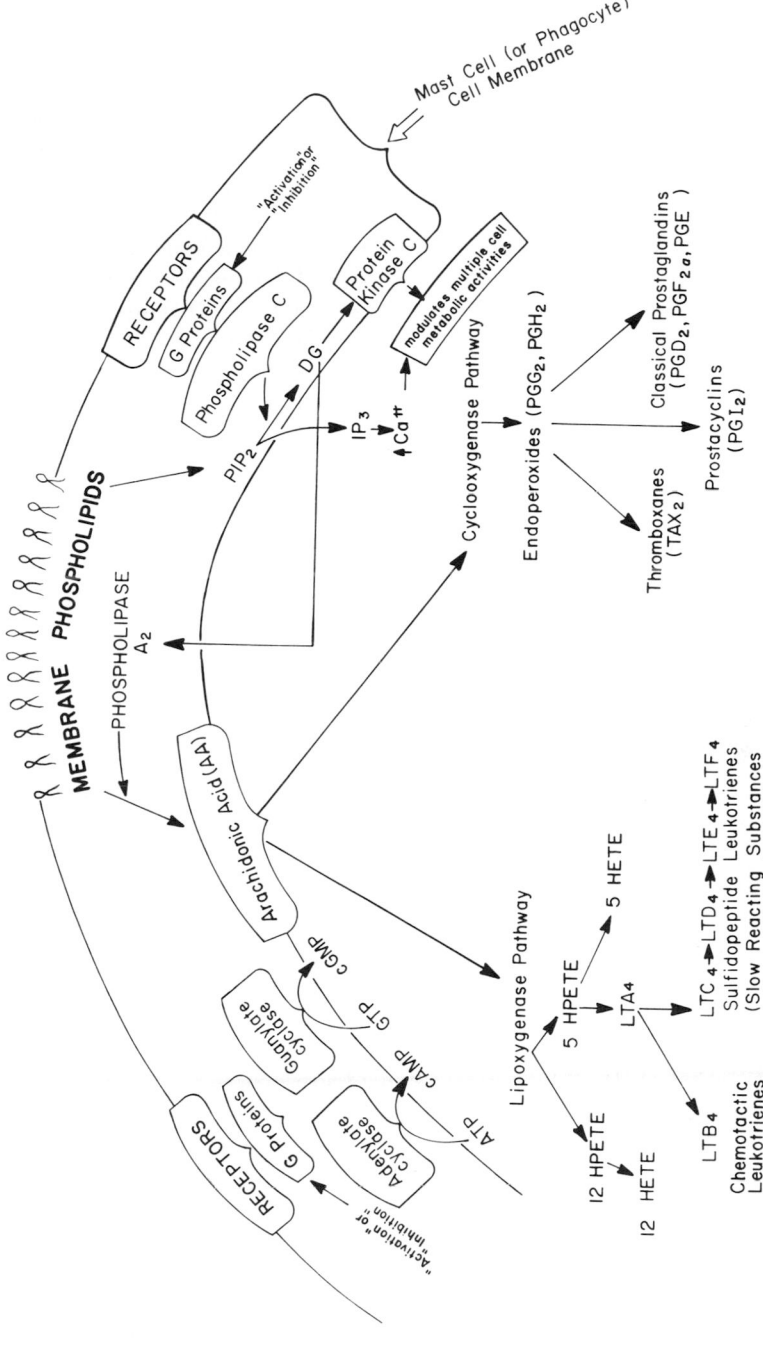

Fig. 3-4. Simplified schematic of mast cell (or phagocyte) membrane "activation" pathways. Receptors are "activated" by numerous substances such as α, β and cholinergic agonists and by non-specific membrane perturbations.

51

recognize that prostaglandins play important roles in the circulation and in kidney and in stomach functions. For example, the discovery that prostaglandins act via a membrane-bound receptor to regulate adenylate cyclase, and thus modulate intracellular cyclic AMP levels, suggests that they could influence a wide variety of airway cell functions. The interactions between prostaglandins and leukotrienes, some in synergy and some in opposition, along with different AA metabolism profiles in individual cells, point to a complex symphony whereby metabolites of AA play a more important role in cellular function than that previously envisioned. The recent disclosure of the synthetic pathways, structure, and airway receptors of the sulfidopeptide leukotrienes opens the way towards new and enlightened study of the pathophysiology and therapy of asthma and other allergic diseases.

It is generally recognized that both mast cells and phagocytes have active biosynthetic systems for the metabolism of AA. Indeed, even isolated cultures of airway epithelial cells have been shown to release metabolites of AA into tissue culture media. It seems probable that AA metabolites play a pivotal role in the pathophysiology of both allergy-related and nonallergy-related inflammation. For example, both mast cell and phagocyte membrane activations result in activations of phosphoinositide hydrolysis with increased phosphatidyl inositol turnover and subsequent activation of phospholipase A_2 and release of AA which has been stored in membrane phospholipid. AA metabolism products via both cyclooxygenase-dependent and lipooxygenase-dependent pathways probably play significant roles as mediators and regulators in numerous allergic, inflammatory, and immune processes. Increasing evidence supports the belief that metabolites of AA can have profound effects upon lung function and that these metabolites may be significant physiologic regulators of airway tone, at least under certain circumstances. Those metabolites which may play a role in causing bronchoconstrictor responses include the endoperoxides, $PGF_2\alpha$, PGD_2, thromboxanes and the sulfidopeptide leukotrienes. Those that may cause a relaxation of bronchial smooth muscle include PGE_2 and PGI_2. (PGI_2 has minimal bronchoactive properties in humans.) Interest in the cyclooxygenase metabolites is high not only because several of this series appear to influence airway tone, but also because several of these prostaglandins (especially those of the PGE_2 series) seem capable of modulating antigen-IgE-induced mast cell mediator release.

AA metabolism has become the main focus of investigators interested in immediate hypersensitivity reactions because of its role in prostaglandin metabolism, sulfidopeptide leukotriene generation, and leukotriene chemotactic activity. This generation of chemostatic factors such as leukotriene B_4 (LTB_4; Fig. 3-4) could not only maintain asthmatic inflammatory stimuli over a period of time, but also reinforces a role for metabolites of AA in nonimmunologic inflammation-related forms of asthma in that all cell types, including respiratory epithelial cells, contain AA as a constituent of their membrane phospholipids. It is likely that AA metabolites contribute to the pathobiology of bronchospastic responses of injured airways, such as that seen following acid aspiration and that seen following overwhelming chemical injury. Further exploration of the cyclooxygenase and lipoxygenase pathways of AA metabolism could represent an important common mechanism by which both immunologic and nonimmunologic mediator releases and metabolic activations result in airway spasmogenesis and inflammation. The concept that allergen-induced and inflammation-induced airway spasmogenesis may be considered to operate through similar mechanisms is further buttressed by the recent demonstration that reactive forms of oxygen (one of the most intensely studied mediators of inflammation at the present time) are capable of activating mast cells and initiating mediator release.

PERSISTENT AIRWAY HYPERREACTIVITY

There is general consensus that airway hyperreactivity to a variety of stimuli represents the cardinal feature of asthma and may be the most basic pathogenic event in the acquisition of the disease. As depicted in Figure 3-5, patients with asthma develop bronchoconstriction in response to a wide variety of physical, chemical, and pharmacological stimuli. Asthmatic patients can be characterized as developing a greater degree of response to smaller doses of various provocative inhalants that do normal subjects.* Whereas immunogenic mechanisms are demonstrable in only 25–50 percent of asthmatic patients, airway hyperreactiviy is detectable in essentially all asthmatics, even during periods of clinical remission. The degree of airway hyperresponsiveness in asthmatic patients seems to vary with the severity of the asthma. Although in some models of asthma the degree of hyperreactivity appears to be associated with the degree of subacute and chronic immune-inflammatory airway pathology, as demonstrated by associations between airway reactivity to provocative challenge and the inflammatory cells and

---

*Hyperreactivity is an abnormally increased response to a stimulus. In the case of airway hyperreactivity, the stimulus (aerosols of chemical mediators or cholinergic agents, noxious gases, allergens, cold or dehumidified air, hypotonic or hypertonic solutions, etc.) is usually inhaled and the response is conventionally a measurement of the mechanical result of airway narrowing. Operationally, three in vivo measurement methods are used in bronchial provocation tests: (1) determination of the smallest stimulus or provocation dose that causes a significant measurable predetermined response, i.e., "threshold"; (2) the slope of the stimulus/response curve, i.e., "sensitivity"; and (3) the measured response to a single quantitative stimulus. A number of factors may play a role in such tests, making it difficult to assess their results. The investigator must pay special attention to a number of potential problems. This attention must include a rigorous assessment of stimulus, including quantitative assessments of the dose and of the location of stimulus deposition in the airways and definitive and reproducible measurement of the stimulus-response relationship. Since aerosol deposition depends not only on the characteristic of the nebulizer but also on the pattern of breathing and the degree of airway obstruction, evaluations of stimulus-responses are somewhat interdependent and not always interpretable.

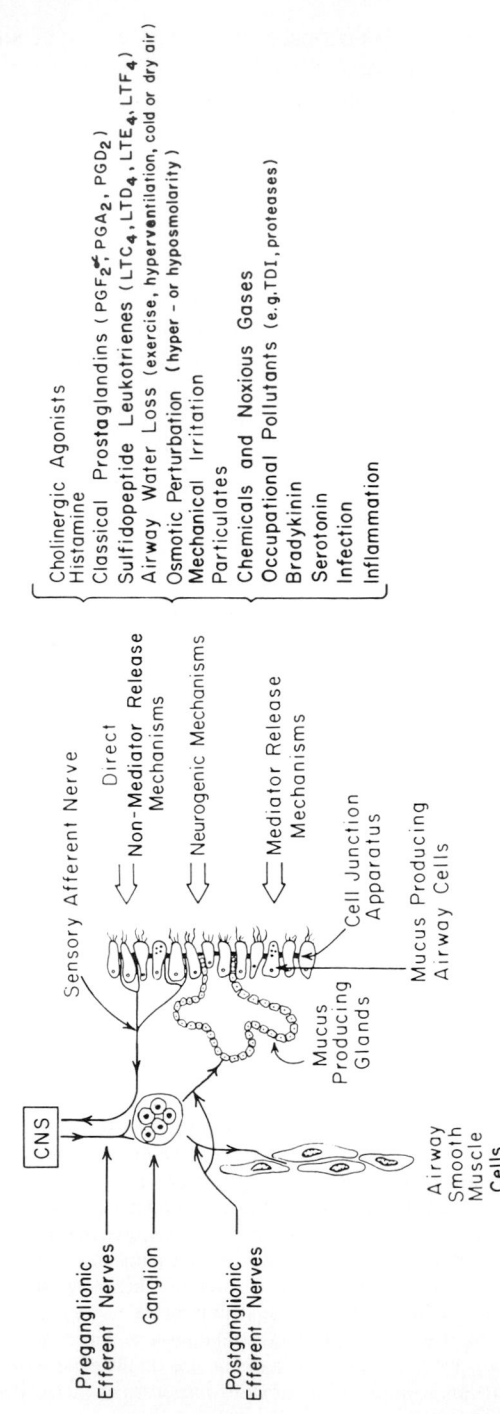

Cholinergic Agonists
Histamine
Classical Prostaglandins (PGF_2^{α}, PGA_2, PGD_2)
Sulfidopeptide Leukotrienes (LTC_4, LTD_4, LTE_4, LTF_4)
Airway Water Loss (exercise, hyperventilation, cold or dry air)
Osmotic Perturbation (hyper- or hyposmolarity)
Mechanical Irritation
Particulates
Chemicals and Noxious Gases
Occupational Pollutants (e.g. TDI, proteases)
Bradykinin
Serotonin
Infection
Inflammation

Sensory Afferent Nerve

Direct
Non-Mediator Release Mechanisms

Neurogenic Mechanisms

Mediator Release Mechanisms

Cell Junction Apparatus

Mucus Producing Airway Cells

Mucus Producing Glands

CNS

Airway Smooth Muscle Cells

Preganglionic Efferent Nerves

Ganglion

Postganglionic Efferent Nerves

Fig. 3-5. Stimuli producing bronchoconstriction in asthmatics.

mediators in bronchoalveolar lavage and/or lung mucosa-submucosa pathology, this correlation does not appear to be invariable and, before accepted, will require more human documentation. In many patients, this hyperreactivity appears to persist even after improvement in antigen-induced bronchial hyperreactivity has been successfully accomplished by specific allergen desensitization procedures or after prolonged removals from known inciting agents.

Although many explanations have been put forth to account for the increased airway reactivity to inhaled irritants and pharmacologic agents that is characteristic of asthma, none fully fits the clinical and experimental data. In fact, the nonspecific airway hyperreactivity that is nearly ubiquitous for asthmatic patients is not specific for those patients alone. Other patients exhibiting airway hyperreactivity include approximately 50 percent of hay fever patients who have never wheezed, some patients with atopic dermatitis, some patients who smoke cigarettes, a minority of patients with cigarette-related chronic bronchitis, and most patients with clinical respiratory tract manifestations of cystic fibrosis. In cystic fibrosis, the degree of bronchial hyperreactivity may undulate with pulmonary exacerbations of the disease. Although some studies have shown that up to 50 percent of patients with chronic obstructive pulmonary disease have bronchial hyperreactivity (defined as an increased response to inhaled histamine or methacholine), the position and shape of the dose-response relationships appear different from the dose-responses of asthmatic subjects with similar degrees of airway obstruction, suggesting that airway hyperreactivity states may be caused by more than one effector pathway.

Individuals with hyperreactive airways appear to exhibit some abnormalities of airway smooth muscle control. For example, after a full inspiration, airway caliber often increases in normals, whereas in asthmatics, bronchoconstriction frequently occurs. This suggests that asthmatics have an impaired ability to reduce bronchomotor tone after lung inflation. The paroxysmal response may provide a clue to the abnormal control of smooth muscle tone seen in asthmatic patients. The failure of cyclooxygenase inhibitors to influence this response makes it unlikely that local inspiration-induced bronchodilatory or bronchoconstrictory releases of prostaglandins could explain this phenomenon. Likewise, the fact that asthmatics have a larger diurnal circadian variation in amplitude of respiratory resistance than do normal individuals remains a pathophysiologic enigma. This increased diurnal variation in lung function appears to be related to the severity of the underlying bronchial hyperreactivity.

Healthy subjects exhibit varying degrees of temporary airway hyperreactivity, such as: (1) during and immediately following upper-respiratory tract viral infections; (2) subsequent to a single exposure to high levels of an irritating vapor, fume, or smoke; (3) following exposures to various air pollutants; and (4) even after routine vaccination with live attenuated influenza virus. This hyperreactivity may last for many weeks following a respiratory tract viral infection and may be persistent for years following overwhelming irritant chemical exposures. This situation pertains to several of the agents that have been associated with occupationally related airway hyperreactivity states. In some instances, such as following inhalant exposure to proteolytic enzymes, the associated bronchial hyperreactivity has been explained by toxic or pharmacological airway epithelial injury (see following), while in other instances the same agent has been shown to elicit more classic immunogenic-related airway inflammatory reactions. For example, in asthmatic conditions associated with both toluene diisocyanate and with platinum, both toxic-pharmacologic and immunologenic mechanisms of pathogenesis have been demonstrated to be present.

Classical concepts of nervous regulation of mammalian airway smooth muscle emphasize the importance of excitatory cholinergic nerves and inhibitory β_2-adrenergic nerves. Thus, cholinergic receptor stimulation produces a bronchoconstriction, while adrenergic stimulation produces a bronchodilating effect, probably due to the relative abundance of dilating β_2-adrenergic receptors and the paucity of bronchoconstricting α_1-adrenergic receptors on airway smooth muscle cells. As with mast cell mediators, considerable differences exist among species with regard to both the types of receptors present on smooth muscle cells and the innervation of these cells.

There is considerable evidence that patients with asthma possess an array of abnormal autonomic airway smooth muscle responses beyond the increased sensitivity to inhaled cholinergic agonists such as methacholine. Some studies have demonstrated that subjects with asthma have increased α-adrenergic as well as increased cholinergic sensitivities. This is consistent with the presence of α-adrenergic receptors in the large airways of primates, although the maximal response by stimulation of these receptors may be only approximately 10 percent of the maximal cholinergic bronchoconstrictive response. The increased sensitivity to inhaled histamine appears to work via neurogenic responses operating through stimulation of afferent airway nerve endings, as both hexamethonium (airway ganglionic blocker) and atropine (cholinergic blocker) appear to abolish the bronchoconstriction elicited by inhaled histamine. This strongly suggests that histamine-induced airway hyperreactivity operates via a cholinergic effector mechanism. In some species, however, and under some experimental conditions, histamine appears to exert its primary effect by a direct bronchoconstrictive effect on airway smooth muscle H_1 receptors. Hexamethonium is not effective in blocking the airway hyperreactivity provoked by cholinergic agonists, suggesting the possibility that in vivo airway hyperreactivity may be due to the responsiveness of airway smooth muscle to contractile agonists.

With abundant evidence showing that airway smooth muscle bronchoconstriction tone is increased in asthma, it is no surprise that numerous investigators have somewhat dogmatically proposed that hypoactive β-adrenergic-receptor bronchodilating activity is the underlying pathophysiologic abnormality. Receptor-binding studies have shown that the concentration of β-adrenergic receptors is higher in the lungs than in other tissues and autoradiograms have confirmed that there is a high density of β-adrenergic receptors in the smooth muscle of the large and small airways. The physiologic role of the β-adrenergic receptors in the airways remain unclarified, however. There are only controversial data suggesting that asthmatic patients possess β-adrenergic defects which could contribute to their airway hyperreactivity. This suggestion is based upon decreased cell membrane receptors for β-adrenergic agonists as demonstrated by several cell types (e.g., lymphocytes) obtained from asthmatic patients. Beta-agonist therapeutic administrations and high levels of endogenous cathecholamines (increased by various kinds of stress, including asthma itself) could themselves cause a decrease in cellular membrane β-adrenergic receptors. For example, the desensitization of β-receptors seen in some patients with depressive disorders has recently been correlated more closely with the severity of the associated psychomotor agitation than with the severity of the depression. This group of patients does not seem hypersusceptible to asthma. Thus, the ultimate validity of the β-adrenergic approach to the etiology of hyperreactive airways pathophysiology seems unconvincing. A more specific analysis of the appropriate human airway smooth muscle receptors should be carried out under appropriately controlled conditions to settle this hypothesis. In fact, there is as yet no conclusive evidence that in vivo airway responsiveness to histamine or carbachol correlates with in vitro airway smooth muscle responses to cholinergic agents, histamine, β-adrenergic agonists, or even agents influencing the smooth muscle adenylate cyclase system.

It was formerly believed that the tonic activity of the parasympathetic and sympathetic nerves alone was the only major determinant regulating the tone of respiratory smooth muscle. Recently, attention has been focused on other types of potentially important innervations in airway smooth muscle; this attention is based on a theory analogous to the current concept that a large number of neurotransmitters operate in the intestinal tract. Unfortunately, knowledge of the action on airways of these peptidergic and nonpeptidergic, noncholingeric, and nonadrenergic pathways is as yet rather fragmentary.

Recent studies of various neuropeptides suggest that local release of these peptides may play an important role in airway responses to injury, including bronchospastic responses. For example, irritant gases, including cigarette smoke, are capable of stimulating vagal afferent neurons in the airway submucosa to release substance P, a substance which has been shown to cause both bronchoconstriction and mucosal edema, an effect that can be at least partially blocked by substance-P antagonists. Thus, substance P released from sensory nerve endings during irritation is capable of potentiating airway immune-inflammatory processes. This hypothesis is strengthened by findings indicating that substance P is a likely mediator of neurogenic protein leakage in many organs, including the skin. Of equal importance is the realization that nonadrenergic inhibitory systems may be even more important than β-adrenergic receptors in modulating normal airway smooth muscle activity. This concept promises to bring about a revision of the traditional ideas which have emphasized cholinergic/adrenergic mechanisms as the sole determinants of airway smooth muscle tone. While the transmitter of this bronchodilation mechanism has yet to be identified with certainty, this system has been found to be operative in airway smooth muscle from the trachea to the smallest peripheral airways. This concept raises important new questions about the process of bronchomotor nerve control and introduces a new complexity into the understanding of airway hyperreactivity states.

The nonadrenergic inhibitory pathway which produces bronchodilation can be elicited by vagal nerve stimulation after muscarinic (cholinergic) receptor blockade with atropine, and is not affected after α- or β-adrenergic blockade with phenoxybenzamine and propranolol, respectively, or after adrenergic neuronal blockade with guanethidine. Activity is likewise unaffected by histamine (H_1) and serotonin receptor blockade. Since the prolonged dilatation response can be abolished by autonomic ganglionic blockade with hexamethonium, the system seems supplied by preganglionic fibers in the vagus. The neurotransmitter involved has not been conclusively identified, although various peptidergic (e.g., vasoactive intestinal peptide, enkephaline) or purinergic (e.g., adenosine) transmitters may be operative. For example, vasoactive intestinal peptide is known to be present in nerves supplying bronchial smooth muscle, glands, and blood vessels. It has been shown to relax segments of airway smooth muscle in vitro and to protect against the bronchoconstrictor action of histamine, PGE_2, LCD_4 and PAF. There are preliminary reports that some human asthmatics respond to inhaled vasoactive intestinal peptide inhalation with bronchodilatation. Conversely, adenosine and AMP are potent bronchoconstrictors when they are administered by inhalation to allergic or non-allergic asthmatic subjects but not to normal subjects. As similar findings have also been reported following exposures to these two purinergic agents in isolated human bronchial smooth muscle derived from airways of normals and asthmatics, it has been suggested that airway smooth muscle has in some way been altered by the airway inflammation seen in both allergic and non-allergic asthmatics.

Although the physiologic significance of the nonadrenergic inhibitory innervation of the airways is unknown, it has been speculated that this system might function as the principal inhibitory pathway for airway smooth muscle. It is recognized that these pathways represent the most important mechanism controlling the relaxation phase of gastrointestinal (GI) tract peristalsis and that the respiratory tract and the GI tract are both endodermic in origin. When the nonadrenergic inhibitory system in the GI tract is abnormal, as in Hirschsprung's Disease or in clinical states involving intramural ganglion cells, the result is loss of inhibitory control and spasm of GI tract smooth muscle. If indeed airway smooth muscle nonadrenergic inhibitory pathways play a correspondingly important role in the regulation of airway muscle tone, a defect in the system could account for the bronchoconstriction caused by β-adrenergic blockade of the remaining functional bronchodilation system in patients with hyperreactive airways. The recent immunoreactive demonstration that abundant vasoactive intestinal peptide is localized in nerve fibers in bronchial walls in locations well situated to influence airway caliber strengthens the analogy that exists between GI tract and respiratory tract smooth muscle innervations. The problem of which bronchodilating neurotransmitter is most important and where it exerts its principal actions (e.g., afferent or efferent nerve endings, airway ganglion cells, airway smooth muscle cells) becomes more difficult to solve because in several instances peptide neurotransmitters occur together with more "classic" transmitters in the same neuron, suggesting significant interactive functions. Whether or not vasoactive intestinal peptide and/or other peptidergic or nonpeptidergic, noncholinergic, nonadrenergic systems that have already been identified in the intestinal tract will prove to be important in modulating overall tone and reactivity threshold in the respiratory tract remains speculative.

It should also be remembered that the variously described neurotransmitters are capable of modulating mast cell receptors and probably capable of influencing a wide variety of different airway cellular receptor sites. It thus may be difficult to ascribe the effects of an administered agent as being due solely to a stimulus on airway smooth muscle receptor sites alone. For example, atropine, a cholinergic agonist which many investigators have used to characterize the role of cholinergic pathways in normal and asthmatic bronchomotor tone, has antihistaminic properties, may effect mast cell mediator release, and has recently been hypothesized to be involved in inhibiting cellular releases of cyclooxygenase products of arachidonic acid metabolism. Adenosine, which may be released from lung purinergic nerve endings, causes bronchoconstriction but also appears to modulate histamine release.

Another confounding feature is that complex adrenergic-cholinergic interactions potentially exist both prejunctionally, at the level of the autonomic nerve terminals, and postjunctionally, at the level of the responding cells themselves. One therefore has to consider not only the direct influences of cholinergic, adrenergic, and various noncholinergic, nonadrenergic neurotransmitters and neuromodulators on receptors on airway smooth muscle cells, but also concomitant potential effects on such interdependent airway structures as mast cells, airway nerves, and airway ganglia. For example, opioid peptides have been reported to cause bronchospasm by central mechanisms or via eliciting histamine release from pulmonary mast cells. These same agents have also been reported to inhibit the medullary bronchoconstrictor center and to inhibit the exocytotic release of acetylcholine from postganglionic parasympathetic neurons innervating airway smooth muscle, thereby modulating bronchomotor tone by inhibiting reflex-induced bronchoconstriction. In addition to modulating mast cell release and intrinsic airway smooth muscle tone, β-adrenergic agonists have been shown to inhibit neurotransmission through the airway parasympathetic ganglia. The recent demonstration that prostaglandin E_2 has an inhibitory effect on cholinergic neurotransmission at a prejunctional site in canine trachealis smooth muscle illustrates the complexities in unravelling the role that specific transmitters potentially play in modulating airway smooth muscle tone.

It should be recognized that just as knowledge of airway smooth muscle innervation is not very far advanced, much basic information concerning airway smooth muscle itself is at a truly rudimentary level. The biochemistry and metabolism of airway smooth muscle has been relatively neglected in contrast to investigation of the contractile systems in intestinal and cardiac smooth muscle. For example, elucidation of mechanisms whereby the various neurotransmitters act on airway smooth muscle cell membrane systems to control intracellular calcium concentration, and knowledge of the sensitivity of calcium and noncalcium-dependent regulatory mechanisms on the muscle contractile apparatus, is little. Although strong neurogenic controls of airway smooth muscle are known to exist, the morphologic and functional correlates responsible for this neurogenic control are poorly understood. Thus, in addition to the probable role of mediator release, it may be that neurogenic mechanisms, alteration of specific membrane receptors, abnormalities in transmembrane signal transduction, or abnormalities in contractile apparatus, could contribute to the phenomenon of airway hyperreactivity.

Increased airway sensitivity is manifested by bronchoconstrictive responses to concentrations of cholinergic drugs, histamine, bronchoconstrictive prostaglandins, leukotrienes, and certain pollutants that are up to several magnitudes lower than amounts necessary to cause equivalent degrees of bronchoconstriction in normal subjects. Although it is generally accepted that asthmatic subjects show a marked hyperreactivity to histamine and methacholine when compared to normal subjects (up to 10–100 times more hyperreactive), there is contradictory information as to whether or not asthmatics exhibit the same degree of increased sensitivity to the sulfidopeptide leukotrienes. The leukotrienes have a longer duration of action and are effective at concentrations from one one-thousandth to one five-thousandth that of both histamine and methacholine in normal subjects.

Precise locations and the cellular basis of airway hyperreactive responses remain surprisingly enigmatic. Although histamine responses appear to be predominantly triggered by stimulation of subepithelial afferent nerve receptors, the specific locus of airway cholinergic hyperresponses seems unsettled. Although airway afferent and cholinergic efferent nerve pathways may play a dominating role in modulating the acute airway bronchomotor responses to inhaled antigens, the precise relative importance of both afferent and cholinergic nerve pathways in the genesis of naturally occurring human asthmatic attacks remains less well clarified.

Increased sensitivity and/or reactivity to inhaled stimuli of afferent receptors lying in the bronchial epithelium represents one mechanism that may be especially important in the pathogenesis of airway hyperreactivity. Airway epithelial cells, like other epithelial surfaces, are tightly "bound" by cell junction apparatus. It is known that various substances, such as mediators of immune-inflammatory phenomena, can influence the "tightness" of the junction apparatus (Fig. 3-3). Although there is not unanimous agreement, it is probable that allergic or inflammatory stimuli influence overall airway permeability via this mechanism, thus facilitating access of airway stimuli (such as histamine) to target receptors, including afferent nerve receptors in the airway submucosa. This mechanism offers an explanation for the heightened airway hyperreactivity seen following airway insults such as those experienced in viral infection, following exposure to sulfur dioxide, nitrogen dioxide, or ozone, or following acute airway exposures to noxious chemicals.

The basic mechanisms for the development of persistent increased airway reactivity remain speculative. In some experimental models, such as following ozone exposure and after antigen-induced, late-phase bronchospastic reactions, the degree of airway hyperreactivity has been shown to be both quantitatively and temporally associated with airway inflammation, as defined by: (1) the presence of inflammatory cells and mediators in lavage fluid; and (2) airway pathology demonstrating a typical inflammatory reaction. In some forms of antigen-induced and exercise-induced asthma, changes in serum chemotactic activity levels and neutrophil complement receptors give further credence to the role of inflammatory reactions in airway hyperreactivity states. In fact, some challenge studies have shown increases in serum neutrophil chemotactic activity to parallel the degree of induced bronchospasm!

The known airway hyperreactivity seen in patients with cystic fibrosis, a condition in which there is chronic airway inflammation, could be explained by the effects of phagocytic immune-inflammatory mediators on respiratory tract mucosa and by the resultant increased access of luminal mediators and antigens to submucosal mast cells, afferent nerve receptors, and airway smooth muscle. Inconsistent with this concept, however, is the fact that most patients with cigarette-induced bronchitis (who also have airway inflammation) do not exhibit airway hyperreactivity. Although it has been speculated that the excessive airway secretions in the bronchitic may provide for a relatively "protective" barrier to inhaled bronchoprovocative agents, patients with cystic fibrosis also have excessive airway secretions.

The recent description of the presence of airway intraluminal mast cells gives further insight into the role that epithelial permeability may play in regulating the transport of substances such as antigens and pharmacologic agents into subepithelial airway tissues. Following exposure to inhaled allergens, activated sensitized luminal mast cell releases of immune-inflammatory mediators not only cause a more generalized airway bronchoconstriction by stimulation of afferent airway nerve pathways, but also presumably enhance the local spasmogenic reaction by causing an increased access of inhaled antigen to subepithelial mast cells via increasing the regional epithelial airway permeability to the antigen (Fig. 3-3). Exercise-induced asthma is especially interesting in this regard. Recent reports have focused not so much upon the thermal exchange or water loss from the airways, but rather on the changing osmolality of the respiratory mucosa as being responsible for exercise-, hyperventilation-, or cold or dry air-induced bronchial hyperreactivity. In vitro mast cell mediator release of histamine has, in fact, been correlated to the osmolality of the respiratory mucosa. However, it remains debatable whether the heightened sensitivity to changing osmolality seen in asthmatics is related to mast cell release, epithelial permeability, or afferent nerve stimulation, or is due to yet another airway target cell effect.

The relationships of airway immune-inflammatory phenomena and heightened airway reactivity are undoubtedly more complex than has been thought. This is not merely a question of the effects of allergic and inflammatory mediators upon epithelial permeability. There are controversial data suggesting that bronchial responsiveness to inhaled antigen is dependent not only upon the degree of antigen sensitivity, but also upon the degree of nonspecific bronchial responsiveness to such substances as histamine and cholinergic agents. This would be consistent with animal models of allergic asthma, which indicate that induction of bronchial hyperreactivity to sensitizing antigens seems to appear almost simultaneously with the induction of nonspecific airway hyperreactivity to histamine or cholinergic stimuli. It should be kept in mind, however, that the magnitude of the mild airway hypersensitivity that can be induced in animals by means of repetitive antigenic challenges does not fully mimic the one- to three-magnitudes-increased airway hyperreactivity that is seen in human asthmatic patients.

Since the ubiquity of calcium-dependent regulator functions in many cell functions is well appreciated, it is not surprising that calcium-dependent processes have been hypothesized to be important in the pathogenesis of asthma at many levels. These levels include such phenomena as stimulus–secretion coupling in mast cells, the physiology of the epithelial cell junction apparatus (epithelial permeability), and cell enzyme systems such as the cAMP, cGMP, and inositol–lipid pathways, which modulate translocations of cell calcium and which effect nerve conduction and transmitter release and excitation–contraction coupling in smooth muscle cells. As with the recent discovery that membrane inositol–lipid pathways are of key importance in regulating a variety of cell functions, including transmembrane calcium transports, there is new and probably important evidence that implicates the intracellular protein calmodulin as a major mediator of intracellular calcium function. However, the case for abnormalities of calcium metabolism in the pathogenesis of asthma, like that for the β-receptor theory, can be considered only speculative. It is perhaps more likely that asthma interrelates with cellular calcium activities in more than one still-to-be-characterized manner. It is intriguing that cromolyn, an inhibitor of mast cell mediator release, has calcium-antagonistic properties (e.g., inhibition of calcium uptake by activated mast cells and possibly other cells) and that smooth muscle calcium antagonists such as nifedipine and verapamil cause bronchodilatation in most asthmatic patients. The specific locus of action of the calcium antagonists is uncertain and may not be solely related to mast cell calcium accumulation or to the modulation of smooth muscle calcium metabolism.

In summary, a number of theories have been advanced to explain the airway hyperreactivity to a variety of stimuli in asthmatic patients. These proposed pathogenic mechanisms include:

1. Increased *release* of mediators (including metabolites of AA) acting directly upon various target cells, including afferent nerve endings, airway ganglia, efferent nervous system receptors, and airway smooth muscle cells.
2. Increased *availability* of mediators to various target cell receptor apparati, including airway afferent nerves (increased epithelial permeability).
3. Increased sensitivity of airway afferent nerve receptors to mediators that cause reflex bronchoconstriction and mucus hypersecretion.
4. Increased central nervous system sensitivity to afferent reflexes that could serve to amplify efferent outputs back to the airways.
5. "Imbalance" of the major efferent motor pathways (e.g., adrenergic, cholinergic, peptidergic, purinergic) to airway ganglion cells and to airway smooth muscles.
6. Increased basal receptor "sensitivity" or intrinsic "tone" of airway smooth muscle cells, which leads to a greater bronchoconstrictor response to otherwise normal stimuli.

As asthma is a heterogenous disorder, there is little reason to believe that only one of the above mechanisms explains all bronchial hyperreactivity states. It seems probable that various combinations of interacting mechanisms are operative.

GEOGRAPHY OF AIRWAY RESPONSES

Considerations of asthma should include recognition that different airway sites may be either preferentially or predominantly affected. Asthma can involve predominant dysfunction of small airways, decreased caliber of large airways, or airway abnormalities at both locations. Recent evidence suggests that the performance of the chest wall may also undergo alterations in asthma, and this may have secondary effects upon airway flow-resistive properties. Such chest wall alterations may include increased inspiratory muscle tone activity, possibly related to increased stimulation of airway vagal afferent nerves, which impact upon central neural outputs to inspiratory muscles and which in turn could influence chest wall mechanics during both inspiratory and expiratory phases of respiration.

The major sites of functional airway changes can be studied using physiologic measurements that will discriminate between large central airway and smaller peripheral airway abnormalities. Changes in airway resistance, specific conductance, or flow increase in helium-oxygen flow-volume loops mainly reflect large airway disease. In contrast, lack of significant flow increases in helium-oxygen, determinations of flow rates at low lung volumes, and/or measurement of frequency dependence of compliance or resistance are believed to more specifically reflect peripheral airflow abnormalities. An illustrative example of this principal was the finding that for the same increase in airway resistance, inhaled ragweed antigen produced less density dependence of flow than did inhaled methacholine, suggesting a preferential effect of antigen on peripheral airways. Many of these tests are relatively easily accomplished in hospital pulmonary function laboratories.

Provocation or bronchodilator agents inhaled as aerosols may effect changes in flow responses in asthmatics by decreasing or increasing flow, according to regional differences in distribution of various receptors, including the patterns of airway innervation and/or mast cell density. The elicited changes in the location of airway flow-resistive properties may, however, also simply reflect the site where the aerosol is deposited (thus reflecting the predominant site of aerosol deposition rather than sites of airway hyperreactivity). Challenge tests properly performed are valuable in determining the degree and site of airway reactivity or bronchospastic reversibility present, but may also be dependent upon the baseline bronchomotor tone and degree of airway obstruction present before the challenge, if for no other reason than that these factors interrelate with aerosol deposition sites: the greater the degree of airway obstruction, the more proximal the airway aerosol deposition of the more commonly used aerosols ($0.5-5\mu$). The magnitude and type of existing baseline functional defects thus present special problems in the interpretation of the effects of constrictor or dilator stimuli in clinical studies. For example, it may be difficult to distinguish strong endogenous bronchomotor stimuli from responses to exogenously administered aerosols.

There is interest in determining the geography of the predominant area of obstruction (larger central or smaller peripheral airways) because this may reflect both pathophysiologic mechanisms and therapeutic approaches. For example, following allergen bronchoprovocation in asthmatics who developed both early-phase and late-phase decrements in FEV_1, early-phase responses (1–30 minutes) have been characterized by flow increases in helium-oxygen flow-volume loops, whereas late-phase responses (4–24 hours) have been associated with a decrease in the density-dependence of maximal expiratory airflows. This is consistent with early-phase neurogenic bronchospastic large airway obstruction and late-phase inflammation-associated small airway obstruction.

Most asthmatic patients exhibit manifestations of airway obstruction in both large central and small peripheral airways. There is evidence, however, that a minority of asthmatic patients manifest airway obstruction principally in only the peripheral airways or in only the central airways. Patients with allergic bronchial asthma with predominant responses in peripheral airways may not experience asthma attacks which are effectively aborted by atropine, as might asthmatics with predominant central airway involvements. This is consistent with studies emphasizing the role of histamine and bronchoconstricting leukotrienes in acting directly upon smooth muscle of peripheral airways and the more abundant afferent nerve distributions available for the induction of neurogenic, reflex-mediated bronchoconstriction in central airways. This is also consistent with the concept that chronic asthma and late asthmatic responses are characterized pathologically by inflammation in small airways, whereas acute and early bronchospastic asthmatic responses probably involve more central airways. The implication for therapy is that these findings provide clues to the types of agents likely to be effective and underline the need to direct interventions to the appropriate region of the tracheobronchial tree.

SUMMARY

The last decade has seen enormous growth in research devoted to airway cell biology. Areas of special attention have included those related to: initiation, transduction, and translation control of such processes as mast cell mediator release; airway epithelial cell function; airway afferent, ganglia and efferent nerve activity; mucus production; airway smooth muscle function; and airway blood flow. Although considerable progress has characterized this research, it is clear that the heterogeneity of cell types, mediators, receptors, transmembrane signal transduction processes, and cell metabolic control systems makes it difficult to develop a coherent picture of the pathophysiology operative in asthmatic patients. Pieces of this gigantic complex puzzle are currently being organized. For example, it seems probable that newly generated lipid compounds are likely to be exceedingly important in relation to allergic bronchial asthma. The stage seems set for the next decade to further refine this new fundamental knowledge concerning airway cellular processes operative in asthma and, importantly, to apply it to the prevention and treatment of the human asthmatic state.

REFERENCES

Aitken ML, Marini JJ: Effect of heat delivery and extraction on airway conductance in normal and in asthmatic subjects. Am Rev Respir Dis 131:357–361, 1985

Aquilina AT: Comparison of airway reactivity induced by histamine, methacholine and isocapnic hyperventilation in normal and asthmatic subjects. Thorax 38:766–770, 1983

Armour CL, Black JL, Bereud N, et al: The relationship between bronchial hyperresponsiveness to methacholine and airway smooth muscle structure and reactivity. Respir Physiol 58:223–233, 1984

Bach MK: Prospects for the inhibition of leukotriene synthesis. Biochem Pharmacol 33:515–521, 1984

Bailey WC (ed): Symposium on asthma. Clin Chest Med 5:555–737, 1985

Bake B, Larsson S, Svednyr N (eds): Asthma: Pathophysiology and treatment. A symposium of Glaxo, Sweden. Eur J Respir Dis 65:Suppl. 136, 1984

Barnes PJ: The third nervous system in the lung: Physiology and clinical perspectives. Editorial. Thorax 39:561–567, 1984

Baumgarten CR, Togias AG, Naclerio RM, et al: Influx of kininogens into nasal secretions after antigen challenge of allergic individuals. J Clin Invest 76:191–197, 1985

Bernstein IL, Boushey HA, Cherniak RM, et al: Summary and recommendations of a workshop on the investigative use of fiberoptic bronchoscopy and bronchoalveolar lavage in asthmatic patients. Chest 88:136–138, 1985

Berridge MJ, Irvine RF: Inositol triphosphate, a novel second messenger in cellular signal transduction. Nature 312:315–321, 1984

Boushey HA, Holtzman MJ, Sheller JR, et al: State of the art: Bronchial hyperreactivity. Am Rev Respir Dis 121:389–413, 1980

Boushey HA, Holtzman MJ: Experimental airway inflammation and hyperreactivity: Searching for cells and mediators. Am Rev Respir Dis 131:312–313, 1985

Brooks SM, Weiss MA, Bernstein IL: Reactive airways dysfunction syndrome: Persistent asthma syndrome after high level irritant exposure. Chest 88:376–384, 1985

Chakrin LW, Bailey DM: The Leukotrienes: Chemistry and Biology. London, Academic Press, 1984, p. 308

Cockcroft DW: Hypothesis: Mechanism of perennial allergic asthma. Lancet II: 253–255, 1983

Dahlen S, Hansson G, Hedqvist P, et al: Allergen challenge of lung tissue from asthmatics elicits to bronchial contraction that correlates with the release of leukotrienes C_4, D_4 and E_4. Proc Natl Acad Sci USA 80:1712–1716, 1983

Delehunt JC, Perruchoud AP, Yerger L, et al: The role of slow-reacting substance of anaphylaxis in the late bronchial response after antigen challenge in allergic sheep. Am Rev Respir Dis 130:748–754, 1984

Durham SR, Carroll M, Walsh GM, et al: Leukocyte activation in allergen-induced late-phase asthmatic reactions. N Engl J Med 311:1398–1402, 1984

Flavahan NA, Aarhus LL, Rinele TJ, et al: Respiratory epithelium inhibits bronchial muscle tone. J Appl Physiol 58:834–838, 1985

Fleisch JH, Rinkema LE, Marshall WS: Commentary: Pharmacologic receptors for the leukotrienes. Biochem Pharmacol 33:3919–3922, 1984

Flint KC, Leung KBP, Pearce FL, et al: Human mast cells recovered by bronchoalveolar lavage: Their morphology, histamine release and the effects of sodium cromoylycate. Clin Sci 68:427–432, 1985

Ford-Hutchsinson AW: Leukotrienes: Their formation and role as inflammatory mediators. Fed Proc 44:25–29, 1985

Gerblich AA, Campbell AE, Schuyler MR: Changes in T-lymphocyte subpopulations after antigenic bronchial provocation in asthmatics. N Engl J Med 310:1349–1352, 1984

Goetzl EJ, Scott WA (eds): Proceedings of a conference on regulation of cellular activities by leukotrienes and other lipoxygenase products of arachidonic acid. J Allergy Clin Immunol 74:310–448, 1984

Hahn A, Anderson SD, Morton AR, et al: A reinterpretation of the effect of temperature and water content of the inspired air in exercise-induced asthma. Am Rev Respir Dis 130:575–579, 1984

Hardy CC, Robinson C, Tattersfield AE, et al: The bronchoconstrictor effect of inhaled prostaglandin D_2 in normal and asthmatic men. N Engl J Med 311:209–213, 1984

Hargreave FE (ed): Airway Reactivity. Mississauga, Canada, Astra Pharmaceuticals Canada Ltd., 1984, p. 238

Hogg JC, Eggleston PA: Is asthma an epithelial disease? Am Rev Respir Dis 129:207–208, 1984

Joseph M, Tonnel AB, Torfier G, et al: Involvement of immunoglobulin E in the secretory processes of alveolar macrophages from asthmatic patients. J Clin Invest 71:221–30, 1983

Juniper EF, Frith PA, Hargreave FE: Long-term stability of bronchial responsiveness to histamine, Thorax 37:288–291, 1982

Juniper EF, Frith PA, Hargreave FE: Airway responsiveness to histamine and methacholine: Relationship to minimum treatment to control symptoms of asthma. Thorax 36:575–579, 1981

Kaliner M, Lemanske R: Inflammatory responses to mast cell mediators. Fed Proc 43:2846–2851, 1984

Karlsson JA, Finney MJB, Persson CGA, et al: Substance P antagonists and the role of tachykinins in non-cholinergic bronchoconstriction. Life Sci 35:2681–2691, 1984

Karlsson JA, Persson CGA: Local anesthetics selectively inhibit non-cholinergic neural contractions in guinea-pig airways. Acta Physiol Scand 120:469–471, 1984

Kay AB: Basic mechanisms in allergic asthma. Eur J Respir Dis:Suppl. 122(63), 9–16, 1982

Kay AB, Austen FK, Lichtenstein LM: Asthma: Physiology, immunopharmacology, and treatment. Orlando, Academic Press, 1984, p. 442

Kikuchi R, Sekizawa K, Sasaki H, et al: Effects of pulmonary congestion on airway reactivity to histamine aerosol in dogs. J Appl Physiol 57:1640–1647, 1984

Kirkpatrick CT: Nervous control of airways muscle tone. Bull Eur Physiopathol Respir 20:389–394, 1984

Krilis S, Lewis RA, Corey EJ, et al: Specific receptors for leukotriene C_4 on a smooth muscle cell line. J Clin Invest 72:1516–1519, 1983

Kuehl FA, DeHaven RN, Pong S-S: Lung tissue receptors for sulfidopeptide leukotrienes. J Allergy Clin Immunol 74:378–381, 1984

Kuehl FA Jr, Dougherty HW, Ham EA: Interactions between prostaglandins and leukotrienes. Biochem Pharmacol 33:1–9, 1984

Laitinen A: Autonomic innervation of the human respiratory tract as revealed by histochemical and ultrastructural methods. Eur J Respir Dis: 66 Suppl. 140, 1–42, 1985

Lee TH, Austen KF, Corey EJ, et al: Leukotriene E_4-induced airway hyperresponsiveness of guinea pig tracheal smooth muscle to histamine and evidence for three separate sulfidopeptide leukotriene receptors. Proc Natl Acad Sci 81:4922–4925, 1984

Leitch AG, Drazen JA: Pulmonary pharmacology of the leukotrienes, in The Leukotrienes, Orlando, Academic Press, 1984, pp. 247–269

Lewis RA, Austin KF: The biologically active leukotrienes: Biosynthesis, metabolism, receptors, functions and pharmacology. J Clin Invest 73:889–897, 1984

Marsh WR, Irvin CG, Murphy KR, et al: Increases in airway reactivity to histamine and inflammatory cells in bronchoalveolar lavage after the late asthmatic response in an animal model. Am Rev Respir Dis 131:875–879, 1985

Mason, R (ed): 27th Aspen Lung Conference: Asthma. Chest:Suppl. 87:1515–2265, 1985

Metzger WJ, Nugent K, Richerson HB: Site of airflow obstruction during early and late phase asthmatic responses to antigen bronchoprovocation. Chest 88:369–375, 1985

Norman PS, Naclerio RM, Creticos PS, et al: Mediator release after allergic and physical nasal challenge. Int Arch Allergy Appl Immun 77:57–63, 1985

O'Byrne PM, Leikauf GD, Aizawa H, et al: Leukotriene B_4 induces airway hyperresponsiveness in dogs. J Appl Physiol 59:1941–1946, 1985

O'Donnell M, Welton AF: Pharmacologic properties of FPL55712 administered by aerosol. Agents Actions 14:43–48, 1984

Patterson R, Bernstein PR, Harris KE, et al: Airway responses to sequential challenges with platelet activating factor and leukotriene D_4 in rhesus monkeys. J Lab Clin Med 104:340–345, 1984

Peters SP, Macglashan DW, Schleimer RP, et al: The pharmacologic modulation of the release of arachidonic acid metabolites from purified human mast cells. Am Rev Respir Dis 132:367–373, 1985

Piper PJ: Formation and actions of leukotrienes. Physiol Rev 64:744–761, 1984

Robinson C, Holgate ST: Mast cell-dependent inflammatory mediators and their putative role in bronchial asthma. Clin Sci 68:103–112, 1985

Rubinfeld AR, Rinard Ga, Mayer SE: Responsiveness of isolated tracheal smooth muscle in a canine model of asthma. Lung 160:99–107, 1982

Russell JA, Simons EJ: Modulation of cholinergic neurotransmission in airways by enkephalin. J Appl Physiol 58:853–858, 1985

Said SI (ed): The Pulmonary Circulation and Acute Lung Injury. Mt. Kisco, NY, Future Publishing Co., 1985, p. 473

Schulman ES, Liu MC, Proud D, et al: Human lung macrophages induce histamine release from basophils and mast cells. Am Rev Respir Dis 131:230–235, 1985

Sheppard D, Rizk NW, Boushey HA, et al: Mechanism of cough and bronchoconstriction induced by distilled water aerosol. Am Rev Respir Dis 127:691–694, 1983

Shore Sa, Bai TR, Wang CG, et al: Central and local cholinergic components of histamine-induced bronchoconstriction in dogs. J Appl Physiol 58:443–451, 1985

Shore SS, Powell WS, Martin JG: Endogenous prostaglandins modulate histamine-induced contraction in canine tracheal smooth muscle. J Appl Physiol 58:859–868, 1985

Simonsson BG (ed): Airway hyperreactivity: A symposium. Eur J Respir Dis 64:Suppl. 131, 1983

Smith LJ, Greenberger PA, Patterson R, et al: The effect of inhaled leukotriene D_4 in humans. Am Rev Respir Dis 131:368–372, 1985

Snapper JR, Brigham KL: Minireview: Inflammation and airway reactivity. Exp Lung Res 6:83–89, 1984

Souhrada M, Souhrada JF: Immunologically induced alterations of airway smooth muscle cell membrane. Science 225:723–725, 1984

Stewart AG, Thompson DC, Fennessy MR: Involvement of capsaicin-sensitive afferent neurons in a vagal-dependent interaction between leukotriene D_4 and histamine on bronchomotor tone. Agents Actions 15:500–508, 1984

Tayler SM, Pare PD, Armour CL, et al: Airway reactivity in chronic obstructive pulmonary disease: Failure of in vivo methacholine responsiveness to correlate with cholinergic, adrenergic, or nonadrenergic responses in vitro. Am Rev Respir Dis 132:30–35, 1985

Tomioka M, Ida S, Shindoh Y, et al: Mast cells in bronchoalveolar lumen of patients with bronchial asthma. Am Rev Respir Dis 129:1000–1005, 1984

Wanner A, Abraham WM: Experimental models of asthma. Lung 160:231–244, 1982

Weiss EB, Segal MS, Stein M: Bronchial Asthma: Mechanisms and Therapeutics. Boston, Little, Brown and Co., 1984, p. 982

Widdicombe J: Control of airway caliber. Am Rev Respir Dis 131:Supp. S33–S35, 1985

Yan K, Salome CM, Woolcock AJ: Prevalence and nature of bronchial hyperresponsiveness in subject with chronic obstructive pulmonary disease. Am Rev Respir Dis 132:25–29, 1985

Adam Wanner

4

Morphologic Basis of Airflow Obstruction

In contrast to other types of obstructive airway disease, in which the pathologic abnormalities observed at postmortem examination can be readily related to the functional derangement in vivo, such a relationship is difficult to establish in bronchial asthma for at least two reasons. First, bronchial asthma is by definition episodic and the morphologic changes associated with the functional abnormalities may follow the same dynamic pattern and hence not be present at autopsy. Second, endoscopic or bronchographic studies which attempt to demonstrate structure-function relationships are rarely carried out because of the morbidity associated with these procedures in patients with bronchial asthma. Therefore, most morphologic examinations have been made in patients who died in or from status asthmaticus. However, the pathologic changes in patients with stable asthma or nonfatal exacerbations of asthma seem to differ only quantitatively from those seen in status asthmaticus.

Despite these methodologic difficulties, a reasonable relationship can be demonstrated between airway morphology and respiratory function on the basis of the available literature.

BRONCHIAL ASTHMA, Second Edition
ISBN 0-8089-1814-1

MORPHOLOGIC CHANGES

Pathologic studies of the lungs in patients with bronchial asthma have been derived from three sources: expectorated sputum, bronchial biopsy, and autopsy material. The typical microscopic features of sputum, such as Curshman's spirals, Charcot-Leyden crystals, and Creola bodies (clumps of epithelial cells), suggest the presence in asthmatics of narrowed airways, abnormal airway secretions, and epithelial damage, respectively. As will be shown, these abnormalities have been clearly confirmed by biochemical and rheologic examinations of sputum and by histologic studies.

Only a few investigations have used bronchial biopsy material from patients with stable asthma; however, by combining these observations with the histologic information derived from postmortem examination of patients who died in status asthmaticus, a fairly completed description of the pathology of bronchial asthma can be given.

At autopsy, the gross appearance of the lung is characterized by overdistention and the failure of the lung to collapse in a normal fashion. There are small areas of atelectasis. The cut surface reveals numerous grey plugs in large and small airways (Fig. 4-1); small areas of cystic bronchiectasis may also be seen. Despite the presence of hyperinflation, the microscopic examination shows no evidence of destructive parenchymal changes and the alveolar walls appear normal. Pathologic findings within the lung parenchyma are restricted to the small areas of atelectasis where accumulations of eosinophils and granulomatous reactions can occur. Since the pathology of asthma seems to spare the alveolar regions, the following discussion will focus on the typical abnormalities involving the wall and lumen of the conducting airways.

NORMAL ANATOMY

Mucosa

The normal respiratory mucosa from the proximal trachea to the terminal bronchioles consists of a pseudostratified columnar epithelium with cilia protruding from the luminal surface of columnar cells (Fig. 4-2). The major cell types found in the respiratory epithelium are basal cells, intermediate cells, nonciliated columnar cells, ciliated columnar cells, and goblet cells. In the larger airways, the major part of the epithelium is ciliated. The ratio of ciliated columnar cells to goblet cells is from five to ten: one, with a relative decrease evident in the number of both cell types from the trachea toward the peripheral airways. The surface of each ciliated columnar cell contains approximately 200 cilia, with an average length of 6 μm and a diameter of 0.2 μm. The thickness of the normal basement membrane is approximately 7

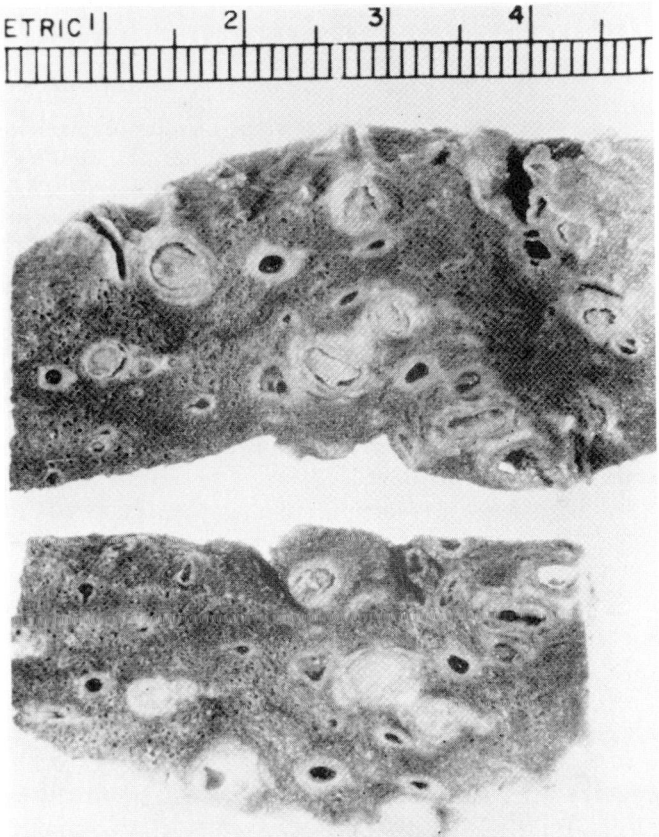

Fig. 4-1. Bronchial obstruction by mucus plugs in a fatal case of bronchial asthma. Scale in cm. (From Rezek PR, Millard M: Autopsy Pathology. Springfield, IL, Charles C. Thomas, 1963, p. 346. Used with permission.)

μm. Tight junctions between adjacent epithelial cells provide a protective barrier against the transport of inhaled agents across the epithelium.

Submucosa

The submucosa is defined as the tissue space contained between the basement membrane of the mucosa and the cartilage. (Fig. 4-3). This space contains submucosal glands, smooth muscle in longitudinal and circular arrangements, and connective tissue which is well vascularized. The cholinergic nervous system and, to a lesser degree, the sympathetic nervous system, innervate the bronchial wall, and both afferent and efferent fibers have been demonstrated. The exact anatomic distribution of the nerve endings

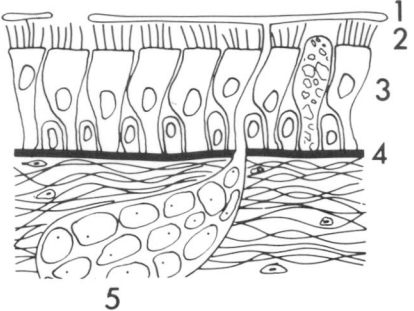

Fig. 4-2. Schematic representation of the normal (N) bronchial mucosa and submucosa. 1 = mucus layer, 2 = periciliary fluid layer, 3 = epithelium, 4 = basement membrane, 5 = submucosa. (From Wanner A: The role of mucociliary dysfunction in asthma. Am J Med 67: 477–485, 1979. Used with permission.)

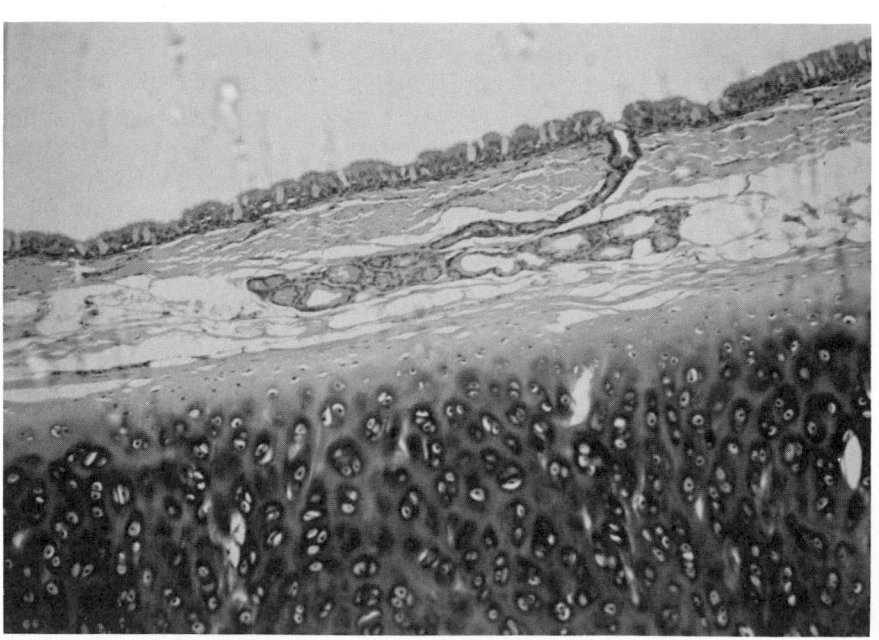

Fig. 4-3. Normal mucosa and submucosa of main bronchus (sheep). Note intact ciliated epithelium, relatively small number of goblet cells, and thin submucosal gland.

within the airway wall has been recently described in detail. Sensory nerve endings have been identified both within the mucosa and in the submucosa. Efferent autonomic nerves have also been detected in the epithelium and in the submucosa, along with corresponding cholinergic, alpha-adrenergic, β-adrenergic and non-cholinergic non-adrenergic receptors in adjacent tissues. These observations have been made primarily in rodents; the distribution of autonomic nerves in the human airway mucosa remains to be described.

The volume of the submucosal glands, which constitute most of the total volume of mucus-producing structures in human airways, has been estimated at approximately 4 ml. The relative volume of the submucosal gland layer in relation to the total volume of the bronchial wall between the cartilage and the luminal surface of the epithelium is less than 15–20 percent under normal circumstances, with a mean value of 13 percent in one study. Using a similar approach, the mean relative volume of the bronchial smooth muscle layer has been reported to be 5 percent, with 11 percent considered as the upper range of normal.

Mucociliary Apparatus

In order to appreciate the significance of the normal morphology of the mucociliary apparatus, this morphology has to be related to the function of the apparatus. The mucosa is a barrier to various inhaled materials and prevents them from making contact with sensitive tissues in the airway wall. In addition, the mucociliary apparatus of the airways serves to remove inhaled particulate matter from the tracheobronchial mucosa, thereby further contributing to pulmonary host defense. This function is dependent upon an optimal interaction between cilia and the mucus that is excreted by submucosal glands and goblet cells. Cilia beat in a fluid layer in a coordinated fashion, so that the exerted force transports mucus cephalad. The resulting surface transport velocity appears to increase from the peripheral airways towards the central airways, with average values in the mammalian trachea of approximately 10 mm/min. The ciliary beat frequency is approximately 1000 beats/min, with a synchronization of effective and recovery strokes among adjacent cilia. The control of ciliary beat in mammals has not been clearly established.

A two-layer concept of respiratory mucus is currently widely accepted. It visualizes a periciliary fluid layer (sol) covered by a mucous layer (gel), which interacts with the tips of the cilia (Fig. 4-2). Controversy exists regarding the continuity of the mucous layer. Some investigators believe that the mucous layer represents a contiguous blanket of 5–10 μm thickness, covering the luminal surface of the tracheobronchial tree, whereas others suggest that mucus is discontinuous, with foci of mucus floating like lilly pads on the periciliary fluid. It is possible to reconcile these two concepts, since the normal amount of mucus decreases from the central airways towards the peripheral airways. Thus, the continuity of the mucous layer cannot be maintained in peripheral airways.

Respiratory secretions consist of mucus, produced by submucosal glands and goblet cells, and tissue fluid. The submucosal glands are predominently under cholinergic control, whereas the goblet cells appear to secrete primarily upon direct irritation. Both goblet cells and submucosal glands are rarely found in peripheral airways. Normal human respiratory secretions consist of approximately 95 percent water. The remaining 5 percent consists of micromolecules (electrolytes, amino acids) and macromolecules (lipids, carbohydrates, nucleic acids, mucins, immunoglobulins, enzymes, albumin). Optimal rheologic properties and volume of mucus are required for normal mucous transport. Studies of the transportability of expectorated sputum obtained from patients with airway disease suggest a direct relationship between elastic recoil, and ciliary transport velocity at relatively low values of elastic recoil, and an inverse relationship at high elastic recoil values. An inverse relationship exists between viscosity and ciliary transport velocity. The influence of elasticity appears to be more important than that of viscosity. Also, mucus seems to propagate fastest at a critical mucus thickness (around 5 μm), with slower motions evident when the mucous layer is thinner or thicker.

ABNORMALITIES IN BRONCHIAL ASTHMA

Mucosa

In status asthmaticus, the mucosa is characterized by edema, separation of mucosal cells, decrease in the number of ciliated cells, increase in the number of goblet cells, and goblet cell metaplasia in peripheral airways (Fig. 4-4). In addition, detachment of superficial epithelial cells can be seen in some areas (Table 4-1).

In stable bronchial asthma, the destructive changes of the epithelium are not as evident as in status asthmaticus, although it has been recently suggested that the integrity of the tight junctions is disturbed. The thickness of the basement membrane is increased to about twice normal. It contains deposits of immunoglobulins G, A, and (predominantly) M. Immunoglobulin has not been demonstrated in or in the vicinity of the basement membrane. Thickening of the basement membrane is not pathognomonic of bronchial asthma, since it can also be observed in patients with chronic bronchitis; it seems to be more severe in bronchial asthma, however (Table 4-2).

Submucosa

The submucosal tissues show edema, dilated capillaries, and cellular infiltration by eosinophils, lymphocytes, plasma cells, and neutrophils. There is also a decrease in the number of mast cells, with partial degranula-

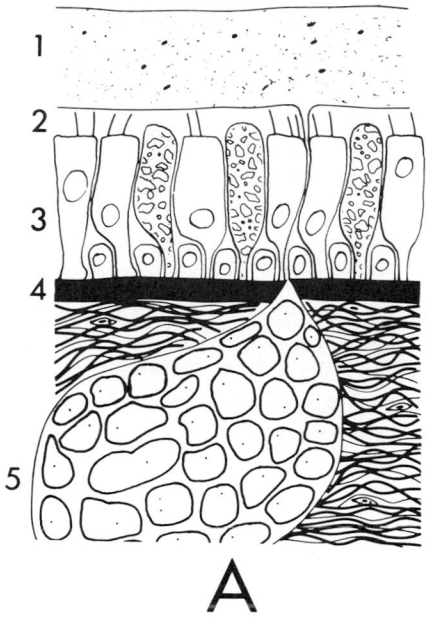

1

2

3

4

5

Fig. 4-4. Schematic representation of the bronchial mucosa and submucosa in asthma (A). See figure 4-2 for explanation. (From Wanner A: The role of mucociliary dysfunction in asthma. Am J Med 67: 477–485, 1979. Used with permission.)

A

tion of those remaining. Although IgE has been demonstrated in lymphocytes and eosinophils within the bronchial wall, its presence is not typical of bronchial asthma; it is also seen in patients with nonspecific bronchial inflammation.

Typically, there is hyperplasia and hypertrophy of the submucosal glands (Fig. 4-5). In one study, the mean relative volume of the submucosal gland layer was 23 percent in bronchial asthma, as compared to 13 percent in normals (Table 4-2). Submucosal gland hypertrophy and hyperplasia is not a

Table 4-1
Pathologic Changes of the Airways in Bronchial Asthma

Submucosa	Hypertrophy and hyperplasia of submucosal glands
	Hypertrophy of smooth muscle
	Edema and infiltration with inflammatory cells
	Degranulation of mast cells
Mucosa	Disruption of epithelium
	Decrease in the number of ciliated cells
	Increase in the number of goblet cells and goblet cell metaplasia in peripheral airways
	Edema
	Thickening of basement membrane
Airway lumen	Increased amounts of airway secretions with occluding mucous plugs
	Inflammatory cells (predominantly eosinophils) and shed columnar cells

Table 4-2

Quantitative Morphology of Airway Wall*

	Thickenss of Basement Membrane (μm)	Volume of Submucosal Glands[a] (% of bronchial wall volume)	Volume of Smooth Muscle[b] (% of bronchial wall volume)
Normal	7 (3)	13 (3)	5 (2)
Chronic bronchitis	9 (3)†	28 (9)†	6 (3)
Bronchial asthma	16 (6)†	23 (5)†	12 (3)†

[a] From Callerame, Condemi, Ishizaka, et al: Immunoglobulins in bronchial tissues from patients with asthma, with special reference to immunoglobulin E. J Allergy 47:187–197, 1971. Used with permission.

[b] From Dunnill, Massarella, Anderson: A comparison of the quantitative anatomy of the bronchi in normal subjects, in chronic bronchitis, and in emphysema. Thorax 24:176–179, 1969. These measurements were made in lungs of patients who died in status asthmaticus. Used with permission.

* mean values with standard deviation in parentheses

† significantly different from normal

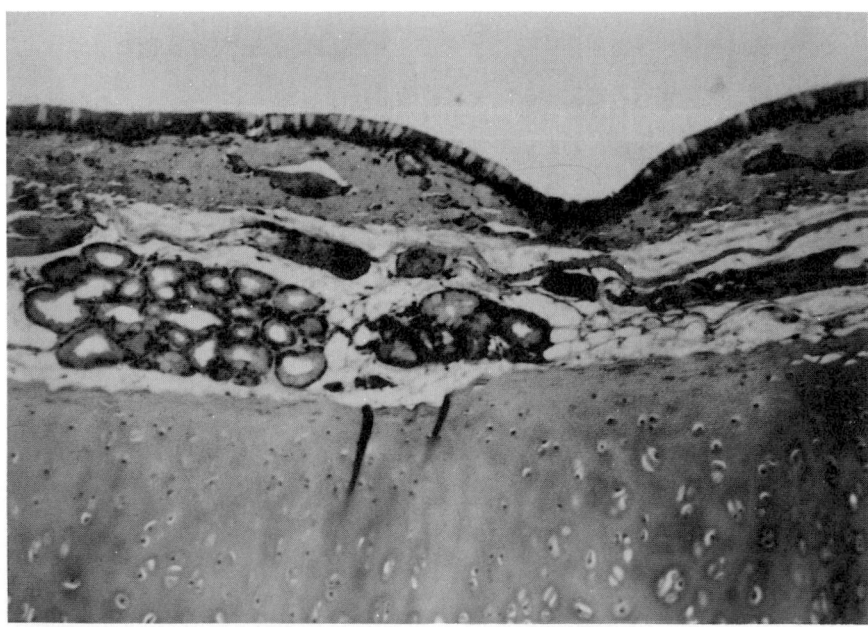

Fig. 4-5. Mucosa and submucosa of main bronchus in sheep with allergic bronchospasm. Note destruction of cilia, increased number of goblet cells, and submucosal gland hypertrophy.

specific feature of bronchial asthma. It is also present in chronic bronchitis; indeed, the submucosal gland volume in patients with chronic bronchitis is usually greater than that in patients with bronchial asthma.

In contrast to the abnormalities of the basement membrane and the submucosal glands, smooth muscle hypertrophy seems to clearly distinguish bronchial asthma from other forms of obstructive lung disease. While the mean values of the relative volume of the bronchial smooth muscle layer for chronic bronchitis (6 percent) and emphysema (6 percent) are not significantly different from that in normal controls (5 percent), the mean value of 12 percent in bronchial asthma is significantly greater (Table 4-2).

Mucociliary Apparatus

Postmortem studies reveal widespread mucous plugging of the airways in status asthmaticus. Recently, peripheral airway obstruction with mucous plugs has also been demonstrated in children with asthma in remission who underwent open-lung biopsy (Fig. 4-6). The intraluminal mucous plugs were mainly present in bronchi greater than 1 mm in diameter, but they were also observed in smaller peripheral airways. The accumulation of airway secretions in bronchial asthma could result from mucus hypersecretion, abnormal mucociliary transport, or a combination thereof. While hypertrophy of mucus-producing structures in the bronchial mucosa suggests mucus hyperse-

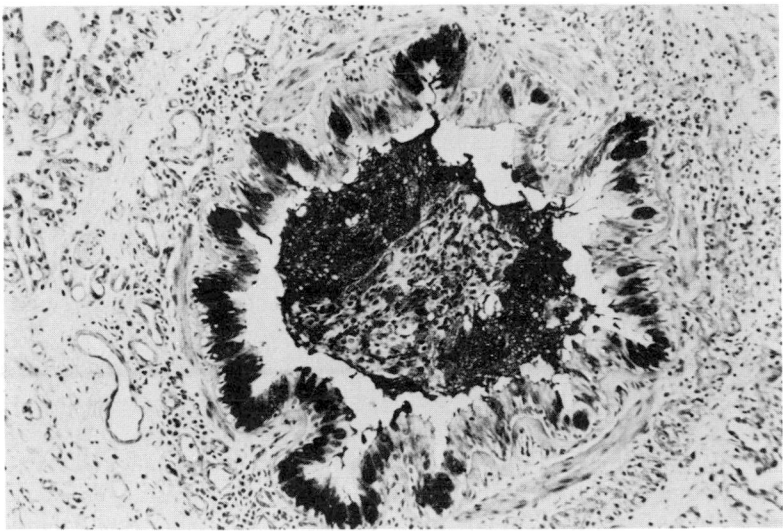

Fig. 4-6. Mucus plug (undergoing organization) in bronchiole (1 mm diameter) of a child with stable bronchial asthma. Note macrophages encased in plug. (From Cutz E, Levison H, Cooper DM: Ultrastructure of airways in children with asthma. Histopathology 2: 407–421, 1978. Used with permission.)

cretion, this has not been confirmed in man by functional studies. In allergic animals, antigen challenge has been shown to produce mucus hypersecretion in the trachea.

A variety of biochemical abnormalities characterize airway secretions in bronchial asthma. Glycoproteins seem to determine the rheologic properties to the greatest extent, especially by means of the cross-linking of glycoproteins. Increased concentrations of unusual polysaccharides and cross-binding between transudated serum proteins and secretory IgA have been found in the sputum of patients with bronchial asthma. Changes in electrolyte concentrations, including increases in calcium, have also been reported, and serum proteins appear to accumulate in the sol phase of asthmatic sputum. Recently, increased amounts of lipids have been found in bronchial mucus obtained postmortem from a patient with fatal status asthmaticus. These lipids seem to be strongly linked to glycoproteins and may possibly contribute to enhanced gel formation. Despite these distinguishing biochemical characteristics and their possible effects on the physical characteristics of mucus, only a few studies examining the rheologic properties of respiratory secretions of patients with bronchial asthma have been reported. In addition, the most relevant observations have been made on expectorated sputum which might not be representative of lower airway secretions. In one study, sputum from asthmatic patients tended to be more viscous than that obtained from patients with other types of obstructive airway disease; a marked increase in viscosity at low shear rates was particularly characteristic of the sputum obtained from asthmatic patients.

In stable asthmatic patients, the transport velocity of mucus in central airways has been shown to be decreased to 10 percent of that seen in young normal controls and to be comparable to that seen in patients with chronic bronchitis. Similar observations have been made regarding smaller airways. Although there seems to be an inverse relationship between mucous transport rate and patient age, the discrepancy between rates for asthmatics and for normals could not be fully accounted for by age, suggesting a true impairment of mucous transport mechanisms in bronchial asthma. This is also supported by the demonstration of a decreased mucous transport velocity in central and peripheral airways of asymptomatic young patients with allergic asthma, as compared to normal, age-matched controls. In the asthmatic patients, bronchial challenge with specific antigen produced a further decrease in mucous transport velocity. Again, animal studies have demonstrated that the decrease of mucociliary transport in airway anaphylaxis is due to the production of qualitatively and quantitatively abnormal respiratory secretions by inflammatory mediators. In addition, other leukocyte products (e.g., eosinophil granule major basic protein of disintegrating eosinophils) and serum factors contained in inflammatory transudates have been shown to be ciliotoxic.

According to these histologic, rheologic, and functional studies, it appears that mucous hypersecretion and abnormal mucociliary transport both contribute to the accumulation of mucus in the airways.

Edema

The pathogenesis of airway edema formation in bronchial asthma has not been elucidated. It is generally assumed that the same mechanisms which are responsible for the edema associated with cutaneous anaphylaxis are also operative in the conducting airways. This has not been tested in man. Animal experiments strongly suggest, however, that certain chemical mediators with vascular effects (e.g., histamine) are capable of augmenting bronchial blood flow and the water content of the airway wall (Fig. 4-7). Thus, chemical mediators of anaphylaxis are likely candidates for edema formation in the airways of patients with bronchial asthma.

STRUCTURE-FUNCTION RELATIONSHIPS

Although bronchspasm is undoubtedly an important cause of airflow obstruction in bronchial asthma, structural changes of the airway mucosa

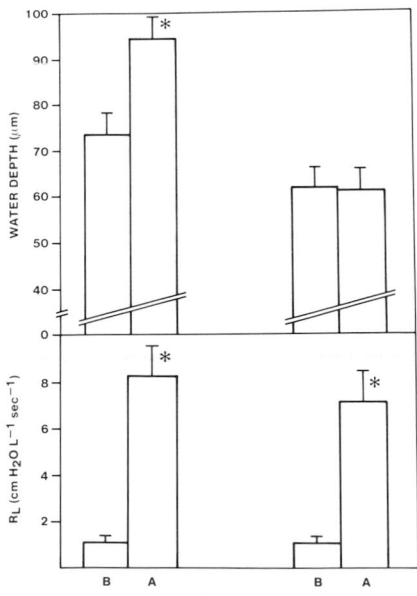

Fig. 4-7. Effects of intravenous histamine or carbachol on measurable tracheal wall water depth and pulmonary resistance in five conscious sheep (mean values with SE in brackets). B = baseline; A = after agonist administration;* = significantly different from corresponding baseline (p < 0.05). Data kindly provided by Dr. Horst Baier, University of Miami.

such as edema and excessive tracheobronchial secretions may play a contributing role. The expected effects of these structural changes on respiratory
function are those on airflow resistance, static lung volumes, gas exchange,
and work of breathing.

Bronchospasm and Pulmonary Hyperinflation

It is generally assumed that the morphologic feature of smooth muscle
hypertrophy in bronchial asthma reflects increased smooth muscle tone in
vivo. Actual measurements of airway dimensions in vivo are difficult to carry
out in patients with bronchial asthma, since endoscopic and bronchographic
techniques may aggravate bronchoconstriction, thereby obscuring the significance of the observation and rendering the patient more symptomatic. In
allergic dogs, the increase in airflow resistance resulting from antigen challenge has been shown to be associated with nonuniform constriction of bronchi as demonstrated by tantalum bronchography. A three to four-fold increase
in airflow resistance was accompanied by a 26 to 49-percent decrease in the
diameter of different-sized airways. Similarly, convolution of the mucosa of
small peripheral bronchi was found in a sheep that died during severe allergic
bronchospasm (Fig. 4-8). In adult patients with stable bronchial asthma,
bronchographic estimates of bronchial dimensions have not been found to
differ from those of normal control subjects; in allergic children, slightly
smaller-than-normal diameters have been demonstrated. In the latter study,
the difference between normals and allergic children was present despite
premedication with atropine, which in the canine experiments blocked the
antigen-induced airway narrowing. This may indicate airway narrowing due
to factors other than bronchospasm, such as mucosal edema and excessive
airway mucus. Thus, airway narrowing can be related to increased airflow
resistance, nonuniformity of gas distribution, and consequent abnormal gas
exchange.

Structure-function relationships are less evident with respect to pulmonary hyperinflation. As mentioned before, morphologic changes in the alveolar wall have not been demonstrated at the light- or electron-microscopic
levels, and although a transient leftward displacement of the static pressure-
volume curve has been reported in acute exacerbations of bronchial asthma,
this cannot fully account for the observed increases in static lung volumes.
Another possible mechanism of pulmonary hyperinflation is persistent inspiratory muscle activity during expiration, which alters the relaxation curve of
the chest bellows. One might also speculate that bronchospasm and excessive
airway secretions with expiratory slowing cause "gas trapping". Several

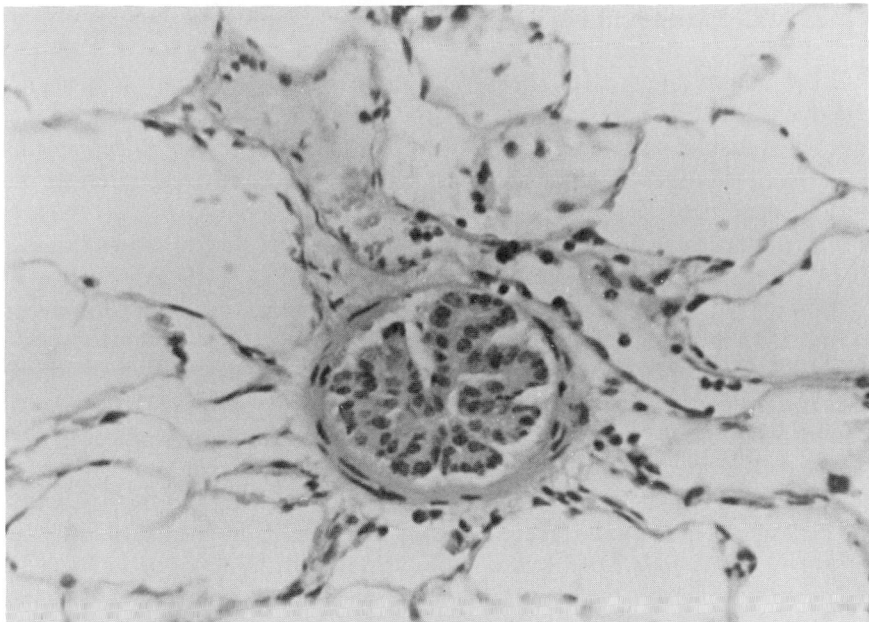

Fig. 4-8. Convoluted epithelium of small bronchiole in a sheep sacrificed during allergic bronchospasm. Note prominent smooth muscle in airway wall.

mechanisms have been suggested for the occurrence of gas trapping in obstructive lung disease. These include the formation of liquid menisci or bubbles within the airway lumen, or airways that close and fail to open during subsequent respiratory cycles. Increased airway mucus could lead to one or more of these results. This would also explain why the lungs fail to collapse completely when the thorax is opened at autopsy in patients who died from status asthmaticus.

Pulmonary hyperinflation appears to have both beneficial and adverse effects on respiratory function. While pulmonary hyperinflation increases airway diameter due to increased retractive forces of the lung tissue surrounding the airways, thus reducing airflow resistance, it has opposing effects on the work of breathing. Although expiratory work is reduced as a result of increased lung elastic recoil, inspiratory work is increased for two reasons, both of which are related to the increase in functional residual capacity. First, the increased functional residual capacity places the inspiratory muscle mechanically at a disadvantage. Second, by placing the tidal volume range near as on the flat portion of the static pressure-volume curve of the lung, the increase in functional residual capacity reduces the dynamic lung compliance.

Airway Edema and Luminal Mucus

The extent to which bronchial edema restricts the airway lumen and contributes to airflow obstruction is unknown. If the increased volume of the mucosa and submucosa due to water accumulation indeed impinges on the cross-sectional area of the airway, one would expect the greatest effect on airflow resistance in peripheral airways.

The endoscopic and radiographic demonstration of mucous plugs leading to atelectasis is not uncommon in patients with bronchial asthma, and it is easily visualized that the widespread mucous plugging found at postmortem examination in patients dying from status asthmaticus caused airflow obstruction. Recently, is has also been suggested that the residual airway dysfunction in patients with bronchial asthma in remission may be related to peripheral airway obstruction. Peripheral airway disease has been morphologically documented in chronic bronchitis, in cystic fibrosis, and in children with bronchial asthma in remission. Although the clinical manifestations and probably the pathogenesis of these three conditions are quite different, the peripheral airways seem to share a common pathologic abnormality: excessive mucus in the airway lumina and the formation of mucous plugs. Asthma in remission is physiologically characterized by abnormalities which have been equated with peripheral airway dysfunction. Thus, frequency dependence of dynamic lung compliance and an alteration in the density dependence of the maximum expiratory flow-volume curve have been reported in asymptomatic asthmatic patients with normal or near-normal spirometry and airway resistance. In addition, it has been shown that these functional abnormalities are not or are only in part reversible with the administration of bronchodilating agents. This implies that the peripheral airway obstruction is not entirely related to an increase in bronchomotor tone. Mucous plugging in the peripheral airways might therefore be contributory in this process.

REFERENCES

Alexander HL: A historical account of death from asthma. J Allergy 34:305–322, 1963

Basbaum CB: Innervation of the airway mucosa and submucosa. Semin Respir Med 5(4):308–313, 1974

Bateman JRM, Pavia D, Sheahan NF, et al: Impaired tracheobronchial clearance in patients with mild stable asthma. Thorax 38:463, 1983

Callerame ML, Condemi JJ, Ishizaka K, et al: Immunoglobulins in bronchial tissues from patients with asthma, with special reference to immunoglobulin E. J Allergy 47:187–197, 1971

Cutz E, Levison H, Cooper DM: Ultrastructure of airways in children with asthma. Histopathology 2:407–421, 1978

Dunnill MS: The morphology of the airways in bronchial asthma, in, Stein M (ed.): New Directions in Asthma. Park Ridge, IL, American College of Chest Physicians, 1975, pp. 213–221

Dunnill MS, Massarella GR, Anderson JA: A comparison of the quantitative anatomy of the bronchi in normal subjects, in status asthmaticus, in chronic bronchitis, and in emphysema. Thorax 24:176–179, 1969

Fraser RG: Measurements of the calibre of human bronchi in three phases of respiration by cinebronchography. J Can Assoc Radiol 12:102–112, 1961

Frazer DG, Weber KC: Trapped gas at maximum lung volume in intact isolated rat lungs. Respir Physiol 37:173–184, 1979

Frigas E, Loegering DA, Solley GO, et al: Elevated levels of the eosinophil granule major basic protein in the sputum of patients with bronchial asthma. Mayo Clin Proc 56:345, 1981

Kessler G-F, Austin JHM, Graf PD, et al: Airway constriction in experimental asthma in dogs: Tantalum bronchographic studies. J Appl Physiol 35:703–708, 1973

Long WM, Sprung CL, Fawall HE, et al: Effects of histamine on bronchial artery blood flow and bronchomotor tone. J Appl Physiol 59:254–261, 1985

Lopez-Vidriero MT, Reid LM: Bronchial mucus in asthma, in, Weiss EB, Segal MS, Stein M (eds): Bronchial Asthma: Mechanisms and Therapeutics, 2nd ed, Boston/Toronto, Little, Brown and Co., 1985, pp. 218–235

Marom Z, Shelhamer J, Bach MK, et al: Slow-reacting substances, LTC_4 and LTD_4, increase the release of mucus from human airways in vitro. Am Rev Respir Dis 126:449–451, 1982

Martin J, Powell E, Shore S, et al: The role of respiratory muscles in the hyperinflation of bronchial asthma. Am Rev Respir Dis 121:441–447, 1980

Rezek PR, Millard M: Autopsy Pathology. Springfield, IL, Charles C. Thomas, 1963, p. 304

Robinson AE: Dimensional response of large airways during bronchography in the pediatric patient. Invest Radiol 8:121–125, 1973

Wanner A: Allergic mucociliary dysfunction. Laryngoscope 93:68–70, 1983

Wanner A: Interpretation of pulmonary function tests, in, Sackner MA (ed): Diagnostic Techniques in Pulmonary Medicine, Part I. New York, Marcel Dekker, 1980, pp. 353–426

Richard E. Kanner
Suetaro Watanabe

5

The Role of the Pulmonary Function Laboratory in Patients with Bronchial Asthma

The pulmonary function laboratory plays an important role in the diagnosis and management of patients with bronchospastic disorders. In this chapter, the use of spirometry and flow-volume tracings, lung volume measurements, the pulmonary diffusing capacity, arterial blood gas measurements, and bronchoprovocation challenge testing will be discussed, since these are the tests that should be readily available to physicians. Although these tests are best performed in a laboratory setting, physicians will also find that an office spirometer is very useful and convenient for patient evaluation.

Spirometry and flow-volume curves are primarily used to assess respiratory flow rates, which usually are decreased in the bronchospastic disorders. Lung volume measurements in these patients demonstrate an increase in certain subdivisions of the total lung capacity. The diffusing capacity can, in some instances, distinguish between airway obstruction due to asthma from that due to emphysema. Arterial blood gas studies are valuable in assessing some of the consequences of bronchospasm. Bronchoprovocation challenge testing can measure airway responsiveness and hyperresponsiveness.

BRONCHIAL ASTHMA, Second Edition
ISBN 0-8089-1814-1

THE "COMPARTMENTS" OF THE LUNG

The lung is subdivided into four volumes and four capacities. By definition, a volume is a compartment which cannot be further subdivided, while a capacity is composed of two or more volumes. Convenient reference points are maximal inspiration and maximal expiration. In addition, there is a resting point to which the lung and thoracic cage return to following a normal breath (Fig. 5-1).

The four volumes are illustrated in Figure 5-1 and are defined as follows: Tidal volume (V_T) is the amount of air or of a gas that is inhaled with a normal inspiratory effort. The additional amount of gas which can be inhaled following this normal inspiratory effort is called the inspiratory reserve volume (IRV). After completing a normal expiratory effort which returns the lung and thorax to the resting position, an additional amount of gas can be exhaled; this is called the expiratory reserve volume (ERV). Thus, the ERV is the amount of gas that can be exhaled when the expiratory effort begins at the resting position and ends at maximal expiration. At the point of maximal expiration, there is still a quantity of gas in the lung that cannot be expelled. This remaining volume is the residual volume (RV).

The four capacities are also shown in Figure 5-1. The total lung capacity (TLC) consists of all four volumes. The inspiratory capacity (IC) is the maximum amount of gas which can be inhaled from the resting position. Thus, the IC is the sum of the V_T and the IRV. After a normal exhalation, the

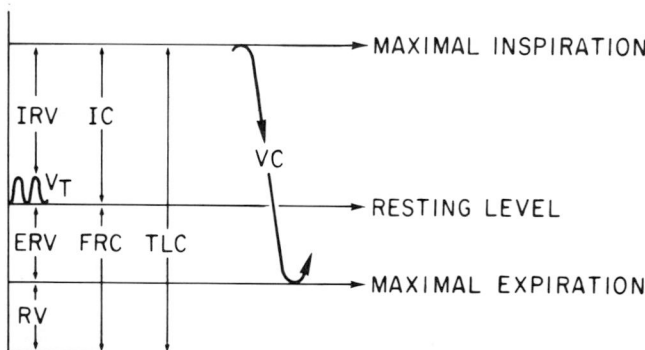

Fig. 5-1. Lung volumes and capacities in relation to points of maximal inspiration and expiration and the resting level. Vital capacity (VC) is an expiratory maneuver. Abbreviations are as follows: IRV—inspiratory reserve volume; V_T—tidal volume; ERV—expiratory reserve volume; RV—residual volume; IC—inspiratory capacity; FRC—functional residual capacity; TLC—total lung capacity.

amount of gas remaining in the lung is the functional residual capacity (FRC), which consists of the ERV plus the RV.

The fourth capacity is the vital capacity (VC). This capacity is by definition measured as an expiratory maneuver and is the amount of gas that can be expelled from the lung when exhalation starts at the maximal inspiratory level and proceeds to the maximal expiratory level. If the VC is measured as an inspiratory maneuver going from maximal expiration to maximal inspiration, it is then called an inspiratory vital capacity, or IVC. Usually the VC is measured as a forced exhalation, in which the subject is asked to inspire to the maximal inspiratory position and then empty the lungs as rapidly and completely as possible. This is termed the forced vital capacity, or FVC. Since the VC measures the change in lung position from maximal inspiration to maximal expiration, it should be considered a measure of the subject's ability to change the size of the thoracic cavity. This is influenced by all the muscles of respiration and their innervation, by the thoracic cage, by lung elasticity, and by the patency of the airways.

The FRC is a physiologic equivalent of a chemical buffer. It enables the individual to maintain a relatively constant level of oxygen and carbon dioxide in arterial blood. Each breath removes carbon dioxide from the FRC and adds oxygen. If the FRC did not exist and each breath completely filled and then emptied the lungs, there would be wide swings in arterial oxygen and carbon dioxide contents, since during inspiration the gases in the lung would have essentially the same pressures as in the atmosphere, while during expiration oxygen and carbon dioxide would be at mixed venous (pulmonary arterial) levels. Since the gases in the blood equilibrate with the gases in the alveoli, these marked changes would be reflected in the blood. The FRC also keeps alveoli and airways patent, which helps to prevent pulmonary arterial-to-venous shunting (through areas of airless lung) and also makes the work of breathing easier, since it takes a greater effort to expand collapsed alveoli than to expand those which are already open. In a chemical reaction, too much buffer can be bad, and this also is true for the FRC. If the FRC is too large, then it cannot adequately be "freshened" by each breath and this can contribute to a decrease in arterial oxygenation and a rise in carbon dioxide tension.

DYNAMIC LUNG MEASUREMENTS—SPIROMETRY AND FLOW-VOLUME TRACINGS

Airflow obstruction or limitation, which is usually present in patients with asthma, is best assessed by dynamic measurements such as flow rates and the timed vital capacity. Spirometry is a simple procedure for obtaining this information. The spirogram is a plot of volume versus time. Another technique which is now in common use in hospital laboratories is the flow-volume tracing. As the name indicates, this is a plot of airflow versus the expired (or inspired) lung volume.

The forced expiratory spirogram is shown in Figure 5-2. In this figure, the subject is breathing normally and the V_T is recorded. The subject is asked to slowly blow all the air out of the lungs and then take a deep inspiration. This allows for the measurement of the ERV, IRV, and IC, as well as the IVC. The subject is then instructed to blow all the air out of the lungs as rapidly and completely as possible. This gives a tracing of the FVC. The FVC can be subdivided into the forced expiratory volume in the first second (FEV_1), the second second (FEV_2), and the third second (FEV_3). These are flows as they are measured as a volume per second. The ratio FEV_1/FVC is often used as an index of airflow obstruction. Predicted normal (reference) values are available for the FEV_1/FVC ratio, as they are for most of the other measurements.

Another way of assessing airflow obstruction with the spirogram is to measure specific flow rates. Different portions of the FVC curve are used. The most rapid flow rates occur early in expiration, when the peak expiratory flow rate (PEFR) occurs. On the spirogram, one can measure the forced expiratory flow from 200 ml to 1200 ml below maximal inspiration ($FEF_{200-1200}$) (Fig. 5-3). These points are used as the subject is overcoming inertia during the initial part of exhalation and, thus, flow during the initial 200 ml is slower than during the peak flow. The $FEF_{200-1200}$ and PEFR are useful measurements in patients with asthma who are trained to perform the maneuver properly. These measurements, however, are very effort-

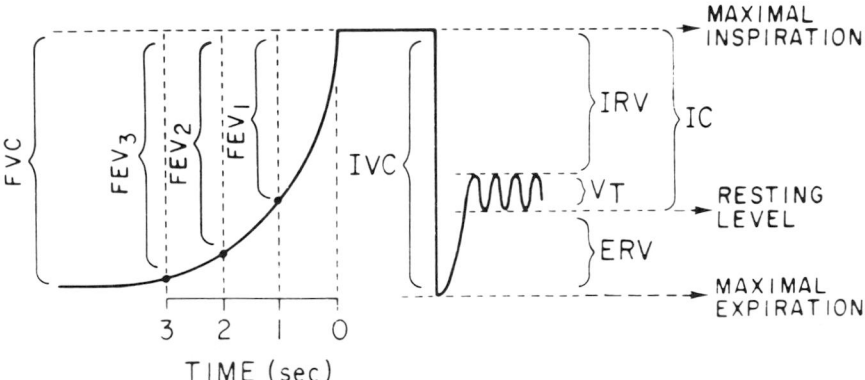

Fig. 5-2. The spirometric tracing demonstrating the lung volumes and capacities which can be measured by this technique. Abbreviations are as given in Figure 5-1, and as follows: IVC—inspiratory vital capacity; FVC—forced vital capacity; FEV_1, FEV_2, FEV_3—forced expiratory volumes in the first, second, and third seconds, respectively.

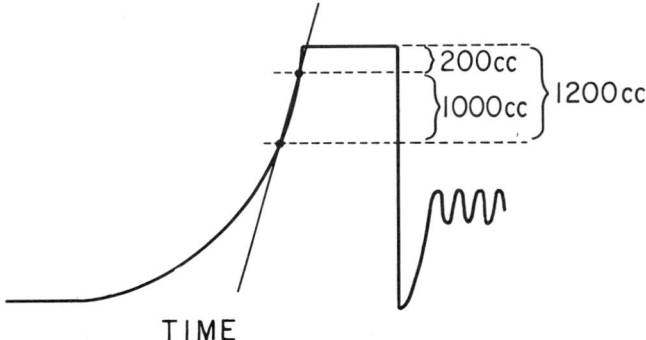

Fig. 5-3. Measurement of the forced expiratory flow from 200 to 1200 ml (FEF$_{200-1200}$). This is the part of the spirometric tracing where the expiratory flow rate is usually maximal.

dependent and an untrained subject may show marked variability in values on repeated efforts.

Another measurement in common use is the forced expiratory flow from 25 to 75 percent of the total FVC. This is termed the FEF$_{25-75\%}$. It is less effort-dependent than is the FEF$_{200-1200}$ and thus is more reproducible. It is shown in Figure 5-4. The volume of air expelled from point A in Figure 5-4 (when 25 percent of the FVC has been expired) to point B (when 75 percent of the FVC has been expired) is measured, as is the time it takes to blow out the air from A to B. This gives a volume per unit time, which is a flow rate.

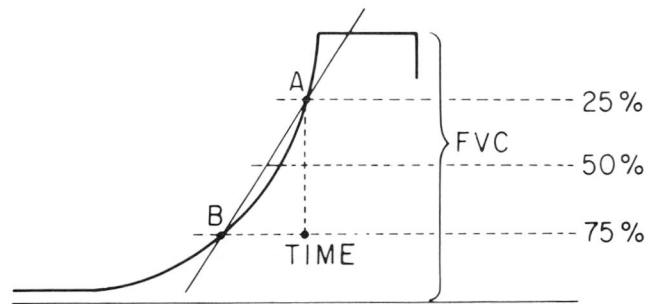

Fig. 5-4. Measurement of the forced expiratory flow from 25 to 75 percent of the forced vital capacity (FEF$_{25-75\%}$). A and B represent the points where 25 percent and 75 percent of the FVC has been expelled. The line connecting these points forms the hypotenuse of a right triangle, of which one arm is volume and the other is time. Thus, the volume per unit time, or flow, during the middle 50 percent of the FVC can be measured.

One should be aware in comparing the $FEF_{25-75\%}$ to a previously obtained value that this comparison can only be made if the FVCs on both tracings are approximately equal. This is because if a tracing has a small FVC, the midpoint of flow is moved up to a point on the curve where flow is normally more rapid. This is shown in Figure 5-5, where the solid-line tracing has a larger FVC than does the dashed-line tracing; the initial flow rates are similar, however. The major difference between the two tracings is that the dashed tracing represents an effort which was prematurely terminated. Thus, it has a steeper midportion, since the slower terminal phase of a complete expiration has been eliminated. This results in a $FEF_{25-75\%}$ which is more rapid than is the value noted when exhalation has been maximal; yet when the two FVC curves are superimposed, it can be noted that the flow rates on both tracings are similar.

An example of what increasing degrees of airflow obstruction does to the appearance of the spirogram is shown in Figure 5-6. Note also that the FRC

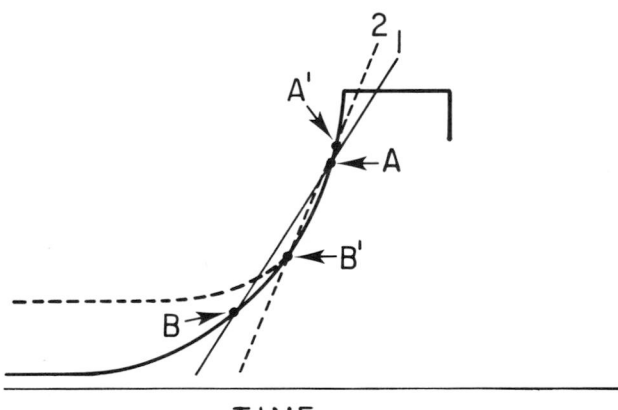

TIME

Fig. 5-5. Demonstration of an artificial increase in the $FEF_{25-75\%}$ due to early termination of the FVC maneuver. A and B on the solid line tracing are the same as in Figure 5-4. Line 1 connecting A and B is used to measure the $FEF_{25-75\%}$. The broken-line tracing is superimposed on and is identical to the solid-line tracing, except that the expiratory effort was prematurely terminated. Thus, A' and B' are on a steeper portion of the tracing and Line 2, which connects A' and B', demonstrates a more rapid $FEF_{25-75\%}$ than does Line 1. Actually, no change in flow rates has occurred. Thus, The $FEF_{25-75\%}$ cannot be used to assess bronchodilator response or patient improvement (or deterioration) unless the measured FVCs of the two studies being compared are within 5 percent of each other or unless the total expiratory times are similar.

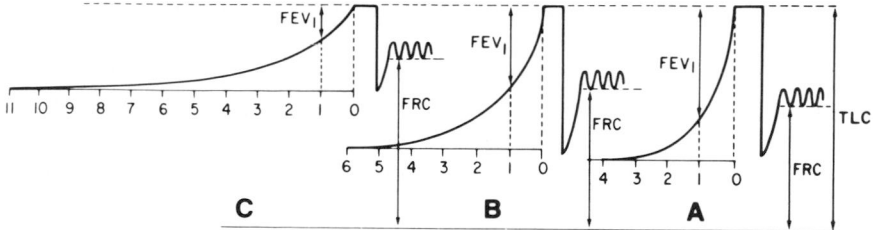

Fig. 5-6. Three spirometric tracings showing a normal curve (A), mild to moderate obstruction (B), and severe airflow obstruction (C). Although the FRC cannot be measured by spirometry, this diagram includes this value to demonstrate the changes in this lung compartment as obstruction increases. Note that the FEV_1 decreases and the FRC increases with increasing degrees of airflow obstruction. The time it takes to complete the maneuver also increases. With severe obstruction (curve C) the FVC has decreased as well.

increases (not measured by spirometry) and that the FEV_1 declines as the obstruction becomes worse. Also, when severe obstruction is present, the FVC is often decreased.

Flow-volume tracings also measure flow rates. The equipment used is usually more costly than is a spirometer, and it is still being argued as to whether or not a flow-versus-volume plot provides more information than does a volume-versus-time plot. An example of a flow-volume plot is shown in Figure 5-7.

The flow-versus-volume tracing relates flow rates to lung volumes. At high lung volumes, the cross-sectional area of the airways is increased, which reduces resistance and allows for higher flow rates. At lower lung volumes, the flow rates are more dependent upon the frictional resistance in the smaller airways. When disease is present, other factors also influence the flow rates. Using the flow-volume tracing, one can determine the flow rate at different lung volumes. At the point where 25 percent of the vital capacity has been

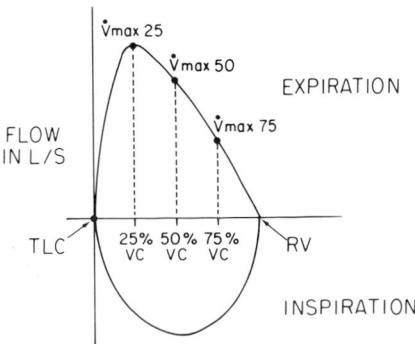

Fig. 5-7. Flow-versus-volume tracing. Expiration begins at the point of total lung capacity (TLC) and ends at residual volume (RV). Flow is measured at the points when 25, 50, and 75 percent of the vital capacity (VC) are exhaled. $\dot{V}_{max\ 25}$ = flow when 25 percent of the VC has been exhaled.

exhaled, this flow rate is termed the $\dot{V}_{max25}$, when 50 percent of the vital capacity has been exhaled it is the $\dot{V}_{max50}$, etc. The inspiratory portion of the curve is helpful in distinguishing large-airway obstruction which occurs above the level of the thoracic inlet from obstruction which occurs below this level. Large airway obstruction above the thoracic inlet results in a "plateau" of the flow rate on the inspiratory portion of the curve, while the expiratory portion is affected when the flow-limiting portion is within the thoracic cavity.

The most useful flow rate is the FEV_1, which is the maximal amount of air exhaled in the first second of expiration. Although the usefulness of this rate is limited by the fact that a poor start which can alter the measurement may occur, this drawback is minor compared to the problems encountered with the other spirometric and flow-volume measurements. The FVC is dependent on a complete exhalation, which may not occur, especially in patients with airflow obstruction. All subjects can produce a maximal effort for at least one second, so this is not a problem in the FEV_1 measurement. The difficulties in using the $FEF_{200-1200}$ and $FEF_{25-75\%}$ have already been discussed. The $\dot{V}_{max75}$ is thought to be very sensitive when used to detect early airflow obstruction, but suffers from having poor specificity—which is to say that it identifies too many normal subjects as being abnormal. Also, $\dot{V}_{max75}$, $\dot{V}_{max50}$, etc. are dependent on the actual volume of air in the lung rather than on the easily determined exhaled percentage of the VC, and this volume is usually not known and may vary in its relation to that particular percentage of the FVC. Thus, the $\dot{V}_{max75}$, etc. has a great deal of both inter- and intrasubject variability. Many pulmonologists find that the flow-volume loop is most useful in identifying upper airway obstruction where the inspiratory portion of the loop is flattened. Also, the flow-volume loop is helpful in identifying poor patient performance, especially in the early phase of expiration. A poor start, a slow rise to the point of maximal flow, and an inadequate effort to produce the maximal flow can be recognized by the technician, who can then instruct the patient on how to produce a better tracing on the next effort.

STATIC LUNG VOLUME MEASUREMENTS

Lung volume measurements are often useful in evaluating patients with asthma. At times, a bronchodilator response may not be evident by spirometry, but may be demonstrated by a decrease in the RV and FRC. Spirometry cannot measure TLC, FRC, or RV. Lung volume measurements are static, and thus will not demonstrate changes in flow rates. They do demonstrate the increases in lung volumes, especially in the RV, the FRC, and even the TLC that may occur secondary to the airway obstruction.

There are two general types of lung volume measurements. These are: the measurement of thoracic gas volume, which is performed in a body plethysmograph or by radiologic techniques; and gas dilution lung volumes, which are determined by measuring the space of distribution of a tracer gas such as helium. Although these two general methods are equally accurate in normal subjects, in the presence of airway obstruction the gas dilution techniques may underestimate lung volume, due to the inhomogeneous distribution of the tracer gas in the lungs. The radiologic method of measuring thoracic gas volume can easily be measured in a physician's office using P-A and lateral chest radiographs. Since the radiographic technique measures the TLC, a VC measured at the same time is necessary in order to allow for determination of the RV. The body plethysmograph method is available in many hospitals in larger communities; although the equipment is expensive, it has the value of providing measurements of airway resistance (R_{aw}) and the reciprocal of R_{aw}, which is airway conductance (G_{aw}).

Gas dilution lung volume measurements are available at most hospitals with a pulmonary function laboratory. Usually such a measurement is performed as the determination of the alveolar volume during the single-breath carbon monoxide diffusing capacity measurement. Also, there is a commonly used re-breathing technique, in which either helium or neon is used as an indicator gas and its space of distribution is measured. Washout of nitrogen from the lungs during 100-percent oxygen breathing is another gas dilution technique. In this method, nitrogen is the indicator gas and it is collected and measured. Since 79 percent of the gas in the lung is nitrogen, the volume of the lung can be determined using the amount of washed-out nitrogen plus corrections for the residual nitrogen in the lung and the quantity washed out of the blood.

Gas dilution measurements of TLC are less useful in measuring true lung capacity in patients with asthma than in normals. This is because the tracer gas is not distributed throughout the lung in a homogeneous fashion, due to the airway obstruction present, and this results in an underestimation of true TLC. Plethysmography is thus a better method of measurement, but with this technique precautions must be taken to avoid overestimating true TLC. In patients with airway obstruction, pressures in the distal airways may not fully equilibrate with pressure at the mouth when the usual methodology is employed. This can lead to the recording of falsely large lung volumes. This can be prevented by having the subject perform the panting maneuver used in plethysmography at slow rates, viz. less than 1/second (less than 1 Hz).

The use of the body plethysmograph has the advantage of measuring R_{aw} and G_{aw} and specific conductance (SG_{aw}), which is G_{aw} divided by the thoracic gas volume at the point where G_{aw} is measured. These values are very sensitive to changes in the larger airways and may demonstrate a bronchodilator effect not seen on routine spirometry.

DIFFUSING CAPACITY

The single-breath carbon monoxide diffusing capacity can be helpful in distinguishing between asthma and other types of obstructive airway disease. The method theoretically measures the ability of the lungs to transfer carbon monoxide from the alveoli to the hemoglobin in the circulating red blood cells. The results are reported as milliliters of carbon monoxide transfered per minute per mmHg pressure. The amount of carbon monoxide in the inspired gas is approximately 0.3 percent. Its space of distribution and, thus, its alveolar partial pressure is determined by the addition of 10-percent helium to the gas mixture on the assumption that the carbon monoxide is distributed throughout the lungs in the same manner as is helium. After a 10-second breath-holding period at TLC, the exhaled gases are analyzed. Since essentially no helium crosses the alveolar capillary barrier, the ratio of $He_{expired}$ to $He_{inspired}$ is used to measure the alveolar volume, which in normals equals the TLC. Also, this ratio is the theoretical dilution of carbon monoxide before this gas crosses into the blood. The volume of carbon monoxide which crosses into the blood can also be determined. Blood carbon monoxide tension is assumed to be zero, since the circulation is a "sink" for small amounts of carbon monoxide. Details of the technique are available in pulmonary laboratory manuals.

ARTERIAL BLOOD GASES

Arterial blood gases are often very useful in assessing the condition of a patient with asthma, especially during an acute episode. The technology for these measurements should be available in any hospital with an emergency room or where acutely ill patients are treated.

QUALITY CONTROL

The value of any study is highly dependent on good quality control. Technicians must be trained not only to perform the various studies but also to troubleshoot problems, to identify poor patient performance and to correct it, and to accurately calibrate the equipment. Even office spirometry requires a well-trained technician and a calibrating syringe if one is to be certain the values obtained are meaningful. Also, the calibrating syringe requires periodic recalibration to be certain it is accurate.

Recognized standards have been developed for obtaining spirometric measurements and for calibrating the spirometer. Lung volume measurements require accurate calibration of the plethysmograph. In the gas dilution technique, the helium meter must be linear. The diffusing capacity measurements require attention to technique and calibration of the meters. Arterial-blood-gas-measuring instruments require frequent checks for accuracy using blood or other solutions with known gas tensions.

Spirometric standards have been developed by the American Thoracic Society at the Snowbird Workshop on Standardization of Spirometry and have been accepted by others for use in both adult and pediatric studies. Standards for the other measurements discussed are being developed at this time. The reference list at the end of this chapter includes currently used quality control methods (Gardner et al., Morris et al., Conrad et al.).

PULMONARY FUNCTION MEASUREMENTS IN ASTHMA

Spirometry and Flow-Volume Studies

The hallmark of airway obstruction is a decrease in flow rates (Figs. 5-6 and 5-8). Thus, in a subject with bronchospasm, a decrease in the rate of air flow is usually noted. In very mild disease, the study may be normal. The spirometric values which are most helpful are the FVC, FEV_1, and the ratio FEV_1/FVC. Using flow-volume tracings, the maximal expiratory flow rates, $\dot{V}_{max75}$, $\dot{V}_{max50}$, etc. are decreased. Usually in asthmatic patients, some reversibility in these measurements of flow is noted following administration of a bronchodilator. The lack of a bronchodilator response may be due to the patient taking medicine prior to the study and thus coming to the laboratory in a maximally bronchodilated condition, or may be due to refractoriness to the drug, or to the fact that the bronchospasm may be occurring in the smaller airways and that lung volume measurements may be a more appropriate test. Also, at times the measurement of R_{aw}, G_{aw}, or SG_{aw} may be more sensitive indices. In some instances, a subject with asthma may have a decreased VC (Figs. 5-6 and 5-8). Since the VC is a measure of one's ability to vary the size of the thoracic cavity, air trapping from the obstructive mechanisms may limit thoracic excursions and cause a fall in VC. Also, airways blocked by inspissated plugs and/or bronchospasm may not conduct inspired air into the alveoli, which also may result in a fall in VC.

Lung Volume Measurements

Lung volume measurements show an increase in the RV, the FRC, and sometimes the TLC. Even when asymptomatic, an asthmatic subject may have an increased RV. When lung volumes are measured by plethysmography, R_{aw}, G_{aw}, and SG_{aw} can also be determined; a change in these three

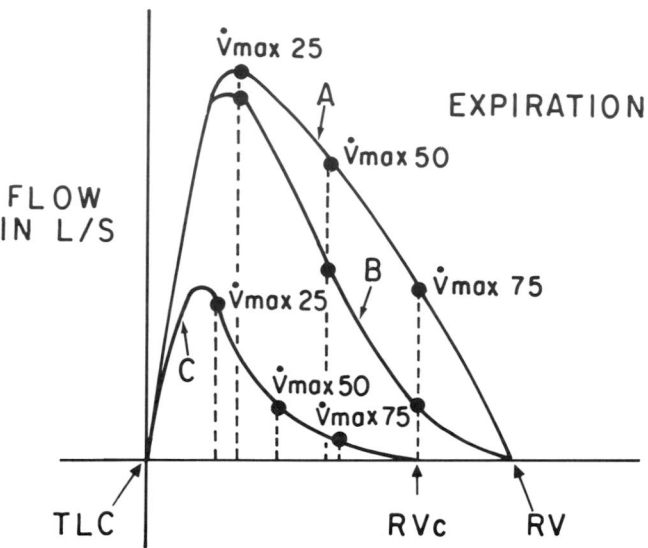

Fig. 5-8. A comparison of expiratory flow volume tracings in a normal subject (curve A), a subject with mild airflow obstruction (curve B), and in a subject with severe airflow obstruction (curve C). Note the decrease in the vital capacity in curve C, with the residual volume point (RV_c) being shifted to the left. This indicates an increase in the RV. Also note in curve C that the points of $\dot{V}_{max\ 25}$, and $\dot{V}_{max\ 50}$, and $\dot{V}_{max\ 75}$ are shifted to the left, and thus correspond to a different lung volume level than in curves A and B.

Table 5-1

Arterial Blood Gas Values in Patients with Asthma

Degree of Severity	Oxygenation	P_{CO_2}	Acid-base State
Mild	relatively normal	decreased	compensated respiratory alkalosis
Moderate	relatively normal to mildly decreased	decreased	compensated respiratory alkalosis
Severe	marked decrease	normal to elevated	respiratory acidosis

values is a very sensitive measure of bronchodilator response, although this is less specific than are changes in the FEV_1.

Diffusing Capacity

The single-breath carbon monoxide diffusing capacity is usually normal but sometimes is increased in patients with asthma. Several explanations have been proposed for this supernormal value, including an increased pulmonary capillary blood volume, which results from the more negative intrathoracic pressures generated during the 10-second breath-holding period which is part of the test performance. Patients with advanced emphysema have a decrease in the single-breath diffusing capacity, so this study is of some help in establishing a diagnosis in certain individuals.

Arterial Blood Gas Measurements

Arterial blood gas values in subjects with asthma are shown in Table 5-1. In cases of mild asthma, the patient usually is able to maintain normal arterial blood oxygen tensions, although the alveolar-arterial gradient may be mildly increased. Hyperventilation is evident as the carbon dioxide tensions are decreased. The carbon dioxide tension is inversely proportional to alveolar ventilation. As the airflow limitation worsens, the alveolar-arterial oxygen gradient widens and the oxygen tension falls. In severe disease, the patient can no longer maintain adequate alveolar ventilation and carbon dioxide levels start to rise. Thus, when the patient has a normal or elevated carbon dioxide level during an acute asthmatic episode, this is a sign of severe disease, since it is evidence that carbon dioxide levels are rising and alveolar ventilation is decreasing. It indicates that the patient should be considered for hospitalization.

INTERPRETATION OF RESULTS

The results obtained from the studies considered in this section must be compared to reference values in order to determine if an abnormality is present, and if so the degree of that abnormality. Normal or reference values are available in the literature and are periodically being superseded by more current studies. Ideally, every laboratory should develop its own normal standards, but this is not realistic. Recently published reference values only include subjects who are healthy lifetime nonsmokers, which is not the case in older series. The better performed studies were done using Caucasians of European ancestry, and thus the data for other populations is either scant or less than optimal. Variations among different racial groups may exist and, thus "normal" is less well defined for these non-Caucasian populations. Normality is usually defined by convention as including 95 percent of a known healthy population—so, by definition, one in twenty persons without any disease will have values outside this normal range. Widening the range of normal will include too many subjects with disease to make the standards useful.

There are few if any ideal studies of arterial blood gases in normal subjects. These results will be affected by altitude, the patient's age, and the position assumed by the subject when the sample was obtained. Reference values are available, but these will need revision as better studies are carried out. The reference list includes a manual with an approach for interpreting the results obtained by spirometry, lung volume measurements, diffusing capacity, and arterial blood gases.

TESTS OF BRONCHODILATOR RESPONSE

When the presence of airflow limitation has been demonstrated, it is important to determine whether or not it is reversible. A therapeutic dose of a bronchodilator aerosol is given by inhalation after baseline spirometry is performed, and the measurement is repeated at an appropriate time (depending on the bronchodilator used—15–30 minutes) after administration of the drug. Bronchodilator medications should be discontinued prior to testing for an appropriate time period in order to avoid the effects on test results of previous medication.

Choice of Bronchodilator

It is desirable to use short-acting bronchodilators such as isoproterenol or isoetharine that act rapidly and lead to a peak response within 10–15 minutes. This will decrease the time between drug administration and the performance of the test. Also, should an adverse drug reaction occur, this will be of shorter duration than is true when a long-acting drug is used. Some of the longer-acting bronchodilators take more than 1 hour to create a maximal response.

CRITERIA FOR DETERMINING A SIGNIFICANT BRONCHODILATOR RESPONSE

Table 5-2 provides an approach to evaluating a patient's response to an inhaled bronchodilator using spirometric values. The criteria presented are based on published studies of the responses of normal subjects to an inhaled bronchodilator and on the maximal differences noted following inhalation of

Table 5-2
Spirometric Response Following Bronchodilator[a]

Category	Ratio of Postbronchodilator/ Prebronchodilator (Post/Pre)		
	$FVC \frac{post*}{pre}$	$FEV_1 \frac{post}{pre}$	$FEF_{25-75\%} \frac{post\dagger}{pre}$
Markedly improved	≥ 1.25	≥ 1.25	≥ 2.00
Improved	1.15–1.24	1.12–1.24	1.45–1.99
Not clearly improved	1.05–1.14	1.05–1.11	1.10–1.44
Not improved	< 1.05	< 1.05	< 1.10

[a] From Morris AH, Kanner RE, Crapo RO, et al: Clinical Pulmonary Function Testing, 2nd ed. Salt Lake City, Intermountain Thoracic Society, 1984 p. 24. Used with permission.
* Expiratory time post/pre must be < 1.10; if not, then FVC cannot be used, since increased FVC might be due solely to the increased expiratory time and not to increased flow.
† If expiratory time post/pre < 0.90 and the FVC post/pre is not between 0.96 and 1.04, then the $FEF_{25-75\%}$ cannot be used, since reducing the expiratory time or the FVC can increase the $FEF_{25-75\%}$ in the absence of any change in flow itself.

a placebo. A patient should demonstrate improvement in the FEV_1 (or other parameter) which is more than 2 standard deviations beyond the mean improvement noted in normal subjects. The FEV_1 is, in most situations, the best parameter to use when considering the response to a bronchodilator. The FVC can be used only if the expiratory time during the postbronchodilator study is approximately equal to or is less than the prebronchodilator expiratory time. Otherwise, any improvement could be due to a longer period of expiration. The FEF_{25-75} also can be used but the wide range of the response in normals means that at least a 45 percent improvement must be seen before the bronchodilator response is considered significant. Also, as has been pointed out previously in this chapter, before the FEV_{25-75} can be used to assess the response to a bronchodilator, the value for the FVC postbronchodilator must approximate the prebronchodilator value. Otherwise, the improvement noted could be due to a shift in position of the middle 50 percent of the FVC to a steeper portion of the curve due to a premature termination of expiration (Fig. 5-5).

Measurement of changes in G_{aw} before and after the inhalation of aerosolized isoetharine in 75 normal persons demonstrated a mean percentage increase (mean $\pm$ S.D.) of 24.3 $\pm$ 14.8. According to these data, normal persons may increase G_{aw} by as much as 53.9 percent and, thus, changes exceeding this value are needed before the response is considered significant. Determining the therapeutic effect of a bronchodilator is more complex. In patients with very low initial values, a 15- or 20-percent improvement may only be 50 or 75 ml, which can be due to the normal variability which can occur in repetitive studies. On the other hand, if the subject has large FVC and FEV_1, a 300-ml improvement may be less than a 10- or 15-percent change. Thus, the interpretation of pre- and postbronchodilator spirometry must always take into consideration clinical information.

A study of the ability of various spirometric tests and body plethysmographic measurements to evaluate the bronchodilator response of five different drug regimens concluded that although the mean percentage improvement after administration of bronchodilators was greater for G_{aw} and $FEF_{25-75\%}$ than for FEV_1, the FEV_1 statistically differentiated between the five regimens best. The reason is that there is less inherent variability in measuring FEV_1 than in $FEF_{25-75\%}$ or G_{aw}. This means that although the FEV_1 is a less sensitive test than the $FEF_{25-75\%}$ or G_{aw}, it is more specific.

At times, a bronchodilator response may not be evident by spirometry, but may be demonstrated by a decrease in the static lung volumes such as the RV, FRC, and TLC, as shown in Figure 5-9. This pattern of bronchodilator response is most apt to occur in severe disease. When lung volume measurements are not available, watch the change in the slow VC (not FVC), since a concomitant change in a slow VC will be seen in most if not all of such cases.

The lack of bronchodilator response may be due to the patient taking medication prior to the test, refractoriness to the drug used, or airflow obstruction due to mechanisms other than bronchospasm, such as mucus plugs.

BRONCHOPROVOCATION CHALLENGE TESTING

Bronchial reactivity or responsiveness to various stimuli is a normal phenomenon in all individuals. When the degree of the responsiveness

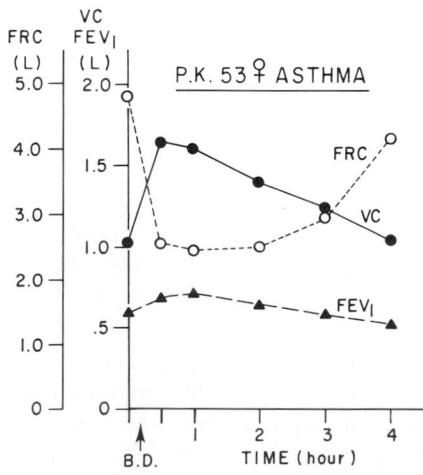

Fig. 5-9. A 53-year-old female with chronic asthma. Note that after two inhalations of fenoterol there is a marked reduction in FRC as measured by body plethysmography and a concomitant increase in VC, with only minimal improvement in the FEV_1. She thus demonstrates a marked response to the bronchodilator despite the lack of a significant effect on the FEV_1.

exceeds that noted in normal subjects, it is termed bronchial hyperrespon-siveness. The demonstration of increased bronchial responsiveness to inhaled biological, physical, chemical, and pharmacologic stimuli can be important in the diagnosis of bronchial asthma. Patients with extrinsic asthma are extremely sensitive to the inhalation of specific allergens as well as to non-specific stimuli. When exposed to these stimuli, the majority of asthmatic patients, including asymptomatic subjects, quickly develop widespread bron-chial smooth muscle constriction. They may also demonstrate bronchial hyperresponsiveness when breathing cold, dry air and/or after strenuous exercise. On the other hand, normal subjects will display only a minimal response when exposed to such stimuli. This is the basis of bronchial provo-cation testing which has been utilized in the diagnosis of asthma. It should be noted that nonspecific bronchial hyperresponsiveness is not unique to asthma and may be seen in some patients with hay fever, chronic bronchitis, and other respiratory diseases. A transient and reversible airway hyperresponsive-ness has been shown to occur in previously healthy persons following acute viral upper respiratory infections. A positive inhalation challenge test itself therefore does not establish a diagnosis of asthma; however, it provides valuable diagnostic information when, (a) a diagnosis of asthma is not obvi-ous from the history, physical examination, and routine pulmonary function tests (for example, in patients with unexplained chronic cough or dyspnea whose pulmonary function tests are within normal limits); and (b) when it is important to determine specific causes of bronchospasm in patients with extrinsic or occupational asthma.

INHALATION BRONCHIAL CHALLENGE

A technique for documenting bronchial hyperresponsiveness in human subjects is to measure the change in expiratory flow rates after the inhalation of increasing concentrations of aerosolized pharmacologic bronchoconstric-tor agents, of specific antigens, or (in some instances) of cold, dry air. Methacholine, a cholinergic agonist, and histamine are the pharmacologic bronchoconstrictor agents most commonly used for nonspecific challenge testing in the United States. The procedures are relatively simple and safe when performed as recommended, and the induced bronchoconstriction can be quickly reversed by the inhalation of a beta-adrenergic agonist. There are no late reactions. It has been shown that the magnitude of the bronchial response to methacholine and histamine correlates well with the severity of clinical asthma. When antigens are used for specific challenge testing, a late bronchospastic response of a severe degree may develop in some patients 1–12 hours after the inhalation of the antigen. Since this late response is not always effectively blocked by beta-adrengeric agonists, patients should be observed for at least 12 hours after the challenge. Thus, antigen challenge may not be suitable for performance in an office outpatient setting.

Detailed methods and procedures for the standardization of inhalation challenge testing have been presented by several groups of investigators. To date, however, a consensus has not been achieved. Two techniques for the generation and delivery of aerosols are the most frequently used. One is an intermittent generation and inhalation of the aerosol using a system consisting of a breath-activated nebulizer (DeVilbiss #42 or #646) and a dosimeter (Rosenthal-French) which is connected to a compressed air tank at a pressure of 20 psi. The time for each aerosol generation is adjusted to 0.6 seconds and a patient takes 5 consecutive slow, deep inspirations starting at the functional residual capacity level. The dosage administered is expressed in terms of breath units. A breath unit equals the concentration of the drug multiplied by the number of inhalations. For example, 1 breath unit equals 1 inhalation of 1.0 mg/ml of drug solution. The second method is one of continuous aerosol generation (with a Wright nebulizer) and continuous inhalation of the aerosol for a fixed duration of time using tidal volume breathing. The dosage is expressed in terms of the concentration of the solution.

INHALATION CHALLENGE TESTING WITH METHACHOLINE AND HISTAMINE

Solutions of methacholine chloride and histamine phosphate are prepared by dissolving these agents in a sterilized diluent containing 0.5 percent NaCl, 0.275 percent $NaHCO_3$, and 0.4 percent phenol (pH 7.0). Concentrations of 5.0 and 25.0 mg/ml solution of methacholine and 5.0 and 10 mg/ml solution of histamine are prepared. These are used to make the various concentrations used for dose-response studies. For the sake of sterility, solutions are passed through a sterilized 0.2-millipore filter into sterile vials.

The test is performed by measuring baseline and control (after inhalation of an aerosol consisting only of the diluent) spirometry followed by inhalations of serially increasing concentrations of methacholine or histamine from the recommended lowest concentration to the highest concentration. Dosing schedules of both methacholine and histamine are shown in Table 5-3. Spirometry is performed 1–5 minutes after inhalations of each concentration. A positive test is a 20 percent or greater reduction of FEV_1 from the control value. This fall in FEV_1 should be sustained for 3 minutes. If the test is negative, the next higher concentration is given. Interpretation of the test results is made by constructing a dose-response curve by plotting the log dose of the inhaled drug on the abscissa in cumulative breath units when an intermittent inhalation technique is used (or in concentration when a continuous inhalation technique is used), and the change in FEV_1 from the control

Table 5-3
Dosing Schedule for Methacholine and Histamine†

Concentration (mg/ml)	Breath Units* per 5 Inhalations	Cumulative Dose (breath units)
0.1	0.5	0.5
0.5	2.5	3.0
1.0	5.0	8.0
2.5	12.5	24.5
5.0	25.0	49.5
10.0	50.0	99.5
25.0	125.0	225.0

* 1 breath unit = 1 inhalation of 1 mg/ml methacholine or histamine solution.
† When histamine is used, do not use a concentration greater than 10 mg/ml because of the frequency of side effects.

value is on the ordinate. The cumulative number of breath units at which the FEV_1 drops by 20 percent is designated as the provocative dose (PD_{20}-FEV_1). When a continuous inhalation technique is used, the concentration that causes a 20 percent fall in FEV_1 is designated as provocative concentration (PC_{20}-FEV_1) (Fig. 5-10). A diagnosis of bronchial hyperresponsiveness can be made using methacholine when PD_{20}-FEV_1 (or PC_{20}-FEV_1) is less than or equal to the highest cumulative value of breath units used in the study (225 breath units) or the highest scheduled concentration (25 mg/ml), since

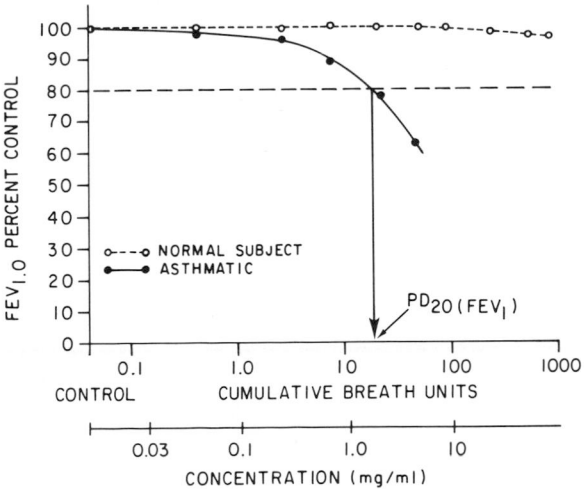

Fig. 5-10. An example of a dose-response curve to the inhalation of pharmacologic bronchoconstrictor agents. Breath units and concentration on the abscissa are expressed as log dose. (Modified from Cropp GJA: Methods of inhalation challenge, in Ellis EF and Wanner A (eds): Interspecialty Focus: Pulmonary Medicine. Morris Plains, NJ, Parke-Davis, Division of Warner-Lambert Inc., 1983, Vol. 1, No. 1, p4. Used with permission.)

the PD_{20}-FEV_1 (or PC_{20}-FEV_1) of the majority of normal subjects are greater than those values. Figure 5-11 shows a positive response to methacholine in a 14-year-old boy who never wheezed, but who complained of easy fatigability and labored breathing associated with a nonproductive cough following mild exercise. The evaluation of his cardiovascular system was normal. Spirometry at rest was within normal limits. Repeated spirometry after mild exercise was not valid because he could not complete a forced expiration due to coughing.

ANTIGEN INHALATION CHALLENGE

Antigen solutions of different concentrations are prepared with the same diluent used for methacholine and histamine. Antigen concentrations are expressed in terms of weight per volume (w/v). An antigen inhalation unit is defined as one inhalation of a 1:5000 w/v dilution of antigen. The dosing schedule is shown in Table 5-4. The challenge usually begins with 5 inhalations of the antigen concentration required to elicit a $2+$ intradermal test (defined as a wheel 5 mm larger than the reaction to the diluent control). A positive response is a 20 percent or greater reduction in the FEV_1 from the

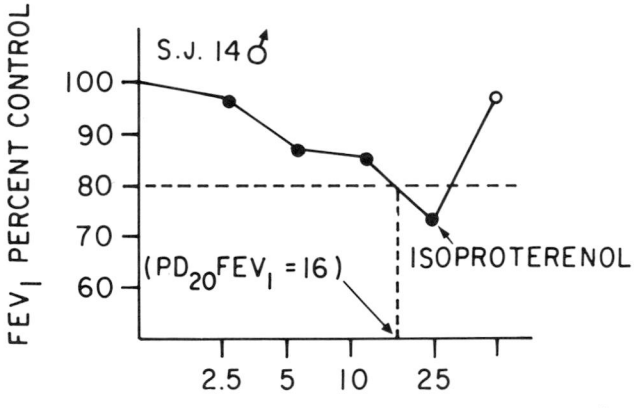

Fig. 5-11. A 14-year-old male who complained of dyspnea and cough but who did not wheeze was challenged with methacholine. Note that his FEV_1 decreased by more than 20 percent after inhaling a relatively low dose of methacholine. This indicates airway hyperresponsiveness and helps establish a diagnosis of asthma. This patient's symptoms were markedly improved by bronchodilator drugs. A subject with normal airway reactivity would demonstrate little change in the value of the FEV_1 with this dose of methacholine.

Table 5-4

Dosing Schedule for Antigens[a]

Antigen Concentration (w/v)	Breath Units* per 5 Inhalations	Cumulative Dose (breath units)
1:1,000,000	0.025	0.025
1:500,000	0.05	0.075
1:100,000	0.25	0.325
1:50,000	0.5	0.825
1:10,000	2.5	3.32
1:5000	5.0	8.32
1:1000	25.0	33.3
1:500	50.0	83.3
1:100	250.0	300.3

[a] From Chai H, Farr RS, Froelich LA, et al: Standardization of bronchial inhalation challenge procedures. J Allergy Clin Immunol 56:323–327, 1975. Many laboratories have modified this schedule. Used with permission.

* 1 breath unit = 1 inhalation of 1:5000 w/v dilution.

control value sustained for 10 or more minutes. If a decrease in the FEV_1 is 15–19 percent wait an additional 5–10 minutes before inhaling the next higher concentration, which is given cautiously with less than 5 inhalations. All patients should be observed carefully for as long as 12 hours for possible late bronchospastic responses.

LABORATORY EVALUATION OF THE THERAPEUTIC REGIMEN

Pulmonary function testing is useful not only in determining the degree of the patient's impairment and the acute response to a bronchodilator, but, in addition, helps in the overall evaluation of the effects of therapy. Pharmacologic agents such as the glucocorticoids can make a patient feel much better by actions other than improving the asthmatic problem. Thus, without objective measurements (or, in selected subjects, a careful physical examination of the chest), the physician may incorrectly believe that significant relief of bronchospasm has occurred, when in fact this is not the situation. A lack of objective improvement in pulmonary function is an indication that the therapeutic regimen may have to be modified. With proper therapy, most asthmatics will demonstrate normal or close to normal pulmonary function. There are a significant number of individuals, however, who, despite optimum therapy, may have to accept some degree of respiratory impairment. If the objective tests indicate that the decrease is chronic and severe enough, the patient may be entitled to disability benefits.

LABORATORY INDICATIONS FOR HOSPITALIZATION DURING AN ACUTE EPISODE OF BRONCHOSPASM

Pulmonary function testing is also a valuable aid in deciding when a patient experiencing an acute asthmatic episode requires hospitalization. Severe hypoxemia and/or carbon dioxide retention are ominous signs which indicate that the individual would best be treated as an inpatient in order to avoid a fatal outcome. A marked decrease in FEV_1 to 1 liter or less also should alert the physician that hospitalization may be necessary.

PROGRESSION OF DISEASE

Pulmonary function studies also can monitor the progression of obstructive lung disease. Although progressive airway obstruction is considered to be a sign of emphysema, there are patients with asthma who demonstrate this problem. No prospective long-term studies are available on a randomly selected group of asthmatics, and in all likelihood, most asthmatics do not have progressive airway obstruction. In a few long-term studies of patients with bronchitis and emphysema, however, a small number of subjects with asthma were included and these few individuals demonstrated marked declines in pulmonary function with time. They may represent a biased sample, but at the same time serve as a warning to physicians that this phenomenon does occur.

REFERENCES

Chai H, Farr RS, Froehlich LA, et al: Standardization of bronchial inhalation challenge procedures. J Allergy Clin Immunol 56:323–327, 1975
Cockcroft DW, Killian DN, Mellon JJA, et al: Bronchial reactivity to inhaled histamine: A method and clinical survey. Clin Allergy 7:235–243, 1977
Conrad SA, Kinasewitz GT, George RB (eds): Pulmonary Function Testing. Principles and Practice. New York, Churchill Livingstone, 1984
Corrao WM, Braman SS, Irwin RS: Chronic cough as the sole presenting manifestation of bronchial asthma. New Engl J Med 300:633–637, 1979
Cropp GJA: Methods of inhalation challenge, in Ellis EF and Wanner A (eds): Interspecialty Focus: Pulmonary Medicine. Morris Plains, NJ, Parke-Davis, Division of Warner-Lambert Inc., 1983, Vol. 1, No. 1, p4
Gardner RM (Chairman): ATS Statement. Snowbird Workshop on Standardization of Spirometry. Am Rev Respir Dis 119:831–838, 1979
Guenter CH, Welch MH, Hogg JC: Clinical Aspects of Respiratory Physiology. Philadelphia, J.B. Lippincott, 1978

Harris TR, Pratt PC, Kilburn KH: Total lung capacity measured by roentgenograms. Am J Med 40:756–763, 1971

Light RW, Conrad SA, George RB: The one best test for evaluating the effects of bronchodilator therapy. Chest 72:512–516, 1977

McFadden ER Jr: Exertional dyspnea and cough as preludes to acute attacks of bronchial asthma. New Engl J Med 292:555–559, 1975

Morris AH, Kanner RE, Crapo RO, et al: Clinical pulmonary function testing. A manual of uniform laboratory procedures, 2nd ed. Salt Lake City, Intermountain Thoracic Society, 1984

Sourk RL, Nugent KM: Bronchodilator testing: Confidence intervals derived from placebo inhalations. Am Rev Respir Dis 128:153–157, 1983

Spector SL (ed): Provocative challenge procedures: Bronchial, oral, nasal, and exercise, vol. I. Boca Raton, FL, CRC Press, Inc., 1983

Watanabe S, Renzetti AD Jr, Begin R, et al: Airway responsiveness to a bronchodilator aerosol. Am Rev Respir Dis 109:530–537, 1974

Woolcock AJ, Read J: Lung volumes in exacerbations of asthma. Am J Med 41:259–273, 1966

Joann Blessing-Moore

6

Differential Diagnosis of the Wheezing Child

Asthma is the most frequent diagnosis in children less than 15 years of age hospitalized in the U.S. for chronic medical problems. It is the number-one cause of school days lost due to a chronic illness, and is the most frequent cause of growth retardation.

In the United States, the prevalence of childhood asthma ranges from 5–19 percent. In 1980, there were 90 deaths in children less than 15 years of age due to this disease. The death rate has been estimated to be 1.5/100,000 in the U.S. and as high as 7/100,000 in New Zealand. New medications have allowed the child with asthma to enjoy a relatively normal childhood. However, this disease accounts for 7.5 million school days lost each year, 11 million days in bed, and 24 million days of restricted activity.

Asthma is one cause of wheezing in children. It is not, however, the only cause of wheezing in children. The differential diagnosis can be considered from an anatomical (Table 6-1), classical (Table 6-2), or pathophysiologic approach (Table 6-3). Each approach offers a unique perspective on this spectrum of illnesses associated with wheezing.

This chapter will: (1) highlight some of the more common causes of wheezing in infancy through adolescence; (2) present relevant new data on this spectrum of illnesses; and (3) review salient clinical findings that will facilitate early diagnosis and treatment.

BRONCHIAL ASTHMA, Second Edition
ISBN 0-8089-1814-1

Table 6-1
Differential Diagnosis of Wheezing: An
Anatomical Systems Approach

Respiratory system
  upper: foreign body
  middle: tumors/masses
  lower: inflammation
        congenital abnormality
        injury
        immunologic process
        other
Cardiovascular system
  cardiac asthma—congenital heart disease
  anomalies of great vessels
  pulmonary embolism
GI system
  esophageal: fistula, foreign body, acalasia
  hiatal hernia/gastroesophageal reflux
CNS
  cerebral palsy, paralysis of palate
  myasthenia gravis
  drug intoxication (ASA)
  metabolic diseases resulting in abnormal breathing (DM)
Psychological illness
  habit cough, diaphragmatic breathing, laryngeal spasms

The chapter will be divided into sections based on a pathophysiologic approach recognizing that many diseases involve more than one process. The individual sections will include a summation of relevant clinical findings, recommendations for the initial work-up, and the chapter will conclude with an overall approach to the work-up of the wheezing child.

WHEEZING DUE TO OBSTRUCTION OF AIRWAY

Foreign Bodies

Tracheobronchial aspiration of a foreign body by children between the ages of 6 months and 5 years is a common occurrence and accounts for approximately 500 deaths/year in the United States. Food particles account for 93 percent of the materials aspirated and, depending on the type of material aspirated and the location, children may be symptom-free for a period of days to months. In a review of 200 cases, Blazer et al. noted that the

Table 6-2
Differential Diagnosis of Wheezing:
A Functional Approach

Developmental/anatomical abnormalities
  upper airway
  great vessels
  middle airway
    trachea/larynx
  lower airway
  gastrointestinal tract
Familial pulmonary diseases
  CF
  primary ciliary dyskinesia
  alpha 1 antitrypsin deficiency
  Williams Campbell syndrome
  immune deficiency diseases
Mechanical obstruction
  intrinsic or extrinsic
Hyperreactive airways
  asthma
  infection
  irritants
  prior pulmonary injury
Associated with other disease
  collagen vascular disease
  cardiovascular disease
  immune deficiency disease
  psychological illnesses
  other—familial dysautonomia

Adapted from Mak H: Recurrent wheezing and massive atelectasis in an adolescent. J Pediatr 102(6): 955–962, 1983.

history was positive in 88 percent of the cases. Chest x-ray and fluoroscopy contributed to the diagnosis in 90 percent, but in 10 percent of all cases the radiologic exam was normal.

The symptoms associated with the aspiration of foreign bodies include wheezing which may be localized to one side, cough, intermittent dyspnea, and cyanosis. Bronchoscopic removal is the treatment of choice. Fiberoptic bronchoscopy allows excellent visualization of the tracheobronchial tree, but with the present instruments available may not be adequate for removal of foreign bodies. Rigid bronchoscopy under general anesthesia is usually the treatment of choice.

Frequently, children will have subsequent wheezing and a second proce-

Table 6-3
Differential Diagnosis of Asthma:
A Pathophysiologic Approach

Obstruction of airway: upper/lower; intrinsic/extrinsic
  foreign body
  tumor
  congenital abnormality
    vascular
    tracheal
    bronchopulmonary
Bronchiolitis
Bronchiectasis
  familial
    cystic fibrosis
    immotile cilia syndrome
    alpha-1-antitrypsin deficiency
  idiopathic pulmonary hemosiderosis
  immune deficiency disease
  secondary to anatomical abnormality or obstruction
Bronchitis
Bronchoconstriction/bronchial hyperactivity
  asthma—IgE mediated
    hyperreactive airways
  bronchopulmonary aspergillosis
    hypersensitivity pneumonitis
  gastroesophageal reflux/sinusitis
  associated with environmental irritants
    cigarette smoke
    household pollution
    gas, wood, kerosene
    ambient pollution
    chemical exposure
  associated with prior pulmonary insult
    near drowning, hydrocarbon ingestion
    RDS/BPD
  associated with infection and/or immunologic process
    BPA
    parasitic or viral disease
Abnormal breathing patterns/psychological factors
  diaphragmatic breathing
  laryngeal "spasms"
  special considerations in the teenager

dure is necessary to rule out residual foreign material in the lungs. Often no other foreign material is noted and the question has been posed regarding whether this procedure itself may induce secondary wheezing. Twiggs followed 58 children after removal of foreign material by bronchoscopy and compared this group to children who had had anesthesia for tonsillectomy and/or adenoidectomy. He found an 11 percent incidence of wheezing in both groups, which compares to the prevalence of wheezing in the general pediatric population.

Foreign bodies in the lung are common and can occur in patients with chronic asthma as well as in the general pediatric population. Esophageal foreign bodies, most commonly coins and buttons, can cause similar symptoms secondary to compression on the trachea. A high degree of suspicion of this cause of wheezing is essential. History, upper airway films, chest x-ray with additional inspiratory, expiratory, and lateral decubitus films, and fluoroscopy can be helpful; however, bronchoscopy remains the essential tool for diagnosis and treatment.

Tumors

Neoplasma of the chest are occasionally the cause of wheezing; they can be divided into pulmonary, mediastinal, cardiac and pericardial, and chest wall and diaphragm.

Primary pulmonary tumors are not common in childhood; however, the mass itself, whether internal or external to the airway and/or the associated lymphadenopathy, can result in wheezing which may proceed to stridor and respiratory distress. Mediastinal tumors such as teratomas, and rhabdomyosarcomas can cause significant wheezing and stridor in the infant and may require immediate surgical intervention. Lymphomas in the teenage population may present as wheezing. These tumors can rapidly expand and cause acute, life-threatening respiratory distress. Radiologic exam, including CT scans of the mediastinum and bronchoscopy, may provide essential initial information.

Congenital Lesions

Congenital lesions may cause life-threatening obstruction of the airways in the young infant as well as contribute to chronic pulmonary disease in the older child. The following discussion will highlight a few of the many congenital anomalies associated with wheezing.

Upper-airway abnormalities such as nasal obstruction and micrognathia-Pierre Robin Syndrome may present as respiratory distress, abnormal inspiratory efforts, apneic spells (glossoptosis-apnea syndrome), oropharyngeal dysphagia, vomiting and/or cor pulmonale. The associated pulmonary findings of upper-airway obstruction may be very similar to those of lower airway obstruction, with: (1) expiratory wheezing; (2) radiographic evidence of hyperexpansion of the chest; and (3) hypoxemia without hypercarbia. Respiratory distress and the glossoptotic-apnea syndrome can be prevented by emergency use of an oropharyngeal cannula. "Acquired glossoptosis" has also been described in children with enlarged adenoids and obstructive sleep apnea. This upper-airway abnormality may also present with lower-airway symptoms.

Midairway lesions include laryngeal, tracheal, and vocal cord abnormalities. Laryngomalacia-congenital stridor accounts for over 75 percent of the laryngeal problems in infancy. The onset is variable and often associated with a viral infection in the first few months of life and occasionally associated with a positive family history. This is usually a mild, self-limiting process. The children characteristically are happy, active, and growing well, and have notable stridor. On repeat bronchoscopy after approximately a year, the epiglottis may be still notably elongated and the arytenoids "bulky" despite a lack of clinical symptoms at the time of follow-up. In some children, this disease may be severe and require a tracheostomy. Bronchoscopy is essential to rule out other causes of laryngotracheal abnormalities such as tracheoesophageal fistulas (H type—with or without Vater's syndrome/abnormalities of the vertebrae), hemangiomas, webs, papillomas, abnormal calcifications (Conradi's disease), and paralysis of the vocal cords.

Vascular rings may be associated with wheezing, stridor, respiratory distress, and vomiting within the first hours to months of life. Children so affected are often small and poorly developed, with notable hyperextension of the neck and head to relieve or reduce tracheal compression. In a 10-year review of admissions of preschool children with this diagnosis, double aortic arch was the most common cause (60 percent), followed by persistent right aortic arch with ligamentum arteriosum, anomalous right subclavian artery, anomalous innominate artery, and anomalous left carotid artery. Barium swallow in addition to the chest x-ray (CXR) often provides the first approach to this diagnosis.

Compression of the airways secondary to lung bud or parenchymal abnormalities may also be a notable cause of symptoms within the first hours to months of life. Congenital lobar emphysema may be associated with wheezing, dyspnea, and cyanosis. On chest x-ray, there is notable hyperlucency of the left upper lobe or, occasionally, right middle lobe with a shift of the mediastinum. Lobectomy provides prompt relief of the associated respiratory distress.

Congenital heart disease with pulmonary edema is the primary cause of extrapulmonary wheezing in the newborn and young infant. The associated symptoms of dyspnea, tachypnea, tachycardia, rales, and cyanosis as shown by the CXR and EKG provide valuable initial information.

Extrapulmonary abnormalities such as thoracic and diaphragmatic abnormalities, muscle weakness, and cerebral palsy are often associated with wheezing as a primary or secondary process.

In summary, internal or external obstruction of an airway due to aspirated foreign material, tumors, or congenital abnormalities can present with acute or chronic, persistent or intermittent wheezing, and associated respiratory symptoms. Upper-airway abnormalities can present with symptoms and clinical findings similar to those seen in lower-airway abnormalities. In all cases of suspected mechanical obstruction, the initial work-up includes radiographic studies and bronchoscopy to rule out a foreign body. Aspirated foreign material should be considered in any and all cases of wheezing in the normal as well as the known asthmatic, as this cause of wheezing can be life-threatening. Sadly, children die each year due to foreign bodies in the lungs.

BRONCHIOLITIS

Bronchiolitis, or inflammation of the bronchi caused by viral infections, is the most common cause of wheezing and hospitalization in children less than 1 year of age. The incidence of this illness is estimated to be 4.2//100 children in the first 2 years, with an attack rate of 29.4 percent. Respiratory syncytial virus (RSV) epidemics last approximately 5 months and peak in November through March. Serum-neutralizing and complement-fixing antibodies are present with infection and may confer small but significant immunity for 1 year, despite lack of control of infection in cell culture with these antibodies. Other viruses of importance that cause wheezing include: (1) Parainfluenza type 3, which is endemic; and (2) Adenovirus (especially types 7 and 21), which is an infrequent cause of bronchiolitis but may be associated with bronchiolitis obliterans.

Clinically, these children often present with upper-airway congestion, nasal discharge, fever, rapid respiration, chest retraction, and significant wheezing which may not be bronchodilator responsive.

The pathology of this disease is characterized by necrosis of the respiratory epithelium, dense plugs of alveolar debris and fibrin, and interstitial pneumonia with edema and lymphocyte infiltration causing increased airway resistance and air trapping. The obstruction and the exaggerated bronchial receptor sensitivity (due to genetic predisposition and/or the virus itself) contribute to the notable wheezing with variable bronchodilator responsiveness.

From studies of hospitalized infants, it has been estimated that 30–50 percent of these infants have subsequent episodes of wheezing which cannot solely be attributed to recurrent "viral bronchiolitis." Certain viruses may actually facilitate allergic sensitization in children who have a positive family history of atopy. Forty-four percent of children diagnosed as having bronchiolitis in infancy may have ongoing intermittent clinical symptoms of wheezing for at least 8 years after the initial episode. Furthermore, in the general population bronchiolitis can be considered to be a causative factor for wheezing in 9.4 percent of children. Therefore, if RSV infections could be prevented in the young child, there would be a notable impact on the overall incidence of wheezing.

Pulmonary function tests postinfection have been noted to be abnormal in 75 percent of infants at ages from 12 months (Stokes) to 8 years (Sims). The children in this latter study did not have wheezing at the time of the follow-up evaluation, despite the decrease in peak flow and increased bronchial lability. An increase in bronchial reactivity with methacholine challenge in children at 10 years after infection has also been noted (Gurwitz). The long-term effects of this infection in children are documented, and data suggest an association of adult respiratory disease with childhood respiratory illness excluding "asthma" (Burrows).

Predictive factors for subsequent wheezing include: (1) increased IgE (greater than 10); (2) positive response to bronchodilators; (3) family history of atopy, asthma, and smoking; and (4) more than 3 episodes of wheezing by 2 years of age. However, no single factor in the history, physical, or laboratory exam has gained consensus opinion as a predictor of future respiratory symptoms.

In summary, young children with bronchiolitis present with wheezing, rales, rhonchi, fever, nasal congestion, irritability, tachypnea, decreased appetite, and fatigue. Dehydration in addition to respiratory distress is the major indication for hospitalization. The initial evaluation includes chest x-ray which may be positive for infiltrates as well as hyperinflation, viral cultures, viral titers, and fluorescent antibody studies for RSV, CBC, and IgE. The clinical evaluation and treatment includes a trial of bronchodilators to assess general reversibility of obstruction.

BRONCHIECTASIS

Bronchiectasis by definition is dilatation of the bronchi and may be caused by infection and/or congenital defects in the supporting structures of the lung; it may also be associated with specific familial diseases.

The onset of symptoms for familial childhood bronchiectasis is usually less than 4 years of age, with most cases recognized in the first 2 decades of life—and in some cases, improvement seen within the third and fourth decades. Cystic fibrosis remains the most common cause of bronchiectasis in children. Other causes are the primary ciliary dyskinesia (PCD), alpha-1-antitrypsin deficiency, idiopathic pulmonary hemosiderosis, immune deficiency syndromes, and causes secondary to anatomic abnormalities or obstruction.

Cystic Fibrosis (CF)

Cystic fibrosis is the most common lethal genetic disease in Caucasians and is the most common cause of brochiectasis in childhood. The frequency of this gene in the population is 1/20, and it is transmitted as an autosomal recessive trait appearing in from 1/1500 to 1/2500 live births. At this time, there is no way to detect the heterozygote carrier state; however, under investigation for newborn screening is the IRT (serum immunoreactive trypsin) assay.

Cystic fibrosis was first described in 1938. Recent work by Knowles and Quinton has revealed epithelial abnormalities of active sodium absorption and chloride permeability in patients homozygous for CF. A unifying hypothesis of underlying epithelial dysfunction has been considered. The defect in chloride permeability is unique to CF and is considered to be responsible for the characteristic high salt content in the sweat associated with this disease.

Forty percent of patients with CF present with respiratory symptoms, which may be associated with gastrointestinal symptoms in 80 percent of the children and with metabolic abnormalities, specifically hypochloremic alkalosis. The lungs appear to be normal at birth. The earliest changes are hypertrophy of the mucous glands and plugging of the peripheral airways by excessive secretions which become mucopurulent with secondary infection. The walls of the airways progressively thicken and the supporting structures of the airways are progressively destroyed, resulting in eventual bronchiectasis and bronchial stenosis secondary to excessive scarring.

Pseudomonas aeruginosa (as well as *Pseudomonas cepacia* and *maltophilia*) in the mucoid form may colonize the lung very early in life. In addition, Staph and other organisms such as *hemophilus influenzae* and Mycoplasma Pneumonia may be prevalent. Pulmonary percussion, antibiotics, and nutritional support are the major elements of treatment. Most centers now report survival beyond 25 years in more than 50 percent of patients.

The chest x-ray in the early stages is characterized by hyperinflation, atelectasis, thickening of the bronchial walls, bronchiectasis, and cystic changes, especially in the right apices. The clinical history of respiratory symptoms with wheeze, cough and congestion with or without malabsorption, positive family history of CF, abnormal chest x-ray, abnormal pulmonary function tests (PFT), and positive sweat chloride test provides necessary information to establish the diagnosis.

Primary Ciliary Dyskinesia/Immotile Cilia Syndrome (ICS)

Primary ciliary dyskinesia or the immotile cilia syndrome is characterized by bronchiectasis, sinusitis, and otitis media with or without situs inversus (Kartagener's syndrome). The ciliary abnormalities as described by electron microscopy include defects in the dynein arm, radial spokes, and microtubular transposition, as well as functional abnormalities with normal ultrastructural organization. The result of the ciliary dysfunction is a decreased clearance of mucous and inhaled particles, resulting in increased infections.

The most characteristic symptoms of primary ciliary dyskinesia are nocturnal cough and wheezing which are of varying severity and may appear in the neonate but most typically are noted in later infancy or childhood. Diagnosis is made by biopsy of the nasal or bronchial mucosa as well as chest x-ray, sinus films, and pulmonary function tests. The prevalence of this disease has been estimated to be twice as high as Kartagener's syndrome, or 1/16,000 children. This disease is probably one of the more significantly underdiagnosed diseases of childhood.

Alpha-1-Antitrypsin (ATT) Deficiency

Alpha-1-antitrypsin deficiency associated with emphysema was first described approximately 20 years ago. Individuals who lack this anti-inflammatory host-defense protein (PiZZ) and who have a partial deficit (heterozygotes or Pi MZ) have an increased risk of early-onset emphysema. The natural history of this disease is not well understood. Buist et al. studied 19 children 3–7 years of age with PiZZ- or SZ-type deficiency and found no gross changes in pulmonary functions in comparison to their normal controls. In Sveger's study of 169 children with ATT, however, 13 (8 percent) of the PiZZ and Pi SZ children at 8 years of age had had asthma or bronchitis with wheezing during the previous year. It remains unknown whether or not these are early symptoms of an ongoing process that will lead to emphysema. Young children of the Pi MZ type have been noted to have a significant decrease in frequency-dependent characteristics of pulmonary function tests, suggesting that the physiologic abnormalities associated with ATT deficiency are present early in life.

Children with severe asthma do not have an increased incidence of this enzyme deficiency when compared to the general population. Conversely, it is known that a few children with severe ATT deficiency (PiZZ) wheeze, and that there is an increased prevalence of Pi variants (46 percent) in nonatopic wheezy children.

IMMUNE DEFICIENCY DISEASES

Respiratory diseases in the immunologically compromised host are typified by either uncommon pathogens or overwhelming infection by organisms of usually low virulence. Such illnesses can present with wheezing, cough, dyspnea, and other respiratory, as well as systemic, symptoms. The four major limbs of the immune system can be considered separately: T lymphocytes, B lymphocytes, phagocytes, and complement system.

Primary or secondary disorders of the T system are characterized by susceptibility to: (1) fungi, such as candida, viruses such as CMV, and parasites such as *Pneumocystis carinii;* and (2) increased susceptibility to malignancies. Infection with HTLV-III/LAV or acquired immune deficiency syndrome (AIDS), as the name implies, is an example of a secondary T cell disorder. As of April 1985, 113 children less than 13 years of age from 17 states have been diagnosed as having AIDS. Fifty-eight percent were under 1 year of age, 68 percent had *P. carinii* pneumonia, 26 percent had other opportunistic infections, and 6 percent had Kaposi's sarcoma.

Patients with B disorders (X-linked agammaglobulinemia and common variable hypogammaglobulinemia) have increased susceptibility to pyogenic infections including *Streptococci, Staphylococcus,* and *H. influenzae.* IgA deficiency is the most common immunoglobulin deficiency, but is infrequently associated with bronchiectasis unless associated with other abnormalities of the immune system (i.e., decreased IgG2 or increased IgE). Quantitative immunoglobulins with IgG subclass studies, isohemaglutinins, and specific antibody titers (i.e., antitetanus and antidiptheria titers in an immunized patient) will provide initial identification of most of these deficiencies.

Phagocytic defects, either primary or secondary (i.e., chronic granulomatous disease, Chediak Higashi syndrome, Job's syndrome, or cyclic neutropenia), result in susceptibility to infections with *Staphylococcus,* gramnegative rods, and fungi. Leukocyte counts, peripheral smears, white cell function studies, and the nitrotetrazolium blue (NBT) test will identify most of these disorders.

Individual complement disorders are generally considered to be inherited in an autosomal recessive manner with codominant expression. The heterozygotes, or "carriers" with one normal gene, have 20–40 percent of the normal concentration of complement which is compatible with normal function and a normal CH50. CH50 is defined as the amount of serum necessary to cause hemolysis of 50 percent of sensitized sheep red blood cells. If any component of the complement cascade is totally missing, there will be no red blood cell (RBC) lysis and the CH50 will be zero. C1q deficiencies are associated with severe combined immune deficiency (SCID) and common variable agammaglobulinemia. C2 deficiencies have a frequency of approximately 1 percent in the general population and have been associated with recurrent *S. pneumonia.* C3 deficiencies are associated with severe recurrent pyogenic infections. No replacement therapy is available for complement deficiencies and early detection of infection is essential.

Bronchiectasis and Developmental Abnormalities

Bronchiectasis may be associated with developmental abnormalities of cartilage such as the Williams Campbell Syndrome. Clinically, these children present with the onset of symptoms in infancy and have a variable course depending on the extent of the airway lesion and associated bronchiectasis secondary to infection. The relationship of this disease to congenital lobar emphysema and bronchomalacia is undefined, but may represent a spectrum of abnormalities of the same basic process.

In summary, the patients with bronchiectasis present with wheezing and associated pulmonary and systemic symptoms. These include cough, dyspnea, respiratory distress, hemoptysis, rales, rhonchi, wheezing, clubbing, chest hyperexpansion, malabsorption, failure to thrive, and sinusitis and situs inversus.

Considered in the evaluation should be radiographic studies, bronchoscopy, CBC, cultures, immunoglobulins, pulmonary function tests, sweat chloride test, ATT level, biopsy of the bronchial or nasal mucosa, and early-morning gastric aspirate for hemosiderin-laden macrophages.

CHRONIC BRONCHITIS

Chronic bronchitis is a notable cause of wheezing in adults. Very little has been known about this disease in children. In a 1978 study of Japanese schoolchildren, the prevalence of this disease was estimated to be 1.4 percent. In a more recent study of schoolchildren from Sydney, the prevalence was estimated to be as high as 20 percent of the general population. Taussig has defined this disease in childhood as a symptom complex of chronic cough of greater than 1 month with intermittent wheezing that may be associated with evidence of airway inflammation and hyperexpansion on CXR. Burrows noted wheezing as the predominant symptom, occurring in 73 percent of the children he evaluated for chronic bronchitis. The pathology of childhood chronic bronchitis closely resembles that of asthma. The adult characteristics are less common, possibly secondary to the shorter duration of this illness.

In children with intermittent wheezing and a history of associated chronic cough, chronic bronchitis should be considered. In addition to the history, pulmonary function tests, chest x-ray, and sputum cultures may be helpful in establishing the diagnosis.

BRONCHIAL HYPERREACTIVITY

The goal of this section is to present diagnostic guidelines that will assist in the differentiation of wheezing due to "asthma" from other, less-common causes of bronchospasm, and will include discussion on:

1. asthma
2. hypcrsensitivity pneumonitis/BPA
3. GER/sinusitis
4. idiopathic pulmonary hemosiderosis (IPH)
5. wheezing associated with
        environmental exposures
        prior pulmonary injury

Asthma

Asthma is characterized by diffuse, reversible pulmonary obstruction caused by two distinct, although often combined, immunologic and pathophysiologic processes: (1) IgE-mediated release of mediators secondary to exposure to specific antigens, often termed "extrinsic" asthma; and/or (2) "intrinsic" hyperreactivity to physical factors such as cold, exercise, and viral infections.

Intrinsic asthma in children often presents in those less than 3 years of age with wheezing secondary to a viral infection. Ninety percent of all children with asthma, intrinsic and extrinsic, and approximately 40 percent of children with allergic rhinitis wheeze with exercise.

Seasonal or extrinsic asthmatic children generally have a later onset of symptoms than do chronic or intrinsic asthmatic children and are usually older than 4 years. However, 76 percent of children with extrinsic asthma will have exacerbation of wheezing with viral infections. In addition to the immediate response to an antigen exposure, children as well as adults may have a significant 5–12-hour delay in onset of symptoms. The delayed response may occur independent of the immediate response. This "ongoing" bronchial hyperreactivity may be a sustaining factor for perennial asthma. Late asthmatic responses in children have been associated with house dust mite exposure and with exercise. The small airways are the primary site of obstruction in these children. Bronchial challenge testing is the most sensitive and specific way to diagnose this entity. Routine prick skin testing may not reveal a positive delayed response.

The differentiation of asthma from other causes of wheezing can be aided by:

1. family history of atopy or chronic lung diseases (CF, emphysema)
2. clinical and PFT evidence of reversibility of bronchospasm
3. evidence of abnormal exercise tolerance, positive methacholine challenge or positive antigen-specific bronchial challenge
4. "normal" chest x-ray with evidence of hyperexpansion with or without peribronchial cuffing and mucous plugging and normal barium swallow
5. normal CBC, normal immunoglobulins (IgG, IgM, IgA), normal sweat chloride

6. increased IgE, positive antigen-specific IgE tests (skin tests or laboratory tests), and eosinophilia
7. 3 or more episodes of wheezing in the first 2 years of life

The differential diagnosis of asthma as a cause of wheezing in childhood can be facilitated by a multifactorial approach as outlined on the preceding page.

Hypersensitivity Pneumonitis/BPA

Hypersensitivity pneumonitis is most commonly associated with dyspnea and cough; however, it may be associated with wheezing in the case of bronchopulmonary aspergillosis and occasionally associated with hypersensitivity due to molds.

Bronchopulmonary aspergillosis (BPA) is primarily diagnosed in patients with chronic asthma or chronic chest disease. The major criteria for BPA include: (1) episodic bronchial obstruction; (2) total IgE often greater than 15,000 ng/ml, specific IgE to *Aspergillus;* and (3) peripheral eosinophilia, immediate skin test reactivity to *Aspergillus,* precipitins to *Aspergillus,* a history of infiltrates, and central bronchiectasis on chest x-ray in advanced disease. Secondary criteria include *Aspergillus* in the sputum, late skin test reactivity to *Aspergillus,* and history of expectoration of mucous plugs. The pulmonary function tests may reveal significant evidence of obstruction with at least partial reversibility and evidence of increased resistance.

The diagnosis involves multiple criteria, since 25 percent of all asthmatics may have a positive immediate skin test reaction to *Aspergillus,* 36 percent a positive late reaction (versus 96 percent with BPA), and 27 percent positive *Aspergillus* precipitin reactions (versus 92 percent with BPA). Because of the lack of specific diagnostic criteria, diagnosis in childhood and in the early stages of this disease is difficult and most often delayed. Significant pulmonary damage has often occurred before the diagnosis has been established and appropriate treatment instituted. This diagnosis is often only considered in patients with other chronic lung disease and probably should be considered earlier in the differential diagnosis of wheezing in childhood.

Hypersensitivity pneumonitis due to environmental/home exposures has been reported in children. Air conditioners and humidifiers contaminated with *Thermoactinomyces* and other organisms can occasionally be a causative factor for wheezing as well as cough and dyspnea in young children. Miller evaluated a 9-year-old girl who had been diagnosed as having asthma with recurrent episodes of pneumonia who was unresponsive to bronchodilator therapy. She was found to have bronchiectasis on bronchogram and responded well to steroids plus removal of a contaminated central home humidifier. Marshall noted in a study of 5 children with hypersensitivity pneumonitis (due to pigeon droppings) unique progression of disease in 4 of 5 children over 3 years, emphasizing the need for early diagnosis and treatment of childhood hypersensitivity pneumonitis to avoid progressive pulmonary fibrosis.

Gastroesophageal Reflux (GER)

Gastroesophageal reflux has been suggested by many authors as a common cause of wheezing with or without chronic asthma. The incidence of GER in infants may be as high as 1/500 live births (Carre, England). By 18 months, 60 percent of children will have improved, and in only 30 percent will symptoms persist longer than 4 years. In 90 percent of the younger children with this diagnosis, vomiting is associated with the respiratory symptoms of wheezing, rales, rhonchi, fever, and dyspnea. Conversely, in a large review of children with gross evidence of reflux or hiatal hernia by barium swallow, 79/507 children had associated pulmonary symptoms.

Recently, 40 children from 5 months to 16 years, with wheezing and in some cases vomiting, who had been referred for evaluation of GER were found to have at least 2/5 diagnostic tests for GER positive. With medical and/or surgical therapy, 6 had complete clearing of symptoms and 92 percent had an improvement in respiratory symptoms, emphasizing the importance of early diagnosis and treatment.

The major diagnostic tests include: (1) extended pH monitoring (modified Tuttle Test), which provides 90-percent accuracy but requires 18–24 hours of hospital monitoring; (2) gastric scintiscan with technetium which detects major aspiration; (3) esophagram; (4) esophagoscopy with biopsy; and (5) the Bernstein Test with 0.1N HCl instilled in the esophagus to induce symptoms. If acid is instilled in the trachea, a significantly smaller quantity will induce symptoms. The chest x-ray in these children may not always reveal evidence of pulmonary infiltrates, consolidation, and atelectasis.

GER can cause wheezing and associated pulmonary symptoms with or without gastrointestinal (GI) symptoms in normal children and may be noted in as many as 16–75 percent of children previously diagnosed as having asthma.

Sinusitis

Acute and chronic sinusitis of children has been described as one of the most frequently overlooked and poorly understood diseases of childhood. Symptoms of this process include nasal discharge associated with persistent nighttime cough, "wheeze," and lower-airway congestion, with or without headache, fever, and face pain. One-third of the cultures obtained from these children will be sterile, 28 percent will grow *S. pneumoniae,* 19 percent *H. influenzae,* and 27 percent *B. catarrhalis.* Abnormal sinus x-rays with normal CXR and normal pulmonary function tests may be helpful. Ethmoid sinusitis can cause significant symptoms in the very young child and may be difficult to diagnose because of the young age. The use of sinus ultrasound for diagnosis is presently under clinical investigation.

Idiopathic Pulmonary Hemosiderosis (IPH)

Idiopathic pulmonary hemosiderosis is an uncommon condition characterized by: (1) hemoptysis; (2) iron deficiency anemia; and (3) infiltrates on chest x-ray secondary to bleeding into the airways. Any acute pulmonary bleeding or aspiration of blood into the lungs can be associated with hemosiderin-laden macrophages which will clear in approximately 1–2 weeks. In IPH, however, there is ongoing, intermittent, low-grade diffuse bleeding and hemosiderin-laden macrophages are notable in the sputum and bronchial or gastric aspirates. Pathologically, IPH can be associated with: (1) Goodpasture's syndrome; (2) diffuse pulmonary hemosiderosis associated with immune complex glomerulonephritis; and (3) Heiner's syndrome or cow's-milk-related pulmonary hemorrhage. The work-up therefore includes: pulmonary function tests, CBC with total eosinophil count, IgE and IgG (precipitins) to milk, renal function tests with antibasement antibody studies, ANA, and immunoglobulins with IgG subclass evaluation.

Three recent reviews of a total of 32 children with IPH followed for maximum of 13 years revealed: (1) an average age of presentation of 4–6 years (range: 7 months–13 years); (2) variability in presenting symptoms, with anemia preceding the pulmonary symptoms by $1\frac{1}{2}$–$2\frac{1}{2}$ years in some patients (Kjellman); (3) variability in course, with 4 deaths at approximately 4 years postdiagnosis (McCloskey, Blessing-Moore); and (4) variability in course despite intermittent or long-term treatment with prednisone, milk-free diet, iron supplements, transfusions, and azothioprine. Prednisone treatment should be considered for the acute episodes but may not be effective in preventing subsequent bleeding. As of this time, there is no known single etiology for this syndrome, which clinically may present as wheezing and may be associated with renal as well as pulmonary involvement. The diagnosis is dependent on the clinical triad of hemoptysis, anemia, and infiltrates on chest x-ray, as well as isolation of hemosiderin-laden pulmonary macrophages.

Cigarette Smoke

The prevalence of wheezing in the general pediatric population is estimated to be 14.8 percent, with a suggested 1.87-fold increased incidence due to cigarette smoke. Numerous studies have associated parental smoking ("passive smoking") with increased respiratory illnesses in children. Initial cross-sectional data studies revealed decreased levels of small-airway function (Forced Expiratory Flaw (FEF) at 25–75 percent of vital capacity) in children as young as 5–9 years of age whose parents smoke. Data from several large longitudinal studies have confirmed the detrimental effects of passive smoking on lung function:

1. decreased small-airway function
2. correlation of the number of packs/day smoked by the mother and the actual FEV 0.75
3. lower-than-expected annual increases in lung function (FEV_1 and FEF 25–75) in children with otherwise normal development
4. greater decrease in small-airway function (FEF 75) in children who were exposed at less than 5 years of age
5. notable decrease in pulmonary function testing that was evident 6 years postexposure
6. associated increase in lower respiratory illnesses

Clinically, lower- as well as upper-respiratory symptoms can be induced by passive exposure to cigarette, marijuana, and clove smoke. Elimination of exposure may alleviate present symptoms and prevent possible long-term effects on lung development. Sixty–75 percent of children may live in homes with one or more smokers, and with two or more smokers, the particle concentrations often exceed federal particle standards set for outdoors.

Approximately 30 percent of high school children 15 years or older smoke. In children who began smoking at less than 15 years of age, a significant decrease in pulmonary functions has been noted when they are 20 years of age, irregardless of the number of cigarettes smoked. The reversibility of such an early insult to the lungs is not well defined as of this time.

Indoor Air Pollution

The relationship of occupational chemical exposure and lung disease has been well studied in adults. Recently, attention has focused on the effect of "household air pollution" on children's lung function.

In the United States, approximately 50 percent of homes use natural gas or liquid propane for cooking. In many homes, measured levels of nitrogen dioxide from combustion have been noted to exceed what are considered to be extremely high outdoor levels. The noted effects on household members, especially young children, have included: (1) increased incidence of lower respiratory symptoms; and (2) decrease in lung function, which is more notable in girls than boys, presumably due to differences in exposure.

Wood-burning stoves and kerosene heaters in poorly ventilated rooms present a potential risk factor for lower-airway symptoms. Honicky noted an increased incidence of wheezing and coughing unassociated with infection in 31 preschoolers exposed to wood stoves.

Furthermore, direct exposure of the infant to particulates such as talcum powder can cause wheezing, dyspnea, and cough and respiratory distress. In our patients, the symptoms have resolved within approximately 48 hours without treatment. A variable course might be predicted based on the exposure.

mbient Air Pollution

he effect of ambient air pollution on children's lung function has been studied by: (1) documenting a decrease in pulmonary function test with exercise in high ambient pollution; and (2) associating the decrease in FEV 0.75 and FVC with increasing levels of total suspended particulates as well as sulfur dioxide. In Japan, 134 preschoolers from a "polluted city" were studied and compared with 49 asthmatic children in a relatively unpolluted city. There was an increase in the number of colds each year, wheezing episodes, and general increased bronchial reactivity associated with high levels of pollution. In a study of 80 asthmatic children over 2 years of age, high levels of pollution and carbon monoxide correlated with an increased duration and severity of attacks in 5–15 percent of the children with hyperreactive airways. Exposure to high levels of air pollution may cause wheezing in the "normal" pediatric population as well as increase in airway reactivity in a small segment of the pediatric asthmatic population.

Chemical and Particulate Exposure

In addition to the previously discussed air pollutants, there are over 115 chemicals used in industry that potentially cause pulmonary symptoms. Formaldehyde from particle board, insulating material, furnishings, and tobacco smoke in the home and school have received significant attention in the pediatric literature. In one evaluation of 13 patients who by history had an onset of wheezing with exposure to formaldehyde, all had a negative bronchial challenge test. Other studies, however, have revealed a small percentage of test-positive patients (12/230) with formaldehyde and (1/4) with urea formaldehyde foam. It was concluded from these studies that formaldehyde is a rare cause of wheezing which is treatable by removal from exposure. This represents the beginning of an awareness of chemical and particulate exposure within the home as well as workplace that may have significant detrimental effects on children's as well as adults' lung function. Precise pulmonary and immunologic studies are essential, since patients may present with polysomatic complaints which may or may not be directly related to environmental exposures.

ANESTHESIA

Bronchial hyperreactivity in children may be the result of an acute pulmonary insult such as hydrocarbon ingestion, near drowning, or smoke inhalation, as well as related to the resuscitation efforts in these cases. Such a history should be considered contributory in nonatopic as well as atopic wheezing children. Other well-studied risk factors include viral infections as previously discussed, bronchopulmonary dysplasia, and possibly anesthesia in children less than 2 years of age.

Respiratory Distress Syndrome (RDS);
Bronchopulmonary Dysplasia (BPD)

Hyaline membrane disease occurs in approximately 1 percent of all deliveries. In addition, approximately 10–15 percent of premature infants who have required mechanical ventilation for respiratory failure will develop progressive pulmonary disease or bronchopulmonary dysplasia (BPD). The exact etiology of BPD is not well defined and is probably multifactorial, including age of gestation, oxygen therapy, patient ductus arteriosus, and other factors. Increased respiratory difficulty, infection, and bronchial hyperreactivity may be notable through the second and third years. Abnormalities in pulmonary function testing may persist for more than 10 years with evidence of obstruction, bronchial hyperreactivity, and abnormal exercise tolerance. Symptoms may be notable in some children with RDS as well as BPD.

In a recent well-controlled study of children born prematurely with or without RDS, it was noted that children with RDS at the time of the 10-year follow-up exam had evidence of airway dysfunction as well as a significant degree of airway hyperreactivity, which was related to the severity of the initial pulmonary disease and the family predisposition to airway reactivity. In prematurely born children without RDS, however, airway reactivity was related to family history and not to their prematurity (Bertrand).

Since lung growth is generally considered to be complete by 6–7 years of age, these studies would suggest that children with RDS as well as BPD may have persistent abnormalities in pulmonary function tests and increased bronchial hyperreactivity. These changes may be even more notable if the family history is positive for atopy or hyperreactive airway disease.

Anesthesia

Anesthesia in children less than 2 years of age was identified as a risk factor for subsequent wheezing in a large study completed in 1970 in Rochester, New York, of children who had had surgery for pyloric stenosis or hiatal hernia and these children were noted to have an 18-percent prevalence of asthma. However, in one controlled study of children exposed to anesthesia before 2 years of age there was no significant difference in incidence of allergy by age 14 years. This corresponds to the Boston study of children undergoing surgery for pyloric stenosis, in which the incidence of allergy and asthma was equal to that of the general pediatric population.

In summary, although asthma is the major cause of wheezing in childhood, bronchial hyperreactivity can be the presenting symptom for a number of diseases besides "asthma": chronic bronchitis, BPA, IPH, GER, and sinusitis. In addition to the present history, chest x-ray and pulmonary function tests, a history of prior pulmonary insult or specific environmental exposures (especially cigarette smoke) may be contributory to the consideration of the differential diagnosis for wheezing.

ABNORMAL BREATHING PATTERNS

This section will focus on the recognition of psychological and additional physiological processes that may present as wheezing. "Atypical asthma" can occur at any age. However, it is noted most frequently in the teenage population. There are several syndromes in this category.

Upper airway obstruction or inappropriate partial closure of the vocal cords can masquerade as asthma. Characteristics include presence of stridorous sounds which are loudest over the larynx, normal expiratory flow, absence of hyperinflation on chest x-ray and absence of positive methacholine challenge. The diagnosis is confirmed by fiberoptic bronchoscopy during an attack. Many names have been applied to this syndrome—Munchausen stridor, emotional laryngeal sneezing, and functional airway obstruction—all of which result in partial glottic closure. Anxiety may not be the sole etiology, but is often a strong contributing factor. Successful intervention has included education, reassurance, and short-term psychotherapy.

In addition, episodes of "status" may be due to dyscoordinate breathing. These episodes are notable for minimal air exchange or wheezing, antidiaphragmatic breathing, and normal pulsus paradoxus. Normal pulmonary function tests are often obtained within 10 minutes of instruction in diaphragmatic breathing and muscle relaxation.

Aside from the "atypical" patterns described above, the teenage asthmatic deserves special consideration. The incidence of death from childhood asthma has increased dramatically over the last few years to 1.5/100,000 (August, 1984) and increase is most notable in children over 10 years of age. In New Zealand, the death rate from asthma in children is 7/100,000. Despite advances in medical management, the hospitalization rate for asthmatic children has increased 3–18 times during 1961–1981 (Washington, DC). The mortality rate due to asthma has also increased. Within our own clinic, we have had 4 recent deaths from asthma. Risk factors in our population involve medical as well as emotional factors. The latter include depression, denial of symptoms and severity of wheezing, and dependence on or abuse of aerosol inhalers.

WORK-UP OF THE "WHEEZING CHILD"

The following is designed to highlight diagnostic techniques that will facilitate an accurate diagnosis as early as possible. Nonetheless, as described throughout this book, there is no substitute for a good history and physical examination.

The radiologic diagnostic work-up in children may be divided into 7 areas:

1. upper airways—lateral and AP neck views

2. barium swallow and esophagram—for diagnosis of abnormalities of swallowing, motility, and aspiration, as well as vascular rings and GER
3. CXR (inspiratory/expiratory, AP, lateral and obliques, decubitus) and conventional tomography—for small parenchymal and rib lesions
4. CT—with or without contrast enhancement for lung parenchymal and mediastinal exam
5. bronchography—for evaluation of bronchiectasis; however, little-used in our institution, given the availability of flexible fiberoptic bronchoscopy
6. angiography—for evaluation of congenital heart disease or vascular abnormalities
7. lung scans (ventilation/perfusion scans, technetium scans)—helpful in evaluating localized pulmonary disease and following the course of such disease

Nuclear magnetic resonance (NMR) or magnetic resonance imaging (MRI) has been described as one of the most exciting developments in diagnostic radiology, since it offers an opportunity to differentiate normal from abnormal early in the diagnostic process without the use of ionizing radiation. Its usefulness in pediatric pulmonary disease is limited by the inherent respiratory motion during the long imaging time required (improved somewhat by respiratory gating) and the poor parenchymal resolution with the low-proton density of the normal air-filled lung. However, this technique is being investigated for use in assessment of the progress of pulmonary disease and the benefits of treatment in patients with cystic fibrosis. The differentiation of atelectasis, mucoid impactions, and peribronchial inflammation from pulmonary vessels is possible with NMR and is superior to CXR and CT. With technical refinement, NMR may be a useful tool in pediatrics as well as adult pulmonary medicine in order to detect pleural fluid, pulmonary nodules, bronchial abnormalities, and soft tissue masses.

Pulmonary function tests are essential in the older child and can often be performed in a child as young as 4 years of age. A simple peak flow meter used before and after a bronchodilator can be used to evaluate the reversibility of the pulmonary process. Repeat peak flow measurements during the day or week can be used to determine the possible effect of environmental exposures. Spirometry with a flow volume loop can provide information about the major airways involved, as well as an indication of extrinsic obstruction, if present.

The laboratory evaluation can be divided in stages (Table 6-4). A CBC with total eosinophil count, immunoglobulins, and total and specific IgE can provide the initial primary information.

Bronchoscopy

Flexible fiberoptic bronchoscopy with the new, small scopes offers the opportunity for direct visualization of the airway. Wood reviewed his evalua-

Table 6-4
Initial Evaluation for Diagnosis

Stage I		

A. *Laboratory*
    CBC, EOS
    immunoglobulins
    IgE, RAST
    cultures
    viral studies
       RSV, paraflu, adeno
       stool O & P
       sputum
	C. *Pulmonary functions*
	    bronchodilator response
	    methacholine and antigen-
	       specific challenge
	
	D. *Radiologic evaluation*
	    upper airway
	       lateral neck films
	    CXR
	    Ba swallow
	    sinus films
		
		fluoroscopy
		CT scan, (NMR)
		V/Q scans
		tomograms
		ultrasound

B. *Skin tests*
    IgE-allergen panel
    T cell delayed panel
    Aspergillus—immediate/
       delayed
	E. *Direct visualization of airway*
	    rhinoscopy
	    laryngoscopy
	    bronchoscopy	

Stage II	
Additional Laboratory Work	
IPH* rectic ct gastric aspergillus milk ppt	BPA¶ aspergillus ppt aspergillus IgE/ST aspergillus/culture/stain

PCD†
Biopsy-EM cilia
    ciliary function studies
	IMMUNE DEFICIENCY
	isohemagglutinins (IgM)
	specific Ab titers
	    antidiphtheria/tetanus

GER‡ Ph probe/Tuttle test	IgG subclasses CH 50 C3, C4, Factor B
CF§ sweat chloride cultures (Ps)	NBT, WBC functions cultures
ATT‖ ATT level	

*IPH = idiopathic pulmonary hemosiderosis
†PCD = primary ciliary dyskinesia
‡GER = gastroesophageal reflux
§CF = cystic fibrosis
‖ATT = alpha-1-antitrypsin
¶BPA = bronchopulmonary aspergillosis

132

tion of 61 children with persistent wheezing: 87 percent of these patients had an abnormality that explained the symptoms, 79 percent had lower airway disease, most commonly tracheomalacia, and 11 percent had a foreign body. The removal of foreign bodies is usually best achieved by a rigid scope under general anesthesia.

The complications noted in 1095 flexible endoscopic procedures in Woods's group of children less than 16 years old were 32/1095, with 8 cases of minor epistaxis and 8 cases of minor transient bradycardia.

In conclusion, the differentiation of "asthma" from other causes of wheezing in childhood can be facilitated by consideration of the pathophysiologic processes that are associated with this symptom: mechanical (intrinsic or extrinsic) obstruction of the airway, bronchiolitis, bronchiectasis, bronchospasm, and abnormal breathing patterns. "All that wheezes is not asthma" and certain causes require immediate attention: foreign bodies and

Table 6-5

Possible Signs and Symptoms Associated with Wheezing

Cough
    infection, foreign body, tumor, environmental irritants, hypersensitivity
      pneumonitis, chronic bronchitis
Failure to thrive
    cystic fibrosis/bronchiectasis, cardiac asthma, immune deficiency disease
Vomiting
    gastroesophageal reflux, tracheoesophageal fistula, vascular ring, foreign body
Excessive sweating
    cardiac asthma
Salty-tasting sweat
    cystic fibrosis
Stridor
    foreign body, vascular ring, tumor/mass
Tachypnea/tachycardia
    cardiac asthma, bronchiolitis
Rales
    bronchiolitis, cardiac asthma, bronchiectasis/cystic fibrosis, idopathic pulmonary
      hemosiderosis
One-sided "wheeze"
    foreign body, pneumothorax, infection with localized infiltrate, congenital
      abnormality causing compression
Dextrocardia
    primary ciliary dyskinesia/Kartagener's syndrome
Clubbing
    chronic pulmonary disease
Anemia
    idiopathic pulmonary hemosiderosis/Heiner's syndrome, collagen vascular disease

Table 6-6
Differential Diagnosis Based on Relative Age at Presentation and Chronicity of Symptoms

Age	Acute	Intermediate	Chronic
Newborn or infant to 1st year	vascular ring congenital lobar emphysema cardiac asthma TE fistula—"H" type	congenital stridor environmental exposures: (smoke/talc)	CNS/CP bronchopulmonary dysplasia
Toddler to school years	bronchiolitis foreign body familial dysautonomia	cystic fibrosis tumor/masses abnormal breathing patterns	chronic bronchitis collagen vascular disease bronchiectasis primary ciliary dyskinesia idiopathic pulmonary hemosiderosis
Teenager	pulmonary embolism spontaneous pneumothorax		

Table 6-7
Relative Value of Work-up for the Diagnosis of Wheezing

DDx of asthma	Diagnostic tools				
	HX	Lab	CXR	PFT	Bronch
Mechanical obst					
intrinsic	*		*		*
extrinsic			*	*	*
Bronchiolitis	*	*	*		
Bronchiectasis		*	*	*	*
CF	*	*	*	*	
PCD			*	*	
IPH		*	*	*	
ATT	*	*	(*)	*	
immune def		*	*		
Bronchitis			*	*	
Bronchoconstriction					
asthma	*	*		*	
environ irritants	*			*	
prior pulm insult	*		*	*	
infection	*	*	*		
Abnormal breathing	*		*		

rapidly enlarging tumors. The challenge for the clinician is to focus the work-up, using the history and clinical exam with radiologic and laboratory assessment to facilitate appropriate early diagnosis and treatment (Tables 6-5, 6-6 and 6-7).

ACKNOWLEDGEMENTS

Appreciation is expressed to Bettina McAdoo, M.D., and Edward Sweeney, M.D., for their review and to Win Vetter for her technical support.

REFERENCES

Altenburger KM: Asthma general evaluation and assessment, in Budstein DA, Strunk RC (eds): Manual of Clinical Problems in Asthma, Allergy and Related Disorders. Boston, Little, Brown and Co., 1984, pp 89–97

Arnaud P, Chapuis-Cellier C, Souillet G, et al: High frequency of P1 deficient phenotypes of alpha 1 antitrypsin in nonatopic asthma of children. Clin Res 24:488A, 1976

Bertrand JM, Riley P, Popkin J, et al: The long-term pulmonary sequelae of prematurity: The role of familial airway hyper-reactivity and the respiratory distress syndrome. N Engl J Med 312:742–745, 1985

Blazer S, Naveh N, Friedman A, et al: Foreign body in the airway. A review of 100 cases. Am J Dis Child 134:68–71, 1980

Blessing-Moore JC, Landon C, Kurland G, et al: Idiopathic pulmonary hemosiderosis in children—Long-term follow-up. Am Rev Respir Dis 123:162, 1981 (abstr)

Boyle J, Tuchman D, Actschuler S, et al: Mechanism for association of GER and bronchospasm. Am Rev Respir Dis 131(5):S16–20, 1985

Brooks J: Tumors of the chest, in Kendig E, Chernick V (eds): Disorders of the Respiratory Tract in Children, W.B. Saunders Co., 1983, pp 565–600

Buist AS, Adams BE, Azzan AH, et al: Pulmonary function in young children with alpha 1 antitrypsin deficiency. Am Rev Respir Dis 122:817–822, 1980

Buist AS, Burrows B, Eriksson S, et al: The natural history of air-flow obstruction in $P_i Z$ emphysema. Am Rev Respir Dis 127(2):S44, 1983

Burrows B, Knudson RJ, Lebowitz MD: The relationship of childhood respiratory illness to adult obstructive airway disease. Am Rev Respir Dis 115:751–760, 1977

Crawford LV: Differential diagnosis of pediatric allergic diseases, in Pediatric Allergic Diseases—Focus on Clinical Diagnosis, New York, Med Exam Publ Co, Inc., 1977, pp 9–40

Davis B, Goodig CA, Lallemand DP, et al: MRI of lung in CF. CF Club Abstracts 26:55, 1985

Davis PB, Hubbard VS, McCoy K, et al: Familial bronchiectasis. J Pediatr 102:177–185, 1983

Day JH, Lee REM, Clarke RH, et al: Asthma relationships to urea formaldehyde foam (UFFI) off-gas exposure. J Allergy Clin Immunol 73(1):122, 1984

Eboriadou M, Chryssanthopoulos C, Sedmak CV, et al: Diagnostic criteria in the early diagnosis of infantile bronchial asthma. J Allergy Clin Immunol 75:171, 1985

Frick OL, German DF, Mills J: Development of allergy in children—Association with virus infection. J Allergy Clin Immunol 63(4):228–241, 1979

Greenberger PA: Allergic bronchopulmonary aspergillosis. J Allergy Clin Immunol 74:645–654, 1984

Gurwitz D, Kattan M, Levison H, et al: Pulmonary function abnormalities in asymptomatic children after hydrocarbon pneumonitis. Pediatrics 62:789–794, 1978

Gurwitz D, Mindorff C, Levison H: Increased incidence of bronchial reactivity in children with a history of bronchiolitis. J Pediatr 98:551–555, 1981

Gyepes M: Diagnostic pulmonary radiology, in Nussbaum E, Galant SP (eds): Pediatric Respiratory Disorders, Clinical Approaches. San Francisco, Grune & Stratton, 1984, pp 251–274

Haddad Z, Kulkarni K: Allergic bronchopulmonary aspergillosis in children, in Nussbaum E, Galant S (eds): Pediatric Respiratory Disorders, Grune & Stratton, 1984, p 45

Hammond KB: Newborn screening for cystic fibrosis. CF Club Abstracts 25:27, 1984

Hasselblad V, Humble CG, Graham MG, et al: Indoor environmental determinants of lung function in children, Am Rev Respir Dis 123:479–485, 1981

Heldt GP, McIlroy MB, Hjansen TN, et al: Exercise performance of survivors of hylan membrane disease. J Pediatr 96:995–999, 1980

Honiky RE, Osborne JS, Akpom A: Symptoms of respiratory illness in young children and the use of wood burning stoves for indoor heating. Pediatrics 75(3):587–593, 1985

Josephs SH: Immunologic mechanisms in pulmonary disease. Pediatr Clin North Am 31:919–936, 1984

Kjellman B: Idiopathic pulmonary hemosiderosis. Acta Pediat Scand 73:584–588, 1984

Knowles MR, Gowen CW, Lawson EE, et al: Fibrosis. CF Club Abstracts 126:7, 1985

Laughlin JJ, Eigen H: Pulmonary function abnormalities in survivors of near drowning. J Pediatr 100:26–30, 1982

Lewiston N: Bronchiectasis in childhood. Pediatr Clin North Am 31:865–878, 1984

Mak H: Recurrent wheezing and massive atelectasis in an adolescent. J Pediatr 102(6):955–962, 1983

Marshall SG, Bierman CW, Shapiro GG, et al: Unique features of hypersensitivity pneumonitis in children. J Allergy Clin Immunol 73(1):126, 1984

McCloskey TJ, Sachs MI, O'Connell EJ: Idiopathic pulmonary hemosiderosis (IPH) in children: A long term follow-up study. Ann Allergy 54:350, 1985

McConnochie KM, Rochman K: Bronchiolitis as a possible cause of childhood wheezing: New evidence. Pediatrics 74:1–8, 1984

Melia RJW, Florey C, Altman DG: Association between gas cooking and respiratory disease in children. Br Med J 2:149–152, 1977

Miller MM, Patterson R, Fink J, et al: Chronic hypersensitivity lung disease with recurrent episodes of hypersensitivity pneumonitis due to a contaminated central humidifier. Clin Allergy 6:451–462, 1976

Morgan W, Taussig LM: The chronic bronchitis complex in children. Pediatr Clin North Am 31(4):851–864, 1984

Nordman H, Keskinen H, Tuppurainen M: Formaldehyde asthma—Rare or overlooked? J Allergy Clin Immunol 75(1):91–99, 1985

Patterson R, Goldstein RA: Clinical and immunologic evaluation of trimellitic anhydride workers in multiple industrial settings. J Allergy Clin Immunol 70:15–18, 1982

Quinton PM, Bijman J: Higher bioelectric potentials due to decreased chloride absorption in the sweat glands of patients with cystic fibrosis. N Engl J Med 398:1185:9, 1983

Rooklin AR, McGeady SJ, Milkadlian DO, et al: The immotile cilia syndrome: A cause of recurrent pulmonary disease in children. Pediatrics 66(4):526, 1980

Schenker MB, Samet JM, Speizer FR: Risk factors for childhood respiratory disease. Am Rev Respir Dis 128:1038, 1983

Schwartz D, VanEss J, Johnstone D, et al: Alpha-1-antitrypsin in childhood asthma. J Allergy Clin Immunol 59:31, 1977

Slechter FG, Hackett P, Rodriguez Q, et al: Illnesses possibly associated with smoking clove cigarettes. MMWR 34(21):297–299, 1985

Sims DC: Downhal maps, study of 8 year old children with history of RSV bronchiolitis in infancy. Br Med J 1:11–14, 1978

Smyth JA, Tabachnik E, Duncan WJ: Pulmonary function and bronchial hyperreactivity in long-term survivors of bronchopulmonary dysplasia. Pediatrics 68:336–340, 1981

Speizer FE, Beris B Jr, Bishop YMM: Respiratory disease rates and pulmonary function in children associated with O_2 exposure. Am Rev Respir Dis 121:3–10, 1980

Stahlman M, Hedvall G, Lindstrom D: Role of hylan membrane disease in production of later childhood lung abnormalities. Pediatrics 69:572–576, 1982

Stokes GM, Milner AD, Hodges IK, et al: Lung function abnormalities after acute bronchiolitis. J Pediatr 98(6):871–874, 1981

Strominger D: Evaluation of the wheezy infant and child, in Korenblat PE, Wedner HT (eds): Allergy Theory and Practice, Orlando, FL, Grune & Stratton, 1984, pp 455–468

Strope G, Stemple D: Risk factors associated with the development of chronic lung disease in children. Pediatr Clin North Am 131(4):757–771, 1984

Sturgess JM, Turner JAP: The immotile cilia syndrome, in Kendig E, Chernick V (eds): Disorders of the Respiratory Tract in Children. W.B. Saunders Co., 1983, p. 623

Sveger T: Prospective study of children with alpha 1 antitrypsin deficiency: Eight year old follow-up. J Pediatr 104(1):91–94, 1984

Swiney PF, Vaeanagh PC, Languth P: Outcome in congenital stridor. Arch Dis Child 52:215–218, 1977

Tabachnik E, Levison H: Infantile bronchial asthma. J Allergy Clin Immunol 67(5):339–347, 1981

Tager IB, Weiss ST, Munoz A, et al: Longitudinal study of the effects of maternal smoking on pulmonary function in children. N Engl J Med 309:699–703, 1983

Taussig LM, Landau LI, Marks M, in Taussig LM (ed): Cystic Fibrosis, New York, Thieme-Stratton, 1984, pp 115–174

Twiggs JT, O'Connell EJ, Yunginger JW, et al: The development of asthma after tracheobronchial aspiration of a foreign body. Ann Allergy 53:407–409, 1984

Vance JC, Hall WJ, Schwartz RH, et al: Heterozygous alpha 1 antitrypsin deficiency and respiratory function in children. Pediatrics 60(3):263–272, 1977

Vedal S, Schenker MB, Samet JM, et al: Risk factors in childhood respiratory disease. Am Rev Respir Dis 130:187–192, 1984

Wang J, Patterson R, Mintzer R, et al: Allergic BPA in pediatric practice. J Pediatr 94(3):376–381, 1979

Wasserman S: Ciliary function and disease. J Allergy Clin Immunol 73(1):17–24, 1984

White MV, Haddad Z, Bellanti JA: Selective IgG 2 deficiency in a patient with skin and upper respiratory tract infections. Ann Allergy 54:498–501, 1985

Wood RE: Spelunking in the pediatric airway: Explorations with the flexible fiberoptic bronchoscope, in Stemple D, Redding GJ (eds): Symposium on Pediatric Airways, Ped Clin North Am 31(4):785–799, 1984

Glen A. Lillington

7

Differential Diagnosis of Asthma in Adults: Bronchial Asthma, Occult Asthma, and Pseudoasthma

Bronchial asthma is customarily defined as a state of bronchial hyperactivity manifested by diffuse airway obstruction which may change in severity over short periods of time, either spontaneously or as a result of therapy. Blood eosinophilia is commonly, but not invariably, present. A number of interrelated syndromes are included in this definition (Table 7-1).

Wheezing is a prolonged, continuous, musical sound detected by auscultation during the respiratory cycle. It is predominantly expiratory, but may also occur during inspiration in many instances. Its genesis depends upon the presence of partial obstruction of one or more airways, combined with airflow of sufficient velocity. Although wheezing is the characteristic clinical manifestation of asthma, it may be absent in certain stages of the disease, particularly if the asthma is very mild or very severe. Conversely, wheezing may be a prominent manifestation of nonasthmatic forms of diffuse or localized airway obstruction.

BRONCHIAL ASTHMA, Second Edition
ISBN 0-8089-1814-1

Table 7-1

Syndromes of Bronchial Asthma

Extrinsic asthma
   atopic, often early-onset
   high levels of IgE in most instances
Intrinsic asthma
   nonatopic, often late-onset
   IgE levels usually normal
Aspirin intolerance asthma
   a subgroup of intrinsic asthma
   nasal polyposis
Exercise-induced asthma
   may be the only clinical manifestation of asthma
   may be intrinsic or extrinsic
Occupational asthma
   mechanisms variable

Conditions to be considered in the differential diagnosis of bronchial asthma may be classified under the headings of occult asthma and pseudoasthma.

OCCULT ASTHMA

This term is applied to patients with bronchial asthma in whom the diagnosis is not apparent or obvious. The main cause is the periodicity and variability of asthmatic wheezing. A typical example is the patient who provides a history of episodic dyspnea, with or without wheezing, but who has no auscultatory evidence of asthma when examined by the physician, and who may even have normal spirometry. In such cases, the asthma may be strictly nocturnal or exercise-induced. In some instances, inhalation challenge testing may be required to document that the patient has hyperreactive airways.

In other instances, the main clinical manifestation of asthma may be chronic or recurrent cough. Spirometric tests may show the presence of diffuse airway obstruction in patients without audible wheeze, but inhalation challenge tests are sometimes required for diagnosis.

PSEUDOASTHMATIC SYNDROMES

There are a number of processes in which diffuse or localized airway obstruction, usually manifested by wheezing on auscultation, is a dominant or occasional feature. For the purposes of this discussion, these conditions are grouped together as pseudoasthmatic syndromes (Table 7-2), and all exhibit the following characteristics:

Table 7-2
Pseudoasthmatic Syndromes

Bronchial inflammatory diseases
  infectious asthma
  bronchiolitis obliterans
  chronic asthmatic bronchitis
  mucoviscidosis
Emphysema and chronic bronchitis
Central airway obstruction
Cardiac asthma
Pulmonary embolism
Aspiration syndromes
Carcinoid syndrome
Hypersensitivity pneumonitis
Pulmonary infiltration with eosinophilia
Sarcoidosis
Psychogenic dyspnea and factitious asthma

1. They simulate bronchial asthma and must be differentiated from it.
2. They respond relatively poorly to standard antiasthmatic therapeutic programs in most instances.
3. They often respond dramatically to specific therapy directed against the basic (nonasthmatic) disease process.

Some processes, such as infectious asthma and chronic asthmatic bronchitis, which are herein classified as pseudoasthmatic syndromes, could, with equal logic, be characterized as variant forms of bronchial asthma. Conversely, many forms of "occupational asthma" should probably be regarded as pseudoasthmatic. The admitted fuzziness of the borders of bronchial asthma remains an unresolved semantic problem and a clinical uncertainty.

In the remainder of this discussion, each of the many pseudoasthmatic syndromes will be described briefly, and the criteria for differentiation from bronchial asthma will be indicated.

INFECTIOUS ASTHMA

In patients with established bronchial asthma, acute respiratory infections may be one of the recognized precipitating factors of asthmatic attacks. In other cases, acute respiratory infections, usually viral, may be the *only* precipitating factors for recurrent attacks of cough and wheezing. In some of these cases of infectious asthma, blood eosinophilia may be absent, but responsiveness to bronchodilator therapy may be clinically apparent nevertheless. This type of infectious asthma is most common in children, and may eventually develop into classical bronchial asthma of either extrinsic or intrinsic types.

BRONCHIOLITIS

In infants and young children, bronchiolitis is an acute infectious process, usually due to respiratory syncytial virus (RSV) and characterized by a diffuse inflammatory process in the bronchioles with hyperinflation of the lungs.

In adults, bronchiolitis fibrosa obliterans may result from inhalation of toxic fumes, the presence of certain "collagen" diseases, as a residuum of pneumonias, and as an idiopathic process. In some cases, the roentgen pattern is reticulonodular, and such patients often show inspiratory crackles, rather than wheezing, on auscultation. In other cases, diffuse hyperinflation, with or without wheezing, may be noted, and such cases may closely simulate asthma. The progressive nature of the disorder and failure to respond to bronchodilator therapy suggest the diagnosis, which requires biopsy confirmation.

CHRONIC ASTHMATIC BRONCHITIS

This is a syndrome rather than a specific disease entity, usually defined as a state of perennial asthmatic wheezing associated with chronic productive cough. It occurs most commonly in older adults and is frequently associated with cigarette smoking.

In many cases, chronic asthmatic bronchitis represents the end stage of prolonged bronchial asthma, extrinsic or intrinsic, particularly in cigarette smokers. Eosinophilia is present in sputum and peripheral blood.

In contrast, some patients with chronic bronchitis but no asthmatic history may eventually develop diffuse airway obstruction which responds to bronchodilators or adrenocorticosteroids in varying degrees. Eosinophilia is sometimes present in chronic asthmatic bronchitis which develops in this fashion. The history of a chronic productive cough which has preceded the wheezing by many years suggests the diagnosis. Emphysema is also present in many instances.

Whether one classifies chronic asthmatic bronchitis as bronchial asthma or as pseudoasthma is relatively unimportant. The critical clinical problem is the recognition that the diffuse airway obstruction that is present is partially reversible by bronchodilators. In some instances, the demonstration of a reversible component requires the use of corticosteroids.

MUCOVISCIDOSIS (CYSTIC FIBROSIS)

The diffuse bronchial obstruction from mucosal swelling and inspissated secretions that occurs in some patients with mucoviscidosis may result in wheezing simulating asthma. Although the disease is congenital, the appearance of clinical manifestations is occasionally delayed until adolescence. Clinical features suggesting mucoviscidosis include early onset, recurrent bronchial infections, poor response to bronchodilators, bilateral pulmonary radiological abnormalities, intestinal malabsorption, and hemorrhoids. The diagnosis is confirmed by sweat chloride measurements. As respiratory allergies and mucoviscidosis may coexist, the presence of eosinophilia and positive skin tests does not rule out the possibility of mucoviscidosis.

EMPHYSEMA

Clinical features which are characteristically present in emphysema but which may also occur in intrinsic asthma or chronic asthmatic bronchitis include exertional dyspnea, expiratory slowing, hyperinflated lungs with hyperresonance and low diaphragms, and evidence of cor pulmonale. Although the auscultatory characteristics of emphysema typically include reduced breath sounds with expiratory prolongation, some patients exhibit wheezing resembling that occurring in asthma. This shows minimal response to bronchodilators, and blood eosinophilia is typically absent.

The presence of anatomic emphysema can be established in several ways: radiographic evidence of bullae and diminished vascularity, and "fixed" airway obstruction with a diminished diffusing capacity measurement on pulmonary function testing. It should be remembered, however, that chronic asthmatic bronchitis often precedes and then coexists with emphysema, and that some patients with "pure" emphysema may eventually develop a reversible "bronchospastic" component superimposed upon the expiratory airway collapse.

It is more important to detect the presence of an "asthmatic" component in a patient with emphysema than to establish the presence of emphysematous lung destruction in an asthmatic. A failure to recognize the asthmatic component may result in the patient being deprived of the important benefits of bronchodilator therapy.

CENTRAL AIRWAY OBSTRUCTION

Partial obstruction of the central airways (larynx, trachea, or both main bronchi) may result in wheezing that can be detected by auscultation over both lungs and that may simulate asthma closely. Clinical features which should suggest central airway obstruction include one or more of the following: hoarseness, inspiratory stridor, brassy cough, masses in the neck, neck vein distension, retrosternal pain, and failure of the wheezing to respond to bronchodilators. In many instances, the lung fields are relatively "silent" on auscultation in comparison with the loud wheeze heard at the mouth, even without stethoscopic aid.

A wide variety of disease processes may give rise to central airway obstruction (Table 7-3). The etiologic multiplicity precludes discussion of the clinical features of the individual disease entities.

If the appearance of one or more of the previously mentioned clinical features suggests the possibility of a centrally located obstructive lesion, the presence, localization, and (often) the etiology of the central airway obstruction can be identified in most cases with the use of one or more of the following diagnostic maneuvers:

1. careful inspection of the tracheal air shadow on the standard chest roentgenograms (Fig. 7-1), and tracheal tomograms
2. CT (computed tomography)
3. mirror laryngoscopy
4. analysis of "flow–volume loops" 5. bronchoscopy
6. mediastinoscopy

Pulmonary function tests may provide considerable assistance in the differentiation of bronchial asthma from central airway obstruction. Spirometry is relatively sensitive and accurate in the detection of the presence of

Table 7-3
Important Causes of Central Airway
Obstruction

Laryngeal
   vocal cord palsy
   epiglottitis
   edema (allergic or inflammatory)
   tumors, polyps
Extrinsic tracheal compression
   mediastinal tumors
   aneurysms
   mediastinal hemorrhage, edema, abscess
   goiters
Intramural tracheal disease
   stricture
   fracture
   tracheomalacia
   tracheopathia osteoplastica
Intraluminal tracheal disease
   tumors, benign or malignant
   tracheitis dessicans
   foreign bodies

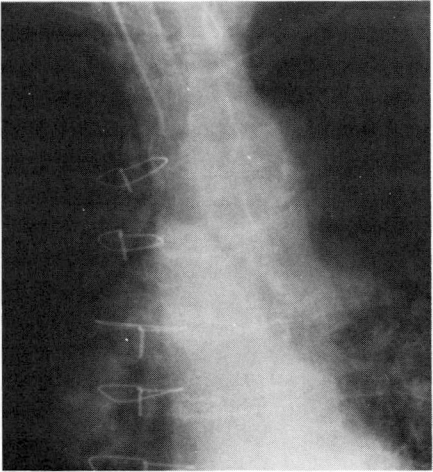

Fig. 7-1. PA chest roentgenogram of a 55-year-old woman with previous cardiac surgery—progressive dyspnea for 2 months, with bilateral wheezing on auscultation. The roentgenogram shows marked narrowing of the air shadows of the trachea and both main bronchi. Bronchoscopy showed a bronchogenic carcinoma at the hilum, causing marked constriction of both main bronchi.

airway obstruction and the degree of reversibility by bronchodilators, but is less precise in the recognition of central obstructions.

Flow-volume loops are particularly helpful in the recognition of central airway obstructions, as the patterns differ from those obtained in patients with asthma and emphysema (Fig. 7-2). With a "fixed" central obstruction (circumferential tumors or strictures), there is marked reduction in both inspiratory and expiratory flows. With a "variable" central obstruction (laryngeal lesions, noncircumferential tumors, strictures, or extrinsic compression), the type of flow restriction will depend upon whether the lesion is extrathoracic or intrathoracic.

CARDIAC ASTHMA

Although pulmonary congestion and edema secondary to left ventricular failure are usually manifested by a "restrictive" breathing pattern (shallow tachypnea and basilar inspiratory rales), confusion with bronchial asthma may occur in two circumstances: paroxysmal nocturnal dyspnea, and cardiac asthma.

If left heart failure is mild in degree, the only clinical manifestation may

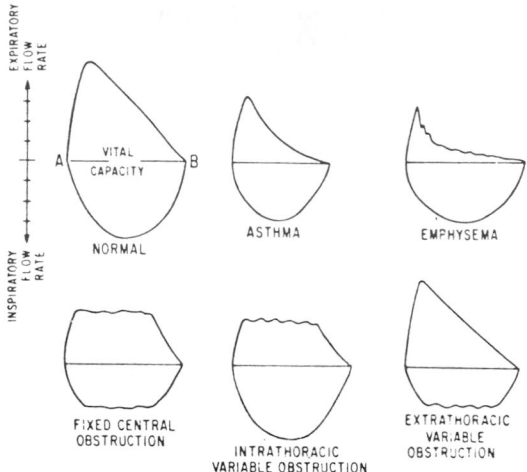

Fig. 7-2. Flow-volume loops. The horizontal axis indicates the volume of air being moved during the vital capacity maneuver. Point A indicates maximum inspiration and point B maximal expiration (residual volume point). Flow rates during inspiration and expiration are shown by the vertical deflection. The "loop" shows the maximal obtainable flows at different lung volumes. The normal loop (upper left) is contrasted with the typical contours in asthma, emphysema, and the various forms of central airway obstruction.

be paroxysmal nocturnal dyspnea brought on by recumbency and relieved by assuming the upright position. The confusion with nocturnal asthma is related to the relative or complete absence of abnormal physical signs during the day in either condition. If the nocturnal dyspnea is not quickly relieved by the change in posture, the possibility of asthma should be considered. In mild left heart failure, the chest roentgenogram often shows subtle changes (cephalization of pulmonary blood flow, Kerley "B" lines, mild cardiomegaly) that are not present in the asthmatic. A trial of therapy (diuretic or digitalis versus bronchodilator) will usually establish the correct diagnosis. The presence or absence of eosinophilia is a valuable diagnostic clue.

Wheezing may occur in some patients with more advanced left heart failure, presumably because bronchial mucosal edema causes diffuse airway narrowing. In such cases of cardiac asthma, reflex bronchoconstriction may also be a factor. Although evidence of left heart failure (roentgenographic changes, rales, gallop rhythm, EKG abnormalities) is usually detectable in cardiac asthma, the differentiation from bronchial asthma may sometimes require a trial of diuretic therapy, or even the use of a Swan-Ganz catheter to measure the pulmonary wedge pressure.

Patients with bronchial asthma or chronic asthmatic bronchitis may develop mild left heart failure which presents clinically as an exacerbation of wheezing. Recognition of this complication is difficult at best. The possible presence of left heart failure should be considered if there are basilar rales as well as wheezes, if there has been recent weight gain, and if there are roentgenographic changes in the absence of such signs of pulmonary infection as fever and purulent sputum.

PULMONARY EMBOLISM

The dyspnea which invariably occurs in patients with pulmonary embolism may occasionally be accompanied by wheezing respirations. If the embolic impaction is not followed by infarction, the combination of wheezing and a relatively normal chest roentgenogram simulates bronchial asthma. If infarction does occur, the possibility that the patient has asthma with bronchopneumonia must be considered in the differential diagnosis.

Clinical features which suggest embolism rather than asthma include:

1.   the presence of predisposing factors for phlebothrombosis
2.   lack of previous history of asthma
3.   wheezing which is disproportionately mild for the degree of dyspnea
4.   a normal blood eosinophil count
5.   pleuritic pain or hemotysis
6.   clinical evidence of acute right heart strain
7.   hypotension and tachycardia
8.   a pleural rub
9.   clinical evidence of phlebothrombosis
10. failure to respond to bronchodilators

Although perfusion defects occur on pulmonary scintiscans in both embolism and asthma, there are usually matching ventilation defects with delayed washout of xenon in the latter condition. The presence of multiple lobar or segmental perfusion defects without matching ventilation defects strongly suggests embolism. Pulmonary angiography is advisable in doubtful cases.

ASPIRATION SYNDROMES

The entry of foreign material, either solid or liquid, into the tracheobronchial tree may result in wheezing respirations which may simulate asthma. There are 3 aspiration syndromes in which wheezing is most likely to occur.

Solid foreign bodies lodging in the trachea may cause sufficient airway obstruction to cause wheezing without lateralizing signs. A foreign body in a lobar bronchus or a main bronchus may be associated with unilateral wheezing. On occasion, a unilateral obstruction is accompanied by bilateral wheezing, presumably due to reflex bronchospasm.

The diagnosis of an aspirated foreign body is usually established from the history, unless the patient is a young child or was obtunded at the time of aspiration. Radio-opaque foreign bodies are usually readily visible on the chest roentgenogram. In the case of radiolucent foreign bodies, a comparison of end-inspiratory and end-expiratory films will help identify the presence of obstruction and aid in the lateralization of the obstructing lesion. Bronchoscopy is almost invariably diagnostic.

Massive aspiration of gastric contents of low pH results in the rapid development of a diffuse acid pneumonitis which resembles acute pulmonary edema roentgenographically. Dyspnea, tachypnea, fever, and cyanosis are usually present, and wheezing occurs in a significant proportion of cases. Even if the history of aspiration of vomitus is unobtainable, the striking roentgenographic changes will enable the clinician to rule out asthma with confidence.

Esophageal disorders (particularly reflux esophagitis, achalasia and Zenker's diverticulum) are often associated with recurrent episodes of aspiration, manifested clinically by recurrent pneumonia, and in some cases by asthma. Asthma may be a reflex response to irritation in the lower esophagus from the acid regurgitate, or may result from actual aspiration into the tracheobronchial tree. The possibility that asthma is due to regurgitant esophagitis should be considered in any older patient, particularly if symptoms such as heartburn or dysphagia are present, and if the attacks are nocturnal. The demonstration by barium studies that regurgitation is occurring does not prove that this is the cause of the pulmonary symptoms. In some cases, a trial of therapy for the esophageal disorder will result in diminution or cessation of the asthmatic episodes.

CARCINOID SYNDROME

Although the carcinoid syndrome may include wheezing among its clinical manifestations, confusion with asthma should rarely occur, as carcinoid syndrome is characterized by a number of striking clinical features which are clearly incompatible with simple bronchial asthma. The manifestations include: (1) recurrent episodes of flushing; (2) chronic watery diarrhea; (3) hypotension; (4) heart murmurs (arising from the tricuspid or pulmonic valves); and (5) hepatomegaly, due to metastatic deposits of tumor. Abdominal carcinoids may show signs of bowel obstruction, while bronchial carcinoids may be associated with unilateral wheezing and hemoptysis. A significant clue to the presence of bronchial carcinoid is the demonstration of atelectasis or a nodular lesion on chest x-ray.

A tentative diagnosis of carcinoid syndrome is easily confirmed by measurement of levels of urinary 5-hydroxyindolacetic acid (5-HIAA). Although spurious elevations of urinary 5-HIAA may occur (certain foods, sprue, Whipple's disease, blind-loop syndrome, ingestion of glyceryl guaiacolate), these elevations are usually less than those occurring in the carcinoid syndrome.

HYPERSENSITIVITY PNEUMONITIS

This syndrome results from a Type III hypersensitivity reaction to a variety of organic antigens, including thermophilic actinomycetes (farmer's lung, humidifier lung), avian proteins (bird-fancier's lung), and many others. Although the symptoms (fever, dyspnea, cough) and signs (rales, interstitial infiltrates) usually begin 4–6 hours after exposure to antigens, there is sometimes an immediate response, characterized by wheezing, which is followed some hours later by the more typical acute restrictive process.

In those cases with a biphasic response, the recognition that the patient does not have simple asthma depends upon a careful analysis of the clinical pattern (including the association with exposure to the specific organic antigen), and the presence of fever, dyspnea without wheezing, and diffuse roentgenographic abnormalities in the delayed phase. Specific serological tests are available in many forms of hypersensitivity pneumonitis.

PULMONARY INFILTRATION WITH EOSINOPHILIA (PIE)

This is a heterogeneous group of conditions characterized by abnormalities on the chest roentgenogram and the presence of eosinophilia in the blood. Asthmatic wheezing may be present in some cases.

Some forms of PIE syndrome develop as complications of well-established asthma. Examples include allergic bronchopulmonary aspergillosis, and some cases of chronic eosinophilic pneumonia and of allergic granulomatosis. In such situations, the diagnosis of asthma has usually been made months or years before the development of PIE syndrome, and the diagnostic problem is the recognition that an additional condition has developed.

In certain other forms of PIE syndrome, wheezing may develop pari passu with the PIE, and the combination of wheezing and eosinophilia may lead to the erroneous conclusion that the patient has bronchial asthma. Conditions in which these circumstances may pertain include tropical eosinophilia, intestinal nematode infestations, and in some cases of allergic granulomatosis and of chronic eosinophilic pneumonia. In all the cases, the presence of roentgenographic abnormalities provides the clue that something more than simple bronchial asthma is present.

Highly specific serological tests have been developed for the identification of many of the diseases which present clinically as PIE syndrome.

SARCOIDOSIS AND OTHER RESTRICTIVE CONDITIONS

Patients with sarcoidosis may occasionally demonstrate diffuse wheezing, associated with spirometric evidence of diffuse airway obstructive disease. The correct diagnosis is suggested by the typical roentgen findings of diffuse reticulonodular disease, often accompanied by bilateral hilar adenopathy, and confirmed by biopsy.

Other conditions which may present with wheezing and with diffuse interstitial patterns on the chest roentgenogram include mucoviscidosis and lymphangiomyomatosis. These conditions have typical clinical features which aid in their identification.

PSYCHOGENIC DYSPNEA, HYPERVENTILATION AND LARYNGEAL ASTHMA

The patient with psychogenic dyspnea may present with a self-made diagnosis of asthma, which is easily accepted by an uncritical physician if the patient is seen during an asymptomatic interval. The true nature of the disorder should be suspected if certain other features are present, such as chest pain, sighing respirations, and bizarre precipitating and relieving factors. The absence of blood eosinophilia and the absence of wheezing or spirometric evidence of airway obstruction during a symptomatic episode will suggest hyperventilation. While most hyperventilation is psychogenic in origin, metabolic causes such as salicylate poisoning, uremia, and diabetic ketoacidosis should be considered.

Two pseudoasthmatic syndromes originating in the larynx have received considerable attention recently. The term "factitious asthma" has been applied to both. In the first, which seems often to be a conversion phenomenon, inspiratory closure of the glottis causes a laryngeal stridor which can be mistaken for asthma. Names for this condition include hysteric croup and laryngismus stridulus. In the second syndrome, called emotional laryngeal wheezing, the glottic narrowing occurs during expiration and is due to a voluntary adduction of the vocal cords combined with forced maximal flows at low lung volumes. Frank malingering may be a factor in some of these cases. A diagnostic clue is the discrepancy between the loud expiratory sound heard at the mouth and the relatively quiet chest.

In many patients with organic asthma, psychogenic factors may precipitate episodic acute attacks of wheezing, a relationship of which the patient may not be aware. It is important that such patients not be labeled as having factitious asthma.

REFERENCES

Allan JD, Moss AD, Wallwork JC, et al: Immediate hypersensitivity in patients with cystic fibrosis. Clin Allergy 5:255, 1975

Bell WR, Simon TL, DeMets DL: The clinical features of submassive and massive pulmonary embolism. Am J Med 62:355, 1977

Churg A: Pulmonary angiitis and granulomatosis revisited. Hum Pathol 14:868, 1983

Corrao WM, Braman S, Irwin RS: Chronic cough as the sole presenting manifestation of asthma. N Engl J Med 300:633, 1981

Dines DE: Chronic eosinophilic pneumonia: A roentgenographic diagnosis. Mayo Clin Proc 53:129, 1978

Ellul-Micallef R: Effect of terbutaline sulfate in chronic "allergic" cough. Br Med J 287:940, 1983

Epler GR, Colby TV: The spectrum of bronchiolitis obliterans. Chest 83:161, 1983

Gross NH: What is this thing called love—Or, defining asthma. Am Rev Respir Dis 121:203, 1980

Hawley PC, Whitcomb ME: Bronchiolitis fibrosa obliterans in adults. Arch Intern Med 141:1324, 1981

Hudgel DW, Langston L, Selner JC, et al: Viral and bacterial infections in adults with chronic asthma. Am Rev Respir Dis 120:393, 1979

Landay MJ, Christensen EE, Bynum LJ: Pulmonary manifestations of acute aspiration of gastric contents. Am J Roentgenol 131:587, 1978

Lehrer S: Understanding Lung Sounds. Philadelphia, W.B. Saunders Co., 1984

Lillington GA: Pulmonary Infiltration with Eosinophilia: A Diagnostic Approach to Chest Diseases, 3rd ed. Baltimore, Wilkins and Wilkins, 1986 (in press)

MacDonnell KF, Chawla SS: Differential diagnosis of asthma, in Weis EB, Segal MS (eds): Bronchial Asthma: Mechanisms and Therapeutics, 2nd ed. Boston, Little, Brown and Co., 1985

Mitsuhashi M, Tomomasa T, Tokuyama K, et al: The evaluation of gastroesophageal reflux symptoms in patients with bronchial asthma. Ann Allergy 54:317, 1985

Owens GR, Murphy DMF: Spirometric diagnosis of upper airway obstruction. Arch Intern Med 143:1331, 1983

Paré PD, Donevan RE, Nelems JMB: Clues to unrecognized upper airway obstruction. Can Med Assoc J 127:39, 1982

Parrish RW, Banks J, Fennerty AG: Tracheal obstruction presenting as asthma. Postgrad Med J 59:775, 1983

Proctor DF: All that wheezes . . . Am Rev Respir Dis 127:261, 1983

Salkin D: Emotional laryngeal wheezing: A new syndrome. Am Rev Respir Dis 128:199, 1984

Wolf PS: Cardiac asthma: Its origin, recognition and management. Ann Allergy 37:250, 1976

Zeitels J, Naunheim K, Kaplan EL, et al: Carcinoid tumors: A 37 year experience. Arch Surg 117:732, 1982

Philip E.S. Palmer

8
Radiologic Considerations of Asthma

Asthma is a clinical diagnosis and it is rare that it will be first recognized radiologically. There is no doubt that the usefulness and the accuracy of radiology depends upon two factors: (1) the age of the patient; and (2) the severity and duration of the asthma. Nevertheless, it is possible to differentiate the chest radiograph of an asthmatic patient from that of a normal person, and to do so with considerable accuracy. The role of radiology in asthma is in the assessment of the severity of the illness, the demonstration of complications (some of which may not be recognized clinically), and the assessment of the progress of the patient during treatment and over the years.

This chapter is based not only upon personal experience but also upon a review of the literature from several countries. These published series total over 2000 patients, in whom the radiographic abnormalities have been carefully assessed by different observers. There is surprising agreement in many of the findings in the different series, and a reliable picture of the accuracy and usefulness of chest radiology in asthmatic patients emerges. Many of these radiologic reports include carefully correlated clinical and pulmonary function studies and are the combined work of radiologists, pulmonary physicians, and pulmonary pathologists.

BRONCHIAL ASTHMA, Second Edition
ISBN 0-8089-1814-1

AGE

Radiographic abnormalities are more frequently seen in children than in adults, and in patients who have suffered from asthma for more than 2 years. Abnormal radiographs are unusual in any patient in whom asthma has developed after the age of 30 years. Neither in children nor in adults do the radiographic changes provide any indication of the duration of the disease.

SEVERITY

In patients classified as having mild asthma, i.e., those with attacks of short duration lasting less than 3 days and with long intervening periods of freedom, the chest radiographs are almost always normal. The most marked and severe radiographic abnormalities will be found in patients, particularly children, who suffer from severe or moderately severe but constant asthma. Those with intermittent symptoms have a variable radiographic picture: at times the chest is normal, even during the asthmatic episode.

WHEN IS A CHEST X-RAY NECESSARY?

Overall, 25–30 percent of all the chest radiographs of asthmatics will be abnormal. (Or, to state it in the opposite way, about 70–75 percent of patients with asthma will have *normal* chest radiographs.) There is agreement on this throughout the published series. What, then, are the indications for chest radiographs and, particularly, should children with repeated attacks of asthma undergo repeated radiologic examination? The simple answer to that question is "no". Clinical judgement must be used in each case, particularly when trying to assess the severity of the attack on each occasion. It is, however, possible to provide some guidelines which indicate when radiographs are likely to be unhelpful, and therefore unnecessary, as well as indicating those children for whom a chest x-ray has a strong possibility of being positive.

Gershel and his colleagues (1983) found that 95 percent of the children who had positive x-rays with the first attack of uncomplicated asthma also had a combination of tachypnea (over 60/minute), tachycardia (over 160/minute), fever, and localized rales or decreased breath sounds. The positive x-ray findings in such children included atelectasis or pneumonia, or both, and, in one patient, pneumomediastinum. They did not include hyperinflation, increased lung markings, peribronchial thickening, or subsegmental atelectasis as findings of importance, particularly as the radiologic criteria for these are very subjective; moreover, even if thought to be present, they would not affect treatment. Brooks and his colleagues, in a different series, came to exactly the same conclusion. In 128 patients, there were only three in whom the radiologic findings altered treatment, and all could have been clinically predicted. In children, therefore, it seems reasonable and generally agreed than an x-ray is indicated only when the child is particularly ill and has definite clinical signs. Other indications include an unsatisfactory response to therapy, or any reason to suspect a different etiology for the asthmatic symptoms (Brooks). While it is true that a clinically unsuspected pneumothorax or pneumomediastinum may occur, in all the published series this is a very rare complication and cannot be reliably excluded by routine radiographs. The clinical indications of the pneumothorax are a change in the quality of the patient's wheezing respiration and the complaint of pain in the chest. Pneumomediastinum may have similar symptoms or be detected by finding palpable emphysema in the neck. Neither, if clinically silent, are likely to be of immediate therapeutic importance, but a severe pneumothorax and pneumomediastinum will have clear clinical signs; if strongly suspected, inspiratory and expiratory and decubitus radiographs will be needed, but these should never be requested without very strong clinical indications. They cannot form any part of a usual x-ray examination. (The word "routine x-ray" has been deliberately avoided; there should probably never be a "routine" x-ray for anything, but especially not for children with asthma.)

The series by Gershel also showed how difficult it is to interpret the radiographs of asthmatic children. When the films were reviewed by radiologists, they agreed in over 97 percent of their findings. House staff, however, both in the pediatric and radiologic departments, in an emergency room situation recognized only half of the positive findings, but added a number of false positives which approximately equaled the true positives.

In asthmatic adults, radiology is seldom helpful, particularly as a means of assessing the severity of the disease or as an indication for admission to the hospital. Petheran and Findlay, in separate series, could find no correlation between the need for hospitalization and the findings on chest radiographs. Findlay showed that acute, uncomplicated asthma in adults, without clinical evidence of pneumonia or other complication, was not an indication for a chest x-ray. Petheran came to much the same conclusion: if there were a severe exacerbation of asthma, an x-ray would affect the management in 9 percent of adults who had pulmonary collapse or consolidation which had not been detected by clinical examination. This series shows, however, that the film need not be taken before admission, and that films taken in the wards will show significant abnormalities. This may be surprising, to suggest that a ward film is as helpful as a film taken in the x-ray department, but during an acute exacerbation of asthma, most of the films will be obtained in almost full inspiration and the abnormalities which are important, pneumonia or collapse, will be clearly seen even if the quality is not optimum. Less significant findings, such as overinflation, bronchial wall thickening, and prominent hilar vessels, correlate well with the clinical findings and lung function studies and are not, therefore, of radiological importance.

In both adults and children, an attack of asthma which does not follow the expected course becomes a firm indication for a radiograph. Clinically unsuspected atelectasis which has not re-expanded, or a slowly resolving segmental infection, particularly when due to the unhappy complication of aspergillosis, may be recognized. If it is necessary in adults to distinguish between chronic emphysema and the sometimes reversible hyperinflation of asthma, this can easily be done radiographically.

It is not likely that there will be any disagreement with these conclusions. It is extremely important that radiation be restricted as much as possible, particularly in children with asthma who are likely to need radiographs more than most of the population. Radiology should therefore only be used when there is a strong likelihood of a significant finding. But at any age, there is no place for a "routine" chest film every time any patient has an asthmatic attack; the productive yield is likely to be low in the absence of strong clinical indications.

PLAIN CHEST RADIOGRAPH IN UNCOMPLICATED ASTHMA

The radiographic abnormalities which will be sought in asthmatic patients are: (1) overinflation; (2) thickening of the bronchial walls; and (3) atelectasis or consolidation.

Overinflation (Hyperinflation)

Overinflation (hyperinflation) may be assessed using either the frontal or lateral projection. Some authorities prefer the lateral view and recommend a subjective estimation of the size of the retrosternal and retrocardiac spaces on a chest radiograph taken at or near full inspiration. Others prefer the use of measurements which permit accurate repetition and comparison with other series; this approach may be preferable for those with less experience in the interpretation of chest radiographs.

The way to measure chest size has been accurately described by Simon and his colleagues (1972) and is shown diagrammatically in Figure 8-1A. The lung length is estimated by using a line drawn horizontally at the level of the tubercle of the first rib and then a perpendicular line through midlung to the top of the right dome of the diaphragm. Lung width is measured across the inside of the rib surfaces where this perpendicular line crosses the right dome of the diaphragm. In normal patients, the lung length should be less than the lung width. This is certainly true from the ages of 5–19 years, and good age-related tables have been published regarding the variations to be expected.

Hyperinflation may also be judged by the height of the diaphragm in full inspiration (Fig. 8-1B): this should normally be between the anterior end of the fifth and sixth ribs or, in a small percentage of patients, halfway between the anterior ends of the sixth and seventh ribs. In normal persons, less than 4 percent of the diaphragms on the right side are below the level of the seventh rib during full inspiration.

It is much more difficult to assess the size of the retrosternal space as seen on the lateral projection (Fig. 8-1C). Measuring 3 cm below the sternal angle, the distance between the sternum and the anterior margin of the ascending aorta is normally between 2 and 3 cm, and should be less than 3.5 cm. This can be an extremely difficult measurement to make, however, particularly in children. Visual assessment of the retrosternal air space, together with that of the retrocardiac space and flattening of the diaphragm as seen in the lateral view, has been used to provide individual indicators and a method of gradation. When all three are increased, the hyperinflation is graded as severe. With experience, this can be a reasonably accurate and reproducible assessment, but it should be emphasized that experience is needed. For the less experienced radiologist, the method of actual measurement of the length compared with the width of the chest in the frontal projection is most reliable.

The cardiac diameter on the frontal erect radiograph has also been used as a sensitive indicator of hyperinflation. The transverse diameter of the heart is measured in the usual way by assessing the maximum width on either side of a vertical line. If the left heart border is almost as near to the midline as is the right, it is recorded as a narrow vertical heart and becomes a significant finding. (No significant variation has been found in the height of children with asthma as compared with the normal height for their age and standard cardiac measurements are applicable.)

Using all or some of these criteria, about 70 percent of the chest radiographs of asthmatics will be normal. About 15 percent will have some degree of overinflation, with long narrow lungs and a narrow vertical heart. The remainder will have additional radiographic abnormalities.

Thickening of the Bronchial Walls

On the chest radiograph of a normal person, it is not possible to recognize the bronchi more than 2–3 cm beyond the region of the hilum. In chronic bronchitis, gross bronchiectasis, and some industrial pneumoconioses, the thickening of the bronchial walls beyond these limits may be recognized on high-quality plain radiographs. At autopsy in cases of bronchial asthma, particularly of those who die in status asthmaticus, thickening of the bron-

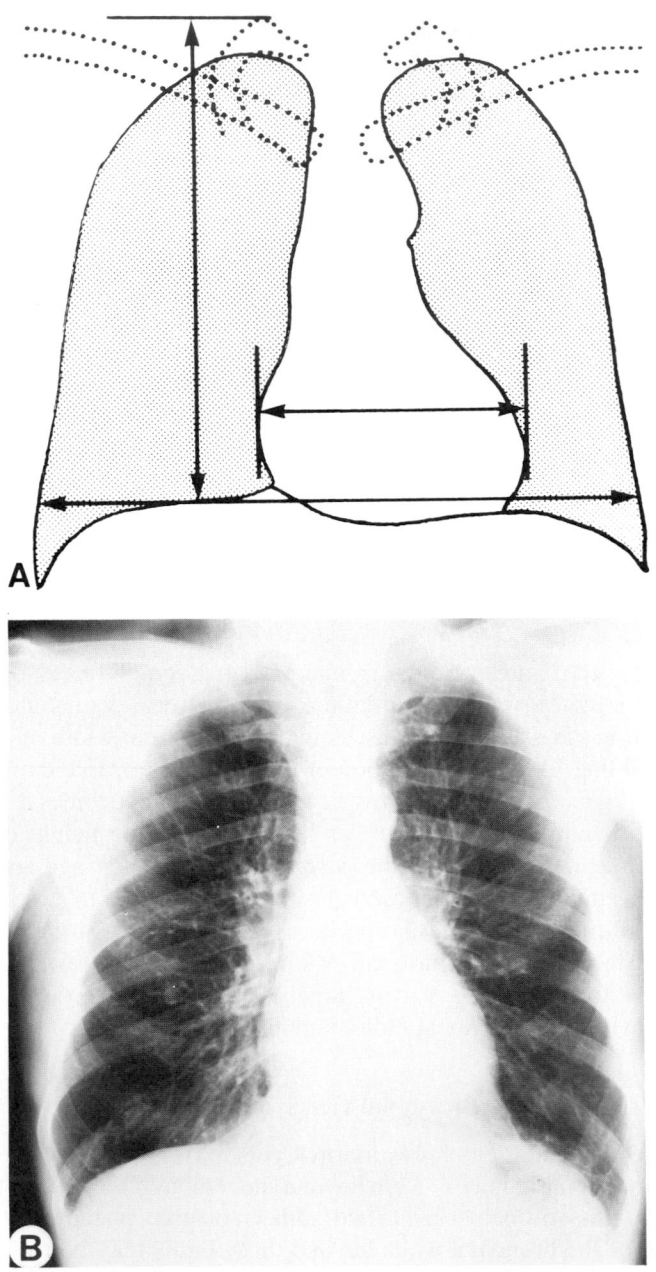

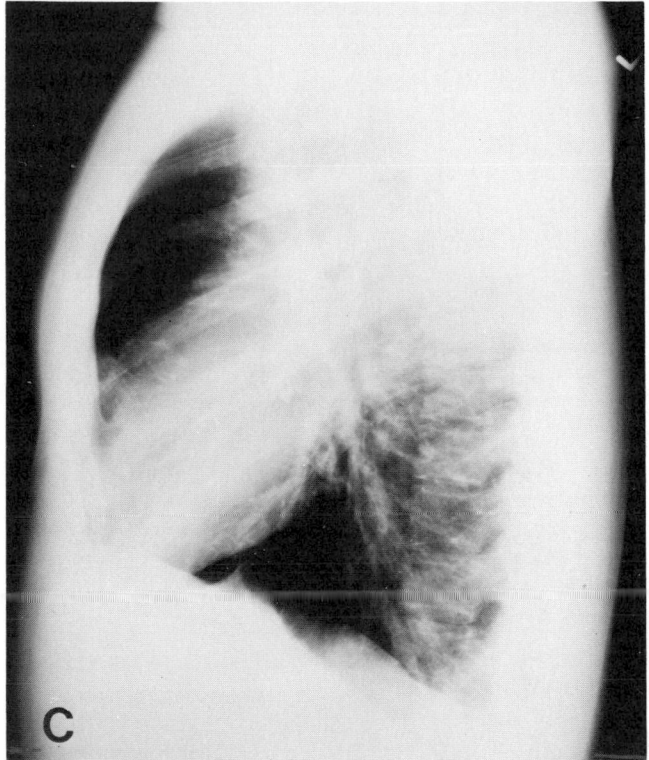

Fig. 8-1. (A) The assessment of pulmonary overinflation. (See also Figures 8-1B and C.) A diagram showing the method of comparing the length and the width of the lungs, and of assessing the cardiac diameter. (B) Hyperinflation as shown on a PA chest radiograph. The top of the diaphragm is level with the anterior end of the seventh right rib. This would occur normally in less than 4 percent of patients. (C) Increased retrosternal and retrocardiac spaces with flattening of the domes of the diaphragm seen in the lateral projection.

chial walls is a very consistent finding. Histologically, there is mucus plugging of the bronchi, eosinophilic infiltration of the bronchial wall, and marked thickening of the basement membranes. When there is an added infective factor, there is also infiltration with lymphocytes and plasma cells, and when the asthma is chronic there will be a thick cuff of fibrous tissue surrounding the bronchi and containing a considerable number of abnormal capillaries. These histological findings can be closely correlated with chest

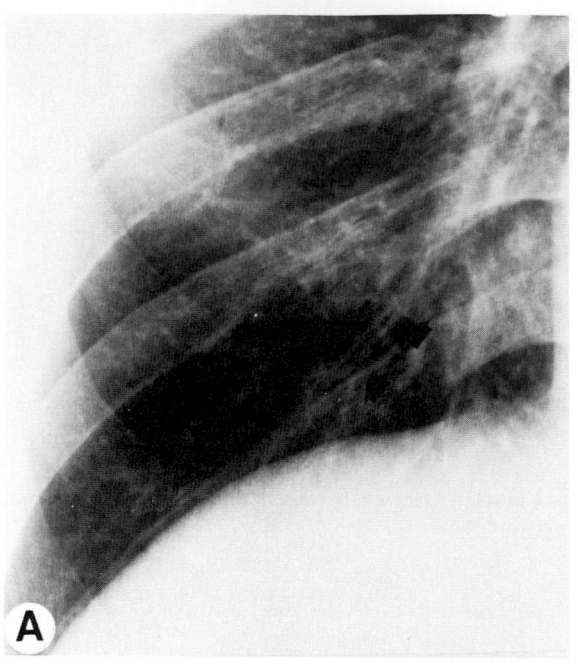

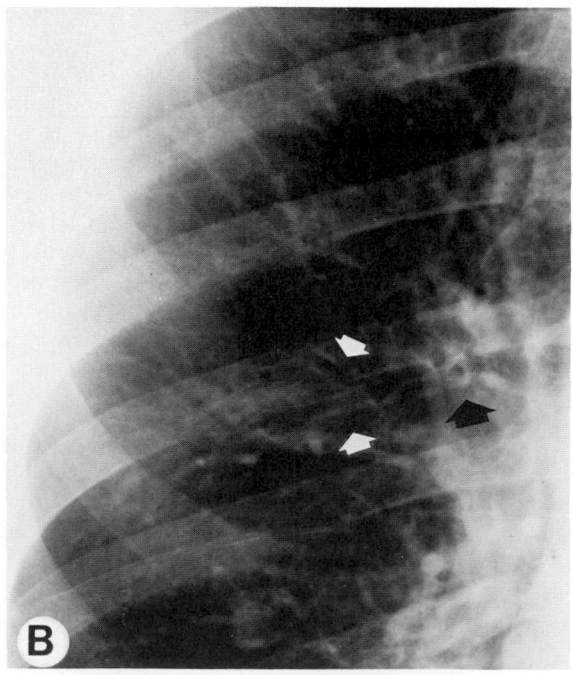

160

radiographs. In patients with asthma graded as of moderate severity (frequent and long attacks, often lasting for several weeks or those with continuous wheezing with superimposed acute exacerbations), thickened bronchial walls will be recognized on two-thirds of the chest radiographs. It must be re-emphasized that in mild asthma thick bronchi cannot be demonstrated and the chest will appear normal.

Radiologically (Fig. 8-2), the bronchi may be recognized as paired parallel lines with a translucent interval, or occasionally as a single, fine line alongside a pulmonary artery, the other bronchial wall being in close apposition to the vessel. These lines should gently taper towards the periphery of the lung and should be in continuity with the shadows of the main bronchi. The peripheral bronchi thus thickened are often visible as far as the secondary or tertiary bronchial divisions. The degree of thickening varies with the severity of the asthma. Visible thickening of bronchi has been recorded in 90 percent of patients with severe asthma in some series. It is important to recognize that the majority of these changes are the result of infection, i.e., of chronic bronchitis superimposed upon the asthma.

There is also good correlation between the plain radiographic findings and the clinical state of the patient: the combination of hyperinflation and thickened bronchi is the most diagnostic of asthma. The thickened bronchial wall seen radiographically will persist in adults once it has developed, although it may vary in visibility and severity, partially due to minimal variations in technique and radiographic quality. In children, it may disappear in response to treatment, particularly in those receiving steroids, and the return of the radiograph to normal matches the relief of symptoms. The identification of these parallel, thickened lines has been shown to be reproducible with experienced observers but the recognition of end-on bronchi and bronchial wall thickening is less reliable among observers. Although the bronchi may be most accurately recognized in high-quality tomography, this is seldom indicated in routine use. No help has been found by comparing films taken in full inspiration with those exposed at the stage of full respiratory expiration.

Fig. 8-2. (A) The thick walls of the bronchi shown as parallel lines in the right lower lobe on the chest radiograph of an asthmatic. (B) The thick walls of an anterior-segment, upper-lobe bronchus seen both end-on and as parallel lines, bifurcating towards the periphery. Bronchi such as these can be recognized in 90 percent of patients with severe asthma and to a varying extent in those with moderate and less severe asthma. This finding always indicates the presence of infection in the bronchial wall and is reversible in children but not in adults.

Pulmonary Vasculature

Although changes in the pulmonary vasculature are described in many of the published series, it is the author's experience, and it is echoed by many other authors, that it is an extremely difficult sign to assess (Fig. 8-3). In the majority of asthmatics, the pulmonary vasculature will be normal. In a small percentage, the peripheral vessels may appear attenuated and the main hilar pulmonary arteries may be prominent. This finding does not correlate with the severity of the attack and it has been noted as being reversible; it has been suggested that it is related to transient pulmonary hypertension, but there is no clinical evidence to support this, nor are there significant changes in the EKG. As the asthma becomes more chronic, the changes in vascularity become uniform throughout the lungs, whereas in the earlier stages some regions of the lung may be more obviously affected than others. Pathologically, the arterial caliber remains normal in asthma as compared with emphysema (with which it may be confused radiologically), in which the medium and smaller branches of the pulmonary artery have disappeared in many segments. When the clinical history is in doubt, such as in middle-aged and elderly patients, tomography has been helpful. In an extensive investigation, Fraser and Bates (1955) showed that only 2 tomographic levels are required, one at the midline and the other 2 cm posteriorly. Both should be in the AP projection and provide good visualization of the upper- and lower-lobe arteries and veins. They emphasize that a minimum of 2 sections is absolutely necessary; one does not suffice. The films should be exposed with the patient in the supine position in quiet inspiration. Assessing the tapering of the third-, fourth-, and fifth-stage branches of the pulmonary artery towards the periphery showed that in their patients with asthma there was no loss of vascularity. In emphysema there was, by contrast, a rapid decrease both in the caliber and in the number of the peripheral pulmonary arteries, occurring at the third- and fourth-stage divisions in particular. Comparison of different zones of the lungs—for example, the upper lung fields as compared with the lower lung fields—made appreciation of the difference in emphysema more easily assessed. Alteration in the caliber of the veins was not found to be of any great help. However, although there is preservation of the pulmonary vascular pattern in spasmodic asthma, it should be noted that in a few patients with emphysema diagnosed clinically and on pulmonary function studies, the plain radiograph will also be completely normal; only tomography clearly demonstrates the vascular destruction.

CHRONIC BRONCHITIS

It is perhaps debatable whether chronic bronchitis should be listed as a complication or as an inevitable part of asthma. Almost all patients, but particularly children in whom the asthma is of moderate or severe degree, will develop concurrent chronic bronchitis. It has been postulated that this infection is the etiology of the asthma rather than a complication, but again this is debatable. The identification of thickened bronchial walls has therefore been listed under the plain radiographic findings, but should be considered further as one of the complications. Bronchography is occasionally requested as a means of identifying a possible focal area of infection that might be treated surgically in patients in whom recurrent attacks of infection either precede or coexist with asthma. It is doubtful whether bronchography should be performed unless the plain radiographs show evidence of bronchial thickening or of localized recurrent zones of consolidation or collapse, suggesting the possibility of a local etiology.

Children should normally be examined under general anesthesia and there is very little risk to bronchography. In the United States, Dionosil oily is the only suitable contrast medium currently available. Elsewhere, Hytrast has been used in children and adults without complications. It should be noted that following bronchography with either of these contrast materials, a pyrexia of 99°–101°F (37.2°–38.3°C) will occur in about 50 percent of all patients. This pyrexia is not of any clinical significance and may indeed not be recognized unless regular temperature recordings are obtained. Should the pyrexia be noted, there is no indication for antibiotic or other treatment; it is a reaction to the contrast material and does not indicate infection.

Bronchography under local anesthetic in older children or adults is also without significant risk. It is good for the psychological benefit of the patient (and perhaps for the radiologist?) to have the patient's favorite antispasmodic agent available, either for injection or inhalation. Use of the inhalation therapy during or following local anesthesia does not alter the radiographic findings or complicate the procedure and is of great moral support. My own preference is for the transtracheal method of bronchography rather than the per oral approach, because many asthmatics are anxious and concerned about the examination and find anesthesia of the nasopharynx unpleasant. No complications have been seen personally during bronchography in many asthmatics, although patient consideration and care in these often-anxious individuals will mean that more time is required for bronchography of the asthmatic than is required for other indications.

The findings in both children and adults have been well described and are illustrated in Figures 8-4–8-8. The most striking finding is of the marked spasm of the bronchi. This is diffuse, with narrow, rapidly tapering bronchi and poor filling of the peripheral bronchioles. This constriction is particularly noted at the bifurcation of a bronchus. It has been suggested that this is related to the constriction of the smooth muscle bundles at these points of division; it is found fairly consistently in asthmatics, but may also be found in other patients with chronic bronchitis who have no evidence of asthma. The

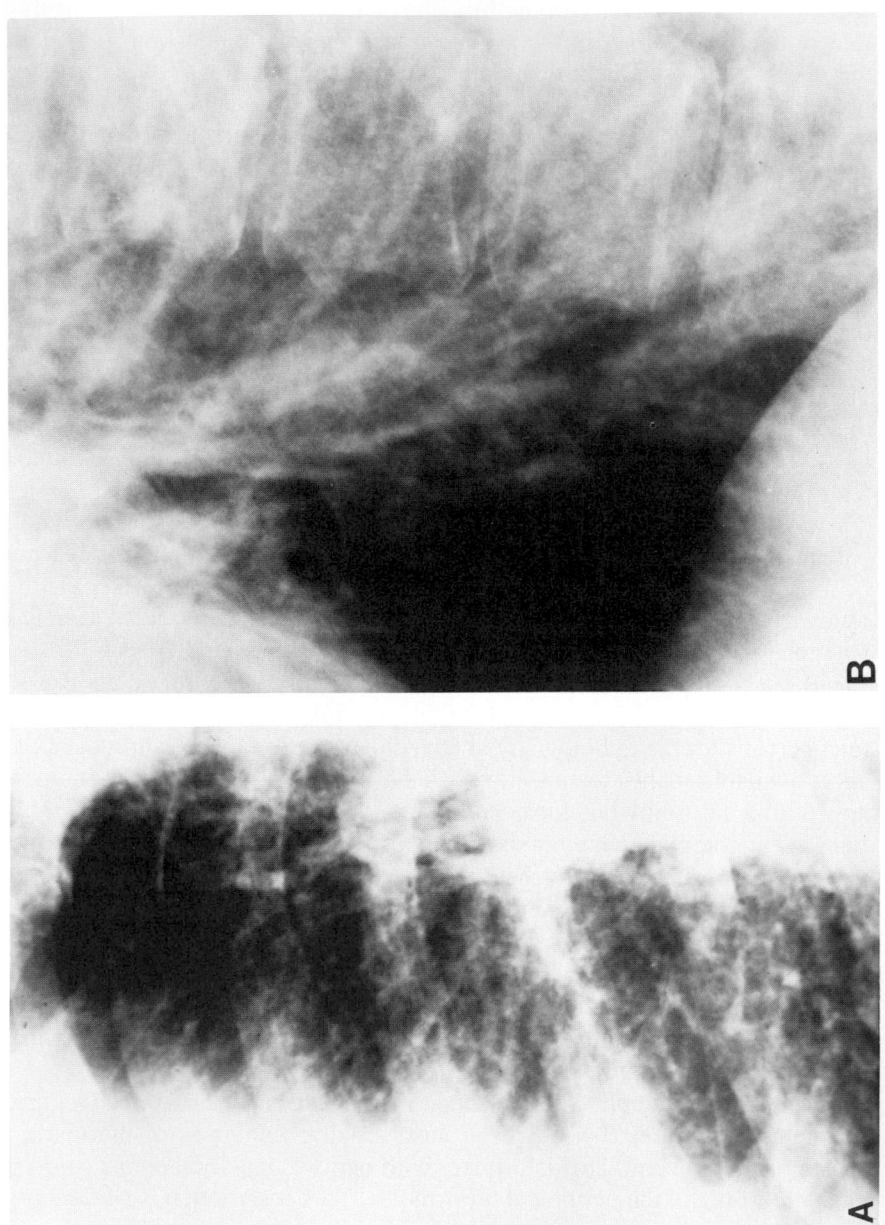

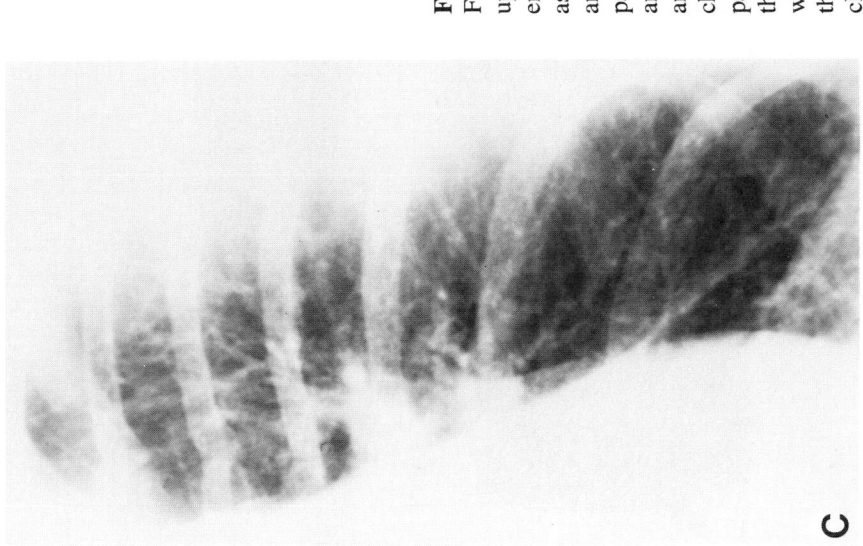

C

Fig. 8-3. (A) The pulmonary vasculature in asthma. (See also Figures 8-3B and C.) Increased vascular markings in the right upper lobe of a patient with long-standing asthma. (B) The lateral view of the lower lobe of another patient with chronic asthma. (C) Increased vascular markings in the left upper lobe and the lingula of a patient with moderate but constant asthma. In patients with chronic asthma, increased vascularity is uniform and well marked. Thickened bronchial walls can also be seen among the pulmonary vessels. In the third patient (C), the changes are more marked in the upper lobe than in the lower parts of the chest; no thickened bronchi are visible. In none of these patients is there any loss of pulmonary vasculature as would occur in emphysema. Tomography may be of help when this differentiation (asthma versus emphysema) cannot be made clinically or with the help of routine radiographs.

165

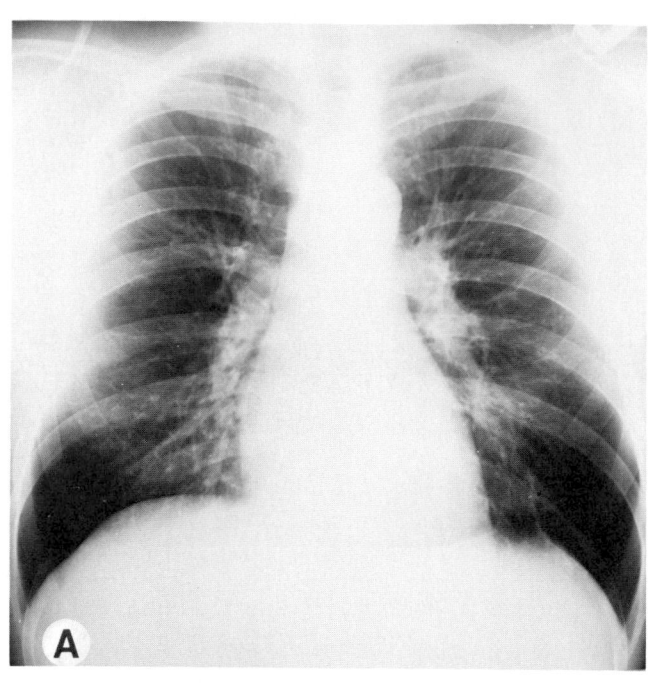

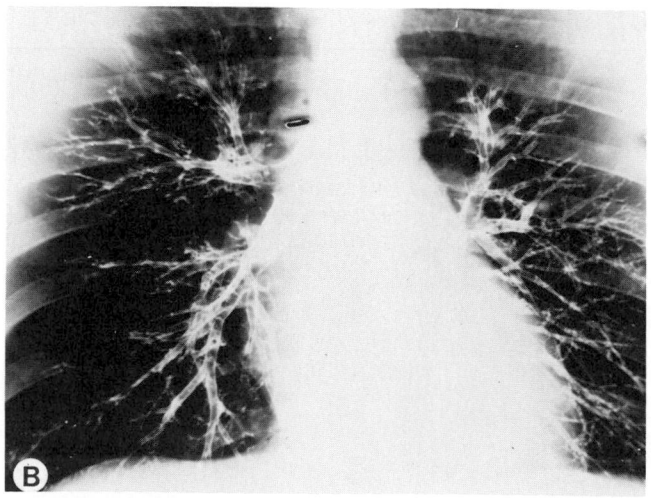

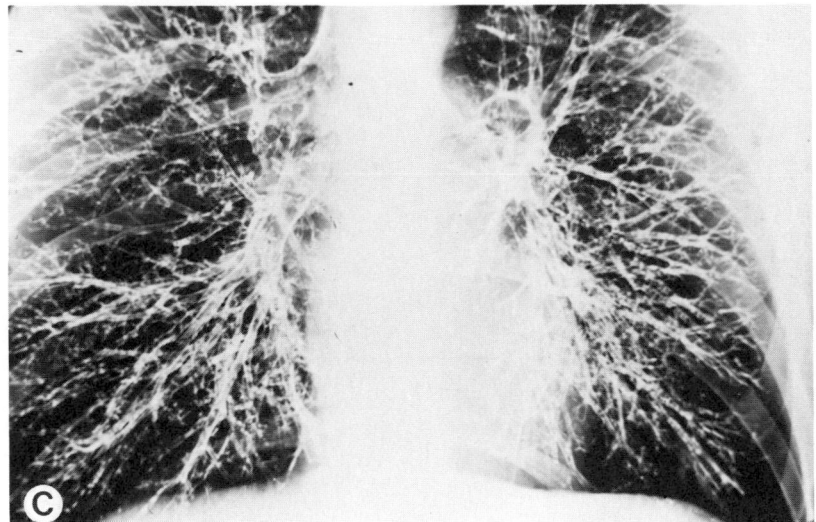

Fig. 8-4. (A) The bronchial tree in asthma. (See also Figures 8-4B and C.) The routine PA radiograph of a moderately severe asthmatic. There is mild hyperinflation and some thickening of the bronchial walls. B shows the bilateral bronchogram of an asthmatic patient; C is a normal bronchogram for comparison, using the same local anesthetic and contrast material. In the asthmatic patient, the bronchi are narrow and there is no filling of the peripheral branches (the "tree in winter" effect), but there is only minimal evidence of bronchitis. This examination shows the result of spasm, and fluoroscopy or cine studies would show that longitudinal extension of the bronchi during full inspiration is considerably restricted.

difference between the normal and abnormal bronchogram is very striking (Figs. 8-4 and 8-5), the "tree in winter" appearance being easily recognized.

Cineradiographic examinations have shown not only spasm of the bronchial walls, causing the marked tapering, but lack of the normal expansion and contraction in the longitudinal diameter of the bronchi (Fig. 8-6). Some contrast materials cause more bronchial spasm than do others: Dionosil aqueous causes quite marked spasm, and Dionosil oily causes spasm to a lesser, but still noticeable, degree. This will be found whether the examination is made under general or local anesthetic. Hytrast causes the least bronchial spasm. Comparison of the two contrast materials, utilizing Dionosil oily in one lung and Hytrast in the other, has confirmed this finding. In the nonasthmatic, even with quite severe chronic bronchitis, cine studies show that on inspiration there is marked elongation of each of the bronchi, so that they stretch outwards as the lung expands. This, of course, must be expected, but is not often visualized. On expiration there is a concertina effect, shortening

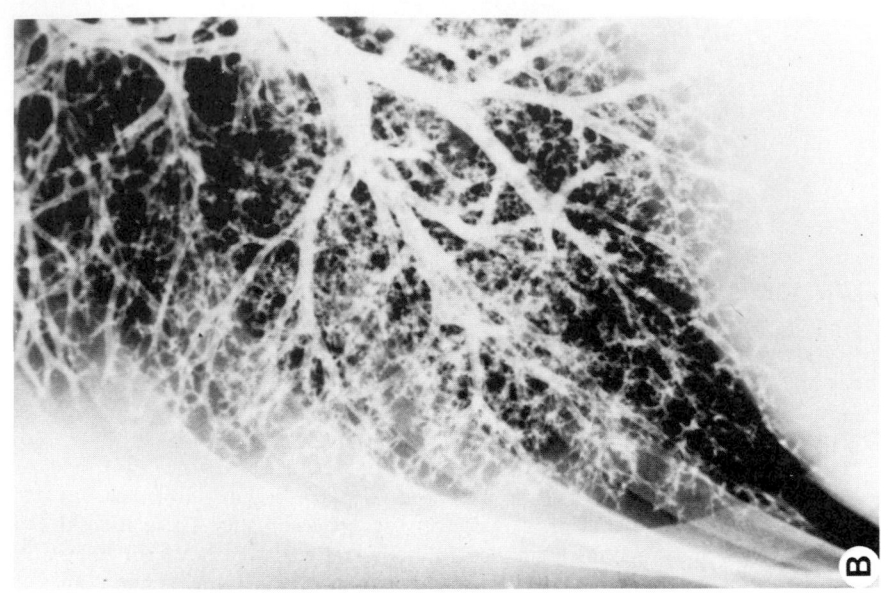

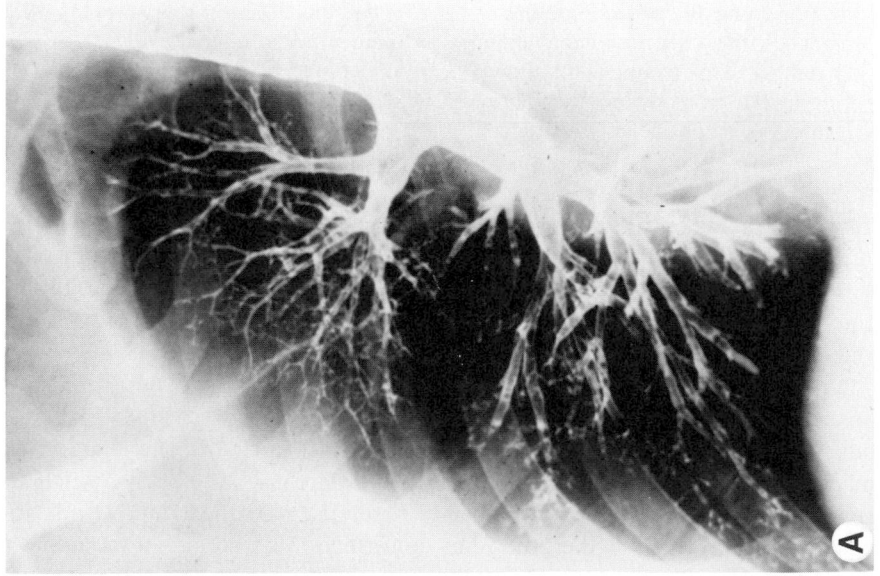

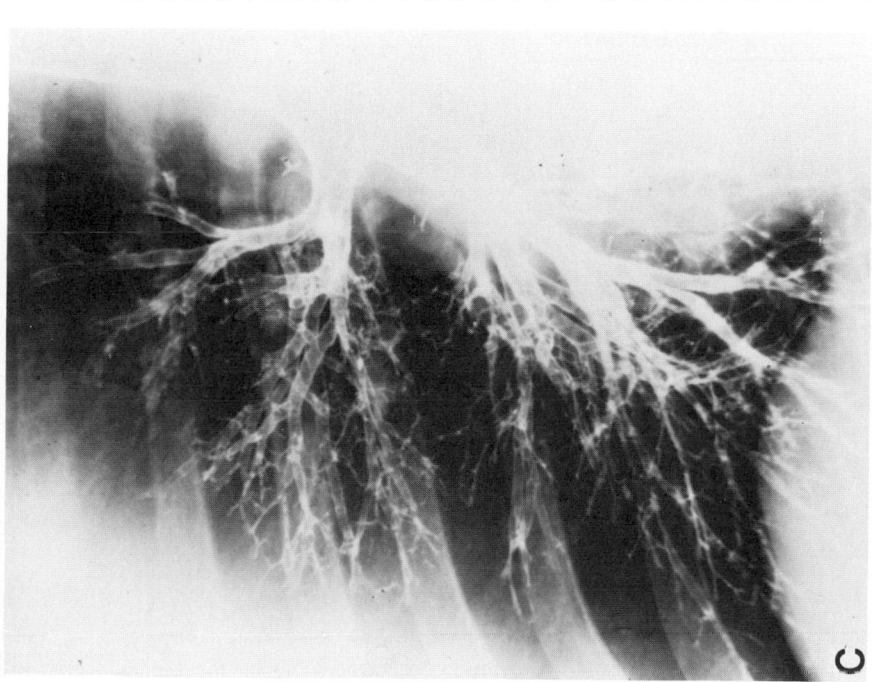

C

Fig. 8-5. (A) Bronchography in asthma. (See also Figure 8-5B.) A bronchogram of the right lung of an asthmatic showing the "tree in winter" effect and the restriction of the bronchi, which do not extend out to the periphery of the lung. (Compare with Figure 8-5B.) In the lower lobe, there is evidence of chronic bronchitis, and in the apical and anterior segments of the right upper lobe there is emphysema. There is more severe bronchitis and emphysema in the basal segments of the lower lobe. B shows a normal bronchogram using the same contrast material and local anesthetic as used in Figure 8-5A. Note that the small bronchi fill out to the periphery of the lung and that there is no part of the lung without adequate bronchial filling. All the bronchi taper smoothly towards the periphery when compared with C, the bronchogram of another asthmatic. In C, there is marked spasm of the lateral basal segment of the right lower lobe and of the right middle lobe in particular. Bronchi are thin and do not taper, the smaller branches have not filled, and the bronchial pattern does not extend to the periphery of the lung. All of these findings are to be expected in severe and chronic asthma.

169

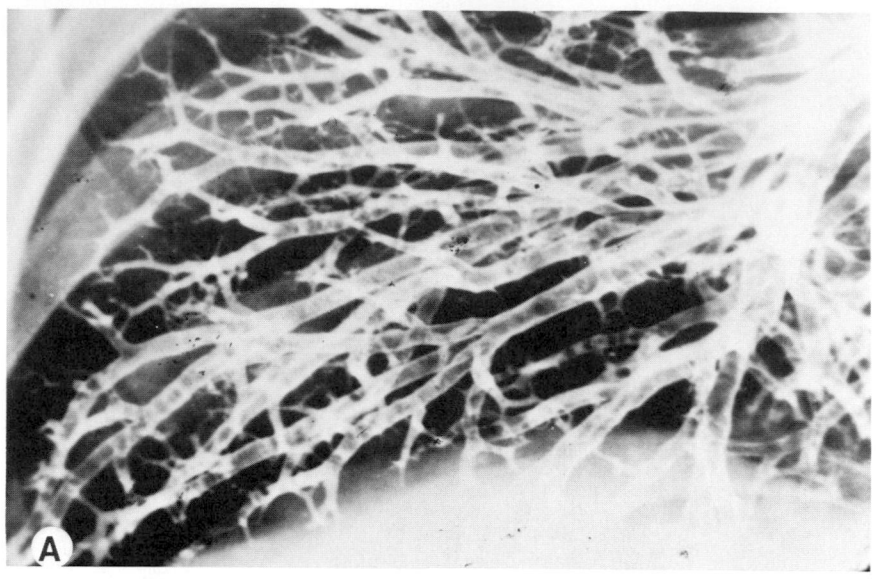

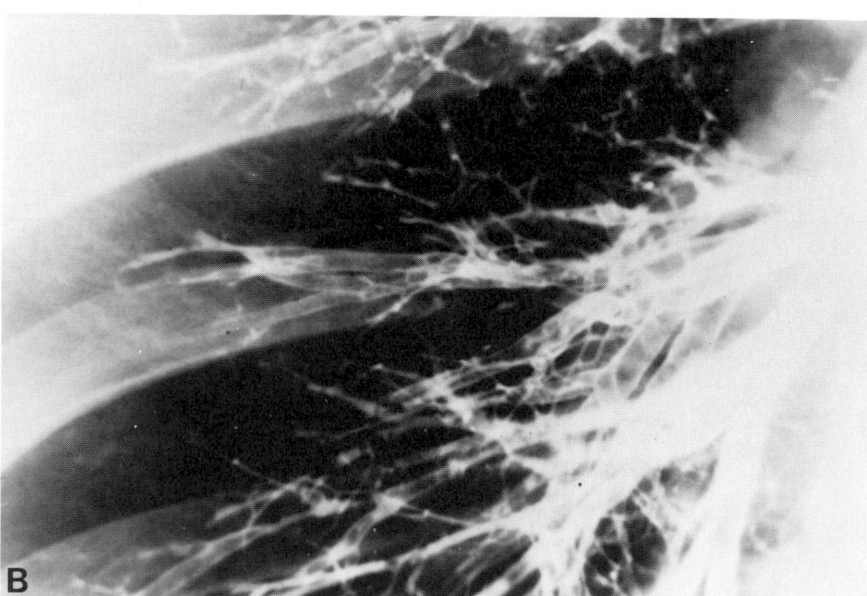

Fig. 8-6. (A) A normal bronchogram. (Compare with Figure 8-6B.) (B) In the asthmatic, the marked spasm of the bronchi is clearly shown, together with the air trapping and the emphysema when compared with the normal pattern. Note that at the top, part of the lung has an almost normal appearance. This patchy distribution is typical of moderate asthma.

the bronchi. In patients with asthma, this expansion and contraction is restricted. The decrease in longitudinal extension on inspiration is very noticeable, and is not dependent upon the extent of chronic bronchial infection or upon other changes. It is found in patients with asthma in whom bronchitis is mild, suggesting that the etiology is related to the spasm of the asthmatic and not to the changes of the superimposed chronic bronchitis.

Most asthmatics will have excess retained secretions as a result of the abnormal and abundant mucus which is found. My own experience suggests that no premedication will alter the amount of mucus in any bronchography patient, and particularly in asthmatics. My own patients are examined without Atropin or any other "drying agent" or antispasmodic premedication. The secretions appear as negative bubbles within the contrast and prevent adequate filling of the smaller bronchi (Fig. 8-7). This alone does not account for the "tree in winter" appearance, but is more significant in the smaller and peripheral branches.

The further progressive changes in the bronchial tree as the bronchitis becomes more severe are indistinguishable from those of any patient with chronic bronchitis (Fig. 8-8). Irregular bronchial dilatation, mucosal irregularity, hypertrophy of the surrounding musculature, and herniation of the mucosa, together with filling of dilated mucus glands along the undersurface of the lobar bronchi, may all be found. While these changes are not of particular diagnostic significance relative to asthma in adults, especially in those who smoke, they are of great significance in children, and may be found with quite marked severity in children under the age of 10 in whom chronic bronchitis would not be expected. The end stage, that of bronchial dilatation to the extent of fusiform bronchiectasis, is likely to occur in long-standing infected asthma. By then, the condition is obviously irreversible.

It has been said with great truth that bronchography offers an excellent means for the study of the pathophysiology of chronic bronchitis in childhood asthma, but only rarely provides new information necessary for specialized treatment (Robinson and Campbell, 1972). Nevertheless, in asthmatics in whom there are plain radiographic findings suggestive of local pathology, bronchography may be both helpful and strongly indicated.

PNEUMOTHORAX AND PNEUMOMEDIASTINUM

A small pneumothorax or pneumomediastinum may be easily missed clinically and can also be missed on plain chest radiographs (Fig. 8-9). It is only of significance if it becomes progressive or if the patient is likely to require intubation and positive-pressure respiration. A tension pneumothorax, however, with shift of the mediastinum to the opposite side,

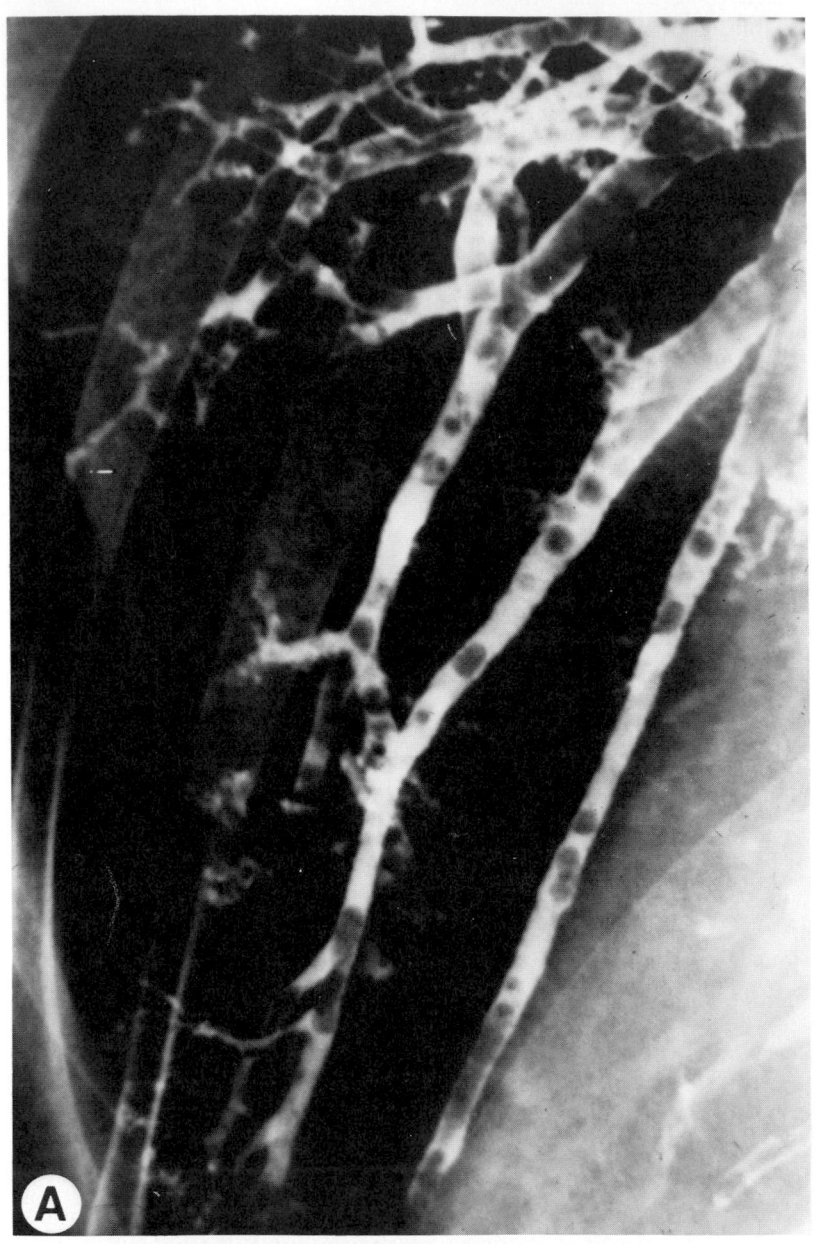

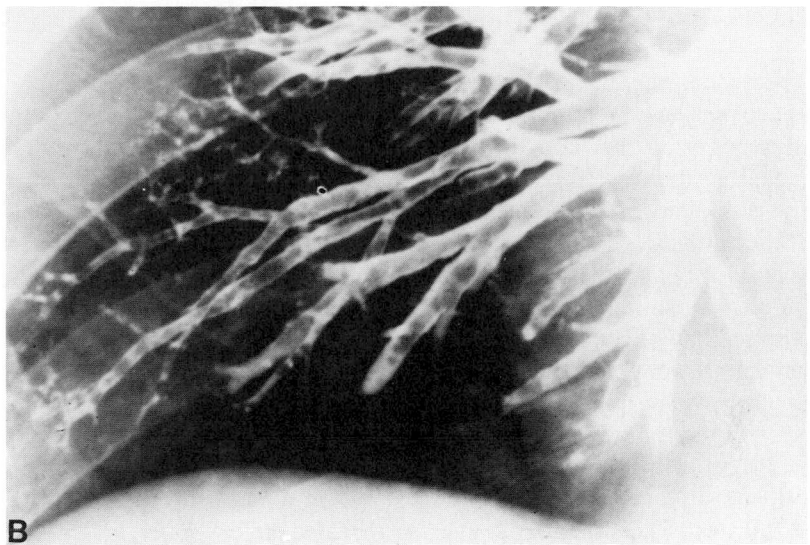

Fig. 8-7. (A) Excess mucus is common in the bronchial tree of patients with asthma. (See also Figure 8-7B.) Negative bubbles of mucus are shown in the lower lobe bronchi. Partially as a result of the excess mucus, there is poor filling of the smaller peripheral branches, although a few may still be seen. The bronchial walls are irregular and do not taper normally. (B) In another patient, many of the ends of quite large bronchi are "cut off" by blockage with mucus and excess secretion. In other parts of the lung, good filling of small bronchi and bronchioles is still obtained.

is of considerable clinical importance. Inspiration and comparative expiration films may accentuate the mediastinal shift, and, by increasing the density of the lung, may also show a shall pneumothorax clearly. It is important to study the lateral projection as well as the frontal view since the pneumothorax may remain beneath the sternum. Pneumomediastinum is a rare complication of asthma, but becomes more common in patients over the age of 10 years; in one series, a frequency of 15 percent has been reported (Eggleston et al.), but other series find this complication much less frequently. My own experience suggests that both pneumothorax and pneumomediastinum are uncommon, but frequently occur together (excluding, of course, cases in which the complication develops as a result of therapy). The distribution and the extent are related to the severity of the asthmatic attack. Air may be seen within the mediastinum at any level, around the hila, the superior mediastinum (particularly anteriorly), or alongside the trachea; dissection into the neck is uncommon from pneumomediastinum in children, but may occur in the older age groups. Recurrence is unusual but not unknown. Anterior chest pain is the only symptom, but the condition may be recognized clinically in some patients because of its severity.

ATELECTASIS (PULMONARY COLLAPSE)

Because of the thick mucus which occurs in asthma, the bronchi may be plugged, particularly in children. In adults, however, such plugging is not easily recognized, nor does it apparently occur so frequently. Clinically, it may well go undetected because of its segmental or subsegmental distribution. The radiologic appearances do not differ from those of collapse due to any other etiology (Fig. 8-10). There is localized increase in density with compensatory overinflation of adjacent lung. The fissures and the mediastinum may be shifted, and if the collapse is severe in the lower lobes, the diaphragm may be apparently higher. The normal vascular landmarks of the upper- and lower-lobe arteries are essential in the recognition of collapse, particularly the normal level of the main pulmonary trunks on the left compared with the right. The loss of the cardiac silhouette may differentiate the middle-lobe or lingular collapse from lower-lobe atelectasis. Bronchography may demonstrate not only the atelectasis, but, in some cases, the etiology due to a local stenosis or irregularity causing repeated atelectasis.

PULMONARY EOSINOPHILIA

In some asthmatics, there is an increase in the eosinophil content of the sputum and in the blood. It may be associated with transient and very variable radiographic densities that have been pathologically found to be due to eosinophil pneumonia. In 80 percent of cases this is probably due to aspergillosis. Asthma may be the presenting sign of parasitic infection when worms (such as *Ascaris* or the *Filaria,* among others) migrate through the lungs, causing the eosinophilia, the variable lung densities, and the clinical condition of asthma.

ASPERGILLOSIS

The frequency of mucoid impaction in the bronchi in patients with asthma results not only in atelectasis or pneumonia, but also in infection with *Aspergillus.* When there is eosinophilia in the blood and sputum, bronchopulmonary aspergillosis is the cause in about 80 percent of cases. Radiologically, the infection may present as either patchy, vague shadowing, lobar consolidation, irregularly shaped shadows of all types, major atelectasis, or even lobar shrinkage (Fig. 8-11). The diagnosis can be confirmed by serology for evidence of *Aspergillus* allergy. It is important to remember that the clinical variation may be minimal: extensive pulmonary consolidation can occur in an asthmatic patient who presents little clinical evidence for the

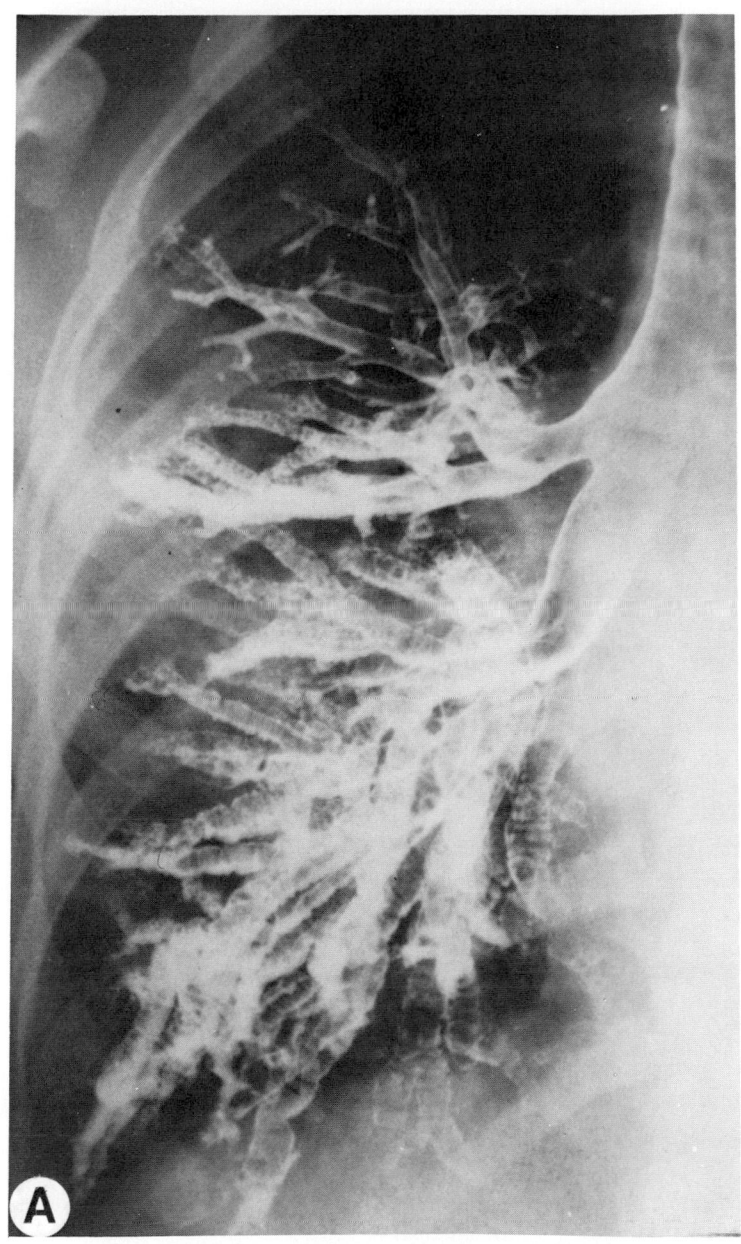

Fig. 8-8. *(Continues next page.)*

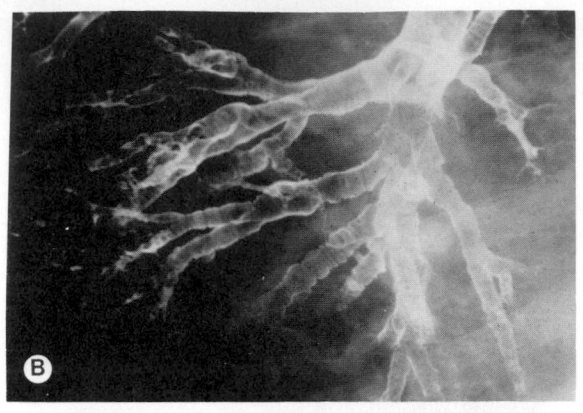

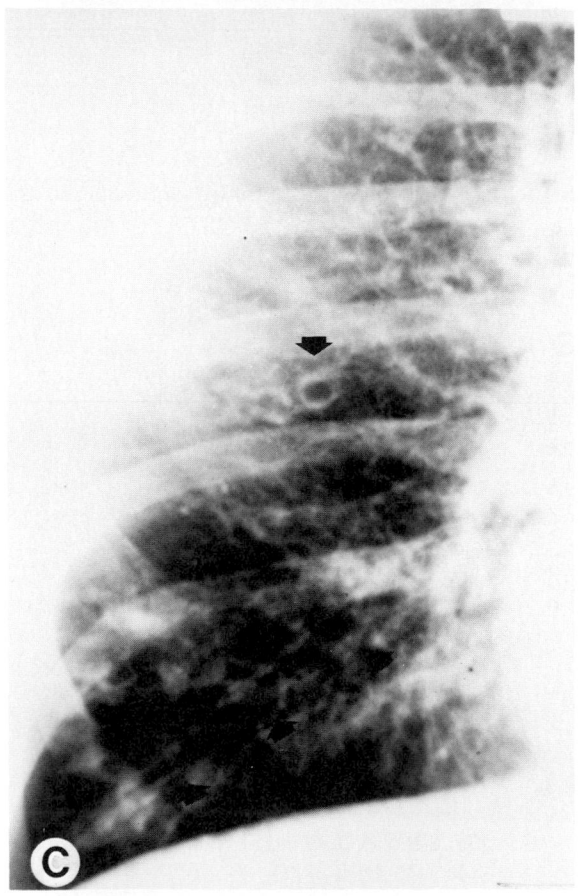

Fig. 8-8. *(Continued.)*

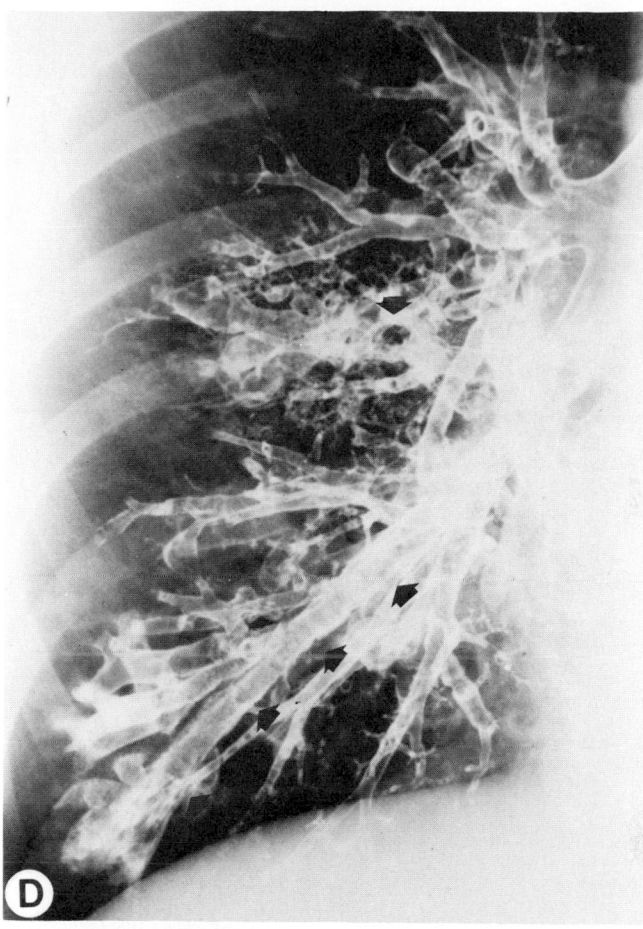

Fig. 8-8. *(Continued.)* (A) The end results of chronic bronchitis in a severe and persistent asthmatic. (See also Figures 8-8A through D.) Bronchography of the right lung shows that all of the bronchi are dilated and irregular, with circular muscle hypertrophy and thickened mucosa. Only a few segmental bronchi in the posterior segment of the right upper lobe even approach normality. (B) The thick irregular bronchial walls are well shown, and some of the smaller bronchi are yet normal in appearance. This fusiform bronchiectasis is found in long-standing infected asthma and is irreversible. (C) The right lower chest of a patient who suffered from asthma for many years, with repeated severe attacks. There is increased vascularity, but thickened bronchial walls can be seen end-on and, in particular, in the long, thick bronchus which slants from the lower hilum down towards the right costrophrenic angle, ending just above the diaphragm. (D) The bronchogram of the same patient. The thickened bronchus is clearly seen, extending with tapering from the right lower lobe bronchus at the hilum peripherally to the costophrenic angle. At the end, there is sacular dilatation. Above it, the variable pattern of thick bronchi is seen in all directions, and yet there are parts of the lung in which the bronchi are relatively normal.

177

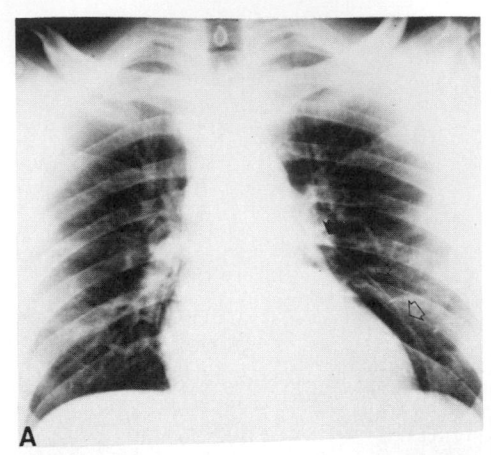

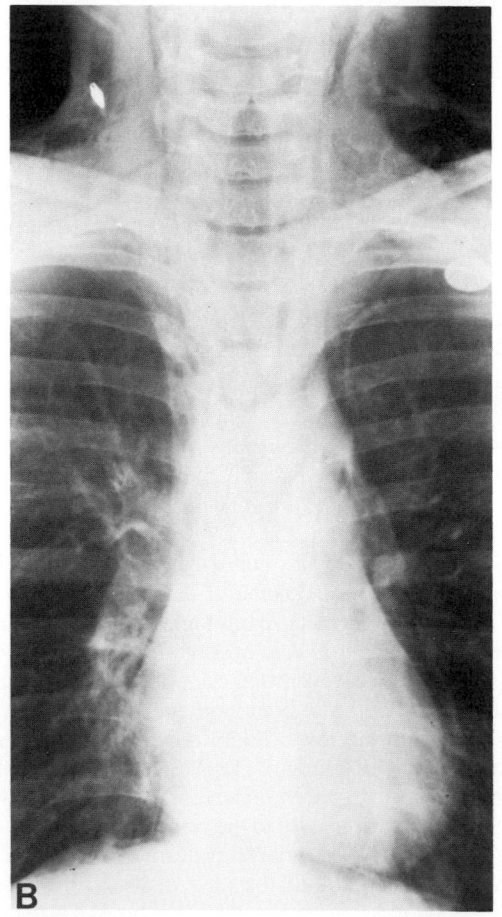

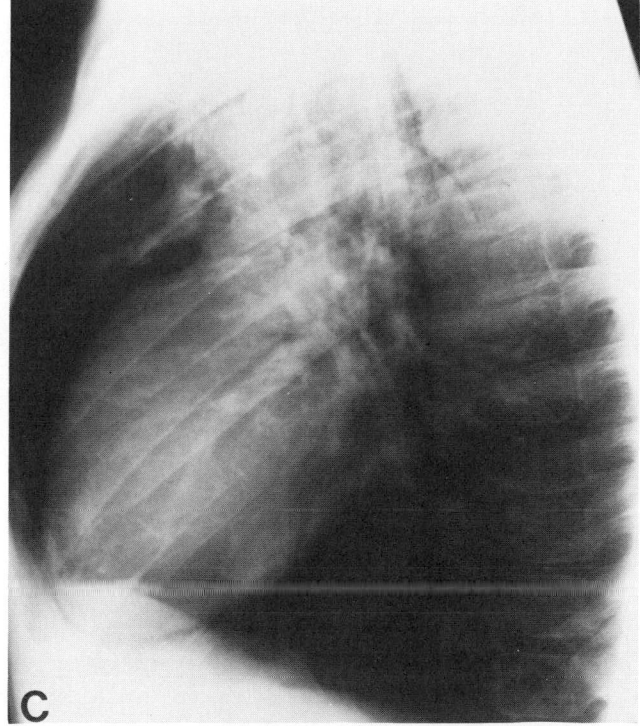

Fig. 8-9. (A) Example of pneumomediastinum occurring in patients during asthmatic attacks. (See also Figures 8-9B and C.) There is air within the pericardium, seen clearly on the left side, but also visible along the right cardiac border. (B) Air in the soft tissues of the neck, on both sides of the mediastinum, and around the heart. In both the PA and lateral projections, the aorta is outlined by air and there is air within the pericardium under the heart. There is a left apical pneumothorax as well. The soft-tissue emphysema was discernible clinically, but the pneumomediastinum, pneumothorax, and pneumopericardium were clinically silent.

infection. Massive consolidation and massive patchy densities occur in over 70 percent of patients who have allergic bronchopulmonary aspergillosis; the lesions may occur bilaterally or on one side only, simultaneously or at different times. Although the shadows appear in different areas, there is a tendency for one part of the lung to be repeatedly affected. Eventually, the consolidation resolves but may leave permanent damage. More clearly defined nodular shadows are seen less frequently, in about 25 percent of infections, and are usually bilateral and in the upper zones of the lungs. Because of the severity

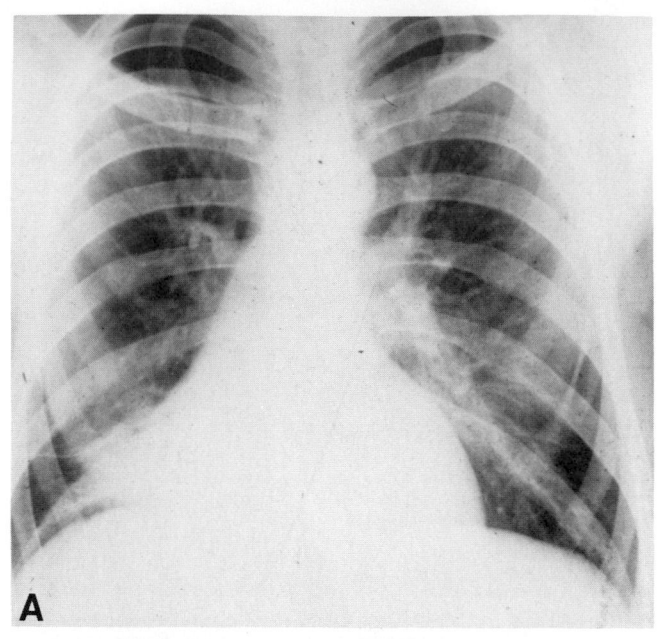

A

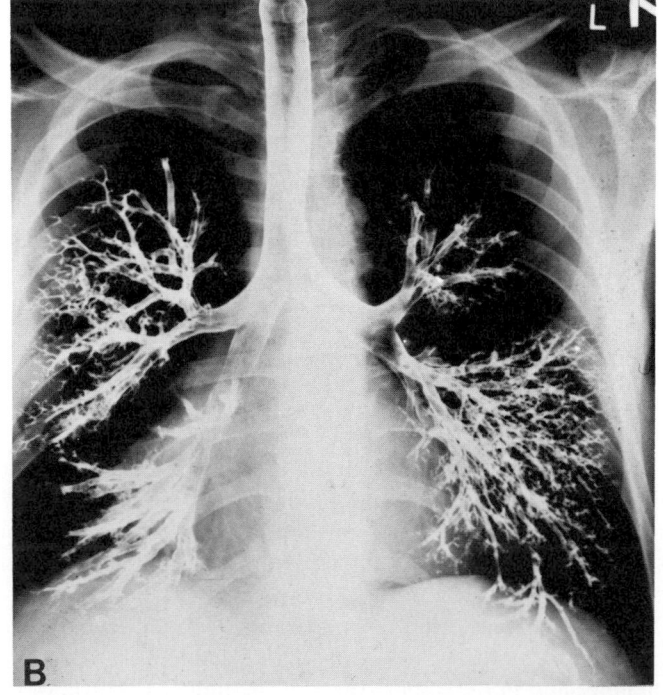

B

180

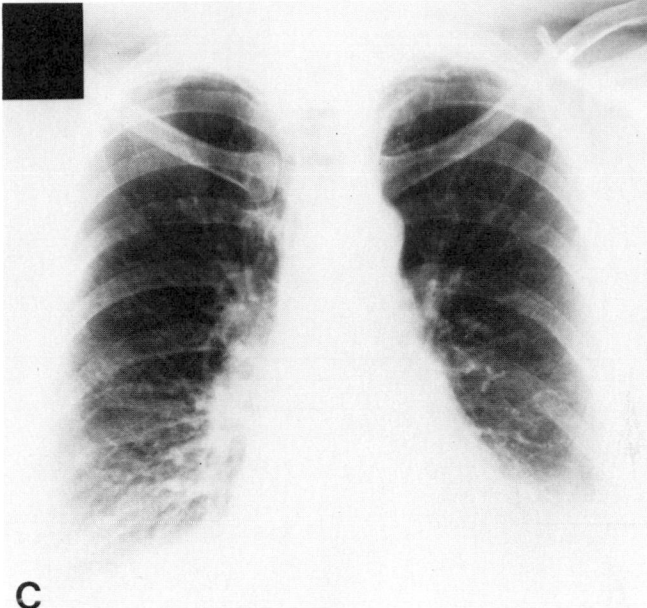

C

Fig. 8-10. (A) Atelectasis (pulmonary collapse) in asthma. (See also Figures 8-10B and C.) The PA radiograph of a patient with moderate and repetitive asthma, showing atelectasis of the right lower lobe. (B) The bronchogram of the same patient. There is obvious crowding of the bronchi in the right lower lobe, with thickening and dilatation of the bronchial walls resulting from repeated infection. The remainder of the bronchial tree is typical of asthma: there is poor peripheral filling, particularly in the upper lobe and the middle lobe. The lingula and the anterior segment of the right upper lobe have filled fairly well. (C) The PA film of a chronic asthmatic with bilateral lower-lobe atelectasis. The right lower lobe is partially collapsed, but the left lower lobe is completely collapsed and obscures the diaphragm on this side. The upper lobes are hyperinflated.

of the asthma, parallel-line shadows (due to thickened bronchi) are seen in a high proportion of patients with aspergillosis. Frequently, the bronchi become dilated as a result of plugging with the *Aspergillus,* the secretions that accumulate become inspissated, and as the surrounding eosinophilic reaction settles, band-like shadows are left, which have been likened to the "fingers of a glove." In the majority of patients, these bronchial contents will be coughed up, but the walls of the bronchi are damaged and remain as bronchiectasis. Bronchography in patients with bronchopulmonary allergic

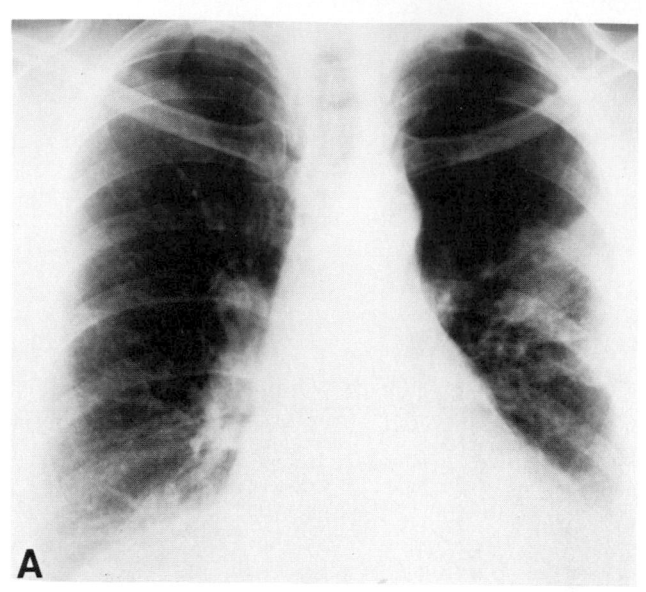

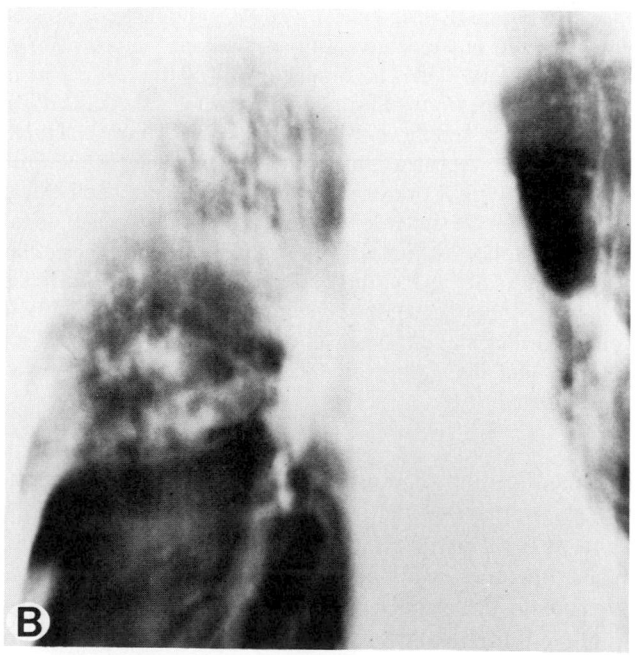

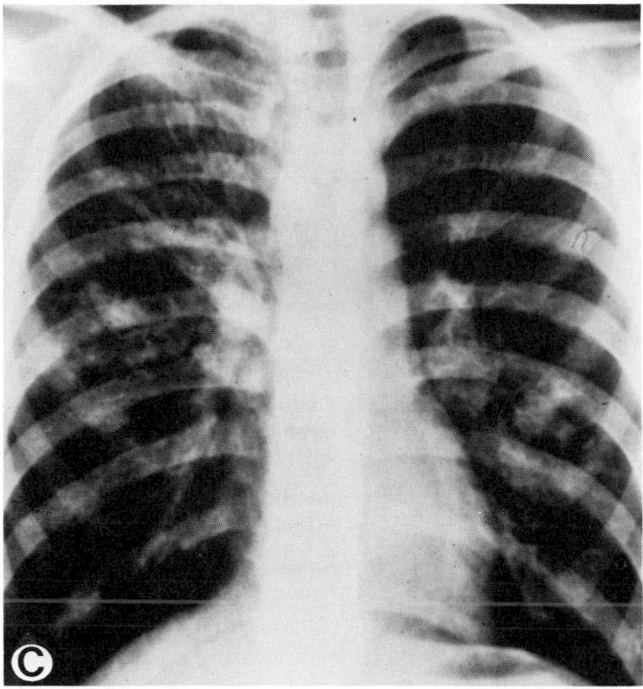

Fig. 8-11. (A) Bronchopulmonary aspergillosis in asthma. (See also Figures 8-11B and C.) The PA radiograph of a chronic, long-standing asthmatic (the same patient as Figure 8-10C). During one of her attacks of asthma, she developed not only bilateral lower-lobe collapse, but also patchy irregular consolidation in the periphery of the left midlung. The raised blood eosinophilia and serology confirmed the diagnosis of aspergillosis. (B) Patchy densities throughout the right upper lobe of a patient with allergic bronchopulmonary aspergillosis. This was unsuspected clinically. (C) The nodular pattern of bronchopulmonary aspergillosis, most marked in the upper half of the right chest but seen also in the lower half of the left chest. In addition, there were thick bronchial shadows, a raised peripheral blood eosinophilia, and, as can be seen, the lungs were overinflated.

aspergillosis demonstrates the local dilatation of bronchi, in every way similar to conventional bronchiectasis, but without occlusion of the distal bronchi beyond the dilatation. Indeed, there may be normal bronchi distal to the damaged area. These local dilatations may be tubular or circular. Eventually, as the aspergillosis progresses, the end result is extensive fibrosis with the typical honeycomb pattern. When the infection occurs in the upper lobes, causing fibrosis and shrinkage, the differential diagnosis from pulmonary tuberculosis may be difficult.

A mycetoma may develop in the damaged lung, perhaps seen most commonly in the mid-zones of the lungs. This occurs in less than 10 percent of patients with allergic bronchopulmonary aspergillosis.

Aspergillosis should be suspected in any patient with blood or sputum eosinophilia, particularly those with a history of recurrent asthma. In the acute phase, the differentiation from bronchopneumonia (also the result of mucus plugging) may be impossible and the blood count and serology are most important.

SINUS AND SINUSITIS

It is accepted that sinus infection often accompanies asthma, but whether this is cause or effect is less certain. Buisinco and his colleagues in Rome studied a series of 80 children, aged 4–14 years, all of whom had asthma. There were 55 who had radiologic (and clinical) evidence of sinusitis. However, the more usually accepted symptoms of sinusitis, e.g., headache, fever, otitis media, and facial pain, were not found in any of the patients. The complaints were of postnasal drip, night cough, and nasal obstruction. Buisinco used the radiologic criteria of more than 2 mm of thickening of the sinus mucosa, opacification of one or more sinuses, or a fluid level in the sinus as indications of sinusitis. In almost all the children, one or more maxillary sinuses were involved, sometimes with others also affected. When the sinus infection was treated, the improvement in the sinusitis was often associated with a decrease in the asthmatic symptoms (in 33 of the 55 children; of these, 20 had considerable decrease in the severity of the asthma).

RADIOLOGIC DIFFERENTIAL DIAGNOSIS OF ASTHMA

In the majority of patients with asthma, the chest x-ray will be normal, and this in itself is an important positive finding. In others, particularly those with severe asthma, the radiologic findings resemble those of emphysema; this may be differentiated, as already described, by tomography and a careful inspection of the pulmonary vasculature. Loss of the peripheral vessels and a rapid diminution in the size of the midlung vessels is important, and in emphysema is seldom throughout the lung. In asthma, the changes, when they occur, are relatively more generalized and symmetrical. Diaphragmatic movement (demonstrated either by ultrasonography, fluoroscopy, or by inspiration/expiration radiographs) is always greatly restricted in emphysema, whereas in asthmatic patients the diaphragms may move normally between attacks.

Clinically, obstructions in the trachea or major bronchi can occasionally cause stridor, which may mimic asthma. For this reason the major bronchi should be sought when looking at the radiographs of all patients with asthma, particularly when it is of clinically late onset. When in doubt, tomography will help. The compression of the trachea due to a retrosternal goiter should not be forgotten. In infants and young children, compression of the trachea due to aortic vascular rings may present as asthma, and in such patients a barium swallow to show the pressure on the posterior part of the esophagus by the vessels is most important. Foreign bodies inhaled in the trachea or major bronchi may provoke an asthma-like attack. Chest radiographs frequently show pulmonary atelectasis or obstructive emphysema, which may be emphasized by an expiratory film. In the majority of patients, this will affect one side or even one segment of the lung only, whereas in asthma the changes are more widespread. Asymmetry is not characteristic of asthma except for the occurrence of atelectasis or differing densities in different parts of the lung. The rapidity with which these changes fluctuate helps to exclude a bronchial blockage due to an inhaled foreign body, which is likely to remain in the same lung segment.

Recurrent chest infection, in some patients with an asthma-like wheeze, may occur in cystic fibrosis and the chest radiographs may be superficially similar to those of severe chronic asthmatics. Parallel lines due to thickening of the bronchi may be seen associated with focal emphysema, and occasionally with peripheral opacities. Small "ring" shadows of bronchi may also be seen. A differentiating feature is the occurrence of peripheral mottling, which is generalized throughout the lungs in patients with cystic fibrosis, and the loss of definition of the vessels around the hilum, neither of which is seen in asthmatics.

In adults particularly, "cardiac asthma" should provide no radiographic difficulty in differentiation. The enlarged heart as compared with the small heart of asthma and the distended vessels, particularly in the upper lobes, and the presence of pulmonary edema and septal lines, should allow a positive diagnosis. Cardiac failure in a severely emphysematous patient may be misleading because the vascular markings may appear to be more normal. The previously attenuated vessels become distended by the cardiac failure. They are well separated, however, are often straightened, and pulmonary edema may be seen in patches around the emphysema when there is associated cardiac failure.

It is important to exclude pulmonary tuberculosis or other infection before using steroids for the treatment of asthma, and when steroid therapy is started the complications must be observed. Multiple pathologic fractures of the ribs and compression fractures of the thoracic vertebrae, with some associated kyphosis, are all possible complications of steroid therapy. Similarly, all patients with asthma in whom aided ventilation is to be initiated should have a chest radiograph in order to exclude a pneumothorax, pneumonia, or pneumomediastinum.

RADIONUCLIDE STUDIES

Isotope studies may be of some help in the diagnosis of patients with asthma, although they are perhaps more of academic than practical importance. Ventilatory studies usually demonstrate an abnormal distribution on single-breath inhalation of ^{133}Xe in a high proportion of cases. This will be found within minutes of the onset of an attack and may be related to bronchial spasm or, less likely, to mucus plugging. When equilibration occurs, there will be symmetrical distribution of the gas. Serial films as the patient breathes room air may demonstrate significant air trapping, as demonstrated by the heterogeneous loss of the radioactive gas from various lung segments.

Perfusion scans also demonstrate heterogeneous distribution of the isotopes. Lack of perfusion is not consistent and different areas of the lung will be involved in different asthmatic attacks. Such perfusion defects usually clear in 24 hours and the etiology is not clearly understood; probably there is vasoconstriction as a result of the focal hypoxia. It has also been suggested that air trapping, causing increased intra-alveolar pressure, may interfere with capillary blood flow. Ventilation-perfusion scans demonstrate the origin of the gas exchange defects in asthmatic patients. Isotope scanning is useful in excluding an acute pulmonary embolus in the differential diagnosis of an acute attack of asthma. The patient with a pulmonary embolus will show a perfusion defect and a normal ventilation scan, whereas asthmatic patients show both perfusion and ventilation defects.

REFERENCES

Brooks LJ, Cloutier MM, Afshani E: Significance of roentgenographic abnormalities in children hospitalized for asthma. Chest 82:315–318, 1982

Buisinco L, Fiore L, Frediani T, et al: Clinical and therapeutic aspects of sinusitis in children with bronchial asthma. Int J Pediatr Otorhinolaryngol 3:287–294, 1981

Eggleston PA, Ward BH, Pierson WE, et al: Radiographic abnormalities in acute asthma in children. Pediatrics 54:442–449, 1974

Findlay LJ, Sahn SA: The value of chest roentgenograms in acute asthma in adults. Chest 80:535–536, 1981

Fraser RG, Bates DV: Body section roentgenography in the evaluation and differentiation of chronic hypertrophic emphysema and asthma. Am J Roentgenol 82:39–62, 1959

Gershel JC, Goldman HS, Stein REK, et al: The usefulness of chest radiographs in first asthma attacks. N Engl J Med 336–339, 1983

Gillies JD, Reed MH, Simons FER: Radiologic findings in acute childhood asthma. J Assoc Can Radiol 29:28–33, 1978

Hodson ME, Simon G, Batten JC: Radiology of uncomplicated asthma. Thorax 29:296–303, 1974

Hungerford GD, Williams HBL, Gandevia B: Bronchial walls in the radiological diagnosis of asthma. Br J Radiol 50:783–787, 1977

Janower ML: Radiographic findings in asthma, in Weiss EB, Segal MS (eds): Bronchial Asthma: Mechanisms and Therapeutics. Boston, Little, Brown and Co., 1976, p. 603

Kerr IH: Radiology, in Clark TJH, Godfrey S (eds): Asthma. Philadelphia, W.B. Saunders Co., 1977, p. 105

Petheran IS, Kerr IH, Collins JV: The value of chest radiographs in severe acute asthma. Clin Radiol 32:281–282, 1981

Rebuck AS: Radiological aspects of severe asthma. Austr Radiol 14:264–268, 1970

Robinson AE, Campbell JB: Bronchography in childhood asthma. Am J Roentgenol 116:559–566, 1972

Simon G, Connolly N, Littlejohns DW, et al: Radiological abnormalities in children with asthma and their relation to the clinical findings and some respiratory function tests. Thorax 28:115–123, 1973

Simon G, Reid L, Tanner JM, et al: The growth of radiologically determined heart diameter, lung width and lung length from 5–19 years with standard clinical use. Arch Dis Child 47:373–381, 1972

PART II

Special Problems

John Mills

9

Respiratory Tract Infections and Asthma

Clinicians have suspected an association between asthma and respiratory tract infections for many years, noting that respiratory tract infections appeared to precipitate wheezing, and that asthmatic individuals seemed to be more susceptible to respiratory infections than were normal subjects. Only recently, however, has clinical data supporting some of these associations become available, along with studies defining a physiologic basis for the associations. This chapter will discuss the interactions between asthma and respiratory tract infections, and in addition will offer practical suggestions for the management and prevention of respiratory infections in the asthmatic patient.

ROLE OF RESPIRATORY INFECTIONS IN THE PATHOGENESIS OF ASTHMA

Numerous prospective clinical studies have documented that respiratory infections may trigger exacerbations of asthma (Table 9-1). This association is particularly evident in children. In many studies, antecedent respiratory infection, especially infection due to respiratory viruses, was the most common factor precipitating worsening of asthma. These clinical studies suggested a pathogenic relationship, because worsening of asthma occurred

Table 9-1

Association of Respiratory Infections
with Precipitation of Bronchospasm in
Asthmatic Patients

Pathogen	Percentage of Infections Causing Exacerbations
Respiratory syncytial virus	80–95%
Parainfluenza viruses 1–3	15–60%
Influenza viruses (A & B)	30–90%
Rhinoviruses	50–70%
Coronaviruses	60–80%
Adenoviruses	10–30%
Group A Streptococci	0–20%

Adapted from Minor TE, Dick EC, Baker JW, et al: Rhinovirus and influenza type A infections as precipitants of asthma. Am Rev Respir Dis 113:149, 1976.

Adapted from McIntosh K, Ellis EF, Hoffman LS, et al: The association of viral and bacterial respiratory infections with exacerbations of wheezing in young asthmatic children. J Pediatr 82:578, 1973.

Adapted from Carlsen KH, Drstovik I, Leegaard J, et al: Respiratory virus infections and aeroallergens in acute bronchial asthma. Arch Dis Child 59:310, 1984.

Adapted from Roldaan AC, Masural N: Viral respiratory infections in asthmatic children staying in a mountain resort. Eur J Respir Dis 63:140, 1982.

more frequently with some agents than with others (Table 9-1), mild viral respiratory infections were less commonly associated with worsening of asthma than were infections with severe symptoms, and selective prevention of one type of viral respiratory infection (influenza) by immunization of asthmatics resulted in a decreased incidence of influenza infection and associated exacerbations of bronchospasm, but no change in the number of asthmatic episodes not associated with influenza. The mechanisms by which respiratory viral infections trigger exacerbations of bronchospasm are complex and numerous (Table 9-2). Several studies have demonstrated that normal subjects with viral respiratory infections may develop airway hyperreactivity (i.e., bronchospasm in response to low doses of inhaled histamine or other irritants) analogous to that seen in asthmatic subjects (Fig. 9-1). This hyperreactivity often persists for as long as 2–6 weeks following the infection. This response may not develop in all subjects, or with every respiratory viral infection, and some studies have failed to show this association. That experimental and naturally occurring infections with respiratory syncytial virus and influenza virus can cause increased airway reactivity is documented fully, however. Airway hyperreactivity appears to be due to

Table 9-2
Mechanisms by Which Respiratory Viral Infections may Trigger
Bronchospasm, Which are Supported by Experimental Evidence

1. Induction of increased airway reactivity (hyperirritability) to nonspecific irritants such as histamine or cold air.
2. Induction of virus-specific IgE; virus-antibody complexes induce mediator release from respiratory tract mast cells.
3. Induction of leukocyte hyporesponsiveness to agonist (e.g., isoproterenol) inhibition of mediator release.

sensitization of rapidly acting vagal airway receptors, as it is blocked by atropine. Viral respiratory infections probably injure airway epithelium and expose (or directly sensitize) airway receptors which produce bronchospasm upon inhalation of irritants. In an asthmatic subject with airways that are already hyperirritable, further sensitization of these receptors may cause bronchospasm with inhalation of very mild irritants or allergens (e.g., house dust or Los Angeles smog) which would not cause bronchospasm in the nonasthmatic subject even during a respiratory infection. This observation also would explain why streptococcal or adenovirus pharyngitis is not associated with triggering of asthma attacks, since these infections tend to involve the pharynx but not tracheal epithelium, and thus would not sensitize vagal receptors. In summary, increased airway reactivity following respiratory viral

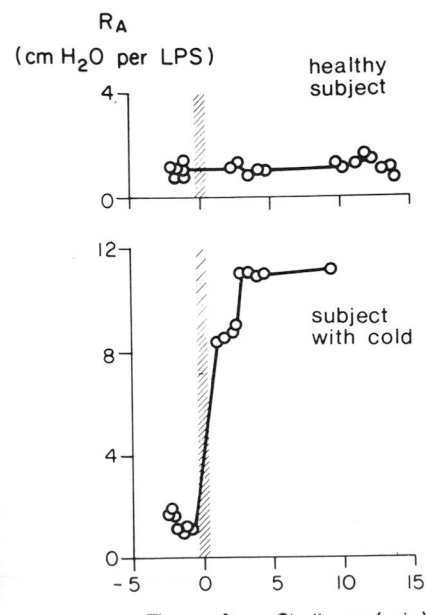

Fig. 9-1. Effect of histamine aerosol on airway resistance (R_A, cm $H_2O/l/sec$) in a normal subject while healthy (upper panel) and during a symptomatic upper respiratory infection (lower panel). Time of histamine challenge is shown as a cross-hatched bar.

infections is common in man, and is likely to be a major mechanism for causing exacerbations of asthma.

Ogra, Welliver, and collaborators have defined an additional potential mechanism by which viruses may induce bronchospasm, that of induction of virus-specific IgE antibody. Children with respiratory syncytial virus bronchiolitis have respiratory syncytial virus-specific IgE in respiratory secretions and bound to respiratory epithelial cells; the amount present is proportional to the severity of the wheezing associated with this infection. Histamine and other mediators presumably released by these virus-IgE complexes can also be detected in respiratory secretions. The presence of immune complexes of respiratory syncytial virus with IgG, however, was not associated with bronchospasm. Similar observations were made by this group in children with croup and bronchiolitis due to parainfluenza viruses. Pauwels et al. have shown that IgE antibodies to bacteria may be of pathogenic importance in some instances. Although these data show an association between pathogen-specific IgE and bronchospasm, direct evidence for their pathogenic role in asthma is lacking.

Busse and collaborators at the University of Wisconsin have shown that patients with viral infections have decreased responsiveness to beta-adrenergic agonists such as isoproterenol, thus resulting in enhanced release of histamine and other mediators of bronchospasm. This phenomenon can be produced in vitro by incubating leukocytes with respiratory viruses (specifically, influenza A and rhinoviruses), and may be mediated, at least in part, by interferon. Interferon itself may induce histamine release from leukocytes. However, evidence is still lacking which clearly links these virus- and interferon-induced abnormalities in leukocyte beta-adrenergic responsiveness and mediator release, which have been demonstrated in vitro, with increased airway reactivity following viral infection in man.

The relationship between viral or other respiratory infections and induction of asthma in a previously well child is not entirely clear. Long-term studies of children following their first episodes of bronchiolitis have generally (although not invariably) shown that 30–60 percent of them go on to develop asthma, as defined by recurrent episodes of reversible airway obstruction. The risk of developing asthma is heightened for older children with bronchiolitis, for bronchiolitis not associated with respiratory syncytial virus infection (e.g., due to parainfluenza viruses), and for children with asthmatic siblings. This does not, however, prove that the infection causes the asthma. It may simply reflect the fact that children destined to get asthma have abnormalities (anatomic, autonomic, allergic, or other) which make it likely that their first episode of respiratory syncytial virus (or other viral) infection will be associated with wheezing.

Although early studies in small numbers of children showed an apparent association between viral infections and development of the atopic state, this has not been confirmed in larger studies. Two large prospective studies (Weiss et al. and Cogswell et al.) failed to show an association between viral infections and development of atopy. This, of course, does not disprove infection as a mechanism in certain patients; it only shows that it is not a common phenomenon. In conclusion, it remains to be proven that an episode of viral respiratory infection in infancy alters the frequency or severity of subsequent reactive airway disorders.

Clinical literature prior to 1960 is replete with cases of severe asthma which improved during severe infections. This was most commonly observed during severe pneumococcal pneumonia and during the fastigium phase of measles and chickenpox. This largely anecdotal information has never been substantiated by prospective studies, and the present rarity of severe measles and untreated pneumococcal pneumonia makes it unlikely that such studies will ever be done. The mechanism by which asthmatic symptoms were relieved is obscure; one may speculate that increased glucocorticoid or beta-adrenergic agonist levels induced by the intercurrent illness may have been responsible for the observed benefits.

PATHOGENESIS AND EPIDEMIOLOGY OF RESPIRATORY INFECTIONS IN ASTHMATICS

Clinical experience would suggest that asthmatics have more respiratory infections than do normal subjects. In this instance, however, the clinician's opinion must be viewed with skepticism. Asthmatics tend to have an exaggerated clinical response to respiratory viral infections (worsening of asthmatic symptoms) which makes them much more likely than normals to come to a physician's attention. Hence, the clinician's impression may represent biased sampling. In some studies purporting to show asthmatics' increased susceptibility to infection, asthmatics have not been clearly differentiated from patients with chronic bronchitis, a condition with chronic airway infection which likely represents somewhat different pathophysiologic mechanisms than asthma. Additionally, IgA deficiency is a common condition which is known to predispose to both respiratory tract infections and to asthma (as well as to other types of allergic disease). Inclusion of IgA-deficient patients in the study population would lead to the erroneous conclusion that all asthmatics have an increased susceptibility to respiratory infection. Therapeutic maneuvers (e.g., steroids, endotracheal intubation) may themselves predispose to infection (see below), and these predisposing factors should not be included in the risk for the whole asthmatic population. Nonetheless, some of the physiologic abnormalities known to be present in asthma, such as inspissated mucus, are known to predispose to infection in other settings.

The only good epidemiologic study of the frequency of respiratory infections in asthmatics was performed by Minor and colleagues in 1972. Interpretation of these data is limited by the small number of subjects studied (16), by the short duration of the study (October, 1971–May, 1972), and because the subjects were preselected to have "infectious asthma" - i.e., asthma known to be precipitated by respiratory infections. In addition, all of the subjects were children. In other respects, however, the study design was excellent and, in particular, sampling bias (due to increased clinical severity of upper respiratory infection in asthmatics) was avoided by doing routine viral and bacterial diagnostic tests on all subjects, regardless of clinical status. This study showed that asthmatic subjects experienced a greater frequency of viral respiratory infection than did their nonasthmatic siblings (5.1 infections/asthmatic patient versus 3.8 for controls) (Table 9-3). The increased incidence appeared to be due largely to rhinovirus infections. The mechanism of this increased susceptibility is obscure. A true increase in susceptibility is difficult to imagine, as a single rhinovirus virion can initiate symptomatic infection in a normal individual. More likely it represents other factors, for example, an increased tendency to put fingers in the nose, thus increasing the likelihood of acquiring rhinovirus infection. The incidence of bacterial respiratory infections (largely streptococcal pharyngitis) was actually lower in the asthmatic population than in the nonasthmatic sibling control population, although this may have been due in part to increased antibiotic usage in asthmatics. Pneumonia was not observed in either patient or control subjects during this study, representing about 20 patient-years of observation.

Table 9-3

Incidence and Etiology of Viral Respiratory Infections in Asthmatic Children and Their Nonasthmatic Siblings, October, 1971–May, 1972

| | Number of Episodes of Respiratory Infection | | | |
| | Asthmatics (N = 16) | | Nonasthmatics (N = 15) | |
Pathogen	Symptomatic	Total	Symptomatic	Total
Influenza A	5	5	4	4
Influenza B	1	1	1	1
Parainfluenza 1–3	2	3	2	3
Respiratory syncytial	0	0	1	1
Rhinovirus	24	30	8	18
Adenovirus	2	4	1	2
Other viruses	7	11	4	6
Unknown etiology	27	27	22	22
Total	68	81	43	57

Adapted from Minor TE, Baker JW, Dick EC, et al: Greater frequency of viral respiratory infections in asthmatic children as compared with their nonasthmatic siblings. J Pediatr 85:472, 1974.

In summary, based upon scanty data, asthmatic patients would appear to have more viral respiratory infections than do normal subjects, but there is no increased risk of bacterial upper respiratory infections. Pneumonia occurs infrequently in asthmatics, and there are no data supporting an increased susceptibility of asthmatics to bacterial or viral pneumonia. Nonetheless, pathophysiologic considerations would a priori suggest at least a slightly increased frequency of lower respiratory infections for asthmatics. Additionally, IgA deficiency is associated both with asthma and with an increased frequency of lower respiratory infections.

Mention should be made of an infection which is relatively unique to asthmatics: allergic bronchopulmonary aspergillosis (and related conditions caused by other types of fungi). This "infection"—actually largely a surface growth of fungi in the bronchial lumen—occurs almost exclusively in asthmatics and is discussed more fully in Chapter 13.

In addition, three of the treatments used for asthma—endotracheal intubation for respiratory failure, inhalation steroids (beclomethasone dipropionate), and systemic steroids—are known to be associated with an increased risk of infection. There is also some theoretical reason to believe that agents that increase intracellular cyclic AMP levels (e.g., beta-adrenergic drugs and theophylline) may be associated with an increased risk of infection.

Endotracheal intubation for respiratory support, used only in severe cases of status asthmaticus, is well known to predispose to bacterial lower respiratory infection. Presumably this occurs for many reasons, including acquisition of hospital bacterial flora by patients cared for in an intensive care unit, and breaching of the normal upper-airway respiratory defense mechanisms. The problem of caring for asthmatics with respiratory failure is covered more fully in Chapters 19 and 21.

Inhalation of nonabsorbable steroids (e.g., beclomethasone dipropionate aerosol) has been associated with an increased frequency of oropharyngeal candidiasis. This complication occurs in 30–60 percent of patients, but is usually only a local infection (i.e., without evidence of tissue invasion) and generally can be managed by topical antifungals (e.g., nystatin mouthwashes and gargles).

Treatment of patients with pharmacologic doses of steroids (i.e., greater than physiologic replacement does, or more than 5 mg prednisone or equivalent each day) may be associated with an increased frequency of infections, often due to unusual pathogens not commonly found in normal patients. The mechanism of this effect is complex and beyond the scope of this chapter. It is important to note, however, that most of the human studies demonstrating an increased frequency of infection with steroids have utilized patients with serious systemic disease (e.g., collagen vascular disease or end-stage renal diseases with renal transplantation), who were treated with very high doses of steroids (over 40 mg prednisone/day), often in conjunction with other immunosuppressive drugs, and often for protracted periods of time. In the case of asthmatic patients, there are no reliable data on the effects of short-term, high-dose steroid therapy on risk of infection; nonetheless, it is a general clinical impression that the risk is low. Asthma patients being treated chronically with steroids seldom require more than 20 mg of prednisone (or equivalent) each day. In one study, 15 allergists were surveyed and they submitted reports on 122 patients with asthma receiving chronic (longer than 6 months) steroid treatment. No patient in this group received more than 20 mg of prednisone (or equivalent) each day; the majority of patients were receiving 5–10 mg/day. Although a large number of corticosteroid side effects were reported (weight gain, moon facies, hirsutism, ecchymoses, etc.), there were no reported infections (and therefore, presumably, no serious infections). Thus it would appear that if low-to-moderate steroid therapy (20 mg or less of prednisone or equivalent/day) is associated with an increased risk of infection, the risk is low and will not be detected unless very large scale studies are done.

There is some laboratory evidence which suggests that administration of beta-adrenergic drugs or theophylline derivatives may predispose to infection. Theophylline derivatives such as aminophylline and beta-adrenergic drugs appear to act wholly or in part by increasing intracellular levels of the "second messenger", cyclic AMP. This is beneficial in allergic patients, since it inhibits IgE-triggered release of the chemical mediators of asthma. However, increased intracellular cyclic AMP levels also inhibit leukocyte phagocytic and microbicidal function in vitro. In mice, administration of large doses of catecholamines or aminophylline produced a dose-related depression of pulmonary antibacterial defenses. It is important to stress that there are absolutely no clinical data to substantiate this effect; however, since nearly all asthmatics with symptoms are treated with beta-adrenergic drugs and/or theophylline, a control population would be nearly impossible to find.

MANAGEMENT OF RESPIRATORY INFECTIONS IN THE ASTHMATIC PATIENT

The principal difficulty in the clinical management of respiratory infections is that of making a precise microbiological diagnosis. Once this has been obtained, treatment is generally quite straightforward. Difficulties in diagnosis occur for many reasons, including the relative inaccessibility of the lower respiratory tract to direct microbiologic examination, presence of contaminating organisms (including potential pathogens) in the upper respiratory tract, through which diagnostic specimens are frequently obtained, and general nonavailability of rapid diagnostic procedures for many important pathogens, including most respiratory viruses and *Mycoplasma pneumoniae.*

Nonetheless, clinical decisions must be made and this section provides one approach to the problem. Since respiratory infections in children are frequently managed differently than in adults, they are discussed separately.

Respiratory Infections in Children

If the clinical syndrome is that of an upper respiratory infection (pharyngitis or rhinitis), a throat culture for group A streptococci should be performed but no further evaluation is routinely necessary. If viral diagnostic facilities are available, it may be clinically important to ascertain if the infection is caused by one of the "asthmagenic" viruses—respiratory syncytial virus, parainfluenza, influenza, or rhinoviruses. No antimicrobial therapy is necessary unless group A streptococci are recovered or highly suspected.

TRACHEOBRONCHITIS

Tracheobronchitis in the child is most commonly due to viral infection (Table 9-4), although occasional patients will have bacterial infection (bacte-

Table 9-4
Common Etiologic Agents of
Lower Respiratory Infections by
Patient Age

Age Group	Common Pathogens
2–8 months	*Chlamydia trachomatis* Respiratory syncytial virus Parainfluenza viruses
9 months–4 years	Respiratory syncytial virus Parainfluenza viruses 1–3 Influenza viruses (A & B) Adenoviruses
5–12 years	*Mycoplasma pneumoniae* Influenza viruses (A & B) Adenoviruses
12–30 years	*Mycoplasma pneumoniae* Pneumococci Influenza virus
Over 30 years	Pneumococci Other bacteria (Group A) Streptococci, influenza Viruses, *H. influenzae*

rial tracheitis); in the setting of serious underlying disease (e.g., cystic fibrosis), bacterial infection is more common. If an uncontaminated sputum specimen can be obtained (see below), this may be helpful to further exclude bacterial infection. Viral cultures are not routinely indicated except (possibly) in patients hospitalized with severe croup. Epiglottitis is invariably a bacterial infection, usually due to *Hemophilus influenzae.*

Pneumonia

Pneumonia in the child also is most commonly due to viruses or mycoplasma (Table 9-4). In infants between 1 and 12 months old, *Chlamydia trachomatis,* respiratory syncytial virus, and parainfluenza virus 1-3 are the most common pathogens, whereas in older children, especially over 5 years of age, *M. pneumoniae* becomes a significant pathogen. Influenza and adenoviruses have also been associated with pneumonia in infants and children. Although bacterial pneumonias are uncommon (representing probably less than 5 percent of all recognized cases of pneumonia), they tend to be devastating illnesses requiring vigorous and appropriate antibiotic therapy as well as supportive care if a satisfactory outcome is to be obtained. The common bacterial pathogens are *H. influenzae,* pneumococci, *Staphylococcus aureus,* and (rarely) group A streptococci.

In the child with pneumonia of mild-to-moderate severity, in whom bacterial infection is considered relatively unlikely (absence of severe toxicity, gradual onset, presence of associated upper respiratory signs and symptoms), antimicrobial therapy is probably not indicated if the child is being observed carefully. The major exception is suspected chlamydial pneumonia in the infant (less than 6 months old), where erythromycin 40 mg/kg/day should be given.

Chlamydial pneumonia has a distinctive clinical picture (lack of fever, barking cough, eosinophilia) that usually leads to a correct diagnosis. High chlamydia IgM titers and positive culture (or direct immunofluorescence test for antigen) confirm the diagnosis. Viral cultures in patients with pneumonia of mild-to-moderate severity may be helpful to confirm the viral etiology and to reassure the responsible physicians that antimicrobial therapy is unnecessary.

If bacterial pneumonia is suspected (severe toxicity, abrupt onset; consolidation, pneumatoceles, or significant pleural effusion on chest x-ray), then the child must be hospitalized. If sputum is being produced, this should be examined microscopically and cultured (see section on diagnosis). If sputum is not being produced, as is often the case with young children, the physician may either obtain blood cultures (often positive) and treat empirically or may attempt to make a specific diagnosis rapidly by performing a pneumocentesis. Pleural fluid, if present, should also be obtained and cultured. Throat cultures for bacteria have *no* value in the diagnosis of bacterial lower respiratory infections.

In children with bacterial pneumonia of unknown etiology, I prefer to initiate therapy with cefuroxime (Zinacef), 100 mg/kg/day in three divided doses, given intravenously. This second-generation cephalosporin is active against all common bacterial pathogens (pneumococci, *S. aureus, H. influenzae*—including ampicillin-resistant strains), and has the additional advantage of being effective for treatment of meningitis. This is particularly important in young children, in whom bacteremia commonly results in meningeal seeding. Once a specific microbiologic diagnosis is available, therapy may be tailored accordingly (Table 9-5).

In children with severe lower respiratory infections thought to be caused by a virus (e.g., croup or bronchiolitis requiring hospitalization because of hypoxia), the physician should attempt to make the diagnosis of respiratory syncytial virus infection as soon as possible. Many laboratories can now identify respiratory syncytial virus antigens on desquamated respiratory epithelial cells using immunofluorescence with commercially available reagents; this test can be performed in 3–4 hours or less (Table 9-6). If respiratory syncytial virus infection is present, therapy with ribavirin aerosol should be considered. At the time of this writing (November, 1985), the drug was experimental in the U.S. and available only from the manufacturer (Viratek-ICN Pharmaceuticals, Newport Beach, California); however, it is expected that the United States Food and Drug Administration will approve it shortly for treatment of severe respiratory syncytial virus infections, since the drug clearly shortens the course of the disease. Follow the manufacturer's instructions for drug administration.

During epidemics of influenza A, lower respiratory infections in children will frequently be due to this virus. Unfortunately, few laboratories can rapidly diagnose influenza A infections, in part because high-quality reagents for antigen detection are not commercially available. Empiric therapy with amantidine is warranted if the child is sufficiently ill to be hospitalized (see Table 9-7 for guidelines).

Respiratory Infections in Adults

Viral upper respiratory infections, although common precipitants of asthmatic attacks, do not require diagnostic procedures and the patient should not receive antimicrobials unless a well-documented complicating bacterial infection (e.g., sinusitis) has occurred. Multiple studies have shown that administration of antimicrobials for treatment of viral upper respiratory infections, or to prevent bacterial complications, is ineffective and potentially

Table 9-5
Antimicrobial Therapy for Common Types of Lower Respiratory Infections

Pathogen	Disease	Appropriate Antibiotic Therapy in Indicated Clinical Setting	
		Child	Adult
M. pneumoniae	Pneumonia	Erythromycin 30–50 mg/kg/day in 4 doses for 14 days; oral preferred	Tetracycline p.o. or erythromycin I.V. or p.o. 0.5 gram qid for 14 days
Pneumococci	Bronchitis or pneumonia	Penicillin G or V, 30 mg/kg/day for 5–7 days; or erythromycin (as above) for 5–7 days	Aqueous procaine penicillin, 1.2 megaunits IM q12h; or penicillin V 500 mg tid; or erythromycin 250 mg p.o. qid; all for 5–7 days
*H. influenzae**	Bronchitis	Amoxicillin 30 mg/kg/day in 4 divided doses for 10 days; or TMP-SMX, 8 mg TMP/kg/day (1 tsp. suspension/10 kg q12h)	Amoxicillin 0.5 gram qid; or TMP-SMX 2 tabs (single strength) bid
	Pneumonia	Ampicillin 200 mg/kg/day in 6 divided doses; or cefuroxime, 100 mg/kg/d I.V. in 3 divided doses	Ampicillin 6–9 gram/day (6 ×/day); or cefamandole 8 gram/day I.V. (2 grams q6h)

* TMP-SMX (trimethoprim-sulfamethoxazole; Bactrim; Septra) cefuroxime and cefamandole are effective against penicillinase-producing (ampicillin-resistant) *H. influenzae*.

harmful. Viral infections do not respond to antimicrobials; bacterial complications are rare (even in asthmatics) and chemoprophylaxis is ineffective and unwarranted.

TRACHEOBRONCHITIS

Tracheobronchitis is a common problem in asthmatics, since acute asthma without intercurrent respiratory infections also results in cough and production of sputum. The primary problem is to differentiate tracheobron-

Table 9-6
Available Methods for Diagnosis of Nonbacterial
Lower Respiratory Infections

		Antigen	
Pathogen	Culture	Detection	Serology
M. pneumoniae	*, †	no	yes
Respiratory syncytial virus	yes	yes	yes
Parainfluenza 1–3	yes	yes†	yes
Influenza A & B	yes	yes†	yes
Adenovirus	yes	yes†	yes
Rhinovirus	yes†	no	no‡
Coronavirus	no†	no	yes†
Enteroviruses	yes§	no	no‡

* Very slow growth (10–20 days) markedly limits clinical usefulness.
† Technically possible—seldom done outside of research setting.
‡ No group-specific antigen; only serologic test is type-specific neutralization
(i.e., a viral isolate is required).
§ Some strains (e.g., Coxsackie A's) don't grow in tissue culture.

chitis due to viruses or asthma from bacterial tracheobronchitis, and, again, microscopic examination of a gram-stained specimen of expectorated sputum is often a helpful diagnostic test. Sputum from patients with viral, mycoplasmal, and asthmatic tracheobronchitis may have leukocytes (polymorphonuclear, mononuclear, and/or eosinophilic), but bacteria should be absent, or present in scant numbers without a predominant organism. Remember that grossly purulent sputum may result from eosinophils alone, without bacteria or polymorphonuclear/leukocytes being present. In contrast, bacterial tracheobronchitis should show inflammatory cells (predominantly polys) and large numbers of bacteria, usually of a single type (see below). Since the organisms which commonly cause tracheobronchitis are limited in number

Table 9-7
Guidelines for Administration of Amantadine for Prevention or
Treatment of Influenza

Consider use in case of:
  1. known epidemic of influenza A, and/or
  2. exposure to virologically documented case

Dosage:
  ADULT   100 mg bid or 200 mg once daily (decrease to 100 mg daily if patient
               is over 65 years of age, or if renal dysfunction is present)
  CHILDREN < 10 years: 5–9 mg/kg/day (< 150 mg/day) in 1–2 divided doses
               ≥ 10 years: 100 mg bid

(*H. influenzae,* pneumococci, rarely others), treatment usually can be initiated solely on the results of a gram stain (see Table 9-5). Culture is seldom necessary.

Asthma is rarely complicated by bacterial tracheobronchitis, and findings suggesting bacterial superinfection should be scrutinized closely in order to verify the evidence for this diagnosis. The clinician almost must differentiate asthma from chronic bronchitis, since this condition has some features resembling asthma (see Chapter 7). Antibiotic therapy for acute tracheobronchitis may be beneficial in patients with chronic bronchitis, even in those with a negative gram stain, but it is not warranted in patients with asthma.

PNEUMONIA

Pneumonia is an unusual complication in adult asthmatics. When it occurs, the common pathogens will be *M. pneumoniae* (especially in patients between 16 and 20 years of age), the pneumococcus, and, uncommonly, viruses (adenovirus, influenza) or, occasionally, other bacteria (*H. influenzae,* group A streptococci, meningococci, *S. aureus*) (Table 9-4). The usual problem is differentiating between bacterial pneumonia and "nonbacterial" pneumonia due to mycoplasma or viruses. Again, as for tracheobronchitis, microscopic examination of a gram-stained sputum specimen is the diagnostic procedure of choice, and it is interpreted as described below. If sputum is not being produced, the clinician must determine if the patient is sufficiently ill to warrant an invasive diagnostic process—e.g., transtracheal aspirate or pneumocentesis (this is almost never the case). If sputum is not being produced (or the specimen is unusable) and the patient is ill enough to warrant antimicrobial therapy but not sick enough for an invasive diagnostic procedure, tetracycline or erythromycin (0.5 gram q.i.d. for 10 days) are the drugs of choice, since they are effective against the major pathogens. If the sputum gram stain is diagnostic, follow Table 9-4.

DIAGNOSIS OF LOWER RESPIRATORY INFECTIONS

Microscopic Examination of Expectorated Sputum

Microscopic examination of sputum is the single most useful test for diagnosis of lower respiratory tract infections; in addition, it is rapid and inexpensive. To be useful, a specimen of lower respiratory tract secretions ("sputum") must be obtained relatively uncontaminated by nasopharyngeal secretions. The presence of alveolar macrophages or bronchial epithelial cells indicates that the specimen came from the lower respiratory tract; the absence of oropharyngeal squamous epithelial cells (less than 25 cells in a 100 x field, and preferably less than 10) indicates relative absence of salivary contamination. The cellular composition of sputum should be classified as: polymorphonuclear leukocytes, mononuclear cells, alveolar macrophages, and/or eosinophils (the latter are usually bilobed, but accurate identification requires a Wright-Giemsa stain). Bacterial lower respiratory tract infections are characterized by the production of purulent sputum containing polymorphonuclear/leukocytes and abundant bacteria, usually of a single type. Viral and mycoplasmal infections produce inflammatory cells, but few or no bacteria are seen microscopically. Asthmatics (without bacterial infection) may produce purulent sputum, but the cells are primarily eosinophils and there are not significant numbers of bacteria.

If an adequate expectorated sputum cannot be obtained, then an invasive procedure should be considered—e.g., transtracheal aspirate or pneumocentesis. This can only be justified in extremely ill patients in whom a 24-hour delay in diagnosis (and institution of appropriate therapy) could be fatal.

Culture of Sputum

Surprisingly, sputum culture is rarely helpful for diagnosis in the setting of community-acquired lower respiratory infections. Most of the bacteria causing community-acquired lower respiratory tract infections (*H. influenzae*, pneumococci, *S. aureus*) are distinctive on microscopic examination of gram-stained material; culture is primarily useful for determining antimicrobial susceptibilities or for confirming the microscopic examination. In some cases (e.g., pneumococcal infections), sputum gram smear may be more sensitive than culture.

Immunodiagnosis

Many lower respiratory tract infections due to viruses and mycoplasma cannot be diagnosed in the community hospital except through the use of acute and convalescent serology (Table 9-6). Sensitive complement fixation (CF) or other serologic tests are available to measure antibodies to *Chlamydia*, *Mycoplasma*, adenovirus, respiratory syncytial viruses, parainfluenza viruses 1-3, and influenza A and B; unfortunately, for technical reasons, serology is impractical for diagnosis of rhinovirus and enterovirus infections. Serologic tests are performed by all state laboratories and by many regional and medical center laboratories. Although serology is not useful for treatment in the acute phase, having a definitive diagnosis later is often helpful.

Haemophilis influenzae and pneumococci in sputum may be identified by the capsular swelling (Quellung) reaction using polyvalent antiserum. This procedure is only useful if there are many organisms (i.e., more than 10 in

each oil immersion field). More sensitive techniques include counterimmu-
noelectrophoresis (CIE), and agglutination of sensitized latex particles
(LPA). Since both CIE and LPA are sensitive, do not require viable organisms, and detect material (capsular polysaccharide) which may persist for
several days after the killing of the bacteria, they are useful tests for the
patient already treated with antibiotics. Sputum, serum, and urine are useful
sources of antigen in patients with serious lower respiratory infections.

Diagnostic Virology

A diagnostic virology laboratory can be a definite asset in the management of infants and children with respiratory illness (Table 9-6). Respiratory
syncytial virus, parainfluenza viruses 1-3, and influenza viruses may be
recovered in tissue culture and a clinical diagnosis available within 3–5 days
in most cases. The cost is similar to that of a bacterial culture, as is the
sensitivity. Even if this is performed too late to be clinically useful, it will
alert clinicians to the activity of the virus in their community. Even more
useful are procedures that detect viral antigens on desquamated respiratory
epithelial cells (e.g., direct immunofluorescence). With these procedures, a
precise diagnosis can be made within a few hours in many cases. Antigen
detection assays have been most useful for respiratory syncytial virus, since it
is the most common virus causing pneumonia in children. It generally causes
severe disease, there is only a single antigenic type, and good reagents are
available commercially.

Although *M. pneumoniae* is easily recovered from patients, its extraordinarily slow growth rate has made culture clinically impractical. Methods for
direct detection of *M. pneumoniae* antigens or nucleic acids in clinical specimens are not yet available.

PREVENTION OF RESPIRATORY INFECTIONS IN
THE ASTHMATIC PATIENT

Epidemiology

Influenza virus and *M. pneumoniae* are spread person-to-person primarily by small-particle aerosol. Rhinoviruses are transmitted primarily through
direct inoculation onto nasal or conjunctival epithelium; this may occur
through direct contact or through intermediary formites (including hands).
The mechanism of transmission of respiratory syncytial viruses and
parainfluenza viruses 1-3 is not completely clear, but probably involves both
aerosol and contact transmission. Many of the agents that cause respiratory
infections are moderately infectious and easily be transmitted person-to-

person, especially in a family or school environment. Respiratory syncytial virus, parainfluenza viruses 1-3, and influenza viruses A and B in particular have been associated with nosocomial outbreaks associated with significant morbidity in staff and patients. There is only a single antigenic type of respiratory syncytial virus, parainfluenza viruses 1-3, and *M. pneumoniae;* however, there are at least four types of coronaviruses and probably more than 100 distinct serotypes of rhinoviruses. Influenza (especially type A but also type B) undergoes periodic antigenic variation.

Prevention of Transmission

Theoretically, respiratory infections can be prevented by interrupting person-to-person transmission—e.g., decreasing personal contact, wearing masks, or increasing ventilation. In practice, transmission of most agents is difficult to prevent other than by the type of strict isolation seen on board a ship or during Antarctic exploration.

Rhinoviruses are an important cause of exacerbations of asthma and there is some prospect of interrupting transmission of these agents. Studies by Gwaltney, Minor, and collaborators have shown that individuals with rhinovirus infection shed large amounts of infectious virus in their nasal secretions. Transmission of infection occurs when as little as one infectious virus particle from these secretions is inoculated onto the nasal or conjunctival mucosa of a susceptible individual. Rhinoviruses can survive for many hours on environmental surfaces such as doorknobs, handkerchiefs, and hands, allowing infection by formites. Volunteer studies have shown that placing small amounts of virus on the hands of a susceptible volunteer quickly results in a respiratory infection, presumably because the virus is inoculated onto susceptible mucosa as the individual rubs the hands on eyes or nose. Because of these data, it would seem prudent for asthmatics to wash their hands frequently (rinsing in water and drying is sufficient), especially after contact with people, to avoid placing their fingers in or on their noses or eyes, and to use disposable tissues for secretions and not to share handkerchiefs with others. Although there are no data demonstrating the effectiveness of these recommendations, they appear logical, and studies with virucidal skin disinfectants have demonstrated reduced transmission of colds. Obviously, these recommendations are difficult to implement in young children.

Recently, it has been demonstrated that impregnation of facial tissues with a virucidal material (a mixture of citric and malic acids with a detergent) results in reduced transmission of colds. If these tissues are used by patients with colds, it results in reduced infectiousness for others (presumably by decreasing the amount of virus on the patient's hands). Test marketing of these tissues (Avert) is underway.

In the hospital, patients with suspected or documented influenza, parainfluenza, or respiratory syncytial virus infections should be placed in respiratory isolation. Although patients with suspected or documented rhinovirus infections (or "common cold") and *Mycoplasma* pneumonia are not usually isolated, it would seem prudent not to place them in close contiguity to asthmatic patients.

Immunoprophylaxis

Of the common respiratory viral pathogens, influenza is the only one for which a vaccine is available. Present preparations of influenza vaccine have been highly purified by zonal centrifugation and contain current strains of influenza A and B inactivated by chemicals. Two vaccine formulations are available: whole virus and split virus. Whole virus vaccines contain intact (but nonviable) virions, while split virus vaccines have been treated with detergents that disrupt the virions into smaller antigenic fragments. Whole virus vaccines are more immunogenic but also more reactogenic than are split virus vaccines, especially in children. For that reason, split virus vaccines are recommended for individuals less than 13 years old. The usual dose is 0.5 ml subcutaneously twice; inoculations 2 weeks apart. Whole virus vaccines are given in a single dose of 0.5 ml subcutaneously. As the vaccine is made in embryonated eggs, immunization is contraindicated in individuals with serious egg (but not feather) allergy. Immunization should be repeated annually for optimal protection.

Influenza vaccines are effective in preventing influenza if the antigenic composition of the influenza strains used to formulate the vaccine is fairly closely related to the strain(s) circulating in the community. Immunization is recommended by the United States Public Health Service for (among others) individuals with chronic respiratory disease (including asthmatics) who are at risk of relatively severe illness with influenza. The few studies that have been done have documented the prophylactic efficacy of influenza vaccine in asthmatics.

Several studies have shown that subcutaneous immunization of asthmatic subjects with influenza vaccines appears to produce transient (1–2 days) worsening of airway obstruction, airway hyperreactivity to methacholine, and an increased requirement for bronchodilator treatment. Clinical exacerbation of severe asthma was very rare. The mechanism of this effect is obscure, since it is not associated with atopy to vaccine components, and immunization of normal subjects does not produce bronchospasm or airway hyperreactivity. Previous studies suggesting that influenza immunization depresses hepatic drug metabolism (resulting, for example, in increased blood levels of theophylline in patients receiving a stable daily dose) have not confirmed the clinical significance of this finding. We recommend no decreases in bronchodilator medication following influenza immunization.

We recommend the routine use of influenza immunization in asthmatics, since they seem to be at increased risk of serious morbidity from influenza infection. Since immunization itself may produce transient, mild worsening of bronchospasm, an increase in bronchodilator medication for 2–3 days after immunization would seem wise. Split virus vaccine, 0.5 ml subcutaneously on two occasions 2–3 weeks apart, is recommended for patients less than 13 years old; whole virus vaccine for older asthmatics need be given only once. Immunization should be repeated annually for best effect. It is contraindicated in patients with severe egg allergy.

Vaccines (both live attenuated and inactivated) against respiratory syncytial virus, parainfluenza viruses 1-3, and *M. pneumoniae* are actively being sought, but to date safe and effective immunogens have not been developed. Some experimental *M. pneumoniae* and respiratory syncytial virus vaccines have been associated with enhancement of disease for uncertain reasons. Experimental rhinovirus vaccines have been effective, but clinical application is limited, since there are probably over 100 serotypes and immunity is type-specific.

Pneumococcal polysaccharide vaccine (Pneumovax®, Pnev-Immune®) containing 23 types of purified pneumococcal polysaccharides is effective in preventing pneumococcal respiratory infections due to the serotypes present in the vaccine. It would seem wise to immunize adult asthmatics with pneumococcal vaccine, although, as discussed previously, there are little firm data to support an increased frequency of pneumococcal respiratory infections in asthmatics. Children with mild asthma are not at greatly increased risk of pneumococcal respiratory infections, and immunization does not seem essential. In addition, children less than 2 years old have a poor immune response to this (and other) polysaccharide vaccines.

Chemoprophylaxis

Prevention of infection with drugs is not practical or possible yet with most of the respiratory pathogens commonly associated with exacerbations of bronchospasm and lower respiratory tract infections in asthmatics. However, for some of the agents (e.g., rhinoviruses), this appears to offer the only practical solution, as immunoprophylaxis in this case (with over 100 serotypes) seems impractical.

Amantadine (Symmetrel, Endo Laboratories) is well established as an effective chemoprophylactic for influenza A infections. Unfortunately, it has several drawbacks. It is active only against influenza A and not against influenza B or other respiratory pathogens. Because of this, it can only be used during documented outbreaks of influenza A. It must be given every day that effect is desired, and some patients develop mild, reversible neuropsychiatric symptoms while on the drug. Despite these drawbacks, we believe that amantadine is a useful drug for prevention of influenza A in asthmatic

Table 9-8
Indications for Amantadine Prophylaxis During Epidemic of Influenza A

Previously immunized individual
1. Vaccine strain not protective against epidemic strain: give for duration of epidemic in the community (generally 4–6 weeks).
2. Close (e.g., household) exposure to active case: give for 10–14 days.

Nonimmunized individual
1. After immunization: give for 14 days (until antibody titers have risen to protective level).
2. Unable to receive vaccine (e.g., egg allergy): give for duration of epidemic (generally 4–6 weeks).

subjects. General guidelines for prophylactic use are given in Tables 9-7 and 9-8. Although not generally recommended, we believe that close household exposure of an asthmatic subject to an active case of influenza warrants short-term amantadine usage, even if the subject has previously been immunized against influenza.

Mycoplasma pneumoniae is susceptible to erythromycin and tetracycline, and chemoprophylaxis of case contacts with these antimicrobials apparently prevents secondary infection (although this has never been rigorously documented). Although *M. pneumoniae* is not considered a major precipitant of bronchospasm, it would nonetheless seem wise to give chemoprophylaxis to asthmatic patients exposed to active cases of highly suspected or documented *M. pneumoniae*. Either tetracycline or erythromycin may be used in the same doses used for treatment (Table 9-5).

REFERENCES

Aquilino AT, Hall WJ, Douglas RG Jr, et al: Airway reactivity in subjects with viral upper respiratory tract infections: The effects of exercise and cold air. Am Rev Respir Dis 122:3, 1980

Bell TD, Chai H, Berlow B, et al: Immunization with killed influenza virus in children with chronic asthma. Chest 73:140, 1978

Bukowskyj M, Munt PW, Wigle R, et al: Theophylline clearance: Lack of effect of influenza vaccination and ascorbic acid. Am Rev Respir Dis 129:672, 1984

Busse WW: The precipitation of asthma by upper respiratory infections. Chest 87:44S, 1985

Buse WW, Anderson CL, Cooper W: Cortisol protection of the granulocyte response to isoproterenol during an in vitro influenza virus incubation. J Allergy Clin Immunol 67:178, 1981

Busse WW, Anderson CL, Dick EC, et al: Reduced granulocyte response to isoproterenol, histamine, and prostaglandin E1 after in vitro incubation with Rhinovirus 16. Am Rev Respir Dis 122:641, 1980

Busse WW, Swenson CA, Borden EC, et al: Effect of influenza A virus on leukocyte histamine release. J Allergy Clin Immunol 71:382, 1983

Campbell BG, Edwards RL: Safety of influenza vaccination in adults with asthma. Med J Austr 140:773, 1984

Carlsen KH, Orstovik I, Leegaard J, et al: Respiratory virus infections and aeroallergens in acute bronchial asthma. Arch Dis Child 59:310, 1984

Centers for Disease Control: Prevention and control of influenza. MMWR 33:253, 1984

Cogswell JJ, Halliday DF, Alexander JR: Respiratory infections in the first year of life in children at risk of developing atopy. Br Med J Clin Res 284:1011, 1982

Davis VS, Earp HS, Stempel DA: Interferon inhibits agonist-induced cyclic AMP accumulation in human lymphocytes. Am Rev Respir Dis 130:167, 1984

Dick EC, Meschievitz CK, Raynor WJ, et al: Interruption of rhinovirus common cold transmission among human volunteers by use of a virucidal facial tissue. Abstract #916, International Conference on Antimicrobial Agents and Chemotherapy, 1984

Drug Committee of the Research Council of the American Academy of Allergy: Side effects of prolonged corticosteroid treatment in patients with asthma. J Allergy 40:88, 1967

Eisen AH, Bacal HL: The relationship of acute bronchiolitis to bronchial asthma—A 4-to-14 year follow-up. Pediatrics 31:859, 1963

Empey DW, Laitenen LA, Jacobs L, et al: Mechanisms of bronchial hyperreactivity in normal subjects after upper respiratory tract infection. Am Rev Respir Dis 113:131, 1976

Frick OL, German DF, Mills J: Development of allergy in children. I. Association with virus infections. J Allergy Clin Immunol 63:228, 1979

Fries JH, Borne S: Remission of intractable allergic symptoms by acute intercurrent infections. Ann Intern Med 38:928, 1953

Glezen WP: Reactive airways disorders in children—role of respiratory virus infections. Clin Chest Med 5:635, 1984

Hall CB, McBride JT, Walsh EE, et al: Aerosolized ribavirin treatment of infants with respiratory syncytial viral infection. N Engl J Med 308:1443, 1983

Hall WJ, Hall CB: Alterations in pulmonary function following respiratory viral infection. Chest 76:458, 1979

Hall WJ, Hall CB: Clinical significance of pulmonary function tests during viral infection. Chest 76:458, 1979

Jenkins CR, Breslin AB: Upper respiratory tract infections and airway reactivity in normal and asthmatic subjects. Am Rev Respir Dis 130:879, 1984

Kaul TN, Welliver RC, Faden HS, et al: The development of respiratory syncytial virus-specific immune complexes in nasopharyngeal secretions following natural infection. J Clin Lab Immunol 15:187, 1984

Liston SL, Gehrz RC, Siegel LG, et al: Bacterial tracheitis. Am J Dis Child 137:764, 1983

McIntosh K, Ellis EF, Hoffman LS, et al: The association of viral and bacterial respiratory infections with exacerbations of wheezing in young asthmatic children. J Pediatr 82:578, 1973

Minor TE, Baker JW, Dick EC, et al: Greater frequency of viral respiratory infections in asthmatic children as compared with their nonasthmatic siblings. J Pediatr 85:472, 1974

Minor TE, Dick EC, Baker JW, et al: Rhinovirus and influenza type A infections as precipitants of asthma. Am Rev Respir Dis 113:149, 1976

Pauwels R, Verschroegen G, Van der Stracten M: IgE antibodies to bacteria in patients with bronchial asthma. Allergy 35:665, 1980

Pullan CR, Hey EN: Wheezing, asthma, and pulmonary dysfunction 10 years after infection with respiratory syncytial virus in infancy. Br Med J Clin Res 284:1665, 1982

Roldaan AC, Masural N: Viral respiratory infections in asthmatic children staying in a mountain resort. Eur J Respir Dis 63:140, 1982

Smith CB, Overall JC: Clinical and epidemiologic clues to the diagnosis of respiratory infections. Radiol Clin North Am 11:261, 1973

Twiggs JT, Larson LA, O'Connell EJ, et al: Respiratory syncytial virus infection: Ten-year follow-up. Clin Pediatr 20:187, 1981

Weiss ST, Tager IB, Munoz A, et al: The relationship of respiratory infections in early childhood to the occurrence of increased levels of bronchial responsiveness and atopy. Am Rev Respir Dis 131:573, 1985

Welliver RC, Kaul TN, Ogra PL: The appearance of cell-bound IgE in respiratory-tract epithelium after respiratory-syncytial-virus infection. N Engl J Med 303:1198, 1980

Welliver RC, Kaul TN, Sun M, et al: Defective regulation of immune responses in respiratory syncytial virus infection. J Immunol 133:1925, 1984

Welliver RC, Wong DT, Middleton E Jr, et al: Role of parainfluenza virus-specific IgE in pathogenesis of croup and wheezing subsequent to infection. J Pediatr 101:889, 1982

Welliver RC, Wong DT, Sun M, et al: The development of respiratory syncytial virus-specific IgE and the release of histamine in nasopharyngeal secretions after infection. N Engl J Med 305:841, 1981

Zoch MS, Schnoll RP, Londou L I: Upper and lower airway hyperreactivity in recurrent croup. Am Rev Respir Dis 121:979, 1980

Gary Incaudo
M. Eric Gershwin

10

Aspirin and Related Nonsteroidal Anti-Inflammatory Agents, Sulfites and Other Food Additives as Precipitating Factors in Asthma

The progression of civilization has heralded a growing list of drugs and other chemicals capable of inducing asthmatic attacks or perpetuating a chronic asthmatic relapse in a susceptible host. The mechanisms by which these adverse reactions occur are as varied as the pathways bronchospasm is suspected to follow. For example, the use of beta blocking agents can enhance latent asthmatic potential or compound an ongoing asthmatic state, depending on the degree of beta-2 blocking activity of the individual drug in question. Similarly, immunologically and nonimmunologically mediated reactions triggered by antimicrobials and macromolecular agents such as vaccines, enzymes, allergenic extracts, and contrast media can induce asthma in an otherwise unaffected host as an accompaniment of an anaphylactic or anaphylactoid reaction. Other chemicals exist which have been shown to induce asthma in a subset of the asthmatic population by mechanisms which remain to be elucidated. ASA and related nonsteroidal anti-inflammatory agents, sulfites, and other food additives are examples in this regard and will serve as the focus for this chapter.

BRONCHIAL ASTHMA, Second Edition
ISBN 0-8089-1814-1

213

ASA IDIOSYNCRASY—A HISTORICAL PERSPECTIVE

Acetylsalicylic acid (ASA) was first synthesized in 1853 by the German scientist von Gerhardt and the clinical application of ASA in rheumatic fever was suggested in Europe in 1899. Reports of side effects such as urticaria, angioedema, and respiratory distress began to appear thereafter. In 1911, one year after ASA was released for use in the United States, the first report of a serious respiratory reaction appeared in the *Journal of the American Medical Association*. Dr. G. Burton Gilbert described the case of a 40-year-old Colorado Springs woman with a history of asthma who took 5 grains of ASA for a headache. She soon developed pruritis, angioedema, and dyspnea. Dr. Gilbert was the physician in attendance and applied cold compresses, injected codeine, epinephrine, and strychnine; he induced vomiting and gave a high enema with eventual recovery of his patient by the following morning. By 1919, enough adverse experience with ASA had accumulated to induce Robert Cooke to write that ASA represented the most common allergic drug reaction he had encountered. He reasoned that allergy was the most likely mechanism involved due to the character of the symptoms these patients experienced upon ASA ingestion and the accompanying peripheral eosinophilia.

The medical literature through the 1940s was marked by reports of adverse reactions to ASA, including some deaths. In addition, two distinct clinical syndromes of ASA intolerance began to emerge. One syndrome was primarily dermatologic, involving an urticarial and angioedematous response. The other syndrome was respiratory, involving primarily the aggravation of a pre-existing asthmatic state, although some upper respiratory symptoms were a common accompaniment. It appeared to be rare for a patient to experience both reactions simultaneously. In 1968, Samter and Beers expanded the definition of ASA intolerance by describing a subgroup of ASA-sensitive asthmatics who presented with a set of clinical findings consistent enough to warrant coining the term "ASA Hypersensitivity Triad." These authors described a clinical sequence of disease which almost invariably began as rhinitis of a vasomotor type, followed by eosinophilic hyperplastic rhinosinusitis, nasal polyposis, and eventually ASA-intolerant asthma.

Despite the fact that Cooke himself could not demonstrate skin test positive reactions in the ASA-sensitive individual, the presumed immunologically based origin to ASA sensitivity remained unchallenged for many years. In 1950, however, Matthews cast serious doubts on the allergic hypothesis. Matthews attempted to demonstrate some immunologic activity by skin testing normal ASA-free subjects, normal subjects receiving ASA, and ASA-sensitive asthmatics with ASA-containing serum from ASA-sensitive subjects, serum from ASA-sensitive subjects, and serum from normal subjects receiving ASA, respectively. In each of these circumstances, there were no significant differences between the reaction caused by the control serum and by the serum containing ASA. Likewise, in vitro attempts to demonstrate ASA-specific antibodies and ASA-induced histamine release and lymphocyte activation in blood samples in ASA-sensitive individuals were unrevealing. Further studies of mast cell mediator release by Stevenson and Wasserman could not support the hypothesis that ASA-induced reactions were an IgE-mediated phenomenon. By the 1970s, it became apparent that there existed little evidence to support an immunologic pathogenesis for ASA-induced asthma. Hence, Dr. Gilbert's original use of the term "idiosyncrasy" over 70 years ago re-emerged as the generally accepted description of these ASA-induced events.

POTENTIAL MECHANISMS OF HYPERSENSITIVITY TO NONSTEROIDAL ANTI-INFLAMMATORY DRUGS (NSAID)

The mechanism or mechanisms by which NSAID induce the respiratory hypersensitivity reaction remain clear. Samter has suggested that ASA intolerance is a "primary connective tissue disease" which enhances autonomic dysfunction of the airways through damaged peripheral receptors for bradykinin and related polypeptides. He hypothesized that ASA acts directly on those altered receptors, inducing bronchospasm exactly as the kinins do. Lasser has suggested that ASA may, in fact, activate the contact-kinin system, directly inducing bronchospasm. Some activation of the kinin system still remains as a viable explanation to ASA sensitivity and is currently being investigated.

The mechanism of the 1970s and 1980s most often put forward to explain the hypersensitivity to ASA-like compounds was the prostaglandin hypothesis. The metabolic pathways of arachidonic acid metabolism in the lung which lead to the generation of prostaglandins and other mediators of inflammation and which may be of relevance in ASA intolerance are shown in Figure 10-1. In 1971, Vane described the inhibition of prostaglandin biosynthesis by ASA and indomethacin, and suggested that the anti-inflammatory properties of these drugs came from the interruption of this pathway. In 1975 and 1976, Szcyeklik and Vane, respectively, suggested that the inhibition of prostaglandin biosynthesis may be responsible for the respiratory symptoms in ASA-sensitive patients.

Various sites of action for ASA have been postulated in the prostaglandin biosynthetic pathway whereby asthma may be induced and are shown in Figure 10-2. The original hypothesis of an imbalance between the bronchodilator PGE-2 and the bronchoconstrictor PGF-2α following ASA ingestion has not been verified. A shunt to the lipoxygenase pathway has also been

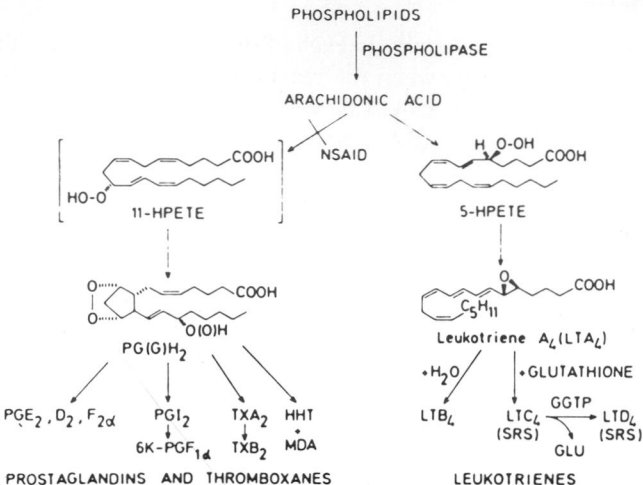

Fig. 10-1. Phospholipid-arachidonate metabolic pathways of probable relevance to aspirin sensitivity in respiratory diseases. Nonsteroidal anti-inflammatory drugs (NSAID) block cyclooxygenase pathways. (From Mathison DA, Stevenson DD, Simon RA: Precipitating factors in asthma: Aspirin, sulfites and other drugs and chemicals. Chest 87:50S, 1985. Used with permission.)

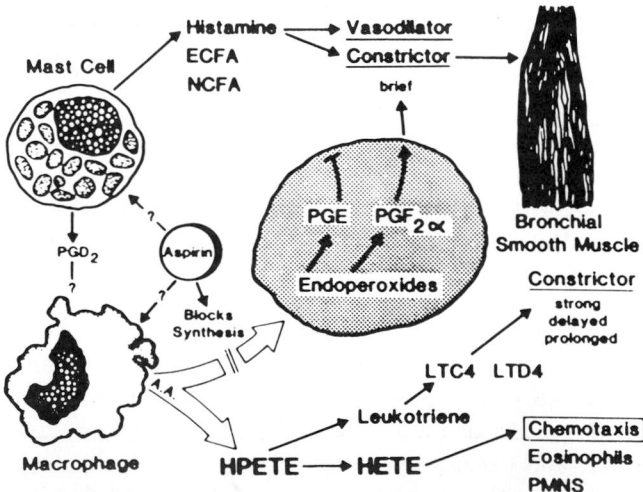

Fig. 10-2. Cellular and mediator pathways affecting bronchoconstriction and inflammation which may be of relevance to aspirin sensitivity in respiratory diseases. (From Mathison DA, Stevenson DD, Simon RA: Precipitating factors in asthma: Aspirin, sulfites and other drugs and chemicals. Chest 87:51S, 1985. Used with permission.)

216

suggested, since an induction of leukotrienes C4, D4, and E4 (slow-reacting substance of anaphylaxis) could theoretically follow. However, benoxaprofen, a NSAID which may inhibit the lipoxygenase pathway of arachidonate metabolism, does not block the ASA-induced reaction. Furthermore, the fact that ASA-sensitive asthmatics develop tolerance to repeated oral administration of ASA poses another problem for the shunt hypothesis, in that continued inhibition of cyclooxygenase should theoretically result in protracted asthma, not tolerance.

A role for other components of inflammation, such as complement, platelet factors, and mast cell mediators through prostaglandin influence, has been suggested. It is known that PGE inhibits the release of histamine and SRS-A from mast cells in the lung. Therefore, a block in PGE generation (e.g., by ASA) may enhance mast cell mediator release. Furthermore, antihistamines and the mast-cell-stabilizing drug cromolyn sodium have the ability to inhibit ASA- and indomethacin-provoked bronchoconstriction in some, but not all, ASA-sensitive patients. Studies to date have failed to demonstrate the presence of mast cell mediators such as histamine and neutrophil chemotactic factors following ASA challenge in sensitive patients. Attempts at measuring variations in complement and Platelet Factor IV have been equally unrewarding. Since the ability of ASA and other NSAID to inhibit cyclooxygenase in vitro correlates closely with the ability of these drugs to induce asthma in a susceptible host, it remains compelling to incriminate the prostaglandin system as the site of asthma induction. However, attempts at demonstrating a defect in the prostaglandin pathway in ASA-sensitive asthmatics remain inconclusive.

INCIDENCE

The prevalence of and clinical clues suggesting ASA intolerance have been extensively studied in adult populations (Table 10-1). The figures, however, vary with regard to the method by which ASA sensitivity is assigned. In general, statistics based on historical data assume a lower incidence than do those based on oral challenge verification. Using historical reviews, the incidence of adverse ASA reactions among a normal adult population is seen to be less than 1 percent. ASA sensitivity among adult asthmatic ranges from 3–7 percent according to historical data. In contrast, studies based on oral ASA challenges indicate that between 8 and 30 percent of asthmatics have ASA-induced asthma. Attempts at assessing the validity of historical data have demonstrated that up to 10 percent of adult asthmatics with no history of ASA intolerance will have a positive ASA challenge. Furthermore, up to 35 percent of asthmatics who are quite certain they have ASA intolerance prove to have a negative ASA challenge at a given point in

Table 10-1

Incidence of Aspirin Sensitivity in Asthma and Rhinosinusitis
Based on Oral ASA Challenge Studies

Age Group	Incidence
Childhood	
asthma < 10 yrs.	infrequent
asthma 10–20 yrs.	10%
Adulthood	
asthma only	8–30%
asthma and no history of ASA intolerance	10%
asthma, rhinosinusitis, and nasal polyposis	30–40%
asthma, rhinosinusitis, and a history of ASA sensitivity	60–85%
NARES syndrome without asthma	unknown

time. Reasons for the discrepancy in incidence figures are not clear. A potential refractory period may alter ASA challenge results if the study did not include an ASA-free time period prior to ASA challenge. There is also data to suggest a possible changing of ASA thresholds in an individual patient as a function of time. Among asthmatic subjects with nasal polyposis and pansinusitis, 30–40 percent prove to be ASA sensitive by challenge. Severity of asthma and corticosteroid dependency appear to be random features in the ASA-intolerant asthmatic. These data suggest that the presence of ASA sensitivity is often unsuspected and occasionally inconsistent in asthmatic patients. In addition, the concurrent presence of paranasal sinusitis and/or nasal polyposis emerges as the only clinical clue to the possible coexistence of ASA sensitivity among asthmatics.

ASA-induced asthma has been less well studied among pediatric patients than among adults (Table 10-1). The available data indicate that ASA sensitivity is as frequent in children over 10 years of age as it is in adult populations. Limited studies suggest that ASA idiosyncrasy is distinctly unusual in children less than 9 years old.

CLINICAL PRESENTATION

The incidence statistics suggest that ASA sensitivity evolves over decades (Table 10-2). The typical ASA-sensitive respiratory syndrome begins as a perennial vasomotor-irritant-aggravated rhinitis, although up to one-third of these patients have evidence of inhalant IgE-mediated disease by skin testing. Increasing nasal congestion and anosmia ensues, generally indicating the presence of hyperplastic mucosal disease with nasal polyposis. Purulent bacterial rhinosinusitis frequently complicates this stage of the illness, especially following upper respiratory tract viral infections. These same infectious

Table 10-2

Clinical Characteristics of ASA-sensitive Rhinosinusitis
and Asthma

1. Age of onset	>20 years
2. Rhinitis	vasomotor (>90%)
	concomitant allergic (approx. 20%)
3. Nasal cytology	Eosinophils (>90%)
	mast cells or basophils (>50%)
4. Sinus radiograph	abnormal (~90%)
5. Asthma	chronic severe (>60%)
	episodic (approx. 20%)
6. Reaction to ASA	nasal and ocular symptoms only (approx. 10%)
	"classic" response (>80%)
7. Cross-sensitivity	nonsteroidal anti-inflammatory agents (>50%)
	dyes, preservatives, flavor enhancers
	(uncertain)

events often herald the onset of a chronic cough as the first symptom of evolving asthma. Intrinsic asthma in its more characteristic form eventually appears. Treatment with corticosteroids almost invariably ensues. Fortunately, as with other forms of eosinophilic respiratory disease, these patients typically prove highly responsive to corticosteroid preparations, although dependency frequently develops.

The clinical expression of ASA sensitivity in asthmatic patients tends to be specific but inconsistent as a function of time and ASA exposure. The most characteristic clinical findings are the appearance of facial or generalized flush, ocular and nasal congestion, and acute and often severe bronchospasm within one-half to several hours following ingestion of a typical dose of ASA or a cross-reacting anti-inflammatory agent. Although dermatologic reactions to ASA such as urticaria and angioedema can occur, their association with adverse respiratory events is distinctly unusual. Limited data suggest that re-exposure to ASA may not predictably induce the same or even any adverse reaction, nor will avoidance of ASA have an effect on the underlying disease process or the likelihood of a repeat reaction on future ingestion.

Variations from the classic pattern of ASA idiosyncrasy have been described. There are individuals with asthma and ASA intolerance who do not demonstrate rhinosinusitis clinically and who do not experience rhinitis on ASA challenge. Lumry has reported that 12 percent of his asthmatic patients experienced a selective naso-ocular response to ASA administration without concurrent bronchospasm. The incidence of ASA sensitivity among patients with chronic eosinophilic nonallergic rhinitis (e.g., NARES) without asthma is unknown.

Physical and laboratory findings most characteristic of ASA sensitivity are related to the examination of the nasal mucosa and secretions. Boggy, pale mucosa is typically seen with a clear mucoid discharge unless secondary infection has intervened. Polypoid growths of white-grey coloration can often be found protruding anteriorly or posteriorly from the middle meatus. Microscopic examination of expelled secretions, or, more consistently, of nasal mucosal scrapings, reveals large numbers of eosinophils, both free within the mucous and embedded within the epithelial cells. Mucosal specimens also commonly demonstrate increased numbers of mast cells or basophils, a distinction which cannot be readily made morphologically using standard Wright-Giemsa staining. Spector and Farr have described the histologic and immunofluorescent findings in sinus tissue from asthmatics with chronic rhinosinusitis, over half of whom were ASA sensitive. The basement membranes of many specimens were thickened, with eosinophilic staining and the deposition of IgD. All tissues examined revealed intense staining for IgE and patchy deposition of IgG, IgA, and IgM. C-3 was also found within a mononuclear cell infiltrate. Their findings can be summarized as demonstrating a nonspecific intense immunologic responsiveness in the sinus tissues of patients with concomitant rhinosinusitis and asthma, the majority of whom were ASA sensitive.

A paranasal sinus radiograph is the only way to accurately define sinus involvement in asthmatic patients with ASA sensitivity. Abnormalities are most typically found in the ethmoid and maxillary sinuses and are best demonstrated on the Waters and Caldwell views. A spectrum of disease changes is seen—from mucosal thickening with or without polypoid shadowing to total opacification.

ASA CHALLENGE-DESENSITIZATION

Since a history of ingesting ASA with or without an adverse respiratory reaction is an unreliable predictor of an individual patient's present risk, an oral ASA challenge remains the "gold standard" for diagnosing ASA idiosyncrasy. The basic procedure for ASA challenge involves the administration of incrementally increasing dosages of ASA with the simultaneous assessment of respiratory symptoms and function. Criteria should also be established at the time of challenge with reference to disease stability and concomitant medications. Since life-threatening reactions to ASA ingestion can occur, challenges should be performed within a setting where emergency resuscitative equipment, an intensive care unit, and trained personnel are readily available. ASA challenges should be performed in the morning hours, so that optimal time and treatment are available to ensure full recovery from any untoward effects which may ensue.

The indications for ASA challenge are varied, but do not include the desire for simple verification or proof of the presence of ASA idiosyncrasy. This exclusion is based on two considerations. Although asthma induced by incremental ASA challenge has been readily controlled and no deaths have been reported in published series, the exacerbation of nasal and sinus disease may last for weeks. Secondly, Matheson has shown that there may be variation in an individual's response to ASA as a function of time. One patient he reported had, on four ASA challenges over a 9-year span, a "classical" oculo-nasal-asthmatic response on the first two challenges, no reaction on the third challenge, and only a nasal response following the fourth challenge. As has been demonstrated from other anaphylactoid reactions, the results of an individual challenge cannot always be used as an accurate predictor of future risks from drug ingestion.

On this basis, the ASA challenge is commonly reserved for research purposes or utilized in conjunction with a desensitization program, in which ASA or an ASA-like drug is necessary for a concomitant disease state. ASA-sensitive asthmatics with musculo-rheumatoid disease inadequately controlled by non-ASA-like drugs, or with vascular disease requiring an inhibitor of platelet aggregation-embolization, would clearly benefit from such an approach. In these circumstances, the individual physician should carefully assess whether the benefit achieved would outweigh the potential risk factors involved.

In Europe and Japan, ASA and NSAID challenge techniques have been developed using inhaled drug. In contrast, oral challenge procedures are used commonly in the United States. An example of an oral incremental ASA challenge-desensitization protocol is shown in Table 10-3. The minimum asthma stability criteria in this example are a symptom-free state for several days, or a FEV1 which is greater than 70 percent of predicted, or the best previously recorded value, at least reaching an absolute minimum of 1.5 liters in an adult. If need be, corticosteroids can be administered for several days prior to the challenge in order to achieve these minimums. All medications except antihistamines, inhaled or oral beta-adrenergic agents, and cromolyn sodium are continued before and during the challenge procedure. Signs and symptoms such as nasal-ocular pruritis, conjunctival injection, nasal congestion, ocular and nasal discharge, chest tightness, cough, and wheezing should be constantly monitored. Pulmonary functions such as FVC and FEV1 are recorded hourly—or sooner if clinically indicated.

The aggressiveness of the incremental dosing schedule should reflect the degree of ASA sensitivity expected. Some groups use two distinct dosage and time schedules with the common endpoint of 650 mg of ASA. In the first and most cautious schedule, asthmatic patients who have a history of a severe ASA reaction are challenged-desensitized over at least a 2-day period with ASA given at 3-hour intervals beginning with 3 mg, as shown. For asthmatic

Table 10-3
Procedure for Oral Aspirin Challenge/Desensitization

1. Asthma absent clinically for several days or a FEV1 >70% of predicted or the best previously recorded and >1.5 liters (adult).
2. Continue all medications except antihistamines, inhaled beta-adrenergic agents, and cromolyn sodium.
3. Administer ASA orally q3h as follows:

Time	Day 1	Day 2
0800 hours	3 mg	150 mg
1100 hours	30 mg	325 mg
1400 hours	100 mg	650 mg
1700 hours	end	end

4. Monitor symptom response continually and PFTs hourly.
5. Minimum criteria for a positive challenge:
   Naso-ocular: nasal and ocular congestion and discharge
   Asthmatic: ≥20% fall FEV1 from the baseline of the best of two consecutive FEMs
   Classical: dual occurrence of naso-ocular and asthmatic response
6. Symptomatic therapy of adverse response ensues after documentation.
7. Maintain desensitization indefinitely with 3–25 mg of ASA daily if desired or with another nonsteroidal anti-inflammatory agent at the desired therapeutic dosage.
8. A refractory period of 1–5 days will ensue after desensitization.

patients who do not present with a history of ASA sensitivity, a 1-day challenge can be safely performed by dosing at 2-hour intervals beginning with 30 mg. Data from Spector and Farr suggest that only patients who present with a history of asthma within 24 hours after ASA ingestion need be approached more cautiously. In their studies, patients with an uncertain history of ASA sensitivity proved no more likely to experience a positive ASA challenge than did those patients with a negative history of ASA idiosyncrasy.

The criteria by which one can judge a positive response can be formalized as shown in Table 10-3. In brief, an increase in nasal, ocular, and/or asthmatic symptoms within 3 hours of a test dose is considered a positive challenge. A positive naso-ocular response is the occurrence of nasal congestion, rhinorrhea, conjunctival injection, and conjunctival discharge. A positive asthmatic response is considered to be FEV1 fall of 25 percent from the baseline represented by the best of two consecutive forced expiratory maneuvers. A classical response is the dual occurrence of the naso-ocular and asthmatic reactions. A negative response is the absence of any subjective or objective findings as noted above. Questionable responses are best repeated with placebo in a double-blind fashion.

Adverse reactions are treated medicinally at the onset of symptoms. A naso-ocular response can be treated with oxymetazoline HCL 0.05 percent nasal spray, 2 sprays in each nostril, and a decongestant-antihistamine eyedrop repeated at 30-minute intervals until symptoms abate. Bronchospasm is promptly treated with inhaled beta-adrenergic agents such as metaproterenol (Alupent®) 0.2–0.3 cc in 2–3 cc of normal saline administered every 15–30 minutes until the FEV1 returns to baseline values. Additional doses of theophylline and corticosteroids can be administered, depending on the clinical status of the patient.

For any patient in whom desensitization is the ultimate goal, the challenge is resumed the following morning, provided baseline stability criteria are met. The starting dose should be that quantity of ASA which provoked the adverse reaction the previous day. Eight or more provoked reactions may be required before a state of desensitization is achieved. Desensitization is defined as the ability to ingest 650 mg of ASA without untoward effects. Refractoriness to the ill effects of ASA generally persists for 1–5 days. As little as 3–25 mg of ASA each day is sufficient to maintain the desensitized status indefinitely. As a general rule, if ASA therapy is suspended for more than 2 days, the patient should be desensitized before resuming treatment. If desensitization to another nonsteroidal anti-inflammatory agent is the ultimate therapeutic goal, that particular medication can be instituted at appropriate doses at this time.

CROSS-SENSITIVITY BETWEEN ASA AND OTHER CHEMICALS

Other nonsteroidal anti-inflammatory agents which inhibit the cyclooxygenase pathway of prostaglandin synthesis can also provoke a respiratory reaction in ASA-sensitive asthmatic subjects. In ASA-sensitive asthma, the potency of bronchospastic induction by an ASA-like agent appears to be directly related to the effectiveness of cyclooxygenase inhibition by that agent. For example, indomethacin is a very potent cyclooxygenase inhibitor. It follows that extreme ASA sensitivity in a subject will usually be accompanied by extreme indomethacin sensitivity (Table 10-4).

It has long been noted that in addition to the anti-inflammatory agents, several unrelated chemical substances can also produce bronchospasm in ASA-intolerant patients (Table 10-5). The most widely studied and still most controversial of these agents is tartrazine. Tartrazine is a coal-tar derivative with a chemical structure very different from that of ASA or indomethacin. It is used in the food industry as a coloring agent under the name of FD&C Yellow #5. Early authors estimated a 0–50 percent incidence of cross-reactivity with tartrazine in ASA-intolerant subjects. Most of the early reports of cross-reactivity between tartrazine and ASA in asthmatic subjects did not

Table 10-4
Relative Cyclooxygenase Inhibition

Agent	Inhibition of Cyclooxygenase IC_{50} (μ mol/l)
Acidic drugs	
Salicylates	
Aspirin	164
Salicylamide	no effect
Diflunisal	2
Polycyclic acids	
a) Indomethacin	0.10
Sulindac	no effect
Sulindac sulphide (metabolite)	2.2
b) Aryl aliphatic acids	
Naproxen	14
Fenoprofen	55
Diclofenac	0.2
Ibuprofen	50
c) Fenamates	
Mefenamic acid	0.25
Flufenamic acid	15
d) Acidic enols	
Phenylbutazone	148
Sulphinpyrazone	700
Nonacidic drugs	
Flumizole	0.10
Nictindole	6.0
Dictazole	540
Amindopyrine	1000
Dipyrone	500
Benzydamine	1000
Diftalone	no effect

employ double-blind placebo controlled methodology in all subjects. More recently, using controlled techniques, Spector found an incidence of 4 percent for tartrazine sensitivity among asthmatics at National Jewish Hospital by using doses up to 50 mg. In contrast, Mathison, using doses up to 75 mg in a double-blind fashion, could not find one tartrazine-positive challenge in over 100 ASA-sensitive asthmatics studied. The discrepancy in published information concerning possible cross-reactivity between ASA and tartrazine in respiratory disorders remains an enigma. Attempts to prove that tartrazine behaves pharmacologically as a "nonsteroidal anti-inflammatory drug" have failed. Suggested possible explanations include a biotransformation of tartrazine in some patients to an active ingredient which induces asthma in a susceptible host. A second possibility suggested by Samter is that the active asthmagenic factor in tartrazine is, in fact, a contaminant variably produced during the synthesis process. The FDA has identified 12 contaminants in the manufactured dye thus far. More double-blind studies are necessary, using a range of tartrazine doses, metabolic products, or contaminants to assess the contribution of tartrazine to asthma.

Conflicting concern has been raised about the relative asthma-inducing potentials of other azo and non-azo dyes, preservatives, and flavor enhancers added to foods. Case reports of potential asthma aggravation from many of these agents have appeared sporadically. The ingestion of monosodium glutamate, sodium benzoate, parahydroxybenzoic acid, parabens, butylated hydroxyanisole (BHA), butylated hydroxytoluene (BHT), potassium sorbate, and of dyes such as amaranth, ponceau, sunset yellow, brilliant blue, erythrosine, and indigotin has been incriminated anecdotally in this regard. Double-blind studies have confirmed up to a 2 percent incidence of adverse respiratory reactions among asthmatic patients, but only to the dyes erythrosine and ponceau and to the preservatives sodium benzoate and parahydroxybenzoic acid. Single-blind studies with monosodium glutamate challenge have suggested the existence of respiratory sensitivity to this flavor enhancer in a small subgroup of asthmatics. These patients are reported to be commonly sulfite-sensitive but infrequently ASA-sensitive, suggesting differing pathways of responsiveness (e.g., a reflex cholinergic response). In contrast to these reports, investigators such as Mathison, using blind controlled challenges, have been unable to confirm the existence of sensitivities to any of the azo and non-azo dyes, preservatives, or flavor enhancers in large populations of asthmatic patients.

The fact that some patients with ASA sensitivity can also experience an adverse reaction to acetaminophen (up to 6 percent) and to sodium salicylate suggests that some caution should be invoked in prescribing these agents to an asthmatic population. Dosages of as little as 37.5 mg of each of these drugs have induced significant bronchospasm in the few cases reported. In general, the more sensitive the asthmatic patient is to ASA, the more likely it is that that patient will experience an adverse reaction to a routine dose of acetaminophen or sodium salicylate. High-dose ASA responders, who are usually those with a negative history of ASA intolerance, and those patients with a negative ASA challenge, tend to not respond adversely to either of these drugs. The mechanism by which these substances produce bronchospasm, their incidence, and their exact relationship to ASA sensitivity and the prostaglandin system remain unknown.

The occurrence of salicylates as a natural or added ingredient in various foodstuffs has provoked some concern among clinicians regarding the question of whether dietary avoidance of salicylates should also be implemented in ASA-sensitive asthmatics. These naturally occurring salicylates and the synthetic salicylate alternatives such as choline salicylate and sodium salicylate lack the acetyl side chain of ASA, but are otherwise chemically similar.

Naturally occurring salicylates are found in almonds, fruits (especially apples, peaches, and plums), most berries, cucumbers, peppers, and the tomato/potato family. Salicylates appear as chemical additives in root beer, wintergreen flavoring, and some packaged cake and frosting mixes. In practice, cross-reaction between these forms of salicylates and ASA-provoked respiratory symptoms has not been demonstrated.

In contract to the case in ASA-sensitive asthma, there is some evidence to suggest a relationship between naturally occurring salicylates and urticaria, but studies to date have been inconclusive. Sodium salicylate has been reported to induce urticaria in up to 30 percent of patients with chronic idiopathic urticaria. However, the role of naturally occurring salicylates in inducing urticaria remains anecdotal and is usually tied to more complex diets which include avoidance of tartrazine and benzoates. Furthermore, some authors have argued that the role of salicylates in foods is most likely limited by the small quantities of salicylates which tend to occur naturally in foods. The role that natural salicylates play in chronic idiopathic urticaria remains controversial and in need of further study.

TREATMENT OF ASA SENSITIVITY

The treatment of ASA-sensitive asthmatics is not different from the many therapeutic approaches one might take to treat asthma in general. Vigorous treatment with bronchodilators and decongestants should be utilized as in any patient with "intrinsic" rhinitis and asthma. Allergy skin testing to help identify potential antigens for avoidance is helpful as a screening procedure. However, immunotherapy, if prescribed, is seldom beneficial in providing symptomatic relief. As with other forms of eosinophilic respiratory disease, corticosteroids are often particularly useful as therapeutic aids and should be utilized early in the treatment program.

One of the more important aspects of the treatment of aspirin-sensitive asthmatics is the recognition of their potential for developing the "Aspirin Hypersensitivity Triad" of clinical problems. Nasal polyps, sinusitis, corticosteroid use, and ASA intolerance are each associated with severe asthma and are, therefore, epiphenomena not necessarily causally related to each other. Nevertheless, the coexistence of the "ASA Hypersensitivity Triad" of clinical problems suggests that patients sensitive to aspirin should be constantly monitored for complicating nasal polyposis and sinusitis, if such are not already evident. Topical nasal corticosteroids such as flunisolide or beclomethasone should be utilized early in the course of the disease, if nasal symptoms are present, in an effort to retard as much polyp growth and preserve as much sense of smell as possible. Although short-term trials have demonstrated a beneficial effect from application of topical nasal corticosteroids in more than 80 percent of patients suffering from nasal polyps, the positive effect this action might have on the natural progression of rhinosinusitis and the need for surgical polypectomy are unknown. Sinus radiographs are nearly uniformly abnormal in aspirin-sensitive asthma, especially once nasal polyps are seen. Radiographs of the paranasal sinuses should be obtained routinely in all asthmatics once aspirin sensitivity is established or nasal polyposis is suspected, in order to assess the degree of sinus involvement and to help direct the aggressiveness of sinus therapy. The sinusitis is typically of an eosinophilic hyperplastic variety, occasionally complicated by a secondary bacterial component as paranasal sinus hygiene is interrupted. The early intervention with antibiotics such as amoxacillin with or without clavulanic acid, tetracycline in adults, or cefaclor should be utilized at the first sign of nasal purulence. Inadequate sinusitis treatment or unrecognized sinusitis in this clinical setting will commonly lead to management difficulties for the accompanying asthma.

Patients with recurrent bacterial sinusitis and nasal polyposis may benefit from surgical removal of the polyps and exteriorization of the sinus cavities in order to enhance proper oxygenation and to provide an avenue for drainage of infected secretions. Topical or parenteral corticosteroids are not a proper substitute for surgical intervention. Rather, these medications are aimed at preventing the formation of polyps and obstructive sinusitis and reducing the frequency of surgical requirements. Reports of asthma being provoked by nasal polypectomy have been cited as a reason to avoid surgical intervention in these cases. In fact, the onset of rhinitis and sinusitis commonly antedates the onset of asthma as a natural course of this disease by months or years. Many investigators feel that it is this natural history of aspirin-sensitive asthma which has led to what is accurately acknowledged as a coincident occurrence of asthma following polypectomy rather than as a true cause-and-effect relationship.

Aspirin avoidance should be recommended to all patients with asthma, especially those with nasal polyposis, rhinosinusitis, or a history of an adverse reaction to aspirin ingestion. A true conscientious effort must be made to avoid aspirin, since over 500 prescription and over-the-counter medications approved for use in the United States contain aspirin. Patients should be instructed to carefully inspect the ingredients listed before purchasing any medications and to ingest only those medications with which they are familiar. Keeping a reference list of aspirin-containing medications provides a false sense of security, since continual updating would be required for true accuracy because of the laxity of governmental control of this medication.

In 1980, Stevenson observed that two patients who had undergone ASA desensitization and continued ASA treatment experienced improvement in their respiratory symptoms. This preliminary observation led to further studies to define the efficacy of ASA treatment in ASA-sensitive asthmatics.

Current data suggest that a significant, but not necessarily indefinite, improvement in rhinosinusitis can be induced in these patients by means of ASA. Two-thirds of ASA-sensitive patients on continuous ASA therapy have reported a subjective improvement in symptoms and required less topical corticosteroids accordingly. Some patients, however, have experienced even greater respiratory symptoms and have consequently been unable to maintain a state of desensitization. The effect of ASA maintenance therapy on asthma stability has been less favorable. In general, patients on maintenance therapy have not experienced statistically significant benefits as judged by pulmonary function testing and concurrent corticosteroid needs, although the subjective data are more encouraging. The role of ASA therapy in ASA-sensitive asthmatics remains experimental and cannot be recommended as a means of disease control at this time.

SULFITING AGENTS (Table 10-5)

Recent studies indicate that as many as 5–10 percent of all asthmatic patients (or from 500,000 to 1,000,000 U.S. citizens) may have some degree of sulfite sensitivity. These figures are based upon a variety of good clinical studies. For example, Sheppard et al., by use of inhalation of sulfur dioxide, have demonstrated conclusively that all asthmatic subjects experience bronchoconstriction after inhalation exposure of from 1 to 5 ppm of sulfur dioxide. The mechanism for this reaction has been shown to be a direct stimulation of parasympathetic afferent receptors in the bronchi by inhaled sulfur dioxide. Whether or not sulfur dioxide is first converted to soluble sulfite in the bronchial mucosal fluid has not been determined in experimental models. Furthermore, other chemicals, such as histamine, are also able to stimulate this nonselective reflex. Yet because of studies in normal subjects, it has been assumed that sulfites are among "safe" chemicals. The Food and Drug Administration has consequently not restricted their use in food and drink other than to prohibit sulfites in certain meats that are a food source of vitamin B_6. This policy, however, is currently coming under intense scrutiny.

In the absence of a ructation and sulfur dioxide formation in the pharynx, the rapid onset of an asthmatic attack after capsule ingestion of sulfite suggests that absorption through gastric mucosa and formation of a sulfite load in the plasma are critical factors in presenting the bronchial mucosa with high concentrations of sulfite radicals. It is tempting to postulate that parasympathetic afferent receptors are the major or exclusive asthmagenic pathway, whether or not HSO_3 or sulfur dioxide is the stimulating agent. In recent studies, 1 mg/ml of atropine (inhaled) appears to protect asthmatic patients from asthmatic attacks after ingestion of sulfite loads previously demonstrated to be asthmagenic. If the suggestions above represent the mechanism

Table 10-5
Maximum Quantity of Sulfur Dioxide in Foods

Food	Maximum Amount of SO_2 (mg/kg)
Beer	25
Cider	200
Cheese mixture and paste	300
Cordials	230
Dyhydrated peas	1000
Dehydrated vegetables (other)	500 to 1500
Fruit juices and soft drinks	115
Gelatine	1000
Glucose—syrup and solid	300
Pickles	750
Raw potatoes (whole, peeled, or sliced)	50
Sausages (and sausage meat)	525
Vinegar	25
Wine	300

of sulfite-sensitive asthma, why do fewer than 10 percent of all asthmatic subjects develop asthma after sulfite ingestion? Special studies of this subgroup suggest that an alternative mechanism may be present. Using fibroblast tissue-culture assays from sulfite-sensitive asthmatics, the presence of sulfite oxidase enzyme has been found to be substantially reduced compared to its presence in normal control patients and in sulfite-insensitive asthmatic subjects. This has been the case in all sulfite-sensitive asthmatic patients to date, suggesting that this enzyme is the critical step in distinguishing these patients.

These data suggest that the vulnerability of sulfite-sensitive asthmatic subjects rests in their enzymatic inability to rapidly clear a sulfite load. Although they have some enzyme activity, the level is insufficient to protect them from the effects of ingestion of large quantities of sulfite, even though they can adequately clear the sulfite generated from their own metabolic sources. By implication, such a theory suggests that the subgroup of sulfite-sensitive asthmatic subjects has parasympathetic bronchial receptors that are at least similar to those of other asthmatic subjects. At least one distinguishing difference, therefore, is their putative inability to prevent HSO_3 from accumulating in bronchial mucosa.

Both the route of sulfite administration and the quantity are important variables when considering asthma provocation potential. Simon and Goldfarb were unable to provoke asthma in sulfite-sensitive asthmatic patients via the subcutaneous route by use of quantities of sulfites found in the usual doses of aqueous epinephrine and common local anesthetics. These dosages, however, were below the asthma-provoking oral dose of sulfite. Concentrations higher than 5–10 mg administered subcutaneously caused intense local pain and thereby usually precluded the administration of larger doses of sulfite. In contrast, Stevenson and Simon were successful in provoking asthma in some subjects using 1–5 mg of sulfite administered subcutaneously. Furthermore, Baker and Allen have reported that the intravenous injection of sulfites can cause severe and immediate asthmatic attacks in sensitive patients.

In a recently published study, Schwartz and Chester presented data demonstrating that sulfite solutions of 5 mg/ml routinely generate 1.2 ppm of sulfur dioxide during standard aerosolization. Eight asthmatic patients with a history suggestive of sulfite sensitivity and 6 patients with positive single-blind oral ingestion sulfite challenges were studied. The authors demonstrated that each of the six latter patients experienced asthma within minutes after inhaling 0.5–5 mg of sulfite solutions. These data support the earlier work of Goldfarb and Simon and of Koepke and associates and further demonstrate the universal cross-reactivity of sulfite sensitivity by inhalation in those asthmatic subjects previously demonstrated to be sulfite-sensitive by ingestion challenge. The subset of asthmatic subjects who react to sulfite when it is presented in an oral capsule is also sensitive to aerosol inhalation at very low concentrations of sulfites. However, a dose-response relationship comparing oral and inhaled sulfite stimulation was not observed in these patients. The most "sensitive" patients by oral challenge were not the most sensitive by inhalation challenge, leaving unclear the significance of and the relationship between these 2 methods of sulfite administration.

REFERENCES

AAAI and NIAID: Adverse reactions to foods. V. Adverse food reactions that do not involve allergic reactions. NIH Publication No. 84:2442, 1984

Baker GD, Collett P, Allen DH: Bronchospasm induced by metabisulfite-containing foods and drugs. Med J Austr 2:614, 1981

Baker GJ, Allen DH: The spectrum of metabisulphite induced asthmatic reactions; their diagnosis and management. Thor Soc Austr 12:213, 1982

Chaff FH, Settipane GA: Aspirin intolerance. I. Frequency in an allergic population. J Allergy Clin Immunol 53:193, 1974

Code of Federal Regulations: Title 21, Food and Drugs parts 10 to 199. Office of the Federal Register, General Services Administration, U.S. Government Printing Office, Washington, D.C., 1976

Dehove RA: La Reglementation des Produits Alimentaires et Non-alimentaires. Paris, Commerce-Editions, 7e ed. 1970

Freedman BJ: Asthma induced by sulphur dioxide, benzoate and tartrazine contained in orange drinks. Clin Allergy 7:407, 1977

Freedman BJ: Sulphur dioxide in foods and beverages: Its use as a preservative and its effect on asthma. Br J Dis Chest 74:128, 1980

Giraldo B, Blumenthal MN, Spink WW: Aspirin intolerance and asthma: A clinical and immunological study. Ann Intern Med 71:479, 1969

Goldfarb F, Simon RA: Provocation of sulfite sensitive asthma. J Allergy Clin Immunol 73:135, 1984 (abstr)

Guill MF, Jamieson D: Metabisulfite reactions on the rise. Allergy Observer 1:5-1, 1984

Hollingsworth HM, Downing ET, Braman SS, et al: Identification and characterization of neutrophil chemotactic activity in aspirin-induced asthma. Am Rev Respir Dis 130:373, 1984

Juhlin L, Michaelson G, Zetterstrom O: Urticaria and asthma induced by food-and-drug additives in patients with aspirin hypersensitivity. J Allergy Clin Immunol 50:92, 1972

Koenig JQ, Pierson WE, Horike M, et al: Bronchoconstrictor responses to sulfur dioxide or sulfur dioxide plus sodium chloride droplets in allergic, nonasthmatic adolescents. J Allergy Clin Immunol 69:339, 1982

Koepke JW, Christopher KL, Chaie H, et al: Dose dependent bronchospasm from sulfites in isoetharine. JAMA 251:2982, 1984

Koepke JW, Selner JC, Dunhill AL: Presence of sulfur dioxide in commonly used bronchodilator solutions. J Allergy Clin Immunol 72:514, 1983

Lockey RF, Rucknagel DL, Vanselow NA: Familial occurrence of asthma, nasal polyps and aspirin intolerance. Ann Intern Med 78:57, 1973

Mathison DA, Stevenson DD: Aspirin sensitivity in rhinosinusitis and asthma. Immunology and Allergy Practice 5:340, 1983

Mathison DA, Stevenson DD: Hypersensitivity to non-steroidal anti-inflammatory drugs: Indications and methods for oral challenges. J Allergy Clin Immunol 64:569, 1979

Mathison DA, Stevenson DD, Simon RA: Precipitating factors in asthma: Aspirin, sulfites and other drugs and chemicals. Chest 87:50S, 51S, 1985

Moneret-Vautrin DA, Andre C: Immunopathologie de l'Allergie Alimentaire et Fausses Allergies Alimentaires, Paris, Masson, 1983, p. 187

Noid HE, Schulze TW, Winkelman RK, et al: Diet plan for patients with salicylate induced urticaria. Arch Dermatol 109:866, 1974

Ough CS: in Branen L, Davidson P (eds): Sulfur Dioxide and Sulfites in Antimicrobials in Foods. New York, Marcel Dekker, 1983, p. 117

Pleskow WW, Chinoweth WE, Simon RA, et al: The absence of detectable complement activation in aspirin sensitive asthmatic patients during aspirin challenge. J Allergy Clin Immunol 72:462, 1983

Pleskow WW, Stevenson DD, Mathison DA, et al: Aspirin-sensitive rhinosinusitis/asthma: Spectrum of adverse reactions to aspirin. J Allergy Clin Immunol 71:574, 1983

Prenner BM, Steven JJ: Anaphylaxis after ingestion of sodium bisulfite. Ann Allergy 37:180, 1976

Rachelefsky GS, Coulson A, Siegel SC, et al: Aspirin intolerance in chronic childhood asthma: Detected by oral challenge. Pediatrics 56:443, 1975

Samter M, Beers RF: Intolerance to aspirin: Clinical studies and consideration to its pathogenesis. Ann Intern Med 68:975, 1968

Schwartz HJ: Sensitivity to ingested metabisulfite—variations in clinical presentation. J Allergy Clin Immunol 71:487, 1983

Schwartz HJ, Chester EH: Bronchospastic responses to aerosolized metabisulfite in asthmatic subjects: Potential mechanisms and clinical implications. J Allergy Clin Immunol 74:511, 1984

Settipane GA, Chafee FH, Klein DE: Aspirin intolerance. II. A prospective study in an atopic and normal population. J Allergy Clin Immunol 53:200, 1974

Settipane GA, Pudupakkham RK: Aspirin intolerance. III. Sub-types, familial ocurrence, and cross-reactivity with tartrazine. J Allergy Clin Immunol 56:215, 1975

Sheppard D, Wong WS, Uehara CF, et al: Lower threshold and greater bronchomotor responsiveness of asthmatic subjects to sulfur dioxide. Am Rev Respir Dis 122:173, 1980

Simon RA, Green L, Stevenson DD: The incidence of sulfite sensitivity in an asthmatic population. J Allergy Clin Immunol 69:118, 1982 (abstr)

Simon RA, Pleskow W, Kaliner M, et al: Plasma mediator studies in aspirin-sensitive asthma: Lack of a role for the mast cell. J Allergy Clin Immunol 71:146, 1983

Spector SL, Farr RS: Aspirin idiosyncrasy: Asthma and urticaria, in Middleton E, Reed CE, Ellis EF (eds): Allergy Principles and Practice. Chapel Hill, SC, The C.V. Mosby Company, 1983, p. 1249

Spector SL, Wangaard CH, Farr RS: Aspirin and concomitant idiosyncracies in adult asthmatic patients. J Allergy Clin Immunol 64:500, 1979

Stevenson DD, Pleskow WW, Simon RA, et al: Aspirin-sensitive rhinosinusitis asthma: A double-blind crossover study of treatment with aspirin. J Allergy Clin Immunol 73:500, 1984

Stevenson DD, Simon RA: Sensitivity to ingested metabisulfites in asthmatic subjects. J Allergy Clin Immunol 68:26, 1981

Stevenson DD, Simon RA: Sulfites and asthma. J Allergy Clin Immunol 74:469, 1984

Szczeklik A, Gryglewski RJ, Czerniawska-Mysik G, et al: Relationship of inhibition of prostaglandin biosynthesis by analgesics to asthma attacks in aspirin-sensitive patients. Br Med J 1:67, 1975

Szczeklik A, Nizankowska E, Nizankowska R: Bronchial reactivity to prostaglandins F_2, E_2 and histamine in different types of asthma. Respiration 34:323, 1977

Tan Y, Collins-Williams C: Aspirin induced asthma in children. Ann Allergy 48:1, 1982

Twarog FJ, Leung DYM: Anaphylaxis to a component of isoetharine (sodium bisulfite). JAMA, 248:2030, 1982

Weber RW, Hoffman M, Raine DA, et al: Incidence of bronchoconstriction due to aspirin, azo dyes, non-azo dyes, and preservatives in a population of perennial asthmatics. J Allergy Clin Immunol 64:32, 1979

Yunginger JW, O'Connell EJ, Logan GB, et al: Aspirin induced asthma in children. Pediatrics 92:218, 1973

Manuel Lopez
John Salvaggio

11

Air Pollution and Asthma

There have been a number of incidents in which severe atmospheric pollution resulting from thermal inversion over industrial areas has been associated with dramatic epidemics of respiratory illness and death. Among the most notorious were those occurring in the Meuse Valley, Belgium (1930); in Donora, Pennsylvania (1948); in London (1952 and 1962); and in New York (1953). The epidemic affecting London and adjacent counties in 1952 was by far the most dramatic. Dense fog enshrouded the city for the 5 days of December fifth through the ninth, during which the temperature was unusually cold. The number of house calls made by family physicians and the number of emergency hospital admissions showed increases of 100–150 percent over the figures normally registered for that time of the year. The death rate for the week ending December 13th showed a similar increase, and overall some 3500–4000 deaths in excess of the norm appeared to be directly attributable to the extreme degree of atmospheric pollution. All age groups were affected. Those above 45 years of age proved to be disproportionately vulnerable (mortality was increased 1.2 times). A particularly high mortality rate was observed in those already disabled by chronic respiratory or cardiac disease. The greatest rise in mortality was associated with bronchitis; certified deaths from this cause increased 8–10-fold compared with the immediately preceeding weeks.

BRONCHIAL ASTHMA, Second Edition
ISBN 0-8089-1814-1

Throughout the 1952 London inversion, atmospheric samples were analyzed daily for their content of smoke particulates and sulfur dioxide. Levels as high as 4.5 mg/m^3 and 1.3 ppm were recorded in some parts of London, and mean concentrations increased seven- to nine-fold. Normal levels were rapidly restored as soon as the fog lifted. The epidemiologic data linking severe air pollution with acute dysfunction of the airways were convincing, and complemented earlier observations made in the Meuse Valley and Donora when concurrent sampling of the atmosphere was not carried out. Although sulfur dioxide concentrations in London reached levels known to be irritative, no attempt was made to incriminate any one specific pollutant as the major provoking factor. The concentrations of both gaseous sulfur dioxide and of particulate smoke showed similar increases, and it seemed probable that the concentrations of all constituent pollutants of the atmosphere had increased in proportion.

Two questions are crucial to the present discussion: Were asthmatic subjects disproportionately represented among those affected? Did their symptoms consist of increased asthma, or were other symptoms or organ systems involved? These questions are not easily answered, for in an epidemic with an appreciable mortality, the minority who are dangerously ill and quickly saturate the health services available provide most of the statistics. It is clear that within this minority in London, the elderly and the infirm were far more conspicuous than were those who were primarily asthmatics. One family practice, celebrated for keeping meticulous records, was able to report that among children (at least) asthmatics were no more affected than were nonasthmatics. It was precisely children, however, who were the least affected overall. A retrospective study of the Donora incident showed that 88 percent of the asthmatic population developed respiratory symptoms, as compared with 43 percent of the general population. It is not evident whether respiratory symptoms were essentially asthmatic or bronchitic in nature. Any distinction is perhaps academic, since the criteria commonly used to identify asthma (airway obstruction that is at least partially reversible) may be applied equally to many cases of "bronchitis."

Less prolonged and severe episodes of acute air pollution have also been associated with significant exacerbations of asthma as measured by emergency room visits or diary records, but correlations were not strong, and this association has not been confirmed by all investigators. It seems possible that cold ambient temperature alone might have been more relevant—a confounding variable not assessed in all studies. Diary records are a sensitive means of monitoring asthmatic attacks of mild-to-moderate severity; only unduly severe attacks influence statistics derived from emergency rooms, house calls, or hospital admissions. The corollary is that aggravating factors of asthma, a disease of high prevalence but low mortality, are unlikely to be recognized from mortality statistics unless they are extremely potent. It is particularly relevant that reports specifically linking deaths from asthma to episodes of air pollution are very uncommon.

RESPIRATORY DISEASE ASSOCIATED WITH CHRONIC AIR POLLUTION

In addition to the relation between acute increases in air pollution and exacerbations of asthma, it appears that some communities chronically exposed to relatively high levels of air pollution show both an increased prevalence of asthma (or bronchitis) and an unusually high frequency of exacerbations. There are many triggering factors in asthma, and many confounding variables have to be considered when longitudinal comparative studies are performed between different communities. In the industrial Kanto plain of Japan, an increased prevalence of cough with airway obstruction was noticed among U.S. military personnel when compared with U.S. servicemen based elsewhere, implying that the responsible factor was environmental rather than genetic. No obvious local allergen could be incriminated, and persistently high levels of air pollution seemed to be the most probable explanation. The disorder became known as Tokyo-Yokohama respiratory disease rather than asthma, largely because industrial pollutants rather than allergens appeared to be responsible, and because cigarette smokers rather than atopic individuals were predominantly affected. In most cases a change in environment brought prompt and lasting recovery, however. Several conclusions can be drawn from these early studies concerning the acute and chronic effects of air pollution. There can be little doubt from clinical and epidemiologic evidence that rapidly developing high levels of air pollution contribute to the morbidity of asthma. Very high levels have been associated with marked increases in mortality from respiratory failure, although acute bronchitis or pneumonia rather than asthma was the usual cause of death, and asthmatic subjects were not disproportionately represented among the dying. Less severe degrees of air pollution have a less certain effect on asthma. Not all epidemiologic studies from mildly polluted environments indicate an excessive asthmatic problem, and when such was demonstrated there were a number of possible confounding variables which were not assessed and which might have been quite relevant—particularly the effect of cold ambient temperature. Recent advances in the understanding of bronchial hyperreactivity suggest that many different factors may both trigger acute asthmatic exacerbations and increase nonspecific bronchial hyperreactivity. The prevalence of asthma and the triggering of exacerbations may thus depend upon complex interactions between many environmental factors. It seems likely that air pollution will prove to be an important factor contributing to these interactions, even if the effect of a given pollutant acting in isolation is comparatively minor.

PHYSICAL AND CLIMATIC CONSIDERATIONS

The Normal Atmosphere

The mixture of gases we call the atmosphere moves with relative ease but in complex patterns over the face of the earth. Except for slight variations in trace components, the composition of dry air is uniform to an altitude of about 50 miles. Nitrogen, oxygen, and argon are the most abundant atmospheric gases, and they constitute 78, 21, and 1 percent by volume, respectively. All other components are minor, and their concentrations are usually expressed in parts per million (ppm). Carbon dioxide is the most abundant of the minor gases. Its concentration averages about 320 ppm. The amount of water vapor in the atmosphere is highly variable. It depends upon geographic location, nearness of water bodies, wind direction, and ambient temperature. It ranges from 0.02 percent (200 ppm) in arid regions to as much as 6 percent (60,000 ppm) in warm, humid climates. The water vapor content of air is generally measured as a percentage of the saturation vapor pressure of water at that temperature and is expressed as percent relative humidity. Other gases present in the earth's atmosphere include helium, neon, methane, krypton, oxides of nitrogen, hydrogen, xenon, and ozone. Their combined contribution to the atmosphere is only 0.004 percent.

Movement of the atmosphere over any given point depends upon two major climatic factors. Differences in barometric pressure from zone to zone produce wind and horizontal flow, while the sun's radiant heat causes vertical flow by convection as the lowest layers of the atmosphere are warmed by the earth's surface. Sometimes, relatively cold layers of the atmosphere are trapped below higher, warmer layers (a thermal inversion), which interrupts the process of vertical flow. If this coincides with widespread stability of barometric pressure, marked atmospheric stagnation results. In an industrial area, high levels of air pollution rapidly follow. These circumstances were responsible for the epidemics described earlier.

The Polluted Atmosphere

Air pollution may be defined as the atmospheric accumulation of substances, usually manmade, to a degree that becomes detrimental to humans, animals, or plants. Pollution is commonly referred to as smog: a combination of the words "smoke" and "fog". There are two main types of pollution.

Industrial smog, the dominant type in large industrialized areas such as New York and Tokyo, results from the combustion of solid or liquid fossil fuels. Photochemical smog, the second type, accumulates in areas such as Los Angeles, with a high density of automobiles and adequate sunlight to permit photochemical reactions. These two types of pollution are not mutually exclusive, and frequently both are present in a given area at the same time. The levels of air pollution are affected by many weather conditions, but the more important meteorologic factors leading to the accumulation of pollutants are temperature inversions, which limit vertical dispersion of pollutants, and low wind velocity, which hinders their horizontal dispersion.

Classification of Pollutants by Physical Characteristics

GASES

Polluted atmospheres are generally associated with man's industrial and domestic activities. Table 11-1 shows typical concentrations of pollutants found in contaminated areas. It can be seen that the proportions of pollutants in polluted air as compared to clean air range from fractional to a thousand-fold.

Carbon monoxide is usually the product of incomplete combustion of carbon and its compounds. It is emitted from fossil fuel combustion in greater quantities than are all other pollutants combined. Though large amounts of carbon dioxide are generated in the same way, this is not generally considered an air pollutant, since it is a normal constituent of clean air. Hydrocarbons are

Table 11-1

Comparison of Trace Gas Concentrations in Clean and Polluted Air[a]

	Clean Air (ppm)	Polluted Air (ppm)	Ratio of Polluted-to-Clean Air
CO	0.1	40–70	400–700
CO_2	320	400	1.3
CH_4	1.5	2.5	1.3
NO_x	0.001	0.2	200
O_3	0.02	0.5	25
SO_2	0.0002	0.2	1000
NH_3	0.01	0.02	2

[a] Adapted from Urone P: The primary air pollutants—gaseous, their occurrence, sources, and effects, in Stern AC (ed): Air Pollution. I. Air Pollutants, Their Transformation and Transport, 3rd ed. New York, Academic Press, 1976, pp. 23–75.

compounds of hydrogen and carbon. They comprise paraffins, olefins, acetylenes, and aromatics. In themselves, the hydrocarbons in air have relatively low toxocity. They are of concern because of their photochemical activity in the presence of sunlight and oxides of nitrogen. Reactions between these produce photochemical oxidants, of which ozone is the most important. These oxidants, which also include peroxyacyl nitrate, are responsible for the plant damage and eye irritation associated with smog. More than 60 hydrocarbons have been identified in smog, most having been emitted from the combustion of oil and gasoline. The total number is possibly much larger, but such a determination is limited by the sensitivity and selectivity of analytical methods. Oxygenated hydrocarbons, like hydrocarbons, include an almost infinite number of compounds. They comprise alcohols, phenols, ethers, aldehydes, ketones, esters, peroxides, and organic acids. Their major sources of emission are automobiles and, to a lesser extent, solvents from chemical, paint, and plastics industries. They are also formed as secondary products from photochemical smog.

Nitrogen forms seven different oxides, though only three, nitrous oxide (N_2O), nitric oxide (NO), and nitrogen dioxide (NO_2) are found in appreciable quantities. The latter two are often analyzed together and referred to as "nitrogen oxides" (NO_x). Nitric oxide is a colorless, odorless, and tasteless gas. As a pollutant, is produced largely by fuel combustion. In Los Angeles smog, nitric oxide levels reach a maximum during the early morning traffic rush hours. The rising sun initiates a series of photochemical reactions which convert nitric oxide to nitrogen dioxide. Within a few hours, nitrogen dioxide reaches a maximum concentration, after which it reacts photochemically to produce ozone (O_3) and other oxidants. At much higher altitudes, ozone is formed naturally by photochemical reactions involving molecular and atomic oxygen.

Sulfur forms a number of oxides, but only sulfur dioxide (SO_2) and sulfur trioxide (SO_3) are of importance as gaseous air pollutants. Sulfur dioxide is a colorless gas with a pungent, irritating odor. Most people can detect it by taste at 0.3–1 ppm. In clean air, it oxidizes slowly to sulfur trioxide. It is oxidized more readily by atmospheric oxygen in aqueous aerosols. In moist air, and in the presence of nitrogen oxides, hydrocarbons, and particulates, sulfur dioxide reacts much more rapidly. Today, sulfur dioxide is one of the major atmospheric pollutants in the United States. Fossil fuel combustion is the main source of emission.

Airborne particulate matter arises from both viable and nonviable sources. Viable particulates are derived primarily from pollens, microorganisms, insects, and the dusts from farming activities. Their respective sizes are given in Table 11-2. Nonviable particulate matter is present in sizes that range from those of small molecules to those of dust particles that are visible

Table 11-2
Size Range of Viable Particulates[a]

Particulate	Stokes' Diameter (μm)
Viruses	0.015–0.45
Bacteria	0.3–15
Fungi	3–100
Algae	0.5
Protozoa	2–10,000
Moss spores	6–30
Fern spores	20–60
Pollen grains	10–100
Plant fragments, seeds, insects, etc.	100+

[a] Adapted from Edmonds RL: in Benninghoff WS, Edmonds RL (eds): Ecological Systems Approaches to Aerobiology Ecology. Ann Arbor, University of Michigan, 1972, pp. 6–11.

to the naked eye. The chemical composition of nonviable particulate matter depends on the local source—industrial combustion of fuel, commercial or domestic furnaces, incinerators, soil dusts, exhaust emissions, and other point sources. The following definitions are used to describe the dispersal of nonviable atmospheric particulates.

Aerosol: This is a dispersion of solid and/or liquid particles of microscopic size in a gaseous medium. The following are all specific examples of aerosols.

Dust: This is a dispersion of solid particles whose size (predominantly greater than 1 μm) allows temporary suspension only in air or other gases.

Fog: This is a visible aerosol in which the dispersed phase is a liquid. Formation by condensation is implied.

Fumes: These are a dispersion of solid particles generated by condensation from the vapor state.

Mist: This is a dispersion of liquid particles, many of which are large enough to be visible to the naked eye.

Smog: This is a mixture of smoke and fog, the former being the result of industrial pollution, the latter of natural climatic factors.

Smoke: This is a dispersion of small particulates resulting from combustion of organic material.

Classification of Pollutants by Physiologic Effects

ASPHYXIANTS

Asphyxiants exert their effects by interfering with the oxidation of tissue. Simple asphyxiants are physiologically inert gases that act by dilution of atmospheric oxygen. Examples are nitrogen, helium, and methane. Chemical asphyxiants or poisons interfere with the delivery or absorption of oxygen from the alveoli, and with its release or utilization in the tissues. Examples include hydrogen sulfide, which causes respiratory paralysis by its action on the nervous system, carbon monoxide, which has greater affinity for hemoglobin than does oxygen, analine, which forms methemoglobin, and hydrogen cyanide, which inhibits tissue oxidation by combining with cytochrome oxidase.

IRRITANTS

Irritant materials may provoke reflex bronchoconstriction by stimulating irritant receptors located in the upper airways. They may also act as corrosives; that is, they inflame and denude mucosal surfaces of the respiratory tract. Their concentration in polluted air is of far greater importance than is the duration of exposure. The solubility of an irritant compound is the most important factor in determining its site of action. Highly soluble materials are quickly absorbed and affect primarily the upper respiratory tract. Examples include ammonia, alkaline dusts, hydrogen chloride, and hydrogen fluoride. Compounds of intermediate solubility, such as ozone and the halogens, affect both the upper respiratory tract and the gas-exchanging tissues. Poorly soluble gases, such as nitrogen dioxide and phosgene, affect primarily the alveoli.

SENSITIZERS

Agents capable of producing an immunologic response are usually foreign proteins. Most are derived from plant, fungal, or animal sources, though more simple chemically reactive agents, such as toluene diisocyanate trimellitec anhydride and formaldehyde, may also induce sensitization in the airways, presumably by acting as haptens or by altering respiratory tract proteins and creating so-called neoantigens.

Deposition and Clearance of Inhaled Particulates

Most suspended particles are removed from inspired air and deposited in the respiratory tract. The site and mechanism of their deposition depends largely upon their size. Particles larger than 10 μm are almost all deposited in the nose, pharynx, and larynx. Most pollen grains falls into this category. Some 30 percent of particles 5 μm in diameter enter the trachea. They are deposited in roughly equal proportions in the airways and alveolar spaces. The inertial forces of these relatively large particles are maximal in the trachea and main bronchi where air flow is greatest, and as a result their deposition in the larger airways occurs by impaction. As the airways divide and their total cross-sectional area increases, air flow and particle inertia decrease. Sedimentation consequently becomes a more important mechanism of deposition as these particles penetrate more deeply into the lung and become less important with respect to provoking asthma. Smaller particles have less inertia than do larger particles, and tend as a result to enter the trachea more readily. They are deposited by sedimentation or even by diffusion in the smaller airways or alveoli. Diffusion becomes the chief means of deposition when particle diameter is less than 0.5 μm, and the alveoli become the main site of deposition.

Once deposited on the walls of the tracheobronchial tree, insoluble particulates are removed by the mucociliary escalator. In normal subjects, clearance is rapid, being quickest in the central airways. Camner and colleagues found the overall biologic half-life of 6-μm particles to be 1–2 hours. A number of factors may impair clearance, and these could play a role in potentiating the effect of asthma-provoking particulates. Narrowing of the airways itself causes increased numbers of particles to be deposited in the central larger airways, while slowed movement is to be expected of the thick, tenacious mucus so characteristic of acute asthmatic attacks. In addition to these unavoidable endogenous factors, cigarette smoke, sulfur dioxide, nitrogen dioxide, and ozone have all been shown to impair mucociliary transport either in humans or in experimental animals. Cigarette smoke is likely to prove the most important factor in such impairment, since the deleterious effects induced by the pollutant gases in laboratory animals required unnaturally high exposures to those gases. On the other hand, minor exposure to cigarette smoke may actually increase mucociliary transport.

SPECIFIC POLLUTANTS

Sulfur Dioxide

Sulfur dioxide is highly soluble in water and is thus readily dissolved in the secretions of the upper respiratory tract. It is also highly reactive, and, with water, generates sulfuric acid. With mild ambient exposure, preferential deposition in the upper respiratory tract protects the alveoli. With more massive exposure, the gas-exchanging tissues are likely to be affected as well as the airways. In one unfortunate industrial accident, sulfur dioxide was accidentally released into a tank in which two maintenance engineers were working. Although they were able to climb out before being overcome, both died of respiratory failure within 5 minutes. Autopsy examination revealed extensive sloughing of the airway mucosa and hemorrhagic alveolar edema. Two other employees working in the vicinity, and a fireman, were exposed to lesser concentrations and all survived. The one with the greatest exposure showed evidence of mild airway obstruction as soon as measurements of lung function could be made. He subsequently developed severe, irreversible obstruction. The one least exposed developed no sequelae, while the third showed normal lung function initially, but subsequently developed mild irreversible airway obstruction.

Sulfur dioxide is present in the air of urban areas as a result of the combustion of solid and liquid fuels. Its atmospheric concentration may average from 0.01 to 0.1 ppm, with occasional peaks of from 1 to 1.5 ppm, such as were rated at the high of the London smog episode in 1952, when concentrations averaging 1.34 ppm over a 48-hour period were detected.

Laboratory experiments in animals have demonstrated increased airways resistance and suppression of mucosal ciliary activity following sulfur dioxide exposure. Nadel and colleagues showed that the mechanism of increased airway resistance in humans is the result of reflex bronchoconstriction, mucosal edema, and increased bronchial secretions. However, these changes occur with concentrations highly irritant to nasal mucosal tissue concentrations, that are from 5 to 10 times the observed levels even in the most polluted areas. Ambient concentrations of sulfur dioxide of less than 1 ppm rarely produce adverse effects. Sheppard and coworkers have shown that asthmatics are more sensitive to the bronchoconstrictor effects of sulfur dioxide than are nonasthmatics. Several recent studies have demonstrated that asthmatics may experience significant bronchospasm if they exercise heavily while exposed to sulfur dioxide at a concentration simulating that experience during ambient pollution episodes (0.5 ppm); stopping the exercise alone reverses the bronchospasm. The amount of bronchoconstriction is not only related to the sulfur dioxide concentration, but is also affected by the amount of exercise, the route of inhalation (nasal or oral), and the degree of airway hyperreactivity.

Epidemiologic studies have implicated sulfur dioxide in the aggravation of respiratory illnesses. The study of Levy and colleagues in a Canadian industrial city demonstrated a significant correlation between ambient sulfur dioxide levels and hospital admissions provoked by acute respiratory illnesses (children) or acute exacerbations of chronic respiratory diseases (adults). The strength of the association was seen to vary inversely with the distance of the particular hospital from the industrial area of the city. The authors speculated that air pollution produced effects on the airways which were additive to those induced by cigarette smoking, and that in chronic bronchitis (at least) both factors were roughly of equal importance. Similar conclusions were reached by Chapman an colleagues in 1973 from epidemiological studies in Utah, Idaho, New York City, and Chicago. Zerdberg an collaborators studied 84 asthmatic patients and found an increased incidence of asthma on days characterized by high sulfate levels. Similar results were obtained by Cohen in a group of asthmatics exposed to pollution from coal-fueled power plants and by Girsh and coworkers, who found an increased asthma rate in children on days of high pollution in Philadelphia. Other studies by Derrick have not been able to correlate sulfur dioxide air levels with asthma symptoms. In general, in these epidemiologic studies it is impossible to separate the effect of other pollutants, so that any correlations found between sulfur dioxide and asthma do not necessarily imply a direct cause-and-effect relationship.

While gaseous sulfur dioxide is predominantly deposited in the upper airways because of its high solubility, sulfur dioxide adsorbed to particulate pollutants is likely to penetrate more deeply. The latter condition (sulfur dioxide absorbed to particulate pollutants) as compared to gaseous sulfur dioxide is perhaps more relevant in city smogs. Scott concluded from his experiences with London fogs that high levels of both particulates and sulfur dioxide were necessary to produce an appreciable effect.

One might conclude that although the sulfur dioxide level in ambient air is commonly used as an index of air pollution, sulfur dioxide is not usually the constituent chiefly responsible for the respiratory sequelae that follow. Sulfur dioxide may, however, make a significant contribution to the overall effect of air pollution when it acts in concert with other air pollutants or viral infections.

Particulates

Particulate pollutants that are suspended in ambient air are generally the product of combustion of fossil fuels, although in industrial zones other particulates are emitted, depending upon the specific industrial process. Because of this, particulates are usually generated along with sulfur dioxide, and variations in ambient concentrations of these two pollutants closely parallel one another. The exact composition of the particulate mixtures varies, as does particle size, although most suspended particles are respirable. They comprise principally mixtures of carbon, soot, and tar; oxides of iron, aluminum, and silicon; sulfates and phosphates; and a variety of organic compounds. Analyses of atmospheric samples conventionally record total concentrations of suspended particles without making an attempt to distinguish component fractions. Particulate pollutants can cause direct adverse effects on the bronchial tree or can act as carriers for other pollutants. It is difficult to separate the effects of inert particles from those of other pollutants, such as sulfur dioxide, that originate from the same source and may have related actions. Cederlof attempted to explain the higher morbidity in London as compared to Scandinavia on the basis of higher inert dust levels, since concentrations of sulfur dioxide were similar in both areas.

Smoke generated from accidental fire may produce hazardous pollutants, depending largely upon the materials burned. Plastics in particular may generate toxic or asphyxiant gases. Particulates may become coated by aldehydes or acids from dissolved oxides of sulfur and nitrogen, and these are chiefly responsible for the irritative effect noted in the upper airways and eyes; they may also induce bronchospasm in asthmatics. Whether repeated exposure to the combustion products of accidental fires (as occurs occupationally in firemen) carries an appreciable risk of asthma or chronic airway obstruction is a matter of controversy. Cigarette smoking is, in any event, a more important threat to airway function, even in firemen, than is smoke from accidental fires.

Photochemical Smog

Photochemical smog is produced by ultraviolet irradiation from sunlight acting on either hydrocarbons or on nitrogen oxides generated from automobile exhaust emissions, which produce ozone, nitric oxide, and other oxidants. These oxidants act on organic substances present in the atmosphere, producing organic radicals that eventually degrade into carbon dioxide, carbon monoxide, water, and ozone. The net result of these reactions is the so-called photochemical smog characteristic of cities with warm and sunny weather and a large number of automobiles.

Ozone

Ozone is the main component of photochemical oxidants and may contribute up to 90 percent of the total oxidant level. According to Jaffe, eye irritation is experienced with levels of 0.1–0.2 ppm. Concentrations of 0.2–0.5 ppm reduce visual acuity, and levels of 0.3–1 ppm cause coughing, choking sensations and severe fatigue.

Exposure of laboratory animals to relatively high concentrations of ozone (0.5 ppm and above) has been shown to produce a variety of anatomic and physiologic effects after a few hours, particularly in the respiratory bronchioles and alveoli. Type I pneumocytes degenerate and are replaced by Type II cells. The latter tend to proliferate and assume a cuboidal form—a nonspecific and common pattern of lung injury at the gas-exchanging level. In addition, macrophage function and mucociliary clearance may become impaired, and an increased susceptibility to infection has been demonstrated.

Pulmonary edema may also occur, and some laboratory animals show high mortality rates when exposure is prolonged for several weeks. In such an experimental setting, ozone has less dramatic effects on the conducting airways (as compared to the above described effects on the aveoli). Of considerable relevance to asthma, however, was the demonstration in dogs that 2-hour exposure to ozone at a concentration of 0.5–1.2 ppm produced increased bronchial reactivity to inhaled histamine. Vagal blockade with atropine or by cooling inhibited this increased reactivity, implying reflex mediation. In half the animals, hyperreactivity persisted for over 24 hours. These important observations have since been confirmed by Golden and Nadel in human volunteers who were exposed for 2 hours to ozone at 0.5–0.6 ppm. The investigators remarked that such a concentration of ozone has been noted in the atmosphere of Los Angeles, though only at times of severe pollution. In six of the eight subjects tested, bronchial reactivity returned to normal after 14 hours, but in the other two, significantly increased responses persisted for over a week. By contrast, in none of the subjects was there a significant effect on baseline (pre-histamine challenge) airway function. In an interesting follow-up study, this induction of bronchial hyperreactivity by ozone was found to be unrelated to atopy.

Human studies by Young and associates, as well as by Goldsmith and Nadel, have demonstrated that exposure of normal subjects to ozone at a concentration between 0.6 and 0.8 ppm produces mild decreases in forced expiratory volume and an increase in airway resistance; Linn and colleagues concluded that exposure to low concentrations of ozone had no detectable physiologic effect on either normal or asthmatic patients. Studies by Folinsbee et al. have shown no significant effect on lung function of healthy volunteers following exposure to 0.2 ppm ozone for 2 hours every day for 5 days. Repeated daily exposures to moderate (0.35 ppm) and high concentrations of ozone (0.5 ppm) were, however, associated with significant degrees of airway obstruction, being greater after the higher dose and maximal on Day 3. Virtually no effect was demonstrated on Day 5. There appears to be a short-term cumulative effect of exposure to ozone on pulmonary function, followed by adaptation. Several conclusions may be drawn from these studies. Exposure to low concentrations of ozone (below 0.2 ppm) appears to be well tolerated by healthy as well as asthmatic individuals. Single exposures of 2–3 hours to concentrations of ozone between 0.2 and 0.8 ppm may induce mild degrees of airway narrowing, which persist for less than 24 hours, and significant increase in bronchial hyperreactivity, which may persist longer. These changes may be observed in normal subjects, but can be expected to be more marked in asthmatics. Exposures to higher concentrations can produce significant changes in pulmonary function, but such concentrations are not likely to be experienced by humans under natural conditions, even during exceptional levels of air pollution. With repeated daily exposures to ozone, a cumulative airway obstruction effect is seen, which reaches its peak after 2–3 days. Thereafter, an adaptive response becomes dominant, and little, if any, immediate effect is evident clinically after 5 days. This is not to say that such repeated exposures are without risk. Adaptation is not synonymous with tolerance, as Mustaffa and Tierney point out, and in subjects who are not fully tolerant, ongoing deleterious effects could occur in the absence of significant airway response.

A possible synergistic interaction between ozone and other air pollutants has been the subject of some controversy over recent years. In 1975, Hazucha and Bates reported that a mixed exposure to ozone (0.37 ppm) and sulfur dioxide (0.37 ppm) produced significant reductions in air flow rates which were not observed after identical exposures to each pollutant separately. Supportive evidence for synergy was reported by Last and Cross in 1978 from biochemical studies of rats exposed to ozone and aerosols of sulfuric acid, while Frolich and colleagues demonstrated increased susceptibility to streptococcal pneumonia when laboratory animals were exposed to both ozone and nitrogen dioxide. In human experiments, however, neither Bell and colleagues nor Bedi and colleagues were able to confirm synergy between ozone and sulfur dioxide, as measured by changes in ventilatory function. Exposure techniques were not identical in all studies, however, and in some of the human volunteers there may have been pre-existing adaptation to the effects of ozone.

Nitrogen Dioxide

Nitrogen oxides are important constituents of automobile exhaust emissions and of tobacco smoke. They are precursors of ozone under conditions favorable for photochemical reactions. Nitrogen dioxide is usually found in urban atmospheres in concentrations less than 1 ppm. Its principal toxic effect as an air pollutant is due to its oxidizing action in photochemical smog. The most widely recognized toxic effect of high concentrations of nitrogen dioxide is the pulmonary disorder produced in farmers working in silos (silo filler's lung). Concentrations of nitrogen dioxide in silos that provoke this disorder are characteristically on the order of hundreds of ppm. The effects of such high concentrations are manifested mostly at bronchiolar and alveolar levels mainly by potentially life-threatening bronchiolitis and pulmonary edema rather than asthma. Complete recovery often follows, though bronchiolitis obliterans or pulmonary edema may occur, and a few occupational deaths result directly from asphyxia.

It is extremely uncommon for nitrogen dioxide concentrations in ambient air to exceed 1 ppm, and in practice the assumed biologic threshold of approximately 0.5 ppm is rarely encountered in nonoccupational settings. The epidemiologic evidence that ambient concentrations of nitrogen dioxide of this order can induce disease of the airways in humans is related to two particular sources of this gas. In the late 1960s, Shy and colleagues reported that schoolchildren living near a nitrogen chemical plant in Chattanooga had both an excess of respiratory illnesses and a significant (though mild) reduction in air flow rates when compared with children living in control areas not contaminated with excess atmospheric nitrogen dioxide. Average nitrogen dioxide concentrations in the contaminated areas were estimated to be 0.08 ppm, and it was peak exposures of 0.15 ppm that were associated with the excess of respiratory illnesses. In 1977, Melia and colleagues noted a similar excess of respiratory illnesses in British schoolchildren who lived in homes where gas rather than electricity was used for cooking. Subsequent studies in Britain and the United States indicate that this domestic source of nitrogen dioxide may raise ambient indoor levels 4–6-fold, though mean levels averaged over 24 hours rarely exceed 0.05 ppm. Nevertheless, the study by Speizer and colleagues involving 6 U.S. cities confirmed that these modest levels were associated with significantly increased risks of respiratory illness and airflow impairment in young children—though of a comparatively minor degree. These associations do not prove a causal relationship, and it remains conceivable that other environmental factors were relevant. Experiments by Davison and coworkers, who exposed rabbits to high concentrations (8–12 ppm) of nitrogen dioxide, induced airway obstruction in these animals. Prolonged exposure may produce bronchiolitis or an emphysema-like picture, illustrating that permanent damage may be induced by inhalation of nitrogen dioxide. It may be emphasized, however, that the concentration of nitrogen dioxide used in these experiments was much higher than the levels in ambient air even with marked degrees of air pollution. In studies involving human subjects, Kerr and colleagues exposed 20 patients with asthma and chronic bronchitis and 10 normal subjects to nitrogen dioxide, 0.5 ppm, for 2 hours in an experimental chamber. Asthmatics developed a significant but mild degree of air trapping, but no significant increase in airway resistance. Orehek and colleagues confined their study to 20 subjects with mild asthma and exposed them for 1 hour to 0.2 ppm nitrogen dioxide. Three developed marked increase in airway resistance, while 13 showed increased bronchial reactivity to inhaled carbacol.

The latter is perhaps the more interesting observation, since it illustrates further the potential importance of interactions between seemingly unrelated environmental triggers in asthma. In this respect, the studies of Utell and colleagues are particularly interesting. They first showed that short-term atmospheric exposures to particulate nitrates had no demonstrable effect on airway function in either normal healthy subjects or asthmatics. They then showed that, with spontaneous influenzal infections in 11 otherwise healthy adults, challenge with sodium nitrate aerosols (but not sodium chloride aerosols) did provoke significant reductions in airway conductance.

Ambient air normally contains a number of oxides of nitrogen, of which nitrogen dioxide and nitrous oxide are by far the most important. Since nitrogen oxide tends to be converted spontaneously to nitrogen dioxide, it is not easy to separate the individual effects of each gas, nor is there much point in doing so. Both gases are soluble in water, though not markedly, and this generates nitrous and nitric acid. It is perhaps not surprising that inhaled particulate nitrates seem to produce effects similar to those of nitrogen dioxide itself. From these and other studies, it appears that in the relatively low concentrations found in urban areas, it is doubtful that nitrogen dioxide has a direct effect on airway resistance. Its possible synergistic relationship with other pollutants and allergens in aggravating asthma remains to be clarified.

Allergens

The relevance of airborne allergens to asthma is discussed more fully elsewhere in this book. It deserves emphasis in this section also because this type of atmospheric contamination may be responsible for exacerbations of asthma of severe degree and of epidemic proportions. The pioneering studies of Blackley in Britain in the 19th century were the first to demonstrate close relationship of seasonal attacks of rhinitis and asthma to concentrations of airborne pollens—especially grass pollens. Grass pollens also contribute to the antigen load of summer air in North America, but ragweed pollen and mold spores of many species provide a greater threat than do grass pollens to atopic subjects. Epidemics of asthma in the city of New Orleans are most easily attributed to natural inhalant allergens acting in seasonal patterns, since the asthmatic population involved is typically atopic, and since the times of peak admissions to hospitals are seasonal and correlate well with high levels of viable particulates and high fungal spore counts. It is interesting that the most severe epidemics occur at times of unusually cold ambient temperature and of atmospheric stagnation. There may consequently be important interactions between climatic and botanic factors.

In more localized environments, many other naturally occurring airborne allergens may be responsible for asthmatic exacerbations in susceptible individuals—particularly those allergens derived from house dust, animals, and insects. In occupational settings, many equally potent, though less natural, allergens may be encountered as described in Chapter 14. Their effects may be experienced well beyond the workplace, not only because the response pattern induced is often one of "late" asthma, but also because a single exposure may provoke ongoing nocturnal exacerbations for several days. Furthermore, these late asthmatic responses may increase the nonspecific reactivity of the bronchi to other triggering factors. This phenomenon was first recorded in 1962, when Sweet described a case in which asthmatic attacks were provoked by house dust and barn dust during convalescence from occupationally induced isocyanate asthma, but not at other times. Several investigators have since measured the degree of bronchial reactivity both before and at intervals after bronchial inhalation challenge testing with occupational agents. Bronchial reactivity increased significantly in subjects showing late reactions to pyrolysis fumes from polyvinyl chloride, dimethyl ethanolamine, Western red cedar, grain, and isocyanates. Thus, airborne allergens, like industrial pollutants, can both provoke asthma directly and increase susceptibility to other triggering factors.

PREVENTIVE MEASURES

From the foregoing discussion, it is clear that air pollution in concentrations found in urban areas can cause irritation of the respiratory tract and may provoke bronchoconstriction. Asthmatic patients as a group are more susceptible to the effects of air pollution than are normals. Air pollutants may also increase bronchial hyperreactivity and hence induce a temporary vulnerability of asthmatic patients to other environmental agents. Several preventive measures could be adopted to reduce the effects of air pollution in asthma. The most obvious involve reducing the emissions of manmade pollutants. Much has been achieved in this respect in recent years, as illustrated by the dramatic abolition of London fogs. High-quality, low-sulfur-bearing coals (e.g., from Colorado) produce less pollution than does coal from, for instance, Appalachia. The electricity generated in a single coal-burning power station can supply domestic heating needs with much less air pollution than can coal-burning fires in each individual home. Sulfur can be removed from oil before it is refined, and the resulting petroleum fuels can be used as alternative, cleaner sources of energy. Atomic power offers the prospect of even purer air, though at a risk some would consider unacceptable. Industrial emissions may be filtered before release, and their site of release can be controlled to some extent by tall chimneys. At a more domestic level, the catalytic converters of modern automobiles diminish the exhaust emissions of hydrocarbons and oxides of nitrogen.

An additional prophylactic approach for the asthmatic subject troubled by air pollutants requires the collaboration of the news media. Several television and radio stations already broadcast data regarding local atmospheric pollen counts and pollution levels, and all give regular meteorological reports. If asthmatics were specifically warned when local climatic conditions were likely to cause rapid increases in pollution levels, they could take advantage of a number of simple preventive measures. Concentrations of air pollutants are much reduced indoors as compared with concentrations in ambient outdoor air, and these concentrations can be diminished further by the use of mechanical filters associated with air conditioning systems or electrostatic precipitators. When the vulnerable asthmatic is obliged to leave a protected indoor environment, a personal respirator could be used. Although face-fit is never perfect with these inexpensive respiratory protection devices, they are reasonably effective and comfortable for short periods of time. Social custom is perhaps the greatest objection to their use in ordinary, albeit polluted, urban environments. More convenient, and probably equally effective, is the obvious and simple measure of increasing appropriate medication prophylactically.

The Weather and Air Pollution Committee of the American Academy of Allergy has published the following guidelines for asthmatic individuals during air pollution episodes:

1. Avoid unnecessary physical activity.
2. Avoid smoking and smoke-filled rooms.
3. Avoid exposure to dusts and other irritants, such as hairsprays and other sprays, paint, exhaust fumes, smoke from any fire, or other fumes.
4. Avoid exposure to persons with colds and respiratory infections.
5. Try to stay indoors in a clean environment. Air conditioning may be helpful, if available, as may charcoal filters and electrostatic precipitators.
6. If it appears that the air pollution episodes will persist or worsen, it may be desirable to leave the polluted area temporarily until the episode subsides.
7. The physician should consider formulation of specific instructions to be followed by the patient in case of an air pollution alert. The patient should know what medication to use, when to call the physician, and when to go to a hospital.
8. The physician's special guidelines should be kept on an instruction sheet in a readily accessible place.

REFERENCES

Bedi JF: Human exposure to sulfur dioxide and ozone: Absence of a synergistic effect. Arch Environ Health 34:233–239, 1979

Bell KA, Lin WS, Hazucha M, et al: Respiratory effects of exposure to ozone plus sulfur dioxide in Southern Californians and Eastern Canadians. Am Indust Hyg Assoc J 38:696–706, 1977

Bethel RA, Epstein J, Sheppard D, et al: Sulfur dioxide-induced bronchoconstriction in freely breathing, exercising, asthmatic subjects. Am Rev Respir Dis 128:987–990, 1983

Boushey HA, Holtzman MJ, Sheller JR, et al: Bronchial hyperreactivity, Am Rev Respir Dis 121:389–413, 1980

Bryant DH, Burns MW: The relationship between bronchial histamine reactivity and atopic status. Clin Allergy 6:373–381, 1976

Camner P, Helstrom PA, Philipson K: Carbon dust and mucociliary transport. Arch Environ Health 26:294–296, 1973

Cederlof R, Friberg L, Johnson E: Morbidity in uniovular twins in relation to smoking habits and residence: Primary report. Nord Hyg Tidskr 45:71–75, 1984

Chapman RS, Shy CM, Finklea JF, et al: Chronic respiratory disease in military inductees and parents of school children. Arch Environ Health 27:138–142, 1973

Cockroft DW, Ruffin RE, Frith PA, et al: Determinants of allergen-induced asthma: Dose of allergen, circulating IgE antibody concentration, and bronchial responsiveness to inhaled histamine. Am Rev Respir Dis 120:1053–1058, 1979

Coffin DL, Stokinger HE: Biological effects of air pollutants, in Stern AC (ed): Air Pollution. II. The Effects of Air Pollution. 3rd ed. New York, Academic Press, 1976, pp. 232–360

Cohen AA, Bromberg S, Benchley RW, et al: Asthma and air pollution from coal fueled power plant. Am J Public Health 62:1181–1188, 1972

Davidson JT, Lillington GA, Hydon GB, et al: Physiologic changes in the lungs of rabbits continuously exposed to nitrogen dioxide. Am Rev Respir Dis 95:790–796, 1967

Dawson SV, Schenker MB: Health effects of inhalation of ambient concentrations of nitrogen dioxide. Am Rev Respir Dis 120:281–292, 1979 (editorial)

Derrick EH: A comparison between the density of smoke in the Brisbane air and the prevalence of asthma. Med J Aust 2:670–675, 1970

DeVries K, Goeli JT, Booij-Noord H, et al: Changes during 24 hours in the lung function and histamine hyperreactivity of the bronchial tree in asthmatic and bronchitic patients. Intern Arch Allergy Appl Immunol 20:93–101, 1962

Edmonds R, Findlay JG, Gardner DE: Effects of repeated exposures to peak concentrations of nitrogen dioxide and ozone on resistance to streptococcal pneumonia. J Toxicol Environ Health 5:631–642, 1979

Edmonds RL: in Benninghoff WS, Edmonds RL (eds): Ecological Systems Approaches to Aerobiology Ecology. Ann Arbor, University of Michigan, 1972, pp. 6–11

Empey DW, Laitinene LA, Jacobs L, et al: Mechanisms of bronchial hyperreactivity in normal subjects after upper respiratory tract infection. Am Rev Respir Dis 113:131–139, 1976

Folinsbee LJ, Bedi JF, Horvath SM: Respiratory responses to humans repeatedly exposed to low concentrations of ozone. Am Rev Respir Dis 121:431–439, 1980

Girsh LS, Shubin E, Dick C, et al: A study on the epidemiology of asthma in children in Philadelphia: The relation of weather and air pollution to peak incidence of asthmatic attacks. J Allergy 39:347–357, 1967

Golden JA, Nadel JA, Boushey HA: Bronchial hyperirritability in healthy subjects after exposure to ozone. Am Rev Respir Dis 118:287–294, 1978

Hackney JD, Linn WS, Bailey MM, et al: Time course of exercise induced bronchoconstriction in asthmatics exposed to sulfur dioxide. Environ Res 34:321–327, 1984

Hazucha M, Bates DV: Combined effect of ozone and sulfur dioxide on human pulmonary function. Nature 257:50–51, 1975

Hetzel MR, Clark TJH: Does sleep cause asthma? Thorax 34:749–754, 1979

Horvath SM, Gliner JA, Matsen-Twisdakem JA: Pulmonary function and maximum exercise responses following acute ozone exposure. Aviat Space Environ Med 50:901–905, 1979

Jaffe LS: The biological effects of photochemical air pollutants on man and animals. Am J Public Health 57:1269–1275, 1967

Kerr HD, Kulle TJ, McIlhany ML, et al: Effects of nitrogen dioxide on pulmonary function in human subjects: An environmental chamber study, U.S. EPA report, April 1978, Washington, D.C., U.S. Government Printing Office, 1978

Kirkpatrick MB, Sheppard D, Nadel JA, et al: Effects of the oronasal breathing route on sulfur dioxide-induced bronchoconstriction in exercising asthmatic subjects. Am Rev Respir Dis 125:627–631, 1982

Last JA, Cross CE: A new model for health effects of air pollutants: Evidence for synergistic effects of mixtures of ozone and sulfuric acid aerosols on rat lungs. J Lab Clin Med 91:328–339, 1978

Levy D, Gent M, Newhouse MT, et al: Relationship between acute respiratory illness and air pollution levels in an industrial city. Am Rev Respir Dis 116:167–173, 1977

Linn WS, Buckley RD, Spier CE, et al: Health effects of ozone exposure in asthmatics. Am Rev Respir Dis 117:835–843, 1978

Linn WS, Shamoo DA, Venet T, et al: Comparative effects of sulfur dioxide exposures at 5°C and 27°C in exercising asthmatics. Am Rev Respir Dis 129:234–339, 1984

Linn WS, Venet TG, Shamoo DA, et al: Respiratory effects of sulfur dioxide in heavily exercising asthmatics. Am Rev Respir Dis 127:278–283, 1983

Melia RJW, Florey C du V, Altman DG, et al: Association between gas cooking and respiratory disease in children. Br Med J 2:149–152, 1977

Mortality and morbidity during the London fog of December 1952. Report on public health and medical subjects, 95. London, Her Majesty's Stationery Office, 1954

Mustafa MG, Tierney D: Biochemical and metabolic changes in the lung with oxygen, ozone and nitrogen dioxide toxicity. State of the art. Am Rev Respir Dis 118:1061–1090, 1978

Nadel JA, Salem H, Tamplin B, et al: Mechanism of bronchoconstriction during inhalation of sulfur dioxide. J Appl Physiol 20:164–167, 1965

Orehek J, Gayrard P, Smith AP, et al: Airway response to carbahol in normal and asthmatic subjects: Distinction between bronchial sensitivity and reactivity. Am Rev Respir Dis 115:937–943, 1977

Orehek J, Massari JP, Gayrard P, et al: Effect of short-term, low-level nitrogen dioxide exposure on bronchial sensitivity of asthmatic patients. J Clin Invest 57:301–307, 1976

Phelps HW: Follow-up studies in Tokyo-Yokohama respiratory disease. Arch Environ Health 10:143–147, 1965

Salvaggio J, Seabury J, Schoenhardt EA: New Orleans asthma. V. Relationship between Charity Hospital asthma admission rates, semi-quantitative pollen and fungal spore counts, and total particulate aerometric sampling data. J Allergy Clin Immunol 48:96–114, 1971

Schoettlin CE, Landau E: Air pollution and asthmatic attacks in the Los Angeles area. Public Health Reports 76:545–548, 1961

Selzer FE, Ferris B, Bishop YMM, et al: Respiratory disease rates and pulmonary function in children associated with nitrogen dioxide exposure. Am Rev Respir Dis 121:3–10, 1980

Sheppard D, Saisho A, Nadel JA, et al: Exercise increases sulfur dioxide induced bronchoconstriction in asthmatic subjects. Am Rev Respir Dis 123:486–491, 1981

Shy CM, Creason JP, Pearlman ME, et al: The Chattanooga school children study: Effects of community exposure to nitrogen dioxide. II. Incidence of acute respiratory illness. J Air Pollut Control Assoc 20:582–588, 1970

Shy CM, Goldsmith JR, Hackney JD, et al: Health effects of air pollution. Am Thorac Soc News 4:22–63, 1978

Smith TJ, Peters JM, Reading JC, et al: Pulmonary impairment from chronic exposure to sulfur dioxide in a smelter. Am Rev Respir Dis 116:31–39, 1977

Sweet LC: Toluene di-isocyanate asthma. Univ Mich Med Center J 34:27–29, 1968

Urone P: The primary air pollutants—gaseous, Their occurrence, sources, and effects, in Stern AC (ed): Air Pollution. I. Air Pollutants, Their Transformation and Transport, 3rd ed. New York, Academic Press, 1976, pp. 23–75

Utell MJ, Aquilina AT, Hall WJ, et al: Development of airway reactivity to nitrates in subjects in influenza. Am Rev Respir Dis 121:233–241, 1980

Von Nieding G, Krekeler H: Pharmakologische Beeinflussung der akuten NO$_2$—Wirkung auf die lungenfunktion von Gesunden und Kranken mit einer Chronischen Bronchitis. Int Arch Arbeitsmed 29:55–63, 1971

Wanner A: Clinical aspects of mucociliary transport. State of the Art. Am Rev Respir Dis 116:73–125, 1977

Zeidberg LD, Pridle RA, Landau E: The Nashville air pollution study. Sulphur dioxide and bronchial asthma. Am Rev Respir Dis 84:489–503, 1961

Simon Godfrey

12

Exercise-Induced Asthma

Sir John Floyer was a 17th-century physician who suffered from asthma and made very detailed observations on his condition, which he reported in his *Treatise on the Asthma,* first published in 1698. He wrote, "all violent Exercise makes the Asthmatic to breathe short" and then went on to relate how different types of exercise had differing potential for causing trouble in the asthmatic. Very little interest was taken in the subject of exercise-induced asthma (EIA) until recent times, although the phenomenon was clearly recognized by clinicians. In some subjects, the EIA was the most prominent feature of their disease and so it was thought by some that EIA was a disease in its own right. Careful clinical and physiological observations have clearly shown that EIA reflects the heightened state of bronchial reactivity found in asthmatics and is not an independent disorder. Although normal subjects can be shown to vary their airway caliber to a minor degree in response to exercise and other stimuli, the significant attack of bronchospasm after exercise which is implied by the term EIA is only seen in asthmatics. EIA merely reflects, however, the state of increased bronchial hyperreactivity of the asthmatic and the difference between the asthmatic and the normal is quantitative rather than qualitative. As will be discussed, not all asthmatics develop EIA, but it is very common in young patients, in whom it may be a very troublesome symptom. Older subjects probably take less exercise as a rule and so notice EIA less.

The ease with which EIA can be provoked and the brevity of the attack coupled with its undoubted similarity to other types of asthma have made EIA

BRONCHIAL ASTHMA, Second Edition
ISBN 0-8089-1814-1

of interest to those seeking a good laboratory model of asthma. Scientific investigation of this subject began with the remarkable pioneering observations by R. S. Jones and his colleagues in Liverpool. These studies clearly showed EIA to be a normal feature of childhood (and young adult) asthma, related the pattern of EIA to clinical severity, and noted persistence of EIA in young adults who had "grown out" of childhood asthma. Other early studies described the diminution of response to further exercise after an attack of EIA—a refractory period. The importance of EIA as a model was shown by studies of the effect of various anti-asthmatic medication. There were some unexplained features of EIA which intrigued investigators at that time, such as the varying responses to different types of exercise and the fact that differences undoubtedly existed between EIA and troublesome, spontaneous clinical asthma. During the mid-1970s, the subject became the center of intense study because of new observations regarding the effect of climate on EIA and because of the isolation of mast-cell-related chemical mediators from the circulation. Some 300 years after Sir John first brought attention to this topic, clinicians are still in the midst of research into EIA.

PATTERN OF LUNG FUNCTION CHANGES IN EIA

The pattern of the response of an asthmatic to exercise is quite consistent and is illustrated in Figure 12-1. Exercise causes an initial mild bronchodilation, which is often maintained throughout the exercise period. After exercise ceases, bronchospasm takes over and lung function reaches its lowest level

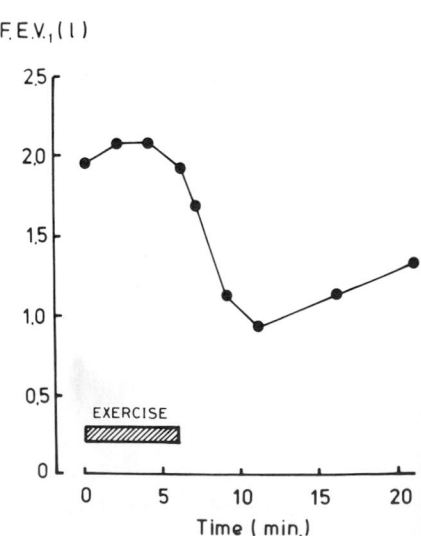

Fig. 12-1. Typical pattern of lung function changes in response to 6 minutes of running by an asthmatic child.

after 3–5 minutes in children and after 5–7 minutes in adults. In order to quantitate EIA, various indices have been proposed, but for the sake of simplicity, those illustrated in Figure 12-2 are widely accepted. The EIA itself is measured by the percentage fall in FEV_1, or ΔFEV_1, as it is usually termed, which is the percentage decrease postexercise from the pre-exercise baseline. The bronchodilation during exercise can similarly be measured by the percentage rise in FEV, while the total exercise-induced bronchial lability is the sum of these two indices. For all practical purposes, the ΔFEV_1, is the only index needed to quantitate EIA. There have been some arguments as to the mathematical validity of such an index, and it is important that, whenever comparative studies are made, the baseline FEV_1 values be as close as possible, in which case all indices are equally valid. In some studies, investigators have used either simpler indices of lung function (such as the peak expiratory flow rate—PEFR) or more complex parameters (such as the specific airway conductance—S_{gaw}), but the general conclusions about the results are usually very close whatever test is used. One variable which is not generally considered is the duration of the attack of EIA, since this can vary from a few minutes to an hour or more. It would seem that a prolonged response should represent more severe EIA than does a brief response, even if the decreases in FEV_1 were to similar levels. This possibility has yet to be fully explored.

When the attack of EIA develops after exercise, there is evidence of generalized airway obstruction with hyperinflation. By using helium/oxygen mixtures, various investigations have attempted to partition the airway obstruction of EIA between large and small airways. These studies have shown considerable variation between individuals, with some apparently having more large-airway and others more small-airway obstruction. Other

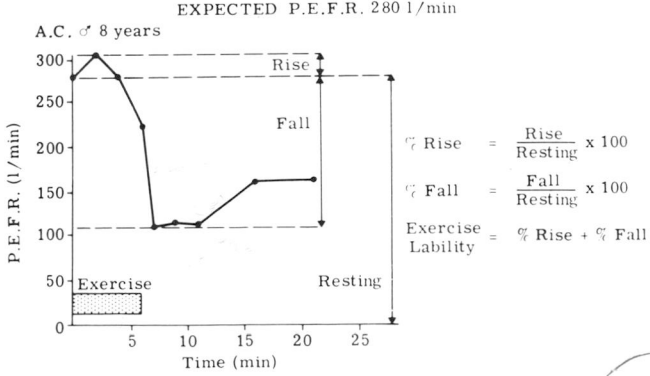

Fig. 12-2. Method of calculation of indices commonly used to quantitate exercise-induced asthma. The % Fall is equivalent to the ΔFEV_1. (From Godfrey S, et al: J Allergy Clin Immunol 52:199, 1973. Used with permission.)

studies have implied that there is widespread airway closure and, in addition, some subjects increased their total lung capacity due to a reduced elastic recoil pressure during the attack of EIA. Loss of elastic recoil would also contribute to the reduction of maximal expiratory flow at low lung volumes. The general and widespread nature of the changes as reflected in the forced expiratory flow volume loop before, during, and after exercise are shown in Figure 12-3.

The effect of exercise on the arterial blood gases of the asthmatic are much as would be predicted from the changes in lung function. During exercise, arterial PO_2 and PCO_2 remain essentially normal, while pH falls due to the accumulation of lactic acid which has been suggested as a triggering factor; comparisons have, however, failed to show any correlation between the pH or lactic acidosis and the severity of EIA. During the attack of EIA, there is moderate arterial hypoxia and occasional hypercapnia. Despite early enthusiasm, it has not been possible to show that changes in blood gases or acid-base balance serve as the triggering factors for EIA.

Until recently, it was generally accepted that exercise resulted in a brief attack of asthma from which the subject recovered over 30–60 minutes. While this closely resembled the immediate type of bronchial response to the inhalation of allergen, it was thought that there was no equivalent after exercise to the late bronchial response which often occurs 4–6 hours following antigen inhalation. The late asthmatic reaction is probably of an inflammatory nature and more closely resembles the asthma which causes persistent, clinically troublesome asthma than it does the acute reactions after either exercise or allergen. Evidence has begun to accumulate which suggests that exercise, like allergen, might induce inflammatory changes in the airways. Some asthmatics develop a late bronchial response to asthma which is accompanied by a second (late) rise in the level of circulating neutrophil

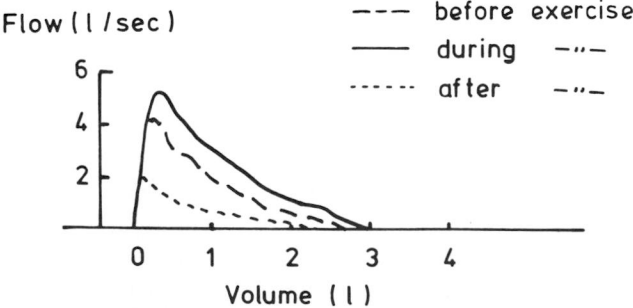

Fig. 12-3. Forced expired flow volume loops before, during, and after exercise in an asthmatic child showing the bronchodilation during exercise and the reductions in flow rates at all volumes after exercise.

chemotactic factor (NCF). Studies of the effect on lung function of breathing a helium/oxygen mixture suggested that the early response to exercise was predominantly in the large airways (flow rates improved with helium), while the late response was predominantly in the small airways (no change with helium). Late responses to exercise are not seen in the majority of asthmatics, but this could be because such responses are mild and easily missed; more studies are clearly needed.

Bronchial Lability of Normal Subjects and of Asthmatics in Relation to Exercise

A number of studies have explored the range of bronchial lability in normal subjects and asthmatics and the reproducibility of EIA. The average improvement in lung function during exercise is about 3–4 percent in both normal children and adults and the maximum postexercise fall is about 9–10 percent. In an investigation of a group of 812 children aged 12 years who were not only healthy themselves but who were not related to asthmatic subjects, 92 percent had a postexercise fall in peak flow rate of less than 10 percent and 98 percent of them had a fall of less than 15 percent. This type of study, based on statistical analysis, is a much more logical method of defining normality (and hence differentiating the asthmatic response) than is the arbitrary selection of a particular ΔFEV_1, as defining abnormality, which has often been used in the past.

The incidence of EIA in asthmatics and the reproducibility of tests of EIA is greatly influenced by the nature of the exercise test and the conditions under which the exercise is performed. Much of this (which will be discussed later) was unknown when studies of incidence and reproducibility were originally undertaken. Although care was taken to standardize exercise, the average coefficient of variation of repeated exercise tests within one week was 21 percent, and this increased as the interval between tests was lengthened. A $\Delta PEFR$ of greater than 10 percent was found in 89 percent of 107 asthmatic children tested. In various other careful studies, the incidence of EIA among unselected asthmatic children and adults has been reported to vary from 71 to 87 percent. It seems likely that all asthmatics can develop EIA if they exercise hard enough under appropriate conditions, but of course many asthmatics, especially adults, never encounter the problem because they take little exercise. Moreover, as will be discussed later, there is now very little doubt that the severity of EIA varies from time to time in the individual.

A somewhat confusing issue is the question of whether nonasthmatic subjects can have increased bronchial lability. This question arose out of the observation that some patients, notably those with cystic fibrosis, could have wide changes in bronchial caliber as a result of exercise. Some of these children were undoubtedly also asthmatic, but in others the confusion arose because their total exercise-induced bronchial lability was indeed increased, but this was due to marked bronchodilation during exercise and not to bronchoconstriction after exercise. A similar pattern of moderately increased total bronchial lability with an improvement of lung function during exercise is sometimes found in the healthy relatives of asthmatic children or in those who had bronchiolitis in infancy. None of these subjects develop significant postexertional bronchospasm unless they happen to be asthmatic, and this type of bronchial lability should not be confused with EIA. Another source of confusion has been the fact that some allergic individuals whose chief complaint is upper respiratory tract allergy have been found to develop EIA, but these patients undoubtedly have asthma, even if it is not very prominent.

CONDITIONS WHICH INFLUENCE THE SEVERITY OF EIA

Since the time of Sir John Floyer, it has been known to both asthmatics and their physicians that some kinds of exercise are more troublesome than others. Formal studies under controlled conditions showed that running caused more asthma than did swimming and that free-range running caused more asthma than did treadmill running, which in turn caused more than did cycling. All these exercise tests were performed at very similar levels of minute ventilation, heart rate, and gas exchange and it did not appear that differences in metabolic rate could account for the differences in asthmagenicity. The difference between running (or cycling) and swimming was so clearcut that it caused several investigators to undertake research with very far-reaching consequences, as will be seen later. Even in the light of these recent developments, there still remains considerable doubt as to whether running, cycling, and other types of exercise carried out under identical conditions are all equally potent stimuli for EIA.

For a given type of asthmagenic exercise, such as running or cycling, the severity of the EIA depends upon the severity and duration of the exercise. Silverman and Anderson showed that the severity of EIA increased with increasing work rate and with increasing duration of exercise up to certain plateau values, as illustrated in Figures 12-4 and 12-5. They had children exercise in random order for various times at constant treadmill settings and with various treadmill slopes for a constant time. The overall conclusion was that the maximum response was seen after 6–8 minutes of running at a gradient of 10–15 percent. It was noted that patients who developed severe EIA after 6–8 minutes often got less asthma after more prolonged exercise— and patients often reported that they could "run through" their asthma. The severity of the exercise usually raised the heart rate to 170–180/minute in children (rather lower in adults). This level of work corresponds to approximately 70 percent of the maximum oxygen uptake of all subjects. The tread-

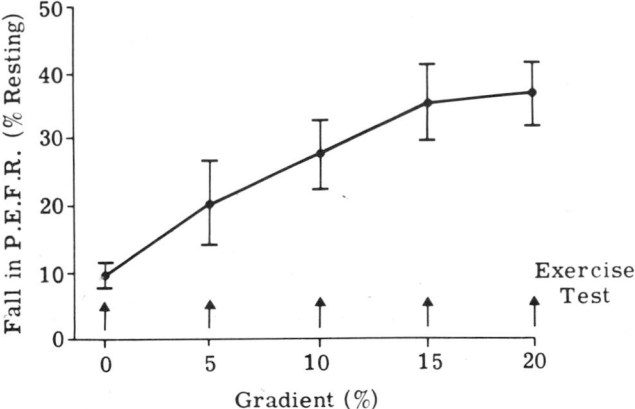

Fig. 12-4. Effect of gradient (work rate) on asthma induced by treadmill running at a constant speed for 6 minutes. Each point represents the mean of tests in 9 children who performed each gradient on a different occasion. (From Godfrey S, et al: J Allergy Clin Immunol 52:199, 1973. Used with permission.)

mill test is particularly useful, since the work performed depends on body weight and hence, at a given setting, such as 3 m.p.h. (5 k.p.h.) and a 10 percent slope, all subjects will be working at a similar relative level. A more recent study essentially confirmed these findings and recommended a test consisting of 5 minutes of continuous treadmill exercise, adjusting slope and speed to produce a heart rate of 90 percent of the predicted maximal heart rate for the age and sex of the subject. In view of the plateau effects seen in

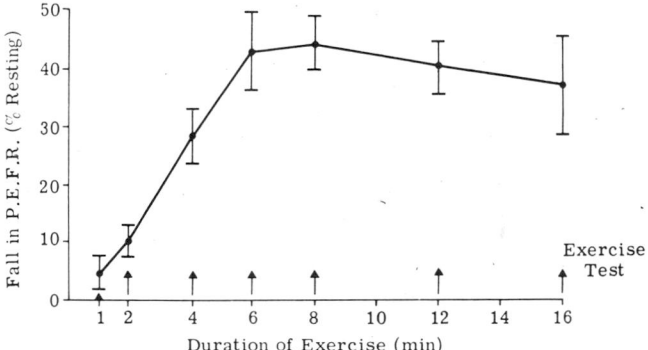

Fig. 12-5. Effect of duration on asthma induced by treadmill running at a constant speed and gradient. Each point represents the mean of tests in 10 children who performed each duration on a different occasion. (From Godfrey S, et al: J Allergy Clin Immunol 52:199, 1973. Used with permission.)

Figures 12-4 and 12-5, it is probably unnecessary to be overly exact about the work rate and time as long as they are close to the values producing the plateaus.

The asthmatic patient often finds that he/she is unable to undertake continuous exercise lasting a few minutes, but is quite capable of playing games such as tennis or football. The reason would seem to be that in most games the exercise is actually brief and intermittent and this allows the mechanism which normally results in bronchospasm to be overcome under the protection of the increased sympathetic drive of exercise. Thus, it has been shown that brief warming-up sprints may markedly diminish the EIA resulting from a subsequent, more prolonged period of exercise. This inactivation of the asthma-provoking mechanism must also account for the well-recognized phenomenon of the refractory period which follows EIA in most subjects. The response to a second exercise challenge is diminished following an attack of EIA and, as can be seen in Figure 12-6, by repeating the exercise the EIA can be almost completely abolished. This refractoriness wears off quite quickly and we were able to show that the half-life of refractoriness was about 1 hour.

Recently there has been a move toward investigating the response to EIA by performing progressively intense, short periods of exercise separated by the measurement of lung function in order to attempt to define the dose-response curve for EIA—akin to that curve used to quantitate the response to methacholine or histamine inhalation. While this would be a desirable advance, it ignores the well-established facts relating to the effect of dura-

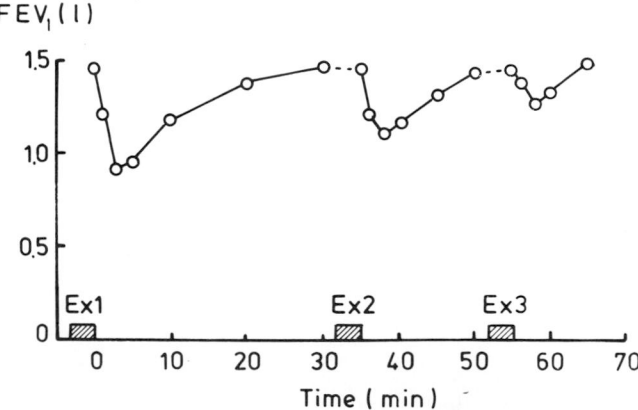

Fig. 12-6. Refractoriness to exercise-induced asthma demonstrated by a decreasing amount of asthma following each of a series of equally severe exercise tests. (From Godfrey S, in Clark TJH, Godfrey S, (eds): Asthma, London, Chapman and Hall Medical, 1983, p. 164. Used with permission.)

tion, severity, and refractoriness on the severity of the EIA. Patients have been studied by both methods and it has been found that the severity of EIA was much greater with the single-level challenge than with the same level during a progressive exercise test.

Not only does the nature and severity of exercise affect the intensity of EIA, but the environmental conditions under which the exercise is performed also have a profound influence on the intensity. Puzzled by the different asthmagenicity of running and swimming, a number of investigators wondered if the answer lay in the humidity of the air breathed and showed that breathing humid air lessened EIA. At the same time, others trying to demonstrate the beneficial effects of a dry climate found exactly the opposite of what they had expected, namely that a humid climate caused subjects to have less EIA than did a dry climate. This research received a great impetus from the studies of McFadden and his colleagues, who developed what has been termed the "respiratory heat loss hypothesis" for EIA. They conceived the idea that the effect of humidity was in reality due to the prevention of cooling of the airways and they soon showed that breathing cold or dry air enhanced EIA. The airways are cooled if inspired air is cold or if it is dry because the air needs humidifying, which requires the latent heat of vaporization to be supplied from the airway mucosa. Contrary to conventionally held beliefs, the upper airway is incapable of fully conditioning inspired air during exercise. The heat loss is reflected by a fall in mediastinal temperature recorded in the esophagus; this phenomenon was similar in normals and asthmatics. This observation from one of our own studies is shown in Figure 12-7, where the time course of the change in esophageal temperature and of lung function can be seen. The very considerable influence of environmental temperature and especially humidity could certainly account for some of the variations in asthmagenicity found in earlier studies of EIA and makes it imperative that

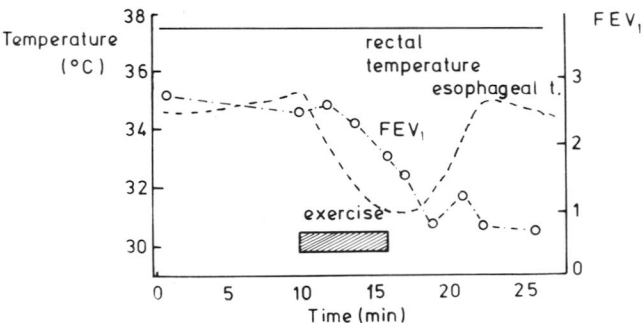

Fig. 12-7. Change in esophageal and rectal temperature before, during, and after 6 minutes of running in an asthmatic subject. The fall in the retrotracheal temperature precedes that in the FEV_1 and returns to baseline while the EIA persists.

environmental factors be standardized in all new studies of EIA. Nevertheless, when we reinvestigated swimming and running by having our patients breathe from a circuit which provided air of the same controlled temperature and humidity for both types of exercise, running still caused some 39 percent more asthma than did swimming. Thus the type of exercise may still be a determinant of the response to some degree.

Effect of Drugs on EIA

It has been long known that various antiasthmatic medications could prevent or curtail EIA and, because EIA is a safe and simple tool, it has frequently been used as a model for testing the effect of various drugs which are used in the treatment of clinical asthma. It was early established that EIA could be inhibited by the prior administration of sympathomimetic agents, but not, apparently, by steroids or antihistamines, while the value of theophylline derivatives and atropine was less certain. As important advance was made when it was shown that cromolyn sodium could also prevent EIA, since this drug was (and still is) believed to act primarily by preventing the release of mediators from mast cells and is not a bronchodilator. Of particular theoretical importance was a study which showed that cromolyn sodium only prevented EIA if given before the exercise, not if given at the end of exercise but before the attack of EIA had developed (Fig. 12-8). This study implied that EIA was due at least in part to the liberation of mediators during the exercise period.

The general pattern of the response of EIA to common antiasthmatic medications is shown in Figure 12-9, which is derived from a study in which each agent was administered to a group of asthmatic children. Because several of the agents were bronchodilators, the results are expressed on an

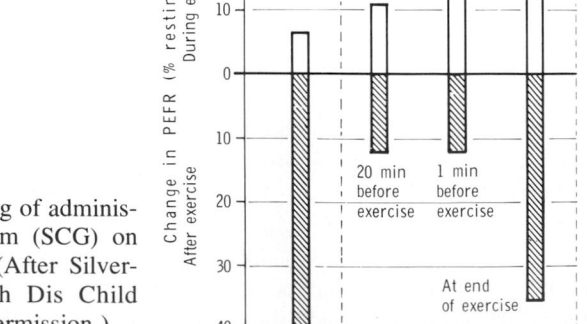

Fig. 12-8. Effect of timing of administration of cromolyn sodium (SCG) on exercise-induced asthma. (After Silverman M, Andrea T: Arch Dis Child 47:419, 1972. Used with permission.)

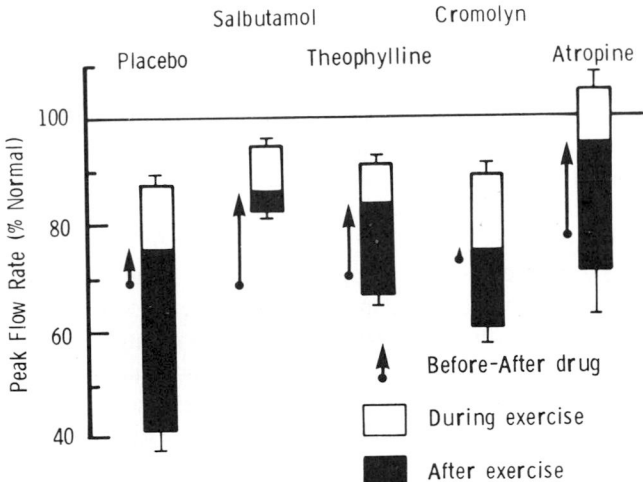

Fig. 12-9. The effect of various drugs on exercise-induced asthma, the results expressed as percentage of the expected normal peak expiratory flow rate for each subject. The arrows indicate the response to the drug at rest before the start of exercise. The bars indicate ±SEM. (After Anderson SD, et al: Br J Dis Chest 61:1, 1975. Used with permission.)

absolute scale of PEFR in order to show the postdrug bronchodilation, the further exercise-induced bronchodilation, and the exercise-induced broncho-constriction. It can be clearly seen that the interpretation of the relative efficacy of the various agents becomes a semantic problem if postdrug, preexercise bronchodilation occurs. Undoubtedly, the absolute postexercise PEFR after atropine and theophylline is better than after placebo and close to pre-drug, pre-exercise values; exercise nevertheless caused a deterioration in lung function from the postdrug, pre-exercise values. The manner of express-ing the result and the problem of judging a response when the baseline lung function is altered is probably responsible for much of the lack of agreement on the efficacy of treatment of EIA with atropine, theophylline, and their derivatives. By contrast, cromolyn sodium does not change baseline lung function and obviously inhibits EIA to a considerable degree, while salbuta-mol, although a bronchodilator, so completely abolishes any postexercise change that there is no doubt as to its efficacy. The question of the effect of steroids on EIA has been reconsidered recently after it was long believed that they did not influence the acute responses following either exercise or antigen stimulation. The regular treatment of asthma with an inhaled steroid has been shown to diminish or abolish EIA, but studies have been complicated by the coincident improvement in baseline lung function which occurred. It remains to be seen whether steroids can influence the immediate response to exercise in the absence of any change in basal airway caliber. The only other agent which has consistently been shown to prevent EIA is the calcium channel blocker, nifedipine, and it is believed to act rather as does cromolyn by preventing the calcium-dependent liberation of mediators from mast cells.

For practical purposes, the most useful way to protect a patient against EIA is to give either an inhaled selective beta-2 sympathomimetic or cromolyn sodium. Both drugs work if given by inhalation immediately before exercise. In absolute terms, the sympathomimetic is the more effective and lasts longer, but the inhalation technique must be perfect; the powder inhaler type of device used to administer cromolyn sodium is rather easier to master. The time until protection falls to about 50 percent of initial protection is about 4–5 hours for salbutamol and 1–2 hours for cromolyn sodium (SCG). There is no logical reason to use theophylline (either short- or long-acting) for the sole purpose of inhibiting EIA and, in any case, it is relatively inefficient. When studying EIA it is best to omit all medications, save perhaps steroids, for 8 hours before the test and to omit long-acting theophylline preparations for at least 24 hours.

THE PATHOGENESIS OF EIA

For a long time, many clinicians believed that it was the exercise itself that triggered EIA in some undefined manner, but there were problems with this idea because, as noted earlier, the same amount of physical exertion performed in different ways could result in different amounts of EIA. With the discovery of the importance of environmental temperature and humidity on EIA, it seemed that much of these differences could be explained and this led to the general concept that the trigger for EIA was the reduction in temperature of the airways which was shown to occur. Of equal importance was the observation that isocapnic hyperventilation also resulted in respiratory heat loss and for the same heat loss it could provoke an attack of hyperventilation-induced asthma (HIA) equal in severity to EIA. This led to the general conclusion that "EIA is probably HIA" and that the exercise itself was not needed to provoke the attack—just the hyperventilation and attendant heat loss. Although very attractive as a unifying hypotheses, there are a few observations which cast some doubt on its universal validity. For instance, asthma should not occur if the subject exercises while breathing warm, humid air which prevents respiratory heat loss, and yet there are occasional subjects who develop as much EIA while breathing warm humid air as while breathing room air, and one investigation showed that as many as half of the subjects developed significant EIA under these conditions, albeit less that that which they developed breathing regular room air. The central role of heat loss as the trigger has also been challenged recently by Anderson and her colleagues, who produced convincing evidence that it was actually the loss of water from the airways and the consequent osmotic changes in the mucosa that triggered the attack of EIA or HIA. In truth, it is a little difficult to separate out the effects of temperature and humidity, and in any case it would appear that the water loss hypothesis suffers from deficiencies similar to those of the heat loss hypothesis, since asthma can be induced in some subjects breathing warm, humid air when neither heat nor water loss occurs. At present, it is known that temperature, humidity, and hyperventilation are important determinants of both EIA and HIA, but researchers cannot be certain exactly what triggers the attack.

While it is generally accepted that exercise or hyperventilation act as stimuli and that bronchospasm is the effect, there is no agreement as to how the stimulus is translated into the effect. One obvious possibility is that EIA is simply the result of a neural reflex mediated via the vagus nerve, the afferent stimulus being the cooling or drying of the airways and the efferent pathway being cholinergic bronchospasm. This seems very unlikely in view of the time course of the changes in temperature and lung function shown in Figure 12-7. The temperature falls soon after the exercise starts and returns to baseline soon after it ends, while the lung function only falls at the end of exercise and returns to baseline some 30 minutes later. An alternative hypothesis is that the exercise stimulus releases chemical transmitters from mast cells, which in turn act directly (or reflexly) on the bronchial smooth muscle to provoke asthma. Originally, this hypothesis was based entirely on circumstantial evidence: the refractory period which follows EIA wears off steadily, with a half-life of about an hour, which would fit very well if refractoriness were due to the need to resynthesize stores of a chemical mediator. Support for the mediator hypothesis was also deduced from the fact that cromolyn sodium inhibits mediator release from mast cells and can prevent EIA if given prophylactically, as illustrated in Figure 12-8. More recently, powerful direct support for the mediator hypothesis has come from the work of Kay and his colleagues, who have been studying the release of a mast cell mediator, neutrophil chemotactic factor (NCF). They have shown that NCF is liberated into the circulation by patients who develop EIA and correlates with the fall in lung function, while both the liberation of NCF and the fall in lung function can be prevented by cromolyn sodium. They did not detect any NCF release with HIA nor in subjects who exercised but failed to develop EIA.

On the whole, it is fairly widely accepted that there is great similarity between EIA and HIA and that, whatever the stimulus, the pathway leading ultimately to bronchospasm is probably the same. There is, however, a fair amount of evidence accumulating to suggest that these unifying hypothesis are too simple. When studying the refractory period after a challenge, it was found, as would be predicted, that isocapnic hyperventilation breathing warm, humid air neither induced asthma nor refractoriness to a subsequent hyperventilation challenge breathing cold, dry air. In a previous study of EIA, it had, however, been found that the majority of subjects did become refractory to a subsequent cold, dry exercise challenge after an initial warm, humid exercise test which did not itself provoke EIA. A similar conclusion can be deduced from a study in which similar (low) levels of EIA were found after a second challenge when the initial exercise challenge consisted of breathing air of 15-, 50-, or 85-percent relative humidity. These results suggest that exercise per se and not respiratory heat (or water) loss is important in the development of refractoriness to EIA but that, in the case of HIA, the climatic condition is all-important. This led to the hypothesis that the trigger site for HIA might lie in the larger, more central airways, whose temperature changes markedly during hyperventilation (or exercise), but that the trigger site for EIA might lie more deeply in the lung tissue and be immune to temperature changes. Support for different trigger sites came from another study, in which it was shown that cromolyn sodium is most effective in preventing EIA if baseline lung function is good, but most effective in preventing HIA if baseline lung function is poor.

There is little doubt that asthmatics do not all respond identically in a particular challenge situation, even when the experimental conditions are carefully controlled. In studies of exercise, hyperventilation, refractoriness to EIA after a warm, humid air challenge, and refractoriness to antigen inhalation after EIA, there were some subjects who responded one way and some another. There is also no doubt that the severity of EIA varies widely from time to time in the same subject—this could be explained by variations in basic airway hyperreactivity. It has been known for some time that reactivity to histamine is considerably increased following antigen challenge and that there is potentiation by exercise of the effect of air pollution (SO_2) on asthmatics. The effect of antigen challenge on EIA has recently been studied and a considerable increase in the severity of EIA has been found during the week following an antigen challenge. Of course, it is possible that antigenic stimulation increases the sensitivity of the receptor site, but it seems very unlikely that EIA and histamine share the same receptors and more likely that it is the effector site that is most responsive.

A model which attempts to combine the established facts about EIA is shown in Figure 12-10. In this model, a combination of exercise intensity, hyperventilation, and environmental factors acts as the trigger which releases mediators from mast cells. At the same time, the increased sympathetic drive during exercise largely prevents bronchospasm as long as the exercise is continuing and, if prolonged enough, this may allow time for the liberated mediator to be metabolized so that EIA does not occur. With the usual 6-minute exercise challenge, the liberated mediator acts on the bronchial smooth muscle to produce the attack of EIA at the end of the exercise period.

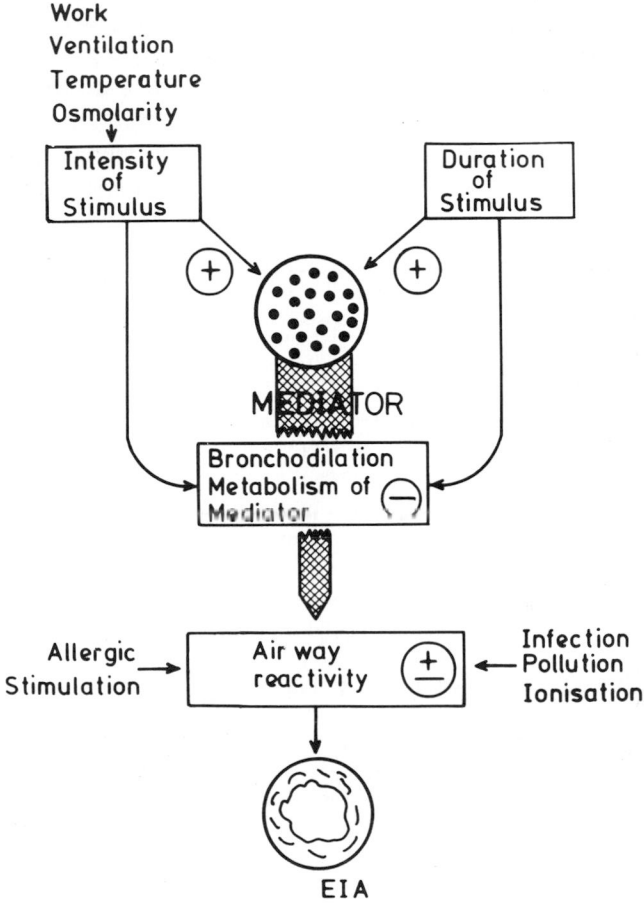

Fig. 12-10. Model of pathways involved in exercise-induced asthma. Various factors are shown influencing the intensity of the stimulus which, together with its duration, determines the amount of mediator released. During exercise, sympathetic drive protects against bronchospasm and causes mild bronchodilation while the amount of mediator is reduced by metabolism. After exercise, the remaining mediator causes asthma by acting on the airways whose intrinsic reactivity is also influenced by external factors.

The severity of the EIA depends not only on the quantity of mediator liberated, which varies with the strength of the stimulus, but also on how much has been destroyed during the exercise and upon the intrinsic hyperreactivity of the airways. This latter is probably governed by the prevailing level of allergenic stimulation as well as by other environmental factors, so that it is well-nigh impossible to predict the severity of EIA in an individual test. Thus, the very variability of EIA which is so troublesome for those studying the subject may help researchers to understand the pathways underlying asthma.

REFERENCES

Anderson SD, Schoeffel RE, Finney M: Evaluation of ultrasonically nebulised solutions for provocation testing in patients with asthma. Thorax 38:284–291, 1983

Anderson SD, Schoeffel RE, Follet R, et al: Sensitivity to heat and water loss at rest and during exercise in asthmatic patients. Eur J Respir Dis 63:459–571, 1982

Anderson SD, Silverman M, Konig P, et al: Exercise-induced asthma. Brit J Dis Chest 69:1–39, 1975

Bar-Or O, Neuman I, Dotan R: Effects of dry and humid climates on exercise-induced asthma in children and adolescents. J Allergy Clin Immunol 60:163–168, 1977

Bar-Yishay E, Gur I, Ben-Dov I, et al: Refractory period following induced asthma: Contributions to exercise and isocapnic hyperventilation. Thorax 38:849–853, 1983

Ben-Dov I, Bar-Yishay E, Godfrey S: Relation between efficacy of sodium cromoglycate and baseline lung function in exercise and hyperventilation induced asthma. Isr J Med Sci 20:130–135, 1984

Ben-Dov I, Bar-Yishay E, Godfrey S: Refractory period following exercise induced asthma unexplained by respiratory heat loss. Am Rev Respir Dis 125:530–534, 1982

Ben-Dov I, Bar-Yishay E, Godfrey S: Exercise induced asthma without respiratory heat loss. Thorax 37:630–631, 1982

Bierman CW, Spiro SG, Petheram I: Characteristics of the late response in exercise-induced asthma. J Allergy Clin Immunol 74:701–706, 1984

Deal EC, McFadden ER, Ingram RH, et al: Role of respiratory heat exchange in production of exercise-induced asthma. J Appl Physiol 46:467–475, 1979

Deal EC, McFadden ER, Ingram RH, et al: Esophageal temperature during exercise in asthmatic and non-asthmatic subjects. J Appl Physiol 46:484–490, 1979

Edmunds AT, Tooley M, Godfrey S: The refractory period after exercise induced asthma, its duration and relation to severity of exercise. Am Rev Respir Dis 117:247–254, 1978

Godfrey S: Controversies concerning the pathogenesis of exercise induced asthma. Eur J Respir Dis, in press

Henriksen JM, Dahl R, Lundquist GR: Influence of relative humidity and repeated exercise on exercise-induced bronchoconstriction. Allergy 36:463–470, 1981

Jones RS, Buston MH, Wharton MJ: The effect of exercise on ventilatory function in the child with asthma. Brit J Dis Chest 56:78–86, 1962

Lee TH, Nagy L, Nakagura T, et al: Identification and partial characterisation of an exercise-induced neutrophil chemotactic factor in bronchial asthma. J Clin Invest 69:889–899, 1982

Mussaffi H, Springer C, Godfrey S: Increased bronchial responsiveness to exercise and histamine after allergen challenge in asthmatic children. J Allergy Clin Immunol 77:48–52, 1986

Sakula A: Sir John Floyer's *A Treatise of the Asthma* (1698). Thorax 39:248–254, 1984

Silverman M, Andrea T: Time course of effect of disodium cromoglycate on exercise-induced asthma. Arch Dis Child 47:419–422, 1972

Weiler-Ravell D, Godfrey S: Do exercise and antigen induced asthma utilise the same pathways? Antigen provocation in patients rendered refractory to exercise induced asthma. J Allergy Clin Immunol 67:391–397, 1981

Harold S. Novey

13

Allergic Bronchopulmonary Aspergillosis

Allergic bronchopulmonary aspergillosis (ABPA) is an inflammatory bronchial and interstitial lung disease that is characterized by tissue and blood eosinophilia and is associated with immunologic responses to bronchial colonization by members of the fungus genus *Aspergillus*. Although most cases have been found in patients with pre-existing asthma, it is being recognized with increasing frequency in cystic fibrosis patients, as well as in some healthy persons. It manifests itself acutely as a febrile bronchitis or pneumonitis, or in a chronic form as a proximal-type bronchiectasis, and rarely as bronchocentric granulomatosis. The disease has been ascribed a taxonomic relation to syndromes associated with: (1) aspergillosis; and (2) pulmonary infiltrates with eosinophilia.

HISTORICAL PERSPECTIVES

In 1952, Hinson, Moon, and Plummer at the London Chest Hospital described 8 cases of ABPA under the title "Broncho-Pulmonary Aspergillosis." Of these, five were considered to have mycetomata containing *Aspergillus* species and were classified as the saprophytic type. The other three, two women aged 45 and 55, and a male aged 37, were described as having recurrent febrile episodes with severe cough productive of a purulent sputum.

The sputum contained plugs with fungal elements, eosinophils, Curschmann's spirals, and Charcot-Leyden crystals. Asthma was said to be definite in two, and wheezing was heard in the other. All had peripheral eosinophilia of over 1000/mm^3. Two had saccular bronchiectasis and the other a mucus plug on bronchoscopy. The male died in status asthmaticus and the pathologic changes in his lungs were briefly described. Each had special exposure to *Aspergillus* through: chicken breeding, gardening using contaminated hog manure, and flour milling. Largely on the basis of the eosinophilias and sputum characteristics, the authors proposed an allergic etiology for these 3 patients. An immune mechanism was not described. These patients were classified under an allergic-type bronchopulmonary aspergillosis. There were no examples for their third type—septicemic or pyemic.

Jack Pepys and his colleagues at the Brompton Hospital, London, are chiefly responsible for elucidating the allergic basis of the disease. They were able to develop antigenic extracts of *Aspergillus* organisms, and with these demonstrated in vitro and in vivo immunologic responses in patients. Scadding, at the same hospital in 1967, described the characteristic proximal or central type of bronchiectasis. Golbert and Patterson in 1970 appeared to passively transfer the disease to Rhesus monkeys using the sera of a patient with reaginic IgE and precipitating IgG antibodies to *Aspergillus*, followed by bronchial challenge to the animals with an extract of the organism.

It is uncertain whether ABPA represents a new disease or a new recognition of an old one. Löffler's syndrome, manifest by transient pulmonary infiltrates with peripheral eosinophilia, had been associated with wheezing since its description in 1932. Variants such as tropical eosinophilia were attributed to allergic reactions to various parasitic protozoans and worms, but not to fungi.

A relationship between asthma and bronchiectasis had been commented upon in anecdotal fashion since the 1920s. Sputum eosinophilia was frequently observed in these cases, but reference to a central-type bronchiectasis or *Aspergillus* in sputum smears or cultures was not found after a search in the literature.

A relationship between fungal spores and asthma can be traced to Sir John Floyer's work in 1726. Dutch and Spanish physicians (Van Leeuwen, Jimenez-Diaz) between 1924 and 1927 ascribed cases of hay fever and asthma to sensitivity to *Aspergillus* spores, and skin testing with extracts of the fungus was begun on a clinical basis. Asthma and pulmonary infection with *Aspergillus* was recognized by Renon, who, in 1897, reported this association in two types of occupational exposure. "Maladie des graveurs" was a chronic respiratory disease in Parisian pigeon-crammers, who force-fed up to 2000 pigeons daily by taking in mouthfuls of grain and water and spitting them into the pigeons' mouths. Wig makers prepared human hair by removing grease with rye flour. The grains used by both groups were contaminated by *Aspergillus*.

DEFINITION AND CLASSIFICATION

In the introductory sentence, ABPA was defined on the basis of its immunopathologic manifestations as an inflammatory bronchial and interstitial lung disease characterized by tissue and blood eosinophilia and associated with immunologic responses to bronchial colonization by members of the fungus genus *Aspergillus*. The salient parts in this rather lengthy definition are that the condition involves: (1) the lungs; (2) *Aspergillus*; (3) eosinophilia; and (4) an allergic mechanism.

There are a host of other disease states that involve the lungs and produce eosinophilia, or involve the lungs and *Aspergillus*. In the paper by Hinson and co-authors, ABPA was considered as part of the second category and a three-part classification was presented, namely: Type I—saprophytic; Type II—allergic; Type III—septicemic or pyemic. Type I included Aspergillomata, invasion of the lung as a terminal event; Type II, ABPA; Type III, multiple mycotic abscesses and granulomata in lungs and other tissues.

Finegold, Will, and Murray, in 1959, classified Aspergillosis as in Table 13-1.

Because it may prove difficult in some cases to determine whether or not there are predisposing factors which will differentiate a primary from a secondary form, the classification in Table 13-2 is proposed based on this definition for Aspergillosis: an invasion, colonization, or allergic reaction in tissues by a member of the genus *Aspergillus*.

An alternative classification is based upon the clinical presentation of pulmonary infiltrates with sputum and blood eosinophilia, or briefly pulmonary eosinophilia. Crofton (1952) proposed 5 groupings as follows:

1. simple (Löffler's syndrome)
2. prolonged—idiopathic and secondary
3. asthmatic
4. tropical
5. polyarteritis and related conditions

Since then, additional syndromes have been described, and the authors favor a revised classification which borrows heavily from Drs. Om P. Sharma, Eric H. Ottesen, and Sheldon G. Cohen (Table 13-3).

Table 13-1
Classification of
Aspergillosis (1959)

Primary	Secondary
localized	localized
invasive	invasive
disseminated	disseminated

Table 13-2

Classification of Aspergillosis with Consideration of Predisposing Factors

I. Noninvasive; allergic
   A. asthma, allergic rhinitis
   B. pulmonary infiltrates with eosinophilia (allergic bronchopulmonary aspergillosis)
   C. hypersensitivity pneumonitis
      example: malt workers' disease

II. Localized infection or colonization
   A. aspergilloma, pulmonary
   B. Non-pulmonary—any other external orifice
      examples: keratitis, otitis, vaginitis, rhinosinusitis
   C. cardiovascular—associated with surgical implants and dissemination by emboli

III. invasive and disseminated infection—associated with immunosuppressed status from neoplasia, radiation, cytotoxic and corticosteroid drugs, chronic granulomatous disease of childhood, and primary and acquired immunodeficiency syndromes

---

Table 13-3

Pulmonary Eosinophilia

I. Primary or idiopathic
   A. localized
      1. Löffler's syndrome
      2. intrinsic asthma with aspirin triad
      3. chronic eosinophilic pneumonia
   B. systemic associations
      1. polyarteritis, Wegener's granulomatosis, variants
      2. lymphoreticular disorders—Hodgkin's, familial reticuloendothelosis, angioblastic lymphoid hyperplasia
      3. sarcoidosis
      4. hypereosinophilic syndrome
      5. immunodeficiency states—Wiskott-Aldrich, selective IgA, hyper E, Nezloff

II. Secondary
   A. localized
      1. allergic asthma
      2. allergic bronchopulmonary aspergillosis
   B. systemic associations
      1. parasitic tissue invasions—helminths, *Pneumocystis carinii*
      2. other infectious diseases—coccidiomycosis, brucellosis, candidiasis, scarlet fever
      3. drugs—sensitizers, mast cell degranulators, beta-adrenergic blockers, aspirin

THE ETIOLOGIC AGENT

The name *Aspergillus* (Latin: "mop") was coined in 1729 by Micheli, the priest-botanist, for its resemblance to the aspergillum, a brush used for sprinkling holy water in the Catholic high Masses (Fig. 13-1). It is a member of the class Fungi Imperfecti, which have asexual spores on specialized hyphae, and shares the family Moniliaceae with *Monilia, Penicillium,* and *Trichoderma,* among others. Over 135 different species of *Aspergillus* have been described.

Pathogenicity

Several dozen species have been involved in human and animal disease. *Aspergilli* are probably the major fungal pathogens in birds and an important one in livestock. Conidia (spores) average about 2.5 micron in diameter, and upon inhalation, can penetrate to the alveoli of mammals, where they germinate rapidly and produce intense inflammatory response. One phenomenon interpreted as resistance to the infecting hyphae has been the formulation of

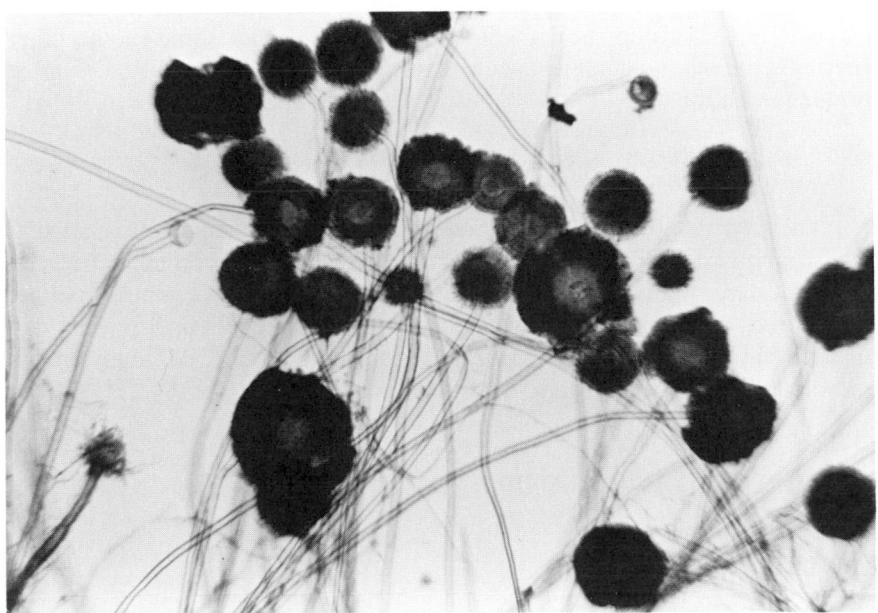

Fig. 13-1. *Aspergillus* organisms showing hyphae terminating in large vesicles containing sterigmata and conidiophores whose conidia (spores) are about 2.5 micron in diameter. India ink wet mount from sputum culture of patient with allergic bronchopulmonary aspergillosis, × 100.

eosinophilic "asteroid" sheaths around the hyphae. Bovine abortion caused by *Aspergillus* is common, but the route to the uterus has not been found. Human cases with pulmonary disease were first reported about the middle of the last century. Monod, in 1951, described the fungus balls in lung cavities, which he called Aspergillomas.

Epidemiology

The greatest number of *Aspergillus* spores in any natural habitat are found in moldy hay and straw; it is these substrates, together with leaf and grass compost, that provide the majority of airborne spores, according to Austwick. Estimations of *Aspergillus* spore concentrations in the outdoor air have ranged from 0 to $600/m^3$, and indoors the range has been from 0.3 to $2300/m^3$ in a hospital room, and from 12 to 21 million/m^3 in a cow shed.

Some data on the amount of lung retention of spores needed to cause animal infection have been gathered. It takes about 16 million retained spores to cause disease in chicks. About one-half of housed dairy cattle have evidence of benign infection in the form of pulmonary lesions containing asteroid bodies and hyphae. The reason *A. fumigatus* is the species most associated with ABPA and human disease (except for malt-workers lung—*A. clavatus* in this group) is not known. They share with some of the other species aerodynamic qualities, such as size, weight, and durability, favorable for lung retention.

Cultural Characteristics

These spores grow well on Sabouraud's blood agar, and simple malt agar media, and best at 37°C. They are fast growing, all have conidophores with expanded large vesicles at their ends giving a sunburst appearance, and are considered the commonest laboratory contaminant. During the 84-day manned Skylab space voyage, *Aspergilli*, together with *Penicillium,* were the prevalent fungal contaminants.

CLINICAL AND LABORATORY FEATURES

Incidence

Shortly after the 1952 report of 3 cases, there followed studies of large series of patients, mainly from the London area, diagnosed as having allergic bronchopulmonary aspergillosis. A group of 59 were reported in 1959, 87 in 1964, and 111 in 1971. Cases gradually were reported from outside England, so that presently the disease appears to have a worldwide distribution.

Although ABPA is undoubtedly the most common cause for pulmonary infiltrates with eosinophilia in asthma, neither its overall incidence nor even its incidence in asthma is known. This lack of knowledge is partly due to the absence of a pathognomic test or universally agreed-upon criteria, as will be discussed under diagnosis. In California, at least 10 new cases have been confirmed annually for 10 consecutive years by one consultation service, while over about a 15-year period, an additional 268 cases were confirmed from 6 other reporting centers in the United States.

More is known about the prevalence of some of the immunological parameters that will be discussed later, than about the disease itself. When comparable studies have been made using similar antigens and test procedures, there is a remarkable degree of concurrence. For example, in different studies using similar antigens, the incidence of positive prick skin reactions to *A. fumigatus* in asthma patients was 21.5 percent in Montreal, 23 percent in London, and 28 percent in Cleveland. The incidence of positive serum precipitins to similar strains of the same organism in asthma patients was 18 percent in Southern California and 22 percent in London. Such immunological findings suggest that sensitization to *Aspergillus*, if not its clinical manifestations, is unaffected by disparate geographic locations.

In cystic fibrosis, one study of 46 patients in the eastern United States detected an incidence of ABPA of 11 percent over a 2-year period. This rate was confirmed from the Midwest, where a study of 100 cystic fibrosis (CF) patients found a 10-percent incidence of ABPA. *Aspergillus* could most readily be found in sputum culture media of these patients if growth of *Pseudomonas* were controlled by incorporation in the media of high concentrations of gentamycin.

Similar to the situation for asthma patients, these and other series of CF patients demonstrated a high incidence of immunologic response to *Aspergillus* antigens. About 20 percent had positive immediate skin reactions, and from 33 to 59 percent had serum precipitins in several series using various *Aspergillus* antigens.

Signs and Symptoms

The original clinical picture described in 1952 was greatly expanded upon in several large series, and it is from these, particularly from the Pepys group, that the clinical manifestations are drawn. Almost all ages have been diagnosed, from infancy to the seventh decade. Most patients are diagnosed between the ages of 20 and 40 years. There does not appear to be a sex predominance. Over 90 percent of reported cases are in patients with existing asthma. The asthma has usually been present since childhood and the majority are considered atopic on the basis of combinations of personal and family history and positive skin tests to common allergens. Dependency on corticosteroids for control of asthma may represent a risk factor. A retrospective analysis of 42 such patients disclosed an incidence of ABPA in that group approaching 14 percent.

Presenting symptoms may be relatively acute or chronic; the acute form is perhaps more common (Table 13-4).

The acute form has some seasonal predilection for the rainy winter months.

Signs include fever of 37°–40°C and sputum that is mostly mucopurulent and often blood-flecked. Occasionally, golden-brown plugs of 2–3 mm in diameter can be separated from the sputum. Physical signs are those of airway obstruction in nearly all patients. Most have generalized wheezes or rhonchi. About one-half will also have localizing signs in the lungs: crepitant rales, dullness to percussion, and evidence of consolidation present mainly over the upper lung areas. Patients with chronic disease may have clubbing of the fingers.

Roentgenographic Findings

During an acute febrile episode of the disease, most persons will develop an abnormal appearing chest film. The types and locations of the abnormalities vary. Some of the more common are large homogeneous densities involving one-half or more of a lobe (Fig. 13-2), triangular infiltrates under a segment in length, and smaller shadows paralleling the lines of large bronchi or rounded, ball-like densities within bronchi that may be diagnosed as mucus plugs.

Patients with chronic disease may have nodular densities, avascular areas, lobar shrinkage and scarring, or atelectasis.

Areas of predilection for these changes are the upper lobes and the hilar areas. Pulmonary tuberculosis, bronchiogenic carcinoma, and lymphomas are commonly entertained radiographic diagnoses.

Most patients in whom bronchograms have been performed have signs of bronchiectasis. Characteristically, the larger proximal bronchi are dilated in

Table 13-4
Presenting Symptoms of ABPA

Acute
asthma worsens
cough and sputum production increases
fever and malaise
pleuritic-type chest pain

Chronic
daily cough with a teaspoon or more of purulent sputum
recurrent febrile episodes resembling bronchitis or pneumonitis

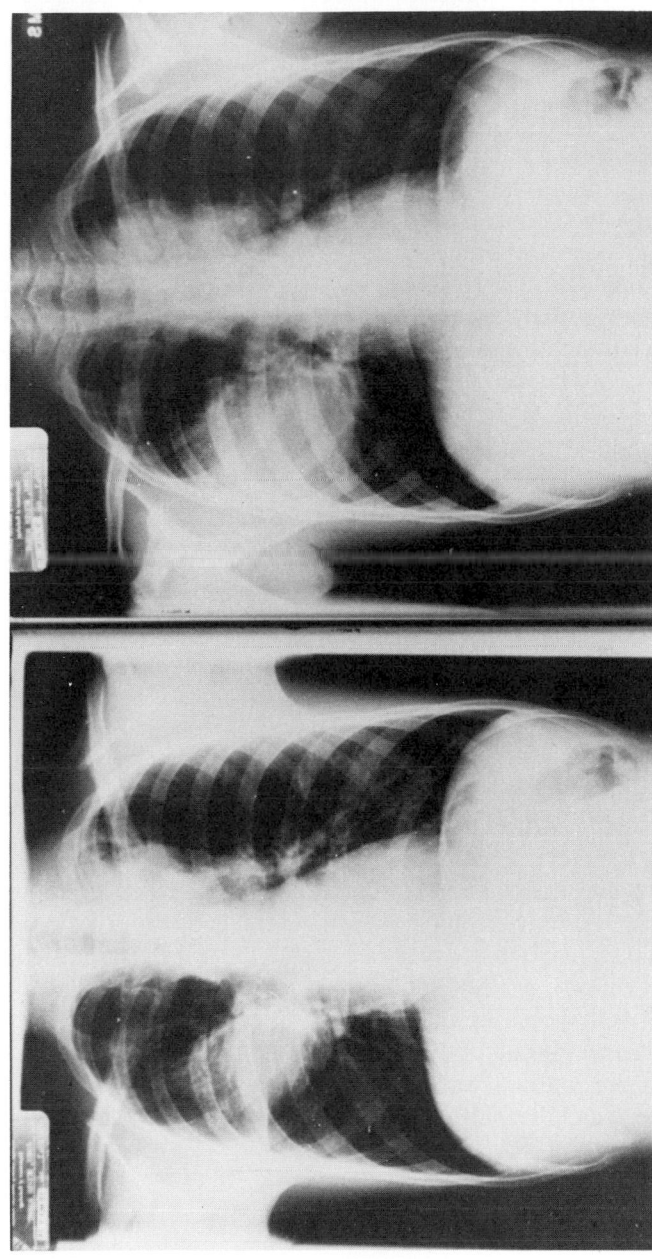

Fig. 13–2. A 12-year-old male with asthma and enlarging infiltrates, peripheral and sputum eosinophilia. Film on right taken 11 days after that on the left. The density involves increasing portions of the right upper lobe, and the left upper mediastinal shadow appears enlarged. A lymphoma was suspected, but allergic bronchopulmonary aspergillosis was later confirmed.

either a saccular or a cystic configuration, while the peripheral portions appear relatively normal. Except for a rare case of pulmonary tuberculosis, this feature is virtually pathognomic of ABPA.

Routine Laboratory Tests

The only consistently abnormal routine laboratory test is the peripheral eosinophil count. The absolute count is invariably over 500 cells/mm³ and often exceeds 1000 cells/mm³, even between acute episodes. The counts increase after pulmonary infiltrates. Patients on daily or high-dose steroids may not be able to manifest an eosinophilia. Nearly all patients will also have sputum eosinophilia, usually exceeding 15 percent of the cells present.

The sedimentation rate and total white cell count may be mildly elevated in acutely ill patients. The rest of the complete blood count is usually normal.

Immunological Tests

IN VIVO—SKIN TESTS

Extracts of *A. fumigatus* or mixes of various *Aspergillus* species can be obtained from commercial sources for skin testing purposes.

A simple prick test with a needlepoint containing a drop of a 1–50 dilution of the extract produces a positive wheal and flare reaction within minutes in some 90 percent of patients with active disease. The test, however, can be positive in patients without ABPA. Like other immunological tests, the skin test denotes an immunologic response which may not be coincident with clinical disease. In addition to the immediate, or Type I, reaction, some patients will later develop another reaction in the same area. About 4–6 hours later, erythema, edema, and tenderness may appear, sometimes over a wider area than that of the first reaction. This reaction, known as an Arthus or Type III immune complex reaction, gradually fades over several hours. If this delayed reaction does not occur after the prick test, an intradermal test with 0.1 ml of a 1–100 dilution of *Aspergillus* extract can be done. The more potent test should be done only if the immediate prick test was relatively small, under 10 mm in diameter, or if the patient is pretreated with an antihistamine preparation. Such a relatively large intradermal test can induce an extensive and discomforting immediate reaction in the susceptible person.

IN VITRO TESTS—RAST, PRECIPITIN, AND
TOTAL IgE

Serum IgE levels are usually two or more times the upper limit of normal in those with active ABPA. The level tends to rise just before or during the phase of pulmonary eosinophilia and drops soon afterward. Thus, levels of 1000 international units (IU) of serum IgE or more are considered both diagnostic and prognostic of acute episodic ABPA when the other criteria are also present.

Similarly, serum precipitins to *Aspergillus* antigens are almost invariably present during the active disease and fade during remission. The precipitins are a more specific finding than total IgE levels, but are less quanitative and may respond more slowly to clinical changes. The tests are generally performed as a double diffusion in agar gel plates (Fig. 13-3). Counterimmune electrophoresis and related techniques are also used. A few commercial laboratories, the Center for Disease Control in Atlanta, Georgia, and some state laboratories will perform the test on request. Commercial kits are available for office laboratory testing. Perhaps most tests are done at university-affiliated research laboratories; these facilities are usually available to interested physicians. Standardized antigens and testing procedures have not been approved by a licensing agency.

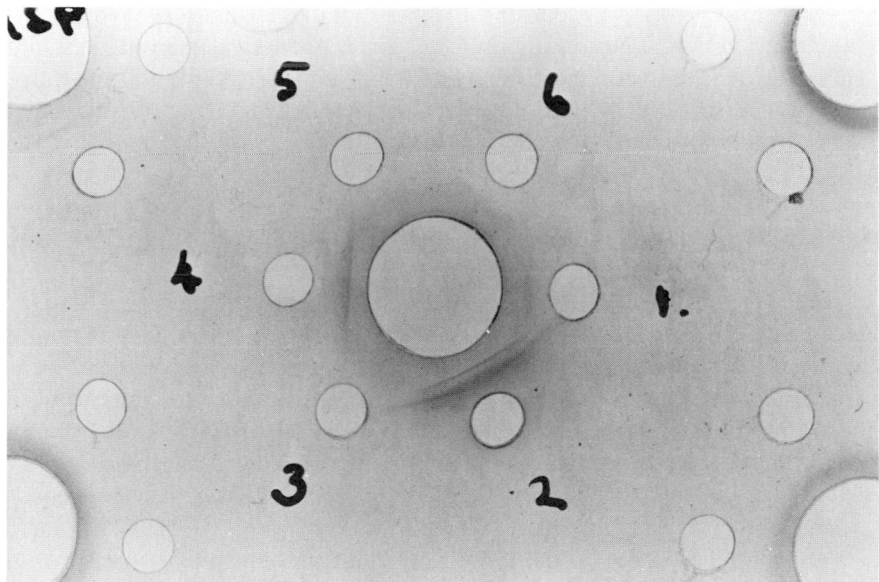

Fig. 13-3. Precipitins to *Aspergillus* extracts as seen in a double diffusion test in agar gel. Central large well contains undiluted serum of patient with ABPA. Antigens in surrounding wells: (1) *Aspergillus* mixture (Hollister-Stier); (2) *A. fumigatus* (U.C. Irvine); (3) *A. ochraceus* (U.C. Irvine); (4) *A. terreus* (U.C. Irvine); (5) *M. faeni* (U.C. Irvine); (6) *C. albicans* (H-S). There is a faint precipitate to the *Aspergillus* mix and a line of identity with it and one of the several precipitant bands to *A. fumigatus* antigens. The patient's serum also reacts with *A. terreus*, but not to the other fungal antigens.

The third test with clinical relevance, the radioallergosorbent test (RAST) for IgE antibodies to *Aspergillus* suffers some of the same availability and standardization problems as does the precipitin test.

Asthma patients with all three serological findings (high IgE levels; precipitating; and specific IgE antibodies to *Aspergillus* antigens) are very likely to have or recently have had ABPA. Aside from technical errors, the most likely cause for false negative results is a high steroid dose, which can decrease immunological synthesis.

Sputum Cultures for *Aspergillus*

Aspergillus is not difficult to grow on blood or maltose agar or on a combination medium, especially when antibiotics are incorporated in order to limit bacterial contamination. Even in proved cases of ABPA, however, the return rate of positive cultures is not much over 50 percent, even with multiple samples. The organism may be growing distal to occluding mucus plugs in the bronchi and thus not be found in expectorates. Conversely, the finding of *Aspergillus* growing in sputum isolates is not diagnostic of in vivo colonization or invasion. Both nasopharyngeal and laboratory contamination with *Aspergillus* is not uncommon. The finding of branching mycelia on microscopic examination of the specimen is likely to mean a viable organism and thus increases the chances of pathologic significance.

DIAGNOSIS AND DIFFERENTIAL DIAGNOSIS

The diagnosis of ABPA is not based upon a single diagnostic criterion. Rather, it results from the assessment of a constellation of symptoms and signs and clinical and laboratory tests. Roy Patterson's group at the Northwestern University Medical School has attempted to promote conformity in diagnosis by presenting a list of criteria. The presence of six of seven primary criteria is considered by them to be highly diagnostic and the presence of all seven is considered to confirm the diagnosis (Table 13-5). The secondary criteria are helpful, but not necessary for the diagnosis.

In using these criteria, the physician should recognize that Number 6 in the table, central bronchiectasis, is not an early finding. In order to improve early case discovery, one should look for recent changes in the course of asthma associated with febrile respiratory symptoms and infiltrates on chest films. A close temporal relationship between the clinical changes and the presence of peripheral eosinophilia and immunological abnormalities is highly diagnostic. Further confirmation would result if the immunological changes reversed in step with clinical improvement. Thus, follow-up immunoserological studies, especially for precipitins and total IgE, are helpful as both diagnostic and prognostic aids.

Table 13-5
Criteria for the Diagnosis of Allergic
Bronchopulmonary Aspergillosis[a]

Primary

1. asthma
2. blood eosinophilia
3. immediate skin reactivity to *Aspergillus*
4. precipitating antibodies against *Aspergillus*
5. elevated serum IgE levels
6. central bronchiectasis (plain films or bronchographic evidence)
7. history of pulmonary infiltrates (transient or fixed)

Secondary

1. mycelia of *Aspergillus* in sputum
2. expectoration of brown plugs or flecks in sputum
3. late skin reactivity (Arthus reactivity) to *Aspergillus* antigen

[a] From Mintzer RA, Rogers LF, Kruglik GD, et al: The spectrum of radiologic findings in allergic bronchopulmonary aspergillosis. Radiology 127:301–307, 1978. Used with permission.

The studies listed in Table 13-6 have been found to be most helpful in evaluating suspected cases of ABPA and in monitoring the course of the disease.

Differential diagnosis would include any of the following conditions: pulmonary infiltrates with eosinophilia (see section on classification), asthma with respiratory infections, bronchiectasis, recurrent pneumonias, and cystic fibrosis. Patients with cystic fibrosis are probably the most common nonasthma group to develop ABPA. Therefore, although the clinical picture of typical cystic fibrosis may closely mimic that of ABPA, especially where there is a bronchospastic component, some of these patients may in fact have developed ABPA as a complication.

In one study of ABPA, the prior diagnoses, based often on radiographic interpretations, were in descending order of frequency as follows: pneumonia, tuberculosis, bronchiectasis, lung abscess, bronchiogenic carcinoma, and pneumothorax. Lymphomas and Hodgkin's disease have also been suspected before the diagnosis of ABPA was established.

ETIOLOGY, PATHOLOGY, AND PATHOGENESIS

Etiology

In simplest terms, the etiology can be said to be: *Aspergillus* and asthma. More specifically, the species *Aspergillus fumigatus* and asthma of moderate degree of severity in the under-40 age group probably account for over 85

Table 13-6
Recommendations for Initial Work-up of Patients with
Diagnostic Impression of ABPA

---

1. History, physical, environmental survey for sources of *Aspergillus* exposure (i.e., mold growth at home or work, contaminated humidifiers or vaporizers, poultry, livestock, silage, mulch or compost, pet birds).
2. Chest films; bronchograms or CAT scans if evidence of bronchiectasis.
3. CBC, total blood eosinophils, quantitative immunoglobulins including IgE.
4. Sputum culture for *Aspergillus* and smear for eosinophils. (Save positive culture for possible extract preparation.)
5. Skin tests: *Aspergillus* mix (Hollister-Stier or comparable), prick with 1:50 W/V. Check for immediate and delayed reactions. If negative for both, retest 0.1 ml., intracutaneous of 1–100 concentration.
6. Immunoserological tests: RAST and immunodiffusion tests for specific IgE and precipitating antibodies to *Aspergillus* antigens.

Follow-up Tests

---

1. Chest films if previously abnormal, or if clinical status worsens.
2. Monthly or every 2 months until stable:
   total blood and sputum eosinophils
   sputum culture for fungi
   immunoserological tests
3. Periodic monitoring of pulmonary function.

---

percent of the confirmed cases of ABPA. The organism is one of the most prevalent fungi in the environment. Most air sampling surveys will find members of the genus *Aspergillus* among the 5 commonest fungi collected. Except for allergic sensitization, none of those other airborne fungal spores are regularly associated with human disease. Asthma is a common disease, with incidence rates of over 4 percent of the total population of the United States with current disease and a rate of 7 percent of the population suffering from asthma sometime in their lives (cumulative incidence). Even after one adjusts for the imprecision of the definition of asthma, it still ranks high in frequency among clinical disorders.

It is evident that more than the juxtaposition of *Aspergillus* and asthma is needed to produce disease, since these are extremely common biological phenomena, while ABPA is relatively uncommon. Immunologic responsiveness to antigenic components of *Aspergillus* is one prerequisite. Since nearly 25 percent of asthmatics show IgE antibody reactivity to *Aspergillus* (see section on incidence), undoubtedly multiple types of sensitization are needed in order to cause disease. As discussed later under immunopathogenesis, two or more major types of immune responses are required before clinical expression occurs.

Some epidemiologic data and individual case histories suggest the importance of degree of exposure to fungal elements. For example, more cases occur in rainy than dry months and relatively more in semi-rural than urban populations. These findings are directly related to quantity of spores present. As with most fungi, common sources of *Aspergillus* are decaying wet vegetation, such as hay, compost, dropped leaves, and straw. Birds and poultry are commonly infested with *Aspergillus*. Among indoor sources of *Aspergillus* are bath tiles and grout, areas around plumbing leaks, and wicker baskets that carry indoor plants or wet laundry (personal communication, Dr. Peter Kozak, Santa Ana, California, regarding wicker baskets).

There are reports of patients who developed ABPA only after relatively high exposure to growths of *Aspergillus*. On the other hand, most case studies have failed to uncover unusual exposures. Bagasse workers exposed to *Aspergillus*-contaminated sugar cane residue have no heightened incidence of ABPA. Thus, it appears that while accidental high exposure to *Aspergillus* may be a precipitant of ABPA, the mechanism in most cases involves a balance between exposure and immunologic response by the host. In any case, knowledge of special sources for exposures will help discover contacts that may be etiologic factors. Table 13-7 lists sources of and activities related to exposure to *Aspergillus*. Most of these activities have been associated with the onset of symptoms in suspected cases of ABPA.

Although the overwhelming number of cases of ABPA have been attributed to one species, *A. fumigatus,* several other species have been incriminated, including, but not limited to, *A. terreus, fischeri* and *ochraceus.* Cole and Samson have suggested that the smaller size and smoother surface of *A. fumigatus* spores when compared to other species of *Aspergillus* promote their deposition into the lower airways.

Pathology

Specimens of tissue affected by ABPA have been obtained from bronchial biopsies and from lung tissue after surgical resection and necropsy (Figs. 13-4, 13-5).

In one series of 7 bronchial biopsies, histopathological findings were those of typical asthma. In addition, mucus plugs were attached to the bronchial walls and some contained fungal mycelial elements compatible with *Aspergillus* species. The walls were infiltrated with polys and eosinophils, and some had granulomatous changes. In areas of consolidation, the alveoli contain numerous eosinophils, giving the appearance of eosinophilic pneumonia.

When W. S. Symmers carefully sectioned and stained bronchial areas involved with ABPA, he found hyphae attached to thickened basement membrane by vesicular structures. On occasion, a mycelial thread penetrated through the membrane into the lamina propria. Riley and his associates described a patient in whom the fungus was found within granulomata in the parenchyma, but in this and other cases, *Aspergillus* could not be grown on

Table 13-7
Sources for Increased Exposure to *Aspergillus*

Activity	Source of Fungal Supply
Outdoors	
gardening	mulch, compost, dead leaves and grass
farming	moldy hay and straw, barns and silos
poultry breeding and chicken farming; pet store owner, bird breeder and fancier, factory worker sorting eggs, zoo worker, poultry agricultural inspector	birds and chickens are commonly infested; found in excreta, tissues, blood
horse riding	stables, corrals
cattle raising	barns, moldy hay
Indoors	
cleaning cages	pet bird
repair work	areas around plumbing leaks, rain leaks
gardening	house plants in wicker baskets
laundry	wicker baskets used to transport wet laundry
smoking	moldy marijuana cigarettes

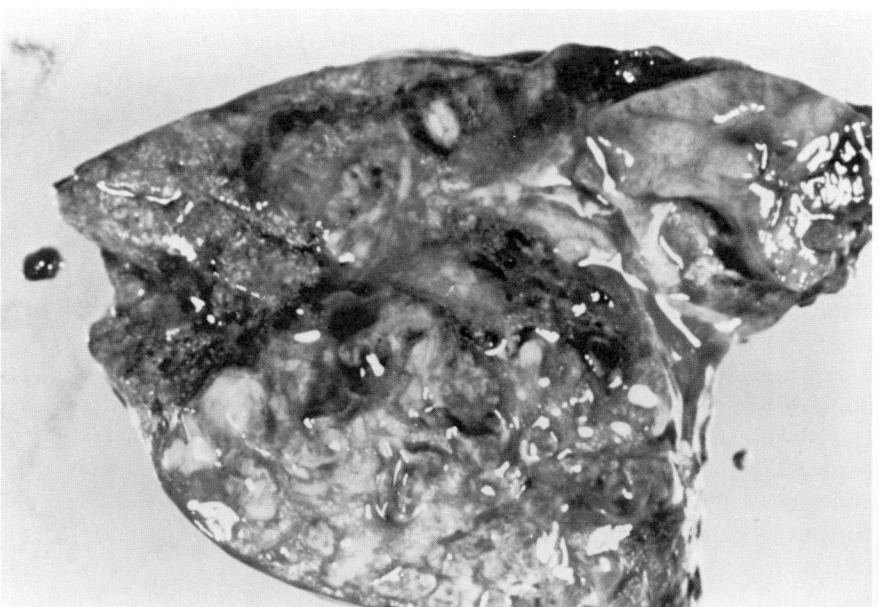

Fig. 13-4. Lung section from lobectomy specimen of patient in Figure 13-2, showing major bronchi on section filled with mucopurulent material. The major portion of the parenchyma was involved by multiple and partially confluent areas of consolidation.

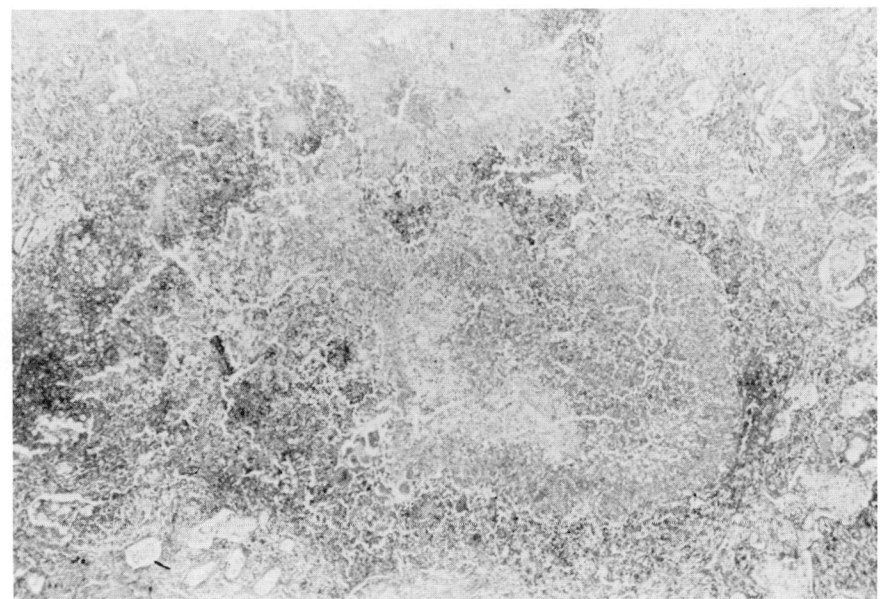

Fig. 13-5. Photomicrogram through a section of the lobectomy specimen (Fig. 13-4) showing a central necrotic area surrounded by a zone of palisading epitheloid and giant cell forms. The area probably involved a bronchus that was destroyed by a necrotizing granulomatous process (× 110). Allergic bronchopulmonary aspergillosis complicated by bronchocentric granulomatosis.

cultures from lung tissue specimens. A prominent feature of ABPA is noncaseating granulomas rich in eosinophilic material. Vasculitis is not in evidence.

Liebow's group has described a particularly devastating form of pulmonary pathology they termed bronchocentric granulomatosis. The primary changes involve a severe necrotizing granulomatous inflammation involving and destroying bronchi with minimal angiitis. Of their first 23 patients, ten had asthma and nine of these had eosinophilia and evidence of noninvasive fungal hyphae. The remaining cases were attributed to other or unknown causes, suggesting multiple etiologic factors for this entity.

In summary, the following changes, in addition to asthma, have been found on histopathological studies of ABPA:

1. ectatic bronchi filled with mucus, fibrin, inflammatory cells, and hyphae of *A. fumigatus*
2. infiltration with mononuclear cells and eosinophils, and noncaseating granulomatous changes in bronchial walls
3. mucoid impactions of the bronchi containing *Aspergillus* hyphae
4. alveoli filled with clumps of eosinophils
5. bronchocentric granulomatosis

Immunopathogenesis

Aspergillus spores, by virtue of their size and shape, are readily deposited into the larger bronchi after inhalation. They sporulate and grow in some persons with asthma (and in some with cystic fibrosis) for reasons not yet determined. They shed antigenic components that are absorbed, and, after contact either with bronchial associated lymphoid tissue or distant lymphoid tissue by systemic circulation or both, elicit an immunologic response. Specific antibodies to *Aspergillus* from all classes of immunoglobulins except D have been found in sera, saliva, and bronchial secretions. Total serum IgE and IgG, as well as all 4 subclasses of IgG, were found to be elevated in one series of 31 patients. Thymus-dependent lymphocytes, on contact with *Aspergillus* antigens, transform to blastic stages and also release various lymphokines in some trials. There is thus evidence for both humoral and cellular immune reactions.

Pepys first proposed that the disease was a result of combined Type I and III immunologic reactions. Support for this proposal comes from the finding of both specific IgE and IgG (as well as other classes of antibodies) in most active cases, from the presence of both circulating and bronchial deposits of immune complexes containing *Aspergillus* antigen, and from the passive transfer of aspects of the disease to primates with sera containing Type I and III antibodies.

This dual mechanism entails initial interaction between *Aspergillus* antigen and IgE antibody attached to bronchopulmonary mast cells. The resultant release of histamine, the leukotrienes, and eosinophilic chemotactic factor could account for bronchospasm, increased permeability of bronchial mucosa, absorption of more *Aspergillus* antigen, and pulmonary and peripheral eosinophilia. The absorbed antigen, reacting with preformed specific IgG antibody, would produce microprecipitates, activate complement, and lead to inflammation of bronchial and peribronchial tissue. Whether these elements could also cause the granulomatous and fibrotic changes is problematical. Several investigators, citing the T lymphocyte sensitization to *Aspergillus* antigen, believe a Type IV immune process also plays a pathogenic role. A unifying hypothesis would have the immune complexes activating killer T cells to attack antibody-coated target cells, a form of antibody-dependent, cell-mediated cytotoxicity.

Of course, immunologic abnormalities alone cannot explain the mechanism for this disease. The bronchial epithelial injuries present in asthma and cystic fibrosis probably encourage deposition, absorption, and persistence of *Aspergillus* components. A unifying proposal for the *Aspergillus*-associated lung diseases is depicted in Figure 13-6.

A genetic component was not found when human leukocyte antigens (HLA) haplotypes were studied in 35 unrelated patients, but in another report a familial effect was suggested when 2 siblings with identical HLA serotypes were found with the disease.

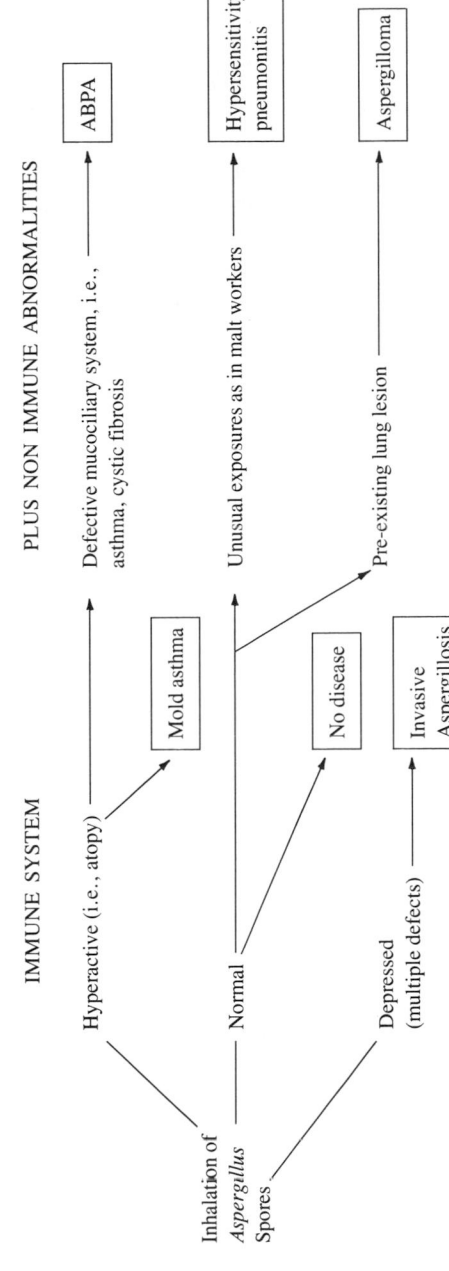

Fig. 13-6. Both immune and nonimmune factors appear to interact in the pathogenesis of most cases of allergic broncho-pulmonary aspergillosis (ABPA). This figure also attempts to place ABPA in relationship with other *Aspergillus* pulmonary diseases.

291

COMPLICATIONS AND SEQUELAE

Presumably as a result of chronic inflammation caused by sensitization to a persisting presence of *Aspergillus* antigen, bronchial, peribronchial, and interstitial lung pathology occurs. Arising from this injury, a number of complications and sequelae of ABPA have been observed. Bronchiectasis has been mentioned in the diagnostic criteria, but should also be considered a complication. Progression to end-stage lung disease manifested by extensive pulmonary scarring and fibrosis and culminating in cor pulmonale and death has been described and is discussed in the section on management. Since the report of Liebow in 1972, an additional 10 cases of bronchocentric granulomatosis in patients with asthma have been published. Several of them had been diagnosed as ABPA. In addition to these sequelae, a summary of the complications of ABPA is listed in Table 13-8.

MANAGEMENT

Treatment has been directed against: (1) the fungal etiological agent; and (2) the inflammatory reaction presumably caused by allergic sensitization.

In the original paper, the first approach was tried on two patients. Hinson's group found no effect on the fungi with iodides or neoarsphenamine. Subsequently, amphotericin B, nystatin, clortrimazole, diiohydroxyquinoline, and other fungicidal agents have been used with mixed results. One study used amphotericin B at 1 mg/5 ml distilled water in a nebulizer on a three-times-daily basis in 6 patients with ABPA. Three experienced dramatic improvement, while the others were unchanged or worsened. One patient with suspected disease cleared his radiographic infiltrates after coughing up mucus plugs. His treatment was limited to bronchodilators and vigorous chest physiotherapy.

Table 13-8
Complications of ABPA

---
1. proximal-type bronchiectasis
2. pulmonary scarring and fibrosis
3. cor pulmonale
4. pulmonary cavitation
5. coexisting opportunistic pathogens such as *Pneumocystis carinii* and atypical mycobacteria
6. bronchocentric granulomatosis
7. invasive pulmonary aspergillosis associated with steroid therapy
8. aspergillomata, pulmonary and cerebral
9. pneumothorax
10. pleural effusion

Thus, it must be recognized that removal of the offending organism and its antigenic load on the patient, while conceptually sensible, is difficult to achieve. Present fungicidal drugs appear inadequate. Attempts at improving airway function by conventional means—bronchodilators, cromolyn sodium, pulmonary toilet—are indicated. Removal of mucus plugs and impaction should be an objective. Whether preventative measures such as removal of unusual sources of *Aspergillus* growth help an existing case is not established. Such measures should lessen the potential antigenic load.

Some patients with asthma or hay fever receive immunotherapy injections with extracts containing *Aspergillus* antigens. Some of them have developed serum precipitins and an Arthus skin reaction after such treatment, but exacerbation of ABPA has not been shown. On the other hand, one child with asthma receiving injections of fungal antigens, including *Aspergillus*, who was exposed to a massive growth of the organism in his bathroom soon afterward developed ABPA and bronchocentric granulomatosis. As a precaution, any patients who are given *Aspergillus* extracts by injection should be monitored by serum precipitin tests. If precipitins and *Aspergillus* should appear, then immunotherapy with these allergens should cease.

Treatment found most successful in shortening the course of an episode of ABPA and in decreasing recurrence has been the use of systemic steroids. Early studies showed that 45 percent of steroid-treated patients cleared their pulmonary densities within 4 weeks, compared to 18 percent of the untreated. In long-term studies, the recurrence rate of pulmonary pathology is less in patients on over 7.5 mg prednisone equivalent daily dose than in those on less or none. Recently, the Patterson group has summarized its experience with the disease by listing specific recommendations for treatment and evaluation (Table 13-9). They have also called attention to the natural and clinical course of the disease by its classification into 5 stages. While most patients probably enjoy a complete remission (stage II) after a single acute episode (I), others are subject to repeated exacerbations (III). These exacerbations in turn result in increasing pulmonary damage until bronchiectasis and steroid-dependent asthma (IV) ensues. Some of those in stage IV progress into fibrotic lung disease (V) and die from cardiac failure.

Preliminary studies suggested that inhaled beclomethasone and triamcinolone could be substituted for the oral preparation in this disease. Subsequently, however, exacerbation of ABPA in patients with asthma and recurrence in patients with ABPA using the steroid aerosols have tempered the initial optimism for such substitutions.

A special caution must be kept in mind about steroid administration in a fungal-related disease. Disseminated aspergillosis is not uncommon in an immunosuppressed patient. There have been at least 2 reports of invasive disease in ABPA patients presumably on high-steroid-dose therapy. Close surveillance of the dose of steroids and of the propensity of the patient to have other infections or a decrease in immune status is in order.

Table 13-9

Suggested Protocol for Management of ABPA[a]

Initial Therapy After Diagnosis

1. 0.5 mg of prednisone per kg of body weight as single daily dose for 2 weeks, then every other day. (Occasionally, longer daily dose therapy is required for complete clearing of chest roentgenograms.)
2. Prednisone is continued at 0.5 mg per kg every other day for 3 months and then tapered and discontinued during a 3-month period.
3. After initial clearing of lung lesions, as determined by roentgenogram, repeated chest films are obtained every 4 months for 2 years, then every 6 months for 2 years, and then annually if no exacerbations have occurred.
4. A total serum IgE concentration is obtained monthly. A decrease in IgE concentration appears in 1–2 months, and a plateau occurs after 6 months. A significant increase in total IgE suggests the presence of asymptomatic infiltrates or a subsequent recurrence of infiltrates and is thus an indication for resumption of prednisone therapy even in the absence of symptoms.
5. After 2 years of observation without evidence of recurrences, total serum IgE is obtained every 2 months.
6. Annual determinations of pulmonary function.

Therapy for a Recurrence of ABPA

1. Resumption of described prednisone regimen.
2. Because recurrences of ABPA appear to cluster in certain patients with ABPA, a recurrence indicates the need for more prolonged, closer observation.

[a] From Wang JL, Patterson R, Roberts M, et al: The management of allergic bronchopulmonary aspergillosis. Amer Rev Respir Dis 120:87–91, 1979. Used with permission.

PROGNOSIS

Although some patients have a single episode of ABPA followed by complete resolution, many are subject to recurring episodes of febrile bronchitis or pulmonary eosinophilic infiltrates with deteriorating pulmonary function. Of course, if complications such as bronchiectasis, pulmonary fibrosis, or bronchocentric granulomatous were present at the time of diagnosis, the outlook for substantial improvement is bleak.

In a 5-year follow-up study of 50 patients by the Pepys group, while daily prednisone dose over 7.5 mg reduced recurrences over those untreated, no treatment regimen completely abolished exacerbations. An important finding, subsequently substantiated by others, is that pulmonary infiltrates could recur and produce pulmonary destruction without symptomatology. Patterson's group evaluated 25 patients over a 1–10-year period, and found that about one-half had no recurrences, while a few had multiple exacerbations. They found that high IgE levels usually preceded these exacerbations and that IgE levels returned to baseline shortly after remission. Neither group could define the patient at greater risk for recurrences and complications. Severity of the underlying asthma did not appear to be a risk factor.

The long-term effectiveness of various treatment programs remains to be established. It is hoped, but still too early to be certain, that early diagnosis and the currently recommended therapy will prevent allergic bronchopulmonary aspergillosis from becoming either a chronic disabling or fatal disease.

ALLERGIC BRONCHOPULMONARY DISEASE ATTRIBUTED TO FUNGI OTHER THAN *ASPERGILLI*

Some patients present with many of the clinical features of ABPA but have immunological and cultural responses to other fungal organisms. Perhaps the most commonly reported of these is *Candida albicans*. A study from India disclosed 13 cases of allergic bronchopulmonary candidiasis. Single case reports have also originated from the United Kingdom, France, and the United States. Other fungi incriminated include *Helminthosporium* and closely related dematiaceous fungi *Curvularia, Drechslera,* and *Stemphylium*. The best-studied of these cases had specific IgE- and IgG-precipitating antibodies to the particular fungal extract and none to multiple species of *Aspergillus*. Most, but not all, of the patients in this category had active asthma.

REFERENCES

Campbell MJ, Clayton YM: Bronchopulmonary aspergillosis: A correlation of the clinical and laboratory findings in 272 patients investigated for bronchopulmonary aspergillosis. Am Rev Respir Dis 89:186–196, 1964

Editorial: Corticosteroids in pulmonary aspergillosis. Br Med J 4:567–568, 1972

Golbert TM, Patterson R: Pulmonary allergic aspergillosis. Ann Intern Med 72:395–403, 1970

Hanson GH, Flod N, Wells I, et al: Bronchocentric granulomatosis: A complication of allergic bronchopulmonary aspergillosis. J Allergy Clin Immunol 59:83–90, 1977

Hinson KF, Moon AJ, Plummer MS: Bronchopulmonary aspergillosis. A review and a report of eight new cases. Thorax 7:317–333, 1952

Imbeau SA, Cohen M, Reed CE: Allergic bronchopulmonary aspergillosis in infants. Am J Dis Child 131:1127–1130, 1977

Katzenstein AL, Liebow AA, Friedman PJ: Bronchocentric granulomatosis, mucoid impaction, and hypersensitivity reactions to fungus. Am Rev Respir Dis 111:497–537, 1975

Malo JL, Longbottom J, Mitchell J, et al: Studies in chronic allergic aspergillosis. III. Immunological findings. Thorax 32:269–274, 1977

McCarthy DS, Pepys J: Pulmonary aspergilloma—Clinical immunology. Clin Allergy 3:57–70, 1973

McCarthy DS, Simon G, Hargreave FE: The radiological appearance in allergic bronchopulmonary aspergillosis. Clin Radiol 21:366–375, 1970

Mendelson EB, Fisher MR, Mintzer RA, et al: Roentgenographic and clinical staging of allergic bronchopulmonary aspergillosis. Chest 87:334–339, 1985

Patterson R, Greenberger PA, Radin RC, et al: Allergic bronchopulmonary aspergillosis: Staging as an aid to management. Ann Intern Med 96:286–291, 1982

Poirier VC, Alfidi RJ: Roentgenographic features of allergic bronchopulmonary aspergillosis. Cleveland Clin Quart 37:171–176, 1970

Riley DJ, Mackenzie JW, Uhlman WE, et al: Allergic bronchopulmonary aspergillosis: Evidence of limited tissue invasion. Am Rev Respir Dis 111:232–236, 1975

Rosenberg M, Patterson R, Mintzer R, et al: Clinical and immunologic criteria for the diagnosis of allergic bronchopulmonary aspergillosis. Ann Intern Med 86:405–414, 1977

Safirstein BH, D'Souza MF, Simon G, et al: Five year follow-up of bronchopulmonary aspergillosis. Am Rev Respir Dis 108:450–459, 1973

Scadding JC: The bronchi in allergic aspergillosis. Scand J Respir Dis 38:372–377, 1967

Slavin RG, Middleton E, Reed CE, et al: Allergic bronchopulmonary aspergillosis, in Middleton E, et al. (eds): Allergy Principles and Practices, vol. 2. St. Louis, C.V. Mosby, 1978, pp. 843–854

Symmers WC: Histopathological aspects of the pathogenesis of some opportunistic fungal infections, as exemplified in the pathology of aspergillosis and the phycomycetoses. Lab Invest 11:1073–1090, 1962

Turner KJ, O'Mahoney J, Wetherall JD, et al: Hypersensitivity studies in asthmatic patients with bronchopulmonary aspergillosis. Clin Allergy 2:361–372, 1972

Wang JL, Patterson R, Roberts M, et al: The management of allergic bronchopulmonary aspergillosis. Am Rev Respir Dis 120:87–91, 1979

Warnock ML, Fennessy J, Rippin J: Chronic eosinophilic pneumonia, a manifestation of allergic aspergillosis. Am J Clin Pathol 62:73–81, 1974

Marc Schenker
Sverre Vedal

14

Occupational Asthma

Occupational asthma may be defined as asthma that is predominantly caused by exposures in the workplace. This definition assumes the commonly, but not generally accepted, definition of asthma as a disorder in which there is intermittent reversible obstruction of the airways. It does not specify the nature of the workplace exposures, which may be specific substances handled at work, incidental exposures, or unknown factors associated with the work environment. There is a great diversity to the mechanisms and causes of asthma due to workplace exposure. Occupational asthma may be immunologic or nonimmunologic in origin and it may be caused by a wide spectrum of small and large molecular weight substances, delivered as gases, fumes, or particles.

The distinction of occupational asthma from asthma of nonoccupational origin may be useful for diagnostic or therapeutic reasons (e.g., removal from the workplace). Another consideration involves compensation, for which it may be important but not always possible to ascertain the etiology or predominant cause in a case of asthma. Furthermore, definitions of *occupational* asthma may vary within different legal contexts or jurisdictions. For the purposes of this chapter, preexisting asthma that is exacerbated by workplace exposures is not considered occupational asthma.

The diagnosis of occupational asthma is important for several reasons beyond the usual considerations in treating a case of asthma:

1. The condition may often be improved or cured by reducing or eliminating exposures at the workplace.

BRONCHIAL ASTHMA, Second Edition
ISBN 0-8089-1814-1

2. Knowledge of sensitization in an individual may affect recommendations for his or her current and future work.
3. Sensitization to new substances introduced in the workplace may signal reactions among other workers.
4. Occupational asthma may be a compensable disorder. In addition, studies of occupational asthma may assist in a better understanding of the causes and mechanisms of nonoccupational asthma.

It is very difficult to estimate the incidence or prevalence of occupational asthma. Many surveys have relied on questionnaire responses only, which may not accurately reflect airway hyperreactivity or its etiology. Cross-sectional studies of workers may also incorrectly estimate asthma prevalence because of preemployment screening to eliminate *sensitive* workers and because of the selective loss of workers who became sensitized at work. This selective loss of workers who become sensitized, one manifestation of the *healthy worker effect*, is often not recorded on work records.

Limited studies suggest that the prevalence of occupational asthma varies with the agent and industry. In industries with exposure to agents such as proteolytic enzymes in the detergent industry and laboratory animals in research facilities, the prevalence of occupational asthma is generally between 2 and 10 percent of workers, but has been reported to be much higher. The prevalence of nonspecific allergic symptoms (e.g., rhinitis, conjunctivitis) is commonly 10–30 percent in these industries. The prevalence and predominant types of occupational asthma in the general population may be affected by the types of industries in the surrounding communities.

MECHANISMS

Exposure to substances found in the workplace can cause episodic respiratory symptoms and airways obstruction by several mechanisms, not all of which result in asthma. Exposure to bronchial irritants such as sulfur dioxide and ozone can result in acute bronchoconstriction and increased airway reactivity. Although workers with preexisting asthma are more sensitive to irritant exposures, all exposed workers will be affected, if the exposure concentrations are high enough.

Another picture results from exposure to extremely high concentrations of toxic agents such as occurs with industrial accidents or spills. After the acute inflammation from such an exposure resolves, workers often continue to have increased airways reactivity and are sensitive to concentrations of bronchial irritants that previously had no adverse effects. This heightened reactivity gradually resolves with time.

In most circumstances, these two examples of airways obstruction would be self-limited and should not be included with occupational asthma. Implications for management and for compensation are considerably different in these instances than in the types of airway hyperreactivity and episodic airway obstruction whose descriptions follow.

Some forms of occupational asthma occur through mechanisms that are identical to those responsible for extrinsic allergic asthma. In these cases, IgE antibody specific for the responsible allergen can be identified either by skin prick testing or by identification of significant serum levels of antigen specific IgE, by either radioallergosorbent testing (RAST) or the enzyme-linked immunosorbent assay (ELISA). Typically, only a small percentage of exposed workers are affected after a latent period during which sensitization occurs. Atopic workers are preferentially affected, although a large percentage of atopic workers will not develop asthma. After sensitization relatively low concentrations of the antigen may trigger bronchoconstriction. In many instances, continued exposure and antigen stimulation result in increasingly severe asthma.

An example of occupational asthma produced through such an immunologically mediated mechanism is that seen in workers employed in the detergent industry, who developed asthma from exposure to proteolytic enzymes derived from *Bacillus subtilis*. Atopic workers are more likely to be sensitized on exposure to these high molecular weight compounds. Specific IgE to the enzymes has been documented both by skin prick tests and by identification of specific circulating IgE using RAST. Late reactions as well as recurrent nocturnal symptoms may be present in addition to the IgE mediated immediate reaction.

Although both large and small molecular weight compounds have been shown to result in immunologically-mediated asthma, many small molecular weight compounds cause occupational asthma, which clinically appears to have an immunologic basis but with features that distinguish it from the immunologic group. These compounds include toluene diisocyanate (TDI), colophony (one cause of asthma in solderers) and plicatic acid (the causative agent in western red cedar). All of these compounds result in asthma in a minority of exposed workers after a latent period of months to years and cause symptoms at low concentrations in sensitized workers. These features are suggestive of immunologically-mediated asthma. However, the demonstration of specific IgE by skin testing or by RAST in workers with occupational asthma, as documented by specific bronchial provocation testing has been inconsistent. For example, no skin test positivity to plicatic acid has been demonstrated in workers with western red cedar asthma, and only 30 to 40 percent of workers with western red cedar asthma have elevated plicatic acid specific IgE antibodies by RAST. Similarly, the RAST for TDI (p-tolyl isocyanate) has failed to identify workers with TDI asthma. Since small molecular weight compounds may act as haptens, it is possible that the correct carrier proteins have not been used in attempting to identify specific IgE. Another possibility is that the asthma is due to nonimmunologic mechanisms in some or all of these cases.

Pharmacologic release of mediators or β-adrenergic blockade and activation of the complement system are potential mechanisms that may produce occupational asthma, and be operative in the immunologic-like asthma seen with some low molecular weight compounds or in occupational asthma that does not have features suggesting an immunologic basis. Both TDI and plicatic acid have β-adrenergic blocking effects, and plicatic acid can activate complement. Neither of these mechanisms, however, is likely to be significant at the low exposure concentrations that can elicit asthmatic reactions in susceptible workers. While the existence of potentially several mechanisms interacting to result in occupational asthma is intriguing, there is no evidence to suggest that these other mechanisms play any role in the actual pathogenesis of occupational asthma.

CAUSES OF OCCUPATIONAL ASTHMA (Table 14-1)

Over one hundred causes of occupational asthma have been described, and there are certainly numerous unidentified causes of this disorder. Some causes have appeared (and have diminished in occurrence) with changes in industrial processes or product formulation. This was the circumstance with the asthma which occurred following the introduction of proteolytic enzymes in the detergent industry. Similarly, a change in the method of meat wrapping to include cutting the polyvinyl chloride film with a heated wire resulted in complaints of mucous membrane and airway irritation. Several irritant or sensitizing agents were found to be released by the new process, although allergic sensitization and asthma have not been demonstrated. It is likely that new causes of occupational asthma will continue to be recognized as industrial processes and exposures change in the workplace.

Etiologic agents of occupational asthma may conveniently be divided into three categories: animal materials, plant materials, and chemicals. This classification allows some generalizations about causal agents and mechanism, although too much is unknown about many substances at the present time to clarify their mode of action or the type of clinical reaction.

Animal Origin Substances

Numerous substances of animal origin may cause allergic reactions or asthma among workers. These substances most commonly contain high-molecular weight compounds, and many have been associated with IgE anti-

Table 14-1
Some Causes of Occupational Asthma

Agents	Occupation(s)
Plant Origin	
Flour (wheat, rye, buckwheat, soybean)	Bakers
Grain dust	Grain elevator operators, dock workers, farmers
Bean dusts (castor, coffee, soy)	Millers, coffee bean workers
Hops	Brewery workers
Vegetable gums (acacia, tragacanth)	Printers, gum manufacturers
Wood dusts (western red cedar, oak, California redwood, mahogany, boxwood, zebrawood, iroko, mulberry, others)	Sawmill workers, carpenters, wood finishers
Plant dusts (green leaf tea, tobacco leaf)	Tea and tobacco workers
Plant enzymes (papain)	Food technologists
Animal Origin	
Laboratory animals	Laboratory workers, veterinarians, animal technicians, zoo workers
Chemical organ extracts (pancreatic, pituitary)	Pharmaceutical workers
Birds	Bird fanciers, poultry workers, feather pickers
Insects (grain weevils, storage mites, moths, silkworms, cockroaches, river flys)	Grainery and dock workers, entomologists, laboratory and outside workers, silkworm cutters
Marine animals (oysters, prawns, pearl shells)	Commercial processors
Chemical Substances	
Metals	
Platinum	Platinum refiners
Nickel	Nickelplaters
Vanadium	Boiler and turbine cleaners
Cobalt	Tungaten carbide grinders
Stainless steel	Welders

Table 14-1
Continued

Agents	Occupation(s)
Chemical Substances continued	
Chemicals	
Chloramine	Brewery workers
Amino-ethyl-ethanolamine	Aluminum solderers
Ethylenediamine	Rubber workers
Pyrethrins	Pesticide applicators
Diisocryanates	Polyurethane foam manufacturers
Pthalic anhydrides	Chemical, epoxy resin workers
Colophony	Solderers
Reactive dyes	Dye manufacturers
Drugs	
Psyllium	Laxative manufacturers
Antibiotics (tetracycline, penicillin, sulfathiazole)	Pharmaceutical workers

bodies. The allergenic molecules may be present in the animal body parts, hairs, dander, excretions (urine, feces), and whole animal or organ extracts (enzyme powders). Exposure to some substances of animal origin has been reported to cause very high prevalences of sensitization (40–70 percent). This may be due to the potency of these antigens and/or to the high concentrations present in some work settings.

One large population of workers at potential risk for asthma or other allergic reactions due to substances of animal origin are animal handlers. This includes veterinarians, pet store workers, laboratory technicians, research investigators, farmers, and zoo workers. Allergic sensitization has been well described among laboratory animal workers, where 10–30 percent of workers will develop rhinitis, conjunctivitis, or other allergic symptoms, and 25–50 percent of these workers will develop asthma. Sensitization and symptoms usually occur within the first 3 years of exposure. Atopy is a predisposing factor for this type of asthma, but many workers with atopy do not develop asthma. Therefore, knowing that a worker is atopic is a poor predictor of his or her risk of developing asthma from laboratory animals.

Proteins with antigenic potential have been demonstrated in the dander extracts, urine, serum, and saliva of laboratory rats and mice. Recent studies have shown increased antigen levels in the air from fear associated urinary voiding, and this may represent an important source of sensitization among laboratory animal handlers that is not controlled by traditional dust suppression methods.

Another group of animal substances that cause asthma occurs among commercial processors of animals or animal products. Examples that have been shown to cause asthma in the occupational setting include wool (sheep), feathers (poultry), oysters, and prawns. As with laboratory animal asthma, these agents may cause immediate or late asthmatic reactions.

Many insects have been described as causes of occupational asthma. Exposure to insects may be incidental in some occupations or the insects may be the primary product of the work. Examples of incidental insect exposures include grainery workers exposed to grain storage mites and river fly sensitization among power plant workers along the Mississippi River. Examples of occupations with asthma due to commercially produced insects include silkworm workers and beekeepers. Finally, insects are often bred for research or teaching, and occupations at risk include entymologists, laboratory workers, teachers, and students.

Several enzymes have been derived from animal extracts, and these may be potent sensitizing agents. Examples include workers handling pituitary and pancreatic extracts, and the enzymes derived from *Bacillus subtilis* species in the detergent industry.

Plant Origin Substances

A large number of plant materials have been reported to cause occupational asthma. While some of the sensitizing agents are high molecular weight compounds, other mediators are organic acids of low molecular weight such as plicatic acid, the cause of western red cedar asthma. As with substances of animal origin, the asthmatic reactions to plant origin materials may be immediate, late, dual, or recurrent nocturnal.

Pulmonary reactions to flour were recognized in 1700 by Ramazzini, and specific asthmatic reactions have now been described for several flours including wheat, rye, buckwheat, and soybean. Asthma has also been described with exposure to the dusts or powders of numerous other foods such as tea leaf, coffee bean, cottonseed, and beer hops. Asthma usually occurs among the commercial producers or handlers of these substances, but may also occur among users of these products such as occurs with sensitization to gum tragacanth and gum acacia among printers.

Numerous woods are known to cause asthma. These include common woods such as western red cedar, California redwood, and oak; rare woods such as mako, mansonia, zebrawood, and boxwood may also cause asthma. Western red cedar asthma has been extensively studied, and bronchial reactivity has been reproduced by bronchial challenge with plicatic acid, the major nonvolatile component of western red cedar. The specific causal agent for asthma from most of these woods is unknown.

Chemical Substances

An increasing number of chemicals are being recognized as causes of occupational asthma. These chemicals may be simple or complex compounds, and most are of low molecular weight (less than 1000 daltons). Some of these compounds have clearly recognized allergic mechanisms, such as trimelletic anhydride, and may cause sensitization at low concentrations. Other chemicals act as irritants and may result in increased airway reactivity but are not associated with demonstrable *sensitization.*

One category of chemical agents are the metallic salts, many of which also cause nonpulmonary allergic reactions. Examples of such metals are nickel and chromium, which cause asthma among metal and chemical workers and are recognized causes of allergic cutaneous sensitization. Other metals that cause asthma include platinum, vanadium, cobalt, and stainless steel (chromium and nickel).

A second category of chemicals includes industrial products and intermediate substances. These include several amines (e.g., chloramine, ethylenediamine), and other chemical compounds (e.g., formaldehyde, diisocyanates, pthalic anhydrides, reactive dyes). Occupational exposure to these agents may occur in primary manufacturing processes or among users of the products.

The diisocyanates are a highly reactive group of chemical compounds used in the production of flexible and rigid foams, synthetic rubber, adhesive, and fibers. The most commonly used diisocyanates are toluene diisocyanate (TDI) and diphenyl-methane diisocyanate (MDI). The isocyanates are known to produce irritation of the skin, eyes, and bronchial tree, and to elicit an asthma reaction on challenge testing that may be immediate, late, or recurrent nocturnal. However, despite the clinical suggestion of an allergic mechanism, it has not been possible to demonstrate an antibody to TDI that correlates with airway reactivity, and it appears that most TDI asthma is nonimmunologic in origin.

A third category of chemical agents known to cause asthma are drugs. Examples of drugs that have caused asthma among manufacturers or formulators include psyllium in laxatives, methyldopa, penicillin, and tetracycline. Many of these drugs are known causes of allergic reactions among users, but the possibility of reactions due to occupational exposures is not generally considered.

DIAGNOSIS (Table 14-2)

There is a general absence of agreement on the definition of asthma, and the diagnosis of occupational asthma is complicated by a lack of uniformly

Table 14-2
Modalities for the Diagnosis of Occupational Asthma

	Ease of Performance	Sensitivity*	Specificity*	Comments
Clinical history	+ + + +	+ + +	+	Important in all cases. May be biased, nonspecific.
Skin prick tests (specific)	+ +	+ + +	+	Poor correlation with bronchial reactivity.
Immunologic tests (RAST, ELISA)	+ +	+ + +	+	Limited assays available. May not know correct antigen for testing. May not correlate with bronchial reactivity.
PEFR, serially	+ +	+ + +	+ +	Useful with other tests. Effort dependent. Can assess effect of intervention.
Bronchial reactivity (nonspecific)	+ + +	+ + + +	+	Very sensitive, standardized. Not specific for etiology.
Bronchial challenge (specific)	+	+ + +	+ + + +	Potentially hazardous. Dose poorly controlled, but reproduces actual exposures.

* Sensitivity and specificity refer to occupational asthma and not to the specific outcome measured by the test (eg. presence of antibody in the serum).

acceptable diagnostic criteria, by different motives for making the diagnosis (treatment, disability), and by the complexity of the industrial environment. For the purpose of medical management, it may be sufficient to document work-relatedness of symptoms. However, since avoidance of exposure would be commonly central to any management plan, the implications of the diagnosis for a worker's livelihood and health are great. A more vigorous pursuit of the diagnosis is therefore often indicated.

Diagnosis of Asthma

As a first step in making a diagnosis of occupational asthma, it is necessary to know that the worker is in fact suffering from asthma. Conditions that might be confused with asthma in this setting include industrial bronchitis and hypersensitivity pneumonitis. Asthma is suggested by episodic symptoms of wheeze, of chest tightness with dyspnea, or of cough or phlegm production. The physical examination may be useful in documenting wheezing during an exacerbation of symptoms. Spirometry may show airways obstruction, which improves after the administration of an inhaled bronchodilator. The presence of eosinophils in the sputum or blood eosinophilia support the diagnosis. However, a normal physical examination, normal spirometry, and the absence of eosinophilia do not rule out the presence of asthma. It is therefore sometimes necessary to try to provoke bronchoconstriction, most commonly with pharmacologic provocation (methacholine or histamine) or with exercise or hyperventilation with subfreezing air. A negative bronchoprovocation test effectively excludes clinically significant asthma.

Although more marked degrees of airway reactivity to specific challenge substances are almost always associated with significant nonspecific bronchial hyperreactivity, one third of TDI asthmatics, for example, may not exhibit nonspecific hyperreactivity. However, those who are sensitive to very low concentrations of TDI (0.001 ppm), almost always have nonspecific airway hyperreactivity. Nonspecific bronchial reactivity also diminishes with time away from exposure. Therefore, increased nonspecific bronchial reactivity does not need to be present to make a diagnosis of occupational asthma.

Some clinical features of occupational asthma may not suggest an initial diagnosis of asthma. If symptoms occur with only exposure at work, the physical examination and spirometry in the physician's office may not be helpful. Also, cough may be the presenting symptom of asthma, and may occur only at night, not immediately suggesting a diagnosis of asthma due to workplace exposure.

Occupational Asthma

Once the causes of respiratory symptoms other than asthma have been excluded, it is important to determine that the asthma is of occupational origin. This may not be easy. Consider the instance of a worker with preexisting asthma who notes that symptoms are worse or occur only at work. The work-relatedness of these symptoms may be due to exposure to nonspecific bronchial irritants at work, by exercise performed in physically demanding jobs, or even potentially by psychological stresses at work. Even more difficult would be the worker who first develops *intrinsic* asthma as an employed adult and also has work-relatedness of his or her symptoms. In these instances and in the case of occupational asthma, appropriate treatment may require removal from exposure. If this were easily accomplished, documentation of the work-relatedness of the symptoms would be all that was required and further refinement of the diagnosis would be unnecessary. It can be appreciated, however, that stopping exposure may not be easy to do, especially if a worker's livelihood is at stake. It has been shown in western red cedar workers that persistence of asthma after stopping exposure was related to the duration of exposure. Thus, diagnosing occupational asthma, rather than work-related exacerbation of asthma, requires that the physician take a more aggressive role in preventing continued exposure than may otherwise be indicated.

There may be clues to an occupational *cause* of asthma from the history. A latent period between the onset of exposure and the development of symptoms suggests sensitization. The length of this latent period is most commonly from months to years, but can rarely occur after only a few weeks or after ten years. Occurrence of symptoms in the evenings after work or at night on work days, although obscuring the temporal relationship with work, is suggestive of late reactions. The late reactions may persist over weekends, further obscuring the relationship, but diminish with longer periods away from work. Symptoms that increase in severity with repeated workplace exposures also suggest an occupational cause, but cannot independently distinguish occupational from nonoccupational asthma. It is useful to know that the patient has exposure to one of the many agents known to cause asthma, since this may simplify the diagnostic process. A detailed history is necessary to identify both substances with which the patient works and substances that are merely present in the work environment, especially in a complex work environment. However, identifying an agent is neither necessary nor sufficient for making the diagnosis of occupational asthma.

One could envision circumstances where a consistent history would make a sufficiently secure diagnosis of occupational asthma. An example would be if removal from exposure entailed no hardship and disability was not an issue, however, such circumstances are unusual. Given the implications inherent in a diagnosis of occupational asthma, more diagnostic data should usually be gathered. Use of serial measurements of peak expiratory flow rate (PEFR) have been proposed as one method to pursue the diagnosis more rigorously. Patient administered tests using either a Wright's peak flow meter, or one of several smaller peak flow meters, are performed every 1–2 hours during the day. While serial peak flow measurements can document the work-relatedness of obstruction during the working day, they are usually inadequate to establish etiology. Another drawback to peak flow testing is that it relies completely on the patient's reliability to be useful.

Recurrent late reactions that resolve after stopping exposure and recur on reexposure are suggestive of an occupational cause of asthma, but it is not known how well this pattern of response distinguishes occupational asthma from asthma with work-related exacerbation. The presence of asthma, a characteristic serial PEFR record, and immunologic evidence of sensitization (skin test, RAST or ELISA) should generally be considered adequate for a diagnosis of occupational asthma. Unfortunately, most cases are not as easily confirmed.

A promising approach is suggested by the observation that the degree of nonspecific bronchial reactivity in occupational asthma increases with continued exposure and declines after exposure ceases. Serial measurements of nonspecific bronchial reactivity using either a methacholine or histamine bronchoprovocation test, performed weekly while the patient is working and during extended periods off work, can document changes in reactivity associated with exposure. It is possible that such serial testing of changes in airway reactivity will be a measure of the occupational cause of asthma, and will reduce the need for testing specific bronchial responsiveness except under uncommon circumstances.

Situations that might require challenge for specific reactivity include testing for an associated occupational cause in patients with preexisting asthma or in patients with adult-onset asthma with a complex pattern of symptom occurrence. It may also be used for identification of a specific causal agent or for confirmation of reaction to workplace substances. If testing of specific reactivity is required, it should be performed by experienced individuals in controlled settings with ready access to hospital facilities. Late reactions produced by challenge can be notoriously resistant to rapid treatment. Patients should, if possible, be off steroids and disodium cromoglycate before testing. Persistent airway obstruction will generally preclude challenge testing. Testing procedures have been formalized by Pepys and Hutchcroft. It is important that a control test also be performed so that nonspecific reactions and the pattern of diurnal variation can be identified.

Reactions seen following specific challenge testing include (Table 14-3): (1) an immediate reaction with fall in FEV_1 occurring within minutes of the challenge and lasting 1–2 hours, (2) a late reaction with the fall occurring several hours after challenge and usually resolving within 24 hours, and (3) dual reactions consisting of both immediate and late responses. Recurrent nocturnal reactions that wane over several nights may occur following late reactions. Other less common reaction patterns have also recently been described.

While it is difficult to control the dose of allergen in specific challenge testing, the patient is exposed to the suspected causal agent in a manner that attempts to reproduce the workplace situation. This may involve activities such as sifting flour in a case of possible baker's asthma, or soldering with exposure to the flux vapors. When possible, the same materials or substances that are used at work should be used in the bronchial provocation test. The duration of exposure will vary with the particular agent and dose, but is usually between 1 and 10 minutes. Initial exposure should be for one minute, with an incremental increase in the duration of exposure if no reaction has occurred in 15 minutes. Highly allergenic substances such as antibiotics and the salts of platinum should be mixed with a vehicle such as dried lactose before being used for challenge testing.

Table 14-3
Types of Bronchial Provocation Test Reactions

Type	Onset	Peak	Resolution	Comment
Immediate	5–15 min	15–30 min	60–120 min	Wheezing usual. No systemic symptoms. Eosinophilia may occur. Inhibited by beta adrenergic agonists and cromolyn sodium.
Late	1–4 hrs	4–8 hrs	24–48 hrs	May resolve in 3–4 hrs. Wheezing often mild. Systemic reactions (fever, malaise) occur. Polymorpholeukocytosis. May recur on successive nights after single exposure (recurrent nocturnal). May be inhibited by corticosteroids and cromolyn sodium.
Dual	5–15 min and 1–4 hrs	—	—	Combination of immediate and late types.

The critical requirement in all bronchial provocation testing is for close monitoring of the patient during the procedure. Spirometry should be repeated every 5 minutes for 1 hour after the exposure, and hourly thereafter for the remainder of the day. Because of the variety of potential reactions, the patient should monitor peak flow in the evening and in the night if awakened with symptoms. A fall of 15 percent or greater in FEV_1 compared with control values is indicative of a positive test.

Identification of circulating antibodies against suspected antigens has only a supporting role in the diagnosis of occupational asthma. RAST or ELISA may detect the presence of IgE, which is specific for the sensitizing antigens. Small molecular weight compounds such as TDI or plicatic acid, which alone cannot act as complete antigens, can sensitize as haptens when conjugated with a carrier protein and can also be detected by RAST or ELISA. However, detection of specific IgE merely determines that sensitization has occurred. Many sensitized workers do not have occupational asthma. The absence of specific IgE in a worker suspected of having occupational asthma from one of the several agents capable of causing immunologically-mediated occupational asthma effectively rules out that agent as the cause of asthma. In suspected occupational asthma due to one of the small molecular weight agents, the absence of a specific IgE is not helpful.

PREVENTION AND TREATMENT

Industrial hygiene controls to reduce exposure in the workplace should be the principal method of preventing occupational asthma. This is particularly important for workplaces with known sensitizing agents. Reduction of exposure by dust suppression and other controls was shown to reduce respiratory symptoms among workers exposed to proteolytic enzymes in the detergent industry. Controls may also be employed to reduce the number of people entering areas with airborne allergens. For example, nonanimal handlers need not enter animal areas in research facilities. Substitution of workplace substances, when possible, is another method to reduce exposures. The use of MDI instead of TDI is an example of the substitution of a less harmful chemical, although some individuals have become sensitized to MDI.

A difficult problem is avoidance of exposure to accidental spills and the consequent exposure to high concentrations of sensitizing agents. Such spills have been associated with occupational asthma among TDI exposed workers. Periodic surveillance of workers with questionnaires, pulmonary function tests or immunologic studies may be the only way to detect the cumulative effects of such exposures.

While reducing exposures may prevent sensitization in some workers, it is more difficult to prevent symptoms in the sensitized worker. In that circumstance even workplaces that meet industrial hygiene standards may not provide adequate protection so that removal from work (and exposure) may be the only available alternative. This is another circumstance in which periodic medical surveillance may detect excessive symptoms or decline in pulmonary function before permanent respiratory impairment occurs.

Personal protection methods such as dust masks or respirators should not be the primary mode of preventing sensitization or of protecting the sensitized worker. Respirators may not provide adequate protection, and effective systems may significantly interfere with work. It is also unlikely that unsensitized, asymtomatic workers will use respiratory protection. However, respirators and protective clothing have been successfully used by laboratory workers to reduce allergic symptoms, and they may be appropriate for some individuals who cannot avoid intermittent exposure to allergen containing environments.

Individuals who develop clinically significant occupational asthma should be removed from exposure to the causative agent. It is preferable to transfer a worker with asthma to another job within the industry, but sometimes a change of industry or of career may be necessary. If permanent removal from exposure is not desirable for career or economic reasons, temporary removal may be tried until pulmonary function has returned to normal. Any return to work, however, should be closely monitored for recurrence of airway hyperractivity and clinical asthma. Serial peak flow measurements (for 1–2 week periods) are a useful method of following such individuals after they return to work.

The drug treatment of occupational asthma is essentially the same as for other types of asthma. Sodium cromoglycate should be tried because of its ability to prevent both immediate and late reactions to some agents. Chronic oral corticosteroids should not be used if removal from exposure will eliminate the requirement for their use. Monitoring of PEFR is also useful to evaluate the effectiveness of medical therapy.

REFERENCES

Bardana EJ, Andrach RH: Occupational asthma secondary to low molecular weight agents used in the plastic and resin industries. Eur J Resp Dis 64:241–251, 1983

Block G, Chan-Yeung M: Asthma induced by nickel. J Amer Med Assoc 247:1600–1602, 1982

Block G, Tse KS, Kijek K, et al: Baker's asthma: Clinical and immunological studies. Clin Allergy 13:359, 370, 1983

Broder I, McAvoy D: Characterization of precipitation reaction between grain dust and normal human serum and comparison of reactive and nonreactive grain handlers. Clin Immunol Immunopathol 21:141, 153, 1981

Brooks SM, Lockey J: Reactive Airways Disease Syndrome (RADS): A newly defined occupational disease. Amer Rev Resp Dis 123:133, 1981

Brooks SM: Occupational asthma, in Weiss EB, Segal MS, Stein M (eds): Bronchial Asthma: Mechanisms and Therapeutics. Second Edition, Boston, Little, Brown, and Company, 1985, pp 461–493

Brooks SM, McGowan K, Bernstein IL, et al: Relationship between numbers of beta-adrenergic receptors in lymphocytes and disease severity in asthma. J Allergy and Clin Immunol 63:401, 406, 1979

Bruckner HC: Extrinsic asthma in a tungsten carbide worker. J Occup Med 9:518–519, 1967

Burge PS, O'Brien IM, Harries MG: Peak flow rate records in the diagnosis of occupational asthma due to colophony, Thorax 34:308–316, 1979

Butcher BT, Hammad YY, Hendrick DJ: Occupational Asthma: Identification of the agent, in Gee JBL. Occupational Lung Disease. New York: Churchill Livingstone, 1984, pp 111–140

Butcher BT, Hendrick DJ: Occupational Asthma. Clin Chest Med 4(1):43–53, 1983

Chai H, Farr RS, Froehlich LA, et al: Standardization of bronchial inhalation challenge procedures. J Allergy Clin Immunol 56:323–327, 1975

Chan-Yeung M: Immunologic and nonimmunologic mechanisms in asthma due to western red cedar (*Thuja plicata*). J Allergy Clin Immunol 70:32, 37, 1982

Chan-Yeung M, Lam S, Koener S: Clinical features and natural history of occupational asthma due to Western red cedar (*Thuja plicata*). Am J Med 72:411, 415, 1982

Chan-Yeung M, Schulzer M, MacLean L, et al: Epidemiologic health survey of grain elevator workers in British Columbia. Amer Rev Resp Dis 121:329, 338, 1980

Davies RJ, Green M, Schofield NM: Recurrent nocturnal asthma after exposure to grain dust. Amer Rev Resp Dis 114:1011, 1019, 1976

DoPico GA, Flaherty D, Bhansali P, et al: Grain fever syndrome induced by airborne grain dust. J Allergy Clin Immunol 69:435, 443, 1982

DoPico GA, Jacobs S, Flaherty D, et al: Pulmonary reaction to durum wheat; a constituent of grain dust. Chest 81:55, 61, 1982

Franz T, McMurrain KD, Brooks S, et al: Clinical, immunologic, and physiologic observations in factory workers exposed to *B. subtilis* enzyme dust. J Allergy 47:170, 180, 1971

Hudson P, Pineau L, Cartier A, et al: Follow-up of occupational asthma due to various agents. J Allergy Clin Immunol 73:174, 1984

Jones RN, Butcher BT, Hammad YY, et al: Interaction of atopy and exposure to cotton dust in the bronchoconstrictor response. Brit J Indust Med 37:141, 146, 1980

Juniper CP, How MJ, Goodwin BFJ, et al: *Bacillus subtilis* enzymes: a 7-year clinical, epidemiological and immunological study of an industrial allergen. J Soc Occup Med 27:3–12, 1977

Karr RM, Davies RJ, Butcher BT, et al: Occupational asthma. J Allergy Clin Immunol 61:54, 65, 1978

NIOSH Criteria for a Recommended Standard. Occupational Exposure to Diisocyanate. US Dept. HEW PHS CDC Publication No. 78:215, September 1978

Olenchock SA, Mull JC, Major P: Extracts of airborne grain dusts activate alternative and classical complement pathways. Annals of Allergy 44:23, 28, 1980

Parkes WR: Occupational Lung Disorders. Second Edition, Boston: Butterworths, 1982, 415–453

Patterson R, Zeiss CR, Roberts M, et al: Human antihapten antibodies in trimellitic anhydride (TMA) inhalation reactions. Immunoglobulin classes of anti-TMA antibodies and hapten inhibition studies. J Clin Invest 62:971, 978, 1978

Pepys J, Hutchcroft BJ: Bronchial provocation tests in etiologic diagnosis and analysis of asthma. Am Rev Resp Dis 112:829, 859, 1975

PART III

Patient Management

Stephen M. Nagy, Jr.

15

Allergic Evaluation and Management Considerations of Patients with Asthma

Although few physicians would debate the role of an immune pathogenesis for most patients with asthma, recent progress in the pharmacologic treatment of asthma has led some physicians to believe that immunologic mechanisms are irrelevant if the patient's disease can be controlled with appropriate drugs. Other physicians take a different view; they regard the identification of relevant sensitizing antigens as paramount to the patient's appropriate treatment. The subset of extrinsic noninfectious asthma is believed to represent 30–50 percent of the total number of patients with reversible obstructive lung disease. The prevalence may be misleading, however. Sensitization, particularly to pollen, requires several seasons of exposure. Immunologic mechanisms are, therefore, infrequently detected in children under the age of four years in whom infections seem to be the predominant triggering event. Between ages 6 and 25 years, a much larger percentage of patients will fall into the latter atopic class of extrinsic asthma; with increasing age, the number steeply diminishes.

The word allergy, a word coined by von Pirquet in 1906 and derived from the Greek *allos,* describes a group of diseases, including extrinsic bronchial asthma, characterized by "altered reactivity or deviation from the behavior of the normal individual in which foreign substances elicit untoward reactions." In 1985, 80 years after von Pirquet and following an understanding of cellular events, allergy now encompasses all untoward physiologic responses based upon immunologic phenomena. Although it continued to be redefined, the original descriptions of allergies are still retained in lay language. Indeed, the layman labels any adverse, unusual, or strange reaction as "allergic." The role of "foreign substances" in evoking asthma has been crudely understood for many years and has been conceptualized as a form of sensitization. In fact, positive skin test responses to offending substances have been described as early as 1873. Prausnitz and Kustner demonstrated the transfer of this sensitivity by a nondialysable component of serum subsequently referred to as reagin. Moreover, a familial predisposition of asthma has long been noted, as well as an increased association with seasonal, nasal, and conjunctival symptoms.

The tools employed in the study and the evaluation of extrinsic asthma are markedly similar to those of 3-score years ago. Rigorous exhaustive histories and accurately performed skin testing are still the backbone of an allergic evaluation. Whereas fiberoptic endoscopy, computerized scanning, and complex biochemical and radioisotope procedures have usurped the tedious and plodding methods of many astute diagnosticians, the detection of elusive exposures, associations, and allergic sensitivities remains a 19th-century Holmesian adventure.

HISTORY

The medical history in a patient with pulmonary complaints always includes a simultaneous search for both diagnosis and etiology. In much of medicine diagnosis and etiology coincide; in allergic disorders they are separate and distinct. The onus on the historian is to pursue the underlying diathesis and to reconstruct all pertinent events and associations just as the sleuth investigates personalities and reinacts the crime. Traditionally, the interview is divided into five areas: social history, family history, past medical history, present illness, and review of systems. Tables 15-1 and 15-2 display a history form on which the ensuing discussion is based. It not only organizes and outlines the ascertained facts, especially in areas not customarily explored, but allows for the rapid retrieval of specific points of information.

The order in which this information is obtained is meaningful. In recent years, budding physicians have been taught to begin the interview with a discussion of the patient's primary complaints, i.e., present illness. Except to indicate an underlying impatience, a rational explanation of this has never been offered. Although every aspect of the history is important, the present illness is the most crucial and outlines critical associations and correlations. The narrative of acute or chronic pulmonary complaints should, therefore, unfold within the perspective of social, genealogical, and past medical rela-

Table 15-1
Patient History Checklist

History	
SH–birthplace	residences
marital status	
occupation(s)	
military service	
tobacco	
Etoh	
pets	
hobbies	bedroom
home	
FH–mother	
father	
siblings	
children	
diabetes, tbc, hypertension, heart disease, arthritis, Ca,	
asthma, hay fever, eczema, food allergies	
PH–operations	
Hospitalization	
Illnesses	
Injuries	
Medications	
allergy	sprays
vits	antibiotics
asa	other
hormones	
Past allergic history—drug reactions	
urticaria	
food sensitivities	
insect stings	
asthma	
hay fever	
eczema	
otitis	

tionships. Symptoms may then be plotted graphically against exposures, drugs, travel, stress, and other factors that relate to alterations of environment.

SOCIAL HISTORY

Asthmatic histories deal in the great majority with a constellation of symptoms that span months, and more frequently, years. In order to properly evaluate the chronology of these symptoms, and especially to be able to relate

Table 15-2
Present Condition Checklist

Present Illness		
Exacerbating Factors	Nasal	Pulmonary

travel
exercise
change in temp.
dust
animals
foods
infection
stress
drugs (ASA)
outside
irritants
smoke

Seasonal Jan. Feb. Mar. Apr. May June July Aug. Sept. Oct. Nov. Dec.
Nasal
pulmonary

Response to Medications—Nasal Sxs
                                   Pulmonary Sxs

System Review

Jan.	Feb.	Mar.	Apr.	May	June	July	Aug.	Sept.	Oct.	Nov.	Dec.
Trees		Olive									
		Grasses									
				Bermuda							
				Weeds							
						Peak of					
						Agricultural Molds					
					Molds						
					Dust		(Peak)				
				Animal Dander							

SEASONAL PATTERNS OF INHALANT-ASSOCIATED ASTHMA

Figure   Several patterns of inhalant-association asthma

them to specific exposures, it is important to know where the patient has resided and for what periods of time. Even moves within a state, and to a lesser extent within a city, may result in significant changes in environment flora. Animal pedigree, number, degree, and length of exposure should all be carefully documented. Small frequently shampooed poodles seldom produce the problems of a German shepherd with the run of the house. Siamese cats, besides being antigenically distinct, are seldom outdoors in spite of protestations to the contrary. Some observations should be made on the nature of the home; its age, heating-air conditioning system, and degree of dampness. The nature of the bedding (i.e., blankets, pillows, and comforters) may be critical and may elucidate a recent or chronic exposure to feathers, wool, or down. Similarly, the occupation of the patient is an important feature. Occupational asthma represents an extrinsic reversible obstructive disease defined more by a peak incidence within specific industries than by biochemical mechanisms. Classically, symptoms remit on weekends or on vacations and then gradually increase with return to work. Rarely, the offending material is introduced into the home by a nonsensitized family member.

The deleterious effects of cigarette smoking and alcohol on bronchial membranes require little emphasis. Recent studies, however, emphasize that asthmatic children of smoking parents present in emergency rooms more frequently than those of nonsmokers. Moreover, the vast majority of non-smoking asthmatics will testify to at least the irritant properties of tobacco smoke. A few will even insist that they are "allergic." In fact, sensitivity to a glycoprotein within smoke has been described in a small minority of patients. Alcohol use, even in moderate amounts, reduces ciliary function and there-fore adversely effects pulmonary clearance mechanisms. In large amounts, chronic aspiration becomes more likely.

FAMILY HISTORY

In clinical studies an extensive pedigree provides an attempt to establish an asthmatic or allergic diathesis. Office genealogic histories are almost always obtained secondhand unless the entire family is under one's care. To establish such facts in family members is difficult. Is grandfather's wheezing due to asthma or chronic bronchitis? Are brother's sinus complaints infectious or allergic in etiology? Possibly the entire exercise is meretricious, for it is still incumbent upon the practitioner to establish the diagnosis in the patient!

PAST ALLERGIC HISTORY

This important subsection undertakes to discuss prior events or illnesses that may have had an immunologic basis, more specifically IgE antibody, and thereby suggest an atopic basis. Primary in this category are reactions to drugs. Indeed, even if the medication responsible for untoward events cannot be identified, the history should still attempt to differentiate the classic types of reactions (i.e., overdose, intolerance, idiosyncracy, side or secondary effect, and vagal) from true IgE-mediated reactions. This latter reaction is usually characterized by signs of histamine release including pruritus, rhinor-rhea, urticaria, and wheezing.

Urticarial episodes are reported by approximately 20 percent of the population at some point during their lifetime. They may be a part of or the sole manifestation of an acute anaphylactic or accelerated reaction and the nature of the offending material is critical. For example, codeine, strawberries, and organic contrast material (IVP dye) induce histamine release by a pharmacologic mechanism not involving an antibody-antigen interaction and thereby would not support an allergic diathesis. Acute systemic reactions of the nonvagal type to stinging and/or biting insects are more common in the atopic patient.

Discussion of food "sensitivities" with patients elicits a myriad of symptoms and syndromes ranging from anaphylaxis to headache, "colitis," and hyperkinetic behavior. Nonetheless, only acute and accelerated food reactions are mediated by specific IgE antibodies. Approximately 6 percent of patients with pollenosis, however, complain of an oral pruritus with melons, bananas, avocados, and some nuts. This ranges from a mild sensation of itching of the palate and pharynx to actual laryngeal swelling and associated hoarseness. At some point, the physician will address the possible association of the patient's asthma with the ingestion of specific foods. Many asthmatics avoid milk, particularly during exacerbations, because they feel it increases the amount and tenacity of both bronchial and pharyngeal mucus. The parents of asthmatic children report the same phenomena and commonly keep the child off of whole milk when they are symptomatic. This phenomenon has never been extensively studied, and the mechanism is unclear. Acute life-threatening exacerbations have been associated with the ingestion of sulfite containing foods; for a more complete discussion and a list of these foods, please see Chapter 10.

Eczema or atopic dermatitis bespeaks a chronic condition of childhood characterized by intense itching and secondary excoriations with a predilection for the anticubital and popliteal fossae and malar areas, although the entire body may be involved. In older children, the extensor surfaces are more affected, and though less frequent in adults, the disease may persist for years. Of the atopic diseases, the highest levels of IgE are found in this one, but paradoxically their role is least understood; however, recent investigations using double-blind challenge techniques have indicated that there is a significant correlation between elevated levels of specific IgE to food and the ability of that food to cause exacerbations of the disease.

PAST MEDICAL HISTORY

A rigorous outline of major medical landmarks (i.e., operations, hospitalizations, and past and current illnesses) is important to obtain the proper perspective with which to view the primary complaints. For example, hypertension, coronary artery disease, valvular heart disease, arrhythmias, migraine headache, and arthropathies may involve the use of certain drugs, (i.e., beta blockers [propanolol, metaprolol, nadolol, atenolol, acebutolol], reserpine, aspirin, and other antiinflammatory compounds). These agents may create *de novo* or exacerbate asthmatic syndromes. Although strictly not allergic, they represent an extrinsic eminently treatable etiology. In fact, new patients should be encouraged to bring a list of all their medications, (i.e., antacids, cold remedies, hormones, analgesics, drops, sprays, vitamins, and laxatives); they frequently provide clues to illnesses poorly understood or simply forgotten. Concomitantly, prior illnesses with similar symptomatologies (i.e., pulmonary emboli, cardiac failure, and/or respiratory infection may all simply have represented recurrent asthma, especially when the diagnosis was made by different physicians. The season and preferably the month these episodes occurred should be noted.

PRESENT ILLNESS

Asthmatic symptoms vary from a mild cough, frequently nocturnal, to severe wheezing, chest tightness, and shortness of breath. It is important for the patient to realize that seemingly insignificant complaints such as chronic clearing of the throat, postnasal drainage, and occasional mild episodes of dyspnea may all respresent asthma. Once defined and understood, such symptoms undergo retrospective and chronologic analysis. A date of onset is approximated, hopefully as to the month, but at least the season. The following questions must then be answered.

1. Has there been a gradual progression from mild cough to severe disabling disease or have symptoms been stable with occasional exacerbations?
2. Are symptoms strictly seasonal with a large hiatus when the patient is quite well, or are they chronic and perennial?
3. Do symptoms remit on travel to climatically different areas?
4. Is asthma associated with specific exposures, situations, or illnesses?

The predilection for nocturnal attacks, never adequately explained, has invariably led to meticulous scrutiny of all items and exposures within the bedroom. Figure 15-1 outlines a schematic to plot these seasonal changes as well as a checklist of various exacerbating factors. A positive response should be accompanied by some approximation of an individual's sensitivity. Severity is, of course, arbitrary. The degree of dyspnea, as well as the intensity and frequency of the cough, are fairly reliable indicators in an acute situation. When attempting to assess the overall disease, however, more substantial and definable landmarks such as frequency of office visits, emergency room visits, hospitalizations, school absences, and/or work disability may represent a more accurate index. The patient's requirement for and response to various medications may be an even more objective assessment. Seasonal asthma adequately treated with an antihistamine is clearly not as severe as that requiring corticosteroids.

It is the rare pollen-sensitive patient whose sole manifestation is wheezing. Nasal congestion, rhinorrhea, sinus tenderness and headaches, sneezing, and watering and itching of the eyes occur with varying intensity. The presence of these complaints provides important clues, not only to establish the diagnosis, but also to provide an additional framework with which to evaluate the seasonal and exposure-related aspects. On the other hand, nasal polyps and infectious sinusitis, both of which may be associated with moderately severe asthma, will present with similar symptomatology in several non-IgE-mediated disorders. Characteristically, such patients do not complain of the classical symptoms of histamine release (i.e., itching and sneezing).

Physical Examination

The examination of the patient should actually begin during the interview. Patients often learn to disguise symptoms that are not socially acceptable; therefore, a chronic cough or such habits as chronic clearing of the throat may be handled very quietly and even denied, but are rather obvious on close observation. An accompanying family member might even attest to the severity and persistence of such symptoms. Children especially might be observed for the distressing habit of rubbing their nose, *allergic salute,* and sniffling (i.e., the voluntary inhalation of nasal secretions).

Overall, the actual examination concentrates on certain specific areas: vital signs, respiratory, cardiac, and integementary systems; for example, pelvic, rectal, and extensive neurologic exams are not usually performed unless indicated by an abnormality in the history. Vital signs should include the patient's weight, temperature, respiratory rate, cardiac rate, rhythm, and blood pressure. The state of the patient's nutrition should be noted; commonly, children with chronic asthma appear somewhat undernourished and small for their age. The pulsus paradoxus has shown some predictive value in terms of asthma severity and should be obtained in patients who are acutely ill and who are old enough to cooperate. The pulsus paradoxus is an accentuation of the normal variation in cardiac output during the respiratory cycle and is increased in several pathologic states, including moderately severe asthma. The skin should be examined for associated atopic disorders particularly urticaria and atopic dermatitis; the latter condition is characterized by erythema, scaling and thickening of the skin; in the acute state, erythema, weeping, and vesiculation will be prominent; in the more chronic form, a dryer, scaling, lichenified eruption develops. Children, characteristically develop a flextural distribution involving the neck, antecubital and popliteal areas, eyelids, and behind the ears. Among older children (i.e., ages 9–12, and teenagers), there is a distinct subset who develop extensor involvement with lesions occurring primarily on the anterior and lateral aspects of the thighs, upper arms, and forearms.

The facies and upper respiratory tract should be examined in some detail. Pigmentation within the infraorbital area, *shiners,* is commonly seen in patients with allergies; overall, it is a sign of chronic nasal congestion and is secondary to chronic lymphedema. A horizontal crease (allergic crease) across the bridge of the nose may be a sign of chronic allergic rhinitis; it is secondary to the patient chronically rubbing the nose; simple upward pressure on the tip of the nose will demonstrate how the crease was produced. An assessment of the tympanic membranes will rule out purulent and serous otitis media in addition to prior ear infections. Allergic upper airway disease predisposes to chronic and acute otitis, particularly in children. The nasal membrane should be described; pale, boggy turbinates imply an allergic diathesis. At times the engorgement and edema may be so severe that a distinction between severe allergic disease and true nasal polyps is impossible. Nevertheless, polyps are usually greyish-white glistening excrescences that may even be mistaken by the untrained observer for nasal mucus; they are commonly seen in patients with asthma and aspirin sensitivity and are also associated with infectious sinusitis, chronic allergic disease, and, in children, cystic fibrosis. The presence of and the nature of the nasal discharge should also be described. Allergic disease produces a clear whitish discharge; purulence implies a possible sinusitis.

Allergic IgE mediated conjunctivities is characterized by tearing and either conjunctival hyperemia or a boggy pale conjunctivae; in its most severe form, the conjunctiva becomes markedly edematous (chemosis), and has a characteristic milky appearance. The disease is usually bilateral, although the exposure of one eye to an inordinate amount of antigen, usually pollen, may produce a unilateral response. Vernal conjunctivitis, a condition commonly seen in atopic patients, is characterized by the presence of giant papillae on the upper tarsal conjunctivae (cobblestone appearance).

The neck should be palpated for the presence of subcutaneous emphysema, an indicator of pneumomediastinum and/or pneumothorax, a complication of severe asthma; adenopathy may be prominent and a sign of chronic infectious sinusitis.

The chest configuration should be noted paying attention to the degree of hyperinflation, pectus deformity, and symmetry of expansion area; chronic asthmatics commonly develop a kyphotic deformity; the use of accessory muscles in respiration should be noted in patients with severe asthma, as their use correlates with the severity of airway obstruction. The lungs should initially be auscultated during quiet respiration; a major characteristic of asthma is the "wheeze," a high pitched piping or whistling sound resulting from partial airway obstruction; it has a musical quality, and most importantly, occurs during both inspiration and expiration, although it usually louder during expiration. The degree and amount of wheezing should be noted as well as the amount of expiratory prolongation (the inspiratory: expiratory ratio), the presence of adventitious sounds, as well as an overall assessment of the adequacy of air exchange. In patients with an essentially normal chest exam, several maneuvers might be helpful: you might ask the patient to breathe deeply 3–4 times in rapid succession; this may initiate paroyoxysms of coughing and indicates excessive secretions within the tracheal bronchial tree. A forced expiration may reveal terminal wheezing, and may also initiate a paroyoxysm of coughing.

In the mild to moderate asthmatic, the cardiac exam should be normal; in severe asthma, a right ventricular heave might be present, as well as prominent pulmonic sound; with severe hyperinflation the liver is displaced downward, and may be palpable although, if the upper border is percussed, it should not be enlarged. The extremities should be assessed for nailbed cyanosis and digital clubbing. In the acutely ill asthmatic, the neurologic exam should focus on the mental status; altered mental states, including confusion, restlessness, irritability, and coma may be signs of respiratory failure.

DIAGNOSTIC PROCEDURES

The *sine qua non* of an allergic diagnosis is the diagnostic challenge. This represents a direct exposure of the target organ (i.e., the bronchi) to the suspected allergen. Bronchial challenge is time consuming, (usually only one antigen can be tested at any one time), both for the patient and physician; the reproduced asthma may be severe and even persistent; and it is quite expensive. For these reasons methods to detect specific IgE within skin (skin testing) or serum (RAST) are commonly employed. Positive results of skin testing and RAST, however, indicate only a presumptive diagnosis because of 2 major assumptions: (1) that the IgE detected in either the skin or the serum is present within the bronchial mucosa; and (2) that challenge with the specific antigen will lead to a significant measureable increase in pulmonary resistance. An extensive literature exists that has assayed the relationship between positive skin tests and provocative data; furthermore, with the introduction of RAST, other studies have indicated excellent agreement between this and more sensitive forms of skin testing. Although the indices of positivity are arbitrary, a concordance rate of approximately 90 percent when using RAST, prick, or intradermal testing has been demonstrated. When high concentrations of antigens are used, however, the concordance rate with intradermal testing may be lower due to increased false-positive skin test responses.

This may be partially overcome by an intradermal titration technique. Scratch testing is a less sensitive method and produces a concordance rate of approximately 75–80 percent.

Skin Testing

The theoretical and practical aspects of skin testing and of *in vitro* testing is discussed in Chapter 16. The antigens chosen should be based upon clinical history, environment, and local flora. Although pollen counts are extremely helpful in determining the major allergens and their periods of pollination, the location of the pollen counter within a community may occasionally miss clinically relevant antigens. Knowledge of local trees and weeds is, therefore, critical. Too often, however, a patient is tested to multiple antigens of dubious significance (i.e., flax, hemp, orris root, or cigarette smoke. Table 15-3 presents a screening list for seasonal and nonseasonal perennial asthma. Testing for various food antigens, although occasionally helpful in acute self-limited anaphylactic or accelerated reactions, is virtually worthless when dealing with asthma. Classical antihistamines should not be taken for at least 48–72 hours and hydroxyzine (Atarax, Vistaril) and hydroxyzine-containing preparations (Marax, Ataraxoid) must be discontinued at least 4 days prior to the testing. Doxepin (Sinequan), an antianxiety agent, should also be discontinued for at least 48 hours; it is not known by what mechanism suppression of skin tests occurs with this latter drug. Corticosteroids, at least in moderate doses, will not effect the immediate response, but will ablate the late-phase reaction. Since anaphylactic reactions, though extremely rare, are a possibility, a physician should be readily available with appropriate supportive facilities. Furthermore, since smooth muscle contraction is initiated by an anaphylactic response, we do not recommend skin testing patients who are pregnant, especially since there are alternative means to assess specific elevations of IgE antibody.

Table 15-3
Common Inhalants

Pollens	Household	Animal Antigens	Molds
Grasses	Dust	Cat	Alternaria
Trees	House mites	Dog	Aspergillus
Weeds	Kapok	Feathers (chicken, goose, duck)	botrytis
		Wool	Cladosporium
		Horse	Fusarium
			Mucor
			Penicillium
			Rhizopus

DIETS

The role of food proteins in various allergic conditions has only recently been more stringently investigated and defined. For many years, the concept that insidious, unrecognized sensitivity to various food proteins was responsible for many poorly controlled steroid dependent asthmatics perpetuated the myth of food antigen testing—a positive test was considered synonomous with relevant sensitivity. Unwitting and inappropriate diagnoses persisted for years as dietary regimens of no proven clinical efficacy. The advent of double-blind challenge testing in an appropriate setting has led to a much more rational approach and certainly to a much better understanding of those foods that are operative in allergic conditions. For example, such studies indicate that the most common response to food is gastrointestinal; skin eruptions such as urticaria and flaring of eczema are second; exacerbations of asthma, a distant third. Furthermore, these same studies indicate that only a small number of foods are responsible for the vast majority of these responses; these include milk, chocolate, egg, soy, wheat, peanut, corn, fish, and tomato, although almost any food at some point may be responsible for a rare, clinically significant sensitivity. The role of food antigen testing has not been adequately evaluated in all of these conditions. In studying children with eczema, it is quite clear that a negative response is almost invariably associated with a lack of clinical sensitivity. On the other hand, a number of false positive responses are noted in allergic patients. That is, although they demonstrate a positive skin test to a food, challenge with that same food will not produce a clinically significant response. Similar studies have not been extensively performed in asthmatic patients, primarily because the pure asthmatic reaction is unusual on food challenge.

For those physicians who, therefore, wish to test the existence of food allergies, an appropriate elimination diet may be prescribed. When one is attempting to assess the role of all ingested substances, a basic diet is preferable (Table 15-4). If one suspects a family of foods (i.e., grains or milk, then a diet (Tables 15-5 and 15-6) specifically eliminating these should be utilized.

One may wish to follow serially a patient's pulmonary function and/or keep a symptom diary so as to assess their requirements for chronic medications. In a disease that has natural and unpredictable periods of relapse, a response, of course, is arbitrary. If it appears that the patient has experienced a positive response, then a gradual reintroduction of suspected offending foods may be accomplished on an open basis.

If that does not prove satisfactory, then a specific challenge utilizing opaque capsules containing the offending food may be accomplished in the physician's office; neither the patient nor the physician should know which food is being challenged in order to eliminate both patient and physician bias. Serial pulmonary funtion studies are utilized to assess flow rates and the

Table 15-4

Basic Elimination Diet

Only these foods are allowed:

Rice and rice cereals
Beets
Lettuce
Asparagus
Sweet potato
Lamb
Chicken
Grapefruit
Cooked peaches and pears (not canned)
Salt
Sugar
Olive oil
Tea with lemon
Water

Table 15-5

Milk-Free Diet

No milk—whole milk, buttermilk, low-fat milk, evaporated milk
No milk products—butter, cheese, yogurt, ice cream, sherbert
No chocolate, cocoa
No creamed soups, vegetables
No pastry or bread containing milk or butter
No food containing whey, casein, sodium (Na) caseinate or non-fat dry milk
   products

Examples: Some margarines, hot dogs, bolognas, other prepared meats, frozen
                    prepared foods.

Table 15-6

Wheat-Free Diet

No wheat cereals
No baked goods including cakes, cookies, crackers, waffles, pancakes, or breads
   containing wheat.
No postum, ale, beer, gin, whiskies
No prepared foods containing grains

Examples: Prepared meats, canned soups, puddings, custards, sherbert, chili,
                    boullion, cheese spreads.

patient's clinical response. Although commonly a fruitless exercise, it is important, at times, to allay a patient's anxiety that specific foods are or are not the root cause of their disease. Food proteins, of course, may not be the only cause of asthma. The sulfite preservatives have been clearly incriminated in acute exacerbations and are discussed extensively in Chapter 10. Until recently, it was presumed that a large number of aspirin-sensitive asthmatics with nasal polyps were also sensitive to a yellow azobenzene dye (FDC #5), a ubiquitous coloring agent in multiple foods. Recent challenge studies with this dye in a number of suspect asthmatics have simply not been able to document that association, although it is still a common practice to initiate a dye-free regimen in such patients.

Other Studies

Although eosinophilia, either in serum or in secretions, has been a hallmark of allergic disease, its value is limited because of its predominance in the sputa of severe intrinsic asthmatics, in nonallergic nasal polyps, and its intermittent appearance in infectious rhinosinusitis. In fact, the most intense eosinophilias are associated with the severely afflicted nonallergic patient.

A total IgE represents a screening tool to detect atopic patients. Not all patients exhibit elevated levels. For example, severe perennial symptomatology might result from an exquisite sensitivity to one antigen (i.e., cat; yet, the total IgE may be normal or only slightly elevated. Mold allergy, in general, also produces very low levels. On the other hand, if skin testing or RAST procedures are contemplated, then the test would be of little value. One occasional exception occurs in children with significant elevations and negative prick tests. In the latter group, more extensive intradermal testing is warranted.

Treatment

The major avenues of therapy are (1) environmental, (2) pharmacologic, (3) immunologic, and (4) prophylactic. While the nonallergic patient must depend entirely upon medications, the prognosis for that subset with extrinsic sensitivities is more sanguine both from the standpoint of management and severity. Severe disabling steroid dependence is the curse of the older nonallergic patient.

While environmental measures will effect a cure in a few and will partially ameliorate the disease in most, other manipulations are usually required to produce the substantial improvement a patient seeks. Allowing for the variability in severity and current pharmacotherapy, an incremental approach is suggested. The benefits of avoidance measures and specific medications cannot be properly observed in a "shotgun" approach. In the initial stages, reinforcement of recommended regimens is essential. In fact, some allergists emphasize home visits to insure that recommendations are carried out. Office visits should be scheduled at appropriate intervals to allow for appropriate compliance, as well as the expected saluatory response. With time and the establishment of a relationship, the final orchestration of all modalities ensue.

Environmental

The classic, and certainly most satisfactory, treatment of an allergic patient is elimination of the offending antigen. The basis for this suggestion was a presumption—and a correct one—that inhalation of the offending protein would induce a demonstrable increase in airway resistance. Recent studies, however, have indicated that such exposures also increase nonspecific bronchial hyperreactivity as measured by bronchial challenge with methacholine or histamine. Moreover, based on the presumption that a reduction in allergenic exposure could decrease bronchial reactivity, a recent study of controlled matched groups of dust sensitive asthmatic children observed for one month revealed that the half being subjected to rigid house dust control not only had fewer symptoms, but also their bronchial sensitivity to histamine was decreased. Although some physicians, particularly pediatricians, institute dust control and removal of epidermal antigens without the benefit of skin testing, the correlation of historial data with skin test positivity allows the practicing allergist an extremely sound foundation for subsequent recommendations. Furthermore, the extent to which antigens are removed may be indexed to the patient's sensitivity, as determined both by the size of the skin test response and/or the concentration at which it occurred. All suggestions must be tailored by severity of the disease, financial considerations, and plain common sense.

Pollen

The vast majority of pollen-sensitive asthmatics do not wish to curtail their outdoor activity during their symptomatic periods. On the other hand, unusually heavy exposures should be avoided. Grass-sensitive asthmatics should not mow the lawn. For those addicted to gardening, the wearing of a simple surgical mask can markedly reduce the amount of inhaled pollen. The removal of offending flora, particularly trees, is frequently considered, but is drastic considering the extremely short pollinating season of any single tree; the presence of neighboring trees of the same species will continue to produce a wide distribution of their windborne pollen. In a rare instance where the sensitivity is exquisite, the symptoms intense, the tree proximal, and the environmental impact minimal, relief may be substantial. Similarly, general airing of a home during pollinating months is a luxury to be avoided. Not infrequently asthmatics feel the need for cool fresh air and sleep with windows fully open, thereby actually increasing their exposure and symptoms. Though pollen is released early in the morning, the actual counts are highest in the late afternoon and early evening. For those willing to alter their daily pattern, outdoor activity such as shopping and exercise might be confined to the morning hours.

Animals

Probably no greater trauma can be heaped upon a family than the knowledge that a well-established pet is the prime cause of moderately severe asthma. In no other area will the physician's judiciousness and resolve be more tested. Although patients with only nasal involvement are frequently willing to tolerate a moderate degree of symptoms, asthma symptomatic enough to warrant a visit to an allergist's office requires more than temporizing measures. The degree to which a particular animal is contributing to an asthmatic problem is based upon historical data as well as the degree of sensitivity. With regards to the latter, titration intradermal skin testing can be an invaluable tool. There are three levels of restriction dealing with offending epidermal antigens.

ABSOLUTE RESTRICTION

When asthma is severe and disabling and the sensitivity exquisite, all animals should be removed from the household. Anything less rigorous will lead to continued symptoms; exposure may occur in outdoor areas, (i.e., the garage or carport), or where the animal seeks shelter. If the family questions the diagnosis and the attachment is close, an alternative is boarding the animal for 2–4 months. Simultaneously rugs should be shampooed, bedding laundered, and even heating and air conditioning ducts vacuumed to remove presistent offending antigens.

MODERATE RESTRICTION

In all cases of epidermal sensitivity, regardless of the severity of the symptoms, it is preferable to remove the animal from the indoor environment and/or greatly restrict assess. This may be sufficient in cases of mild-to-moderate sensitivity.

MINIMAL RESTRICTION

In some households simply removing the pet from the patient's bedroom will amount to a major achievement. Well-established poodles and declawed cats are found to have more privileges than family members. Although it is the least desirable solution, restricting the animal to a room or an area of the home that can be easily cleaned may be all that can be accomplished.

Other animal proteins include feather (down) pillows, comforters, sleeping bags, wool blankets, carpets, carpet pads, horsehair furniture, and stuffed animals. Proscription of these items on general principles is generally unwarranted. The degree of sensitivity and their proximity to the patient should be taken into consideration. For example, a feather pillow in a sibling's room should produce no untoward reaction; likewise, a small oriental carpet in the living room. Even a down pillow to which a patient is quite attached may be encased in impermeable material.

Dust

The preparation and maintenance of a dust-free environment has been a perennial trademark of the allergist's practice. Although initially based upon clinical associations as well as positive skin tests to house dust extracts, more recent studies have indicated that the allergenic properties of dust are related to the presence of house mites (*Dermatophagoides farinae* or *pteronyssinus*). Although these insects are found throughout homes on a worldwide basis, it is still not clear whether the mite antigen plays as great a role in the United States as it does in some other countries. They breed optimally at 85 percent relative humidity and 25°C; the major source seems to be the mattress. Dust elimination, therefore, involves either vacuuming the mattress thoroughly once a month or encasing it with nonallergic material. Whether the mites will colonize waterbeds still awaits the efforts of researchers. Other precautions to reduce the accumulation of dust within bedrooms consist of the removal of dust-collecting objects, minimizing the amount of furniture, and frequent vacuuming. Generally, cleaning should be done while the patient is not at home. If the patient must clean, a surgical mask is helpful. Increasingly, the families of allergic patients have become interested in installing filtration systems. Both electronic precipitators and HEPA filters are commercially available and are quite effective at reducing particulate matter in ambient air. They are usually attached to central heating or air conditioning units; however, portable machines are available and may, in fact, be preferable for the renter or teenager going to college. In the experience of this author and other allergists, a large majority of those installing these systems report substantial improvement.

Molds

Sensitivity to fungi frequently accompanies both seasonal and perennial allergic disorders. The extent to which the physician both investigates and recommends is again based upon the type of mold, the degree of sensitivity, and the clinical history. This requires some knowledge of aerobiology. At the risk of over-simplification, allergists have frequently classified these antigens on the basis of of indoor and outdoor contamination. Although all species of fungi flourish in a moist outdoor habitat, the spores of the darkspored deuteromycetes (e.g., *Alternaria* and *Cladosporium* species) frequently predominate in outdoor samplings with specific elevations seen in agricultural areas, particularly with increases in wind velocity and decreases in relative humidity. Spore counts seem to be lowest when the snow covers the ground. In the Eastern and Midwestern United States peak counts occur in the late summer and early fall, whereas in the Great Valley of California, there is minimal seasonal variation with occasional high levels, usually during the windy summer months.

Although any fungus can colonize an indoor area, endogenous growth within homes seems dominated by the small-spored deuteromycetes, primarily *Penicillium, Aspergillus, Rhizopus,* and *Mucor.* Increases in humidity within the home will certainly facilitate such growth and, for this reason, allergists are frequently ambivalent when recommending central humidification. Portable vaporizers are commonly contaminated with various species. In the presence of a good clinical history and supportive skin test data, documentation of excessive exposure is essential. Unfortunately, sampling procedures are rather crude and depend upon gravitational settling of the spores on exposed media. Growth usually takes 1–2 weeks and the number of colonies is considered a gross index of contamination. If a source is identified, it should be removed. Occasionally, even a wall or subflooring may have been invaded. Old, overstuffed furniture may be laden with mold. Foam pillows attract and hold moisture and are a prime source of mold growth. Otherwise, general measures to reduce mold growth include repair of leaky pipes and appliances, rigorous use of bathroom ventilation, and dehumidifers, particularly in basements and humid climates. Occasionally, a fungicide may be required. Trioxymethylene (crystalline paraformaldehyde) is an inexpensive and convenient preparation. Five to ten grams (about 1–2 teaspoonfuls) are allowed to sublimate in an open dish in the various rooms of the home. A slight smell of formaldehyde occurs that may be slightly irritating to asthmatics. This usually clears with adequate ventilation, however. Excellent inhibition of mold growth has been reported with this method.

Immunotherapy

Leonard Noon, a brilliant English physiologist whose major work involved immunity to tetanus, began the saga of injection treatment for atopic disorders with his "Prophylactic innoculation against hay fever" in 1911. Even today this 2-page article with its hand-drawn graphs is remarkable for the accuracy of its presumptions, clinical correlations, and educated speculations. Working with grass-pollen sensitive patients with detected precipitating antibody to pollen extracts, Noon presumed that a "satisfactory result would be expected from the induction of an active immunity." A patient's sensitivity was approximated by titrating the concentration of grass–pollen that would provoke a moderate conjunctival reaction. Subsequent injections, "immunization," produced a significant reduction in the patient's sensitivity as determined by the concentration required to reproduce the reaction. Although Noon presumed that he was producing an "antitoxin" to a "toxin" liberated by grass pollen, the concept that he ameliorated the condition by producing an antibody against an offending protein has stood the test of 75 years. His further observations of an increased sensitivity during the initial states of immunotherapy, and systemic reactions with high doses, have also been documented. When Cooke and Vander Veer suggested that the atopic diseases were a form of human sensitization, the "immunization" of Noon became desensitization. The vast majority of clinical allergists probably still refer to it in these terms; however, academic semanticists are now asking us to return to the term "immunotherapy." The term "desensitization," when applied to human disease, now refers to the transient depletion of reaginic antibodies by the administration of sublethal doses, as in penicillin sensitivity.

The immunologic events that occur as a result of the injections of gradually increasing doses of pollen extract have been elucidated and well defined over the past 20 years. Unfortunately, the majority of these studies involve patients with allergic rhinitis. Many such studies deal with ragweed pollen because of its potency, the severity of clinical symptoms, and most important, the lack of other major seasonal inhalants during the time of its pollination. In multiple double-blind control studies using placebo groups, the saluatory effects of this mode of therapy is no longer questioned provided that a specific cumulative antigenic dose is achieved.

The following immunologic mechanisms have been associated with the beneficial effect achieved with immunotherapy. They are not completely understood, and at the moment one simply assumes that they may be responsible for the improved symptoms.

1. Antigen injections lead to the production of IgG blocking antibody, which combines with antigen and partially or completely prevents the PK reaction. By competing for antigen with antigen-specific cell-bound IgE, it thereby reduces the effective concentration of antigen. Although the concentration of blocking antibody is found to correlate with the quantity of antigen administered, the level of blocking antibody does not correlate statistically with the degree of reduction in symptoms in the vast majority of studies. This is to say that although treated patients have an expected higher level of blocking antibody within the treated group, the higher antibody titers do not correlate with those patients experiencing the greatest relief of symptoms.

2. In untreated patients levels of specific IgE tend to remain stable for

years, with an increase during and after the pollen season, which then gradually tapers to baseline levels. Numerous studies have indicated that injection therapy is associated with an initial brief rise in antigen-specific IgE titers. If initiated prior to the appropriate season, a blunting of the typical seasonal rise is seen with a gradual reduction in total IgE over several years of therapy. This data, however, is not confirmed by all studies.

3. After injection therapy, circulating basophils (presumably analogous to human lung mast cells) become less responsive to antigen. Other studies have indicated that in untreated patients, the dose response to antigen remains relatively constant.

4. After immunotherapy, diminished lymphocyte proliferation and diminished production of two lymphokines, macrophage migration inhibition factor and lymphocyte mitogenic factor, were observed in response to ragweed antigen E. This decreased response was antigen specific in that neither lymphocyte proliferation nor lymphokine production was unchanged after challenge with an unrelated antigen.

5. Allergen-specific IgE and IgA in nasal secretions increases with allergy immunotherapy.

6. In some studies, immunotherapy has been associated with decreased levels of IgM-bearing B cells and increased T-suppressor cells bearing Fc receptors for IgG. The significance of these changes remains to be determined.

In the past, this data has been extrapolated and applied to allergic bronchial asthma; that is, asthmatic patients have continued to be immunized, presuming a similar saluatory response. Fortunately, recent studies focusing on both the immediate and late phases of the asthmatic reaction, support a role for an immune pathogenesis and immune intervention. The pathophysiology of this response has been discussed elsewhere in this volume; nevertheless, the following critical observations need to be made in view of recent controversies surrounding the use of immunotherapy in bronchial asthma.

1. The occurrence of symptomatic bronchial asthma (as opposed to asymptomatic small airways disease), in association with florid spring or fall pollenosis on the East Coast is an unusual occurrence. In contrast, in the Great Valley of California, asthma is a frequent severe complication of pollen sensitivity. Therefore, initial clinical trials to study immunotherapy in pollenosis, when conducted east of the Mississippi, did not usually encompass patients with bronchial asthma as well.

2. The extrinsic asthmatic is afflicted with two major variables, the asthmatic diathesis and an IgE mediated triggering event. Though the sensitivity of each may be grossly approximated by histamine and/or methacholine challenge in the former, and bronchial challenge with spe-

cific antigen in the latter, the modulating influence of each on the interrelationship has only recently been investigated; that is, as noted previously in this chapter, chronic antigen exposure probably increases bronchial hyperreactivity, whereas reduced antigen exposure will lead to a concomitant decrease. Nevertheless, for the scrupulous researcher, the matching of patients become a major problem and hence the difficulty with acceptable clinical trials.

In spite of these handicaps, controlled studies of immunotherapy in extrinsic asthma have been carried out in pollen-sensitive, dust-sensitive, and cat-sensitive patients. There is, when the studies are reviewed, a body of data, not as clean as one would like, that suggests substantive efficacy for immunotherapy in selected asthmatic patients. Although none would argue that treatment should not be utilized if an antigen can be easily avoided, there is much quibbling in those patients who require intermittent or regular medications. Furthermore, since a large number of these patients also suffer from symptoms of allergic rhinitis and conjunctivitis, a decision to use this mode of treatment must encompass their response in these areas as well. With these uncertainties in mind, the following guidelines are suggested.

1. Evidence of significant levels of specific IgE antibody directed against antigens to which the patient has a known exposure.
2. Satisfaction that these sensitivities are clinically relevant. As an example, a child with primarily late fall and winter asthma is found only to be sensitive to grass pollen. Specifically, relevant antigens such as weeds, household inhalants, and molds are negative. Immunotherapy with grass–pollen would be inappropriate.
3. Inability or unwillingness to avoid incriminated antigens, (i.e. veterinarians), or to alter their relationship with a well-established pet.
4. Although virtually all asthmatics can be controlled by pharmacologic agents, this means may not always be either desirable or appropriate. For pollen-sensitive seasonal asthmatics, theophylline and terbutaline might produce undesirable side effects; sodium cromolyn might be ineffective or tedious; and corticosteroid usage and toxicity may be extensive. The indications for immunotherapy in the perennial allergic asthmatic are usually more compelling, even in the presence of adequate control with various drugs. In recent years, more patients seem unwilling to take daily medications whose long-range effects are not known.
5. Asthmatics with chronic allergic aspergillosis should be excluded from treatment, most particularly with mold antigens.
6. Although long-term retrospective analysis of patients on allergy immunotherapy has indicated that it is eminently safe and has not been associated with the development of any "immunologic" disorders, there have been sporadic reports of possible associations between it and increased

incidence of collagen vascular diseases; this has led to a certain reluctance to initiate treatment in those with "immune complex" disorders.

7. We do not recommend initiating allergy immunotherapy in pregnant patients, primarily because of the risk of anaphylaxis with administering increasing doses of antigen; on the other hand, we do not recommend discontinuing allergy immunotherapy in an asthmatic female who becomes pregnant. This has been studied by a retrospective method, and the incidence of prematurity, toxemia, abortion, neonatal death, and congenital malformation is no greater than for the general population. We do, however, recommend reducing the maintenance dose to reduce the risk of systemic reaction.

8. Bacterial vaccines have also been widely advocated by some, however, based on several well controlled trials, there is no justification for their use.

The final choice of antigens used for hyposensitization is based upon skin tests, clinical history, and environmental considerations. Identified sensitivities that will subsequently be avoided should not be included. One should also avoid immunizing a patient with an allergen to which they are not allergic. The testing procedure should therefore, be as specific as possible in defining the patients various sensitivities. The eccentricities that color the mixing process are, at times, a tribute to man's ingeniousness. Some physicians prefer placing all the antigens in one vial, whereas others are adamant that a vial should contain no more than several antigens and use as many as eight or ten vials. Injections are begun at an appropriate dilution based in part upon the patient's sensitivity and are given once or twice weekly with appropriate increments as determined by the amount of local reaction and a continued absence of systemic symptoms. They should be given in a setting where both a physician as well as appropriate drugs and equipment to treat anaphylaxis are readily available. Although anaphylactic or accelerated reactions should be distinctly uncommon, the patient is asked to wait at least 20 minutes after the injection. Finally, beta blockers, which are now employed with increased frequency not only to treat arrhythmias, but also hypertension and vascular headache, reduce a patient's sensitivity to epinephrine and other beta agonists. Patients taking these medications are at increased risk when developing anaphylaxis; in fact, some deaths have been reported in this subset. These patients should therefore, be clearly identified as they would require increased amounts of epinephrine to overcome the pharmacologic blockade; furthermore, one should be more conservative in attempting to achieve an arbitrary maximum dose.

A substantial clinical response is usually not seen for 3–5 months, after which the frequency of the injections may be gradually reduced. Perennial (year-round) treatment is the current recommended form, but many seasonal patients whose injections have been reduced to every 4–6 weeks may require additional preseasonal booster therapy. There is no general agreement as to when to terminate injection therapy. Many patients, of course, make the decision for the physician. Nevertheless, it certainly should be terminated in that patient who has not benefited clinically after one year of uninterrupted maintenance therapy. Quantification of symptoms is difficult and it is probably best to rely on more objective measurements such as the patient's requirements for and the potency of various medications, and/or pulmonary function data obtained at the same time of the year for patients with known seasonal disease. In pure hay fever, if the patient is totally asymptomatic without a requirement for medication for 2 seasons, then a trial off of allergy immunotherapy might be attempted. Similar guidelines could be applied to asthmatics, although most physicians would treat asthmatics for a longer period of time. Controlled double-blind trials in hay fever patients have indicated the effects of immunotherapy may last for as long as 2 years after it has been discontinued. Therefore, symptoms recur with increasing intensity in a certain subset of patients, which may require the reinstitution of immunotherapy. A similar sequence of events is quite common in the asthmatic population as well.

Although there are multiple allergen preparations available for use in hyposensitization, most of them are soluble or adjuvant extracts with alum or tyrosine. Unfortunately, there is very little standardization of these extracts except for weight/volume or protein/nitrogen assessment, which does not assay the biologic potency. The recent thrust of current research has been to attempt to identify and purify the active antigens. For example, antigen E (not to be confused with IgE) was isolated by King and Norman from ragweed pollen and, on a weight/volume basis, is approximately 200 times more potent than the whole extract. Although immunization with this provides no more efficacy than the crude extract, it offers a standard by which to measure the potency of all ragweed extract. The methodology to apply these techniques to all antigens is available and it is only a matter of time before well characterized standards for most antigens will be developed.

Various attempts have been made to delay the absorption of the antigen and thereby reduce the local reaction and the need for frequent injections. An aqueous antigen-mineral oil emulsion enjoyed a vogue some years ago, but was discontinued because of the late local reactions such as sterile abscesses and granulomata. Alum-precipitated pyridine-extracted pollen extracts (Allpyral) are available for a wide variety of antigens, however, control studies have not yielded consistently satisfactory results.

Finally, the future may well lie with the development of altered antigens; chemical modification of allergens by formalin, urea, or ultraviolet light produce *allergoids,* reducing their allergenic properties, but maintaining their immunogenicity. Similarly, the polymerization of allergen proteins by glutalderhyde treatment has produced a preparation that is as clinically effective as the aqueous preparation but much less allergenic; none of these preparations is currently available for current use.

Prophylactic

Prospective asthmatic parents will frequently consult a physician regarding the chances that their child will be asthmatic; furthermore, they will want to know whether there is something they can do to prevent that. At this point in time, there seems to be no way to alter the development of bronchial hyperreactivity, or at least the capacity to become asthmatic. On the other hand, there is a substantial body of evidence that has continued to build over the last 10 to 15 years, which indicates that the onset of allergic symptoms can be prevented or delayed in infants and young children by not only a dietary regimen during pregnancy, but also exclusive breast-feeding and the avoidance of allergenic foods during the first year of life. For example, a large Finnish study performed prospective follow-up on 256 children from birth to five years of age. Clearly, the incidence of atopic eczema and food sensitivity were clearly inversely proportional to the length of exclusive breast-feeding. Such studies are only in their infancy and whether such differences will be seen in the occurrence of allergic hay fever and allergic asthma, which classically occur after the age of four, is yet to be determined. Nevertheless, based on these studies, we currently suggest that the allergic parents of potentially allergic offspring consider the following recommendations.

1. During the last trimester, the mother should avoid foods to which she is allergic, as well as markedly reduce her intake of cow's milk and eggs.
2. The child should be breast-fed exclusively for the first 6 months; if supplements are required then a soy or casein hydrolysate should be used.
3. The introduction of solid foods should be postponed until 6 months of age, at which time only cooked fruits and vegetables should be used.
4. The introduction of the classically allergenic foods, (i.e., fish, nuts, chocolate, milk, tomatoes, eggs) should be postponed until one year of age.
5. The child's environment should be hypoallergic; the presence of inhalants that commonly cause sensitivity, (i.e., mold, feathers, house dust, animal danders) should be limited.

REFERENCES

Aas K: Hyposensitization in housedust allergy asthma. Acta Paediatr Scand 60:264–268, 1971

Aas K, Johansson SGO: The radioallergosorbent test in the *in vitro* diagnosis of multiple reaginic allergy. A comparison of diagnostic approaches. J Allergy Clin Immunol 48:134–142, 1971

Bruun E: Control examination of the specificity of specific desensitization in asthma. Acta Allergol 2:122, 1949

Canonica GW, Mingari MC, Moretta L, et al: Imbalances of T cell subpopulations in patients with atopic diseases and effect of specific immunotherapy. J Immunol 123:2669, 1979

Colldahl H: Study of provocation tests on patients with bronchial asthma. Acta Allegol 5:133–154, 1952

Cooke RA, Vander Veer A Jr. Human sensitization: J Immunol 1:201, 1916

Cooper PJ, Darbyshire J, Nunn AJ, et al: A controlled trial of oral hyposensitization in pollen asthma and rhinitis in children. Clin Allergy 14:541–550, 1984

Dolovich J, Hargrave FE, Chalmers R, et al: Late cutaneous allergic responses in isolated IgE-dependent reactions. J Allergy Clin Immunol 52:38, 1973

Frankland AW, Augustin R: Prophylaxis of summer hay fever and asthma: Controlled trial comparing crude grass-pollen extracts with isolated main protein component. Lancet 1:1055–1057, 1954

Friedlaender E, Friedlaender AS: Effectiveness of a portable electrostatic precipitator in elimination of environmental allergens and control of allergic symptoms. Ann Allergy 12:419, 1954

Gatien JC, Merler E, and Colten HR: Allergy to ragweed antigen E: Effect of specific immunotherapy on the reactivity of human T lymphocytes in vitro. Clin Immunol Immunopathol 4:32, 1975

Ishizaka K, Ishizaka T: Identification of IgE antibodies as a carrier of reaginic activity. J Immunol 99:1187, 1967

Johnstone DE: Study of the role of antigen dosage in the treatment of pollenosis and pollen asthma. J Dis Child 94:1–5, 1957

Johnstone DE, Dutton A: The value of hyposensitization therapy for bronchial asthma in children—A 14 year old study. Pediatrics 42:793, 1968

King TP, Norman PS: Isolation studies of allergens from ragweed pollen. Biochemistry 1:709, 1962

Kohler PF: Circulating immune complexes and the practicing allergist. J Allergy Clin Immunol 63:297–299, 1979

Kranz P: Indoor air cleaning for allergy purposes. J Allergy 34:155, 1963

Levy DA, Lichtenstein LM, Goldstein EO, et al: Immunologic and cellular changes accompanying the therapy of pollen allergy. J Clin Invest 50:360, 1971

Lichtenstein L, Norman P, Winkenwerder W: Clinical and in vitro studies on the role of immunotherapy in ragweed hay fever. Am J Med 44:514, 1968

Lieberman P, Patterson R: Immunotherapy for atopic disease 19:391–411, 1974

Marsh DG, Lichtenstein LM, Campbell DN: Studies on allergoids prepared from naturally occurring allergens. I. Assay of allergenicity and antigenicity of formalized rye group I component. Immunology 18:705, 1970

Metzger WJ, Donnelly BA, Richardson HB: Modification of late asthmatic responses (LAR) during immunotherapy for Alternaria-induced asthma (abstract). J Allergy Clin Immunol 71:119, 1983

Murray AB, Ferguson AC: Dust-free bedrooms in the treatment of asthmatic children with house dust or house dust mite allergy: a controlled trial. Pediatr 71:418, 1983

Noon L: Prophylactic innoculation against hay fever. Lancet 1:1572–1573, 1911

Norman PS, Winkenwerder WL, Lichtenstein LM: Trials of alum-precipitated pollen extracts in the treatment of hay fever. J Allergy Clin Immunol 50:31, 1972

Ohman JL Jr, Findlay SR, Leitermann KM: Immunotherapy in cat-induced asthma. Double-blind trial with evaluation of in vivo and in vitro responses. J Allergy Clin Immunol 74:230–239, 1984

Ortolani C, Pastorello E, Moss RB, et al: Grass pollen immunotherapy: a single year double-blind, placebo-controlled study in patients with grass pollen-induced asthma and rhinitis. J Allergy Clin Immunol 73:283–290, 1984

Patterson R, Suszko IM, McIntire FC: Polymerized ragweed antigen E. J Immunol 110:1402, 1973

Platts-Mills TAE, Michel EB, Nock P, et al: Reduction of bronchial hypersensitivity during prolonged allergen avoidance. Lancet 2:675–678, 1982

Price JF, Warner JO, Hey EN, et al: Controlled trial of hyposensitization with adsorbed tyrosine Dermatophagoides pteronyssinus antigen in childhood asthma: in vivo aspects. Clin Allergy 14:209–219, 1984

Pruzansky JJ, Patterson R: Histamine release from leukocytes of hypersensitive patients. II. Reduced sensitivity of leukocytes after injection therapy. J Allergy 39:44, 1967

Rocklin RE, Sheffer AL, Greineder DK, et al: Generation of antigen-specific suppressor cells during allergy desensitization. New Eng J Med 302:1213, 1980

Saarinen UM, Kajosaari M, Backman A, et al: Prolonged breast-feeding as prophylaxis for atopic disease. Lancet ii:163–166, 1979

Smith AP: Hyposensitization with Dermatophagoides pteronyssinus antigen: Trial in asthma induced by house dust. Br Med J 4:204–206, 1971

Spector SL, Farr RS: Bronchial inhalation procedures in asthmatics. Med Clinic North Am 58(1):71–84, 1974

Taylor WW, Ohman JL, Lowell FC: Immunotherapy in cat-induced asthma. J Allergy Clin Immunol 42:283–287, 1978

Valovirta E, Koivikko A, Vanto T, et al: Immunotherapy in allergy to dose: a double-blind clinical study. Ann Allergy 53:85–88, 1984

Voorhorst R, Spieksma FTM, Varekamp H, et al: The house dust mite (Dermatophagoides pteronyssinus) and the allergens it produces: identity with the house dust allergen. J Allergy 39:325, 1967

Georges M. Halpern
M. Eric Gershwin

16

Use and Relevance of the Clinical Laboratory

The laboratory aides to diagnosis in allergic bronchial asthma have progressed vigorously in the past decades as a result of the elucidation of the nature of the responsible immunoglobulin, IgE, by the Ishizakas. This progress was materially advanced by the discovery of several IgE myelomas as by the diagnostic technology that was largely developed by Johansson, Bennich, and Wide.

IgE is a monomeric immunoglobulin molecule produced by plasma cells and, like IgA, is found within tissues exposed to heavy antigen contact. The major reservoirs, therefore, include lung, gut, and skin. In general, very low levels of IgE are normally found in the circulation. Of particular importance is the binding of IgE to specific receptors residing on the surface of mast cells and basophils. Contacts with antigens (allergen) and attachment to these cells result in sensitization. Moreover, repeated contacts with allergen result in rapid (15–20 min) discharge of vasoactive amines stored within the granules of these cells, and synthesis of mediators in their membranes (arachidonic acid derivatives, platelet activating factor).

Vasoactive amines are responsible for the significant amplification of these reactions in comparison to the minute amount of antigen contacted. These chemical mediators and their properties are discussed in Chapter 2.

Several techniques are currently available for evaluating the allergic responsiveness of a patient to a specific potential allergen. The most widely

341

employed is skin testing. Here, introduction of a dilute solution of the suspected allergen via a prick or intradermal technique results in development of local skin reactions of a wheal and flare nature. The concentration of the allergen that results in a positive reaction and the intensity of that reaction are roughly correlated with the degree of sensitivity in the patient. Multiple studies have confirmed the close association between a high degree of skin test reactivity to an allergen and the severity of symptoms caused by that allergen. The test results correlate more closely with rhinitis symptoms than with development of asthma or bronchial reactivity. However, in some well studied systems, such as ragweed- or cat dander-induced bronchial reactivity, skin test reactivity and symptom production are in close agreement with results obtained from direct antigen challenge, suggesting that for some allergens the skin test can also reflect bronchial reactivity.

Skin testing, which has been used for the diagnosis of allergy disorders for over 5 decades, is a powerful tool. It is, however, almost universally misused in that standardized antigens are not yet employed, and little effort is made to quantify the results. Positive skin tests reactions to common inhalant allergens may occur in patients who have no clinical disease when high concentrations are used. It is, therefore, necessary, in order for these tests to be useful, to use either endpoint or midpoint titrations. The dilute solutions of allergens that are commonly used for testing are readily denatured or absorbed in glass in the absence of a protective material such as Tween or protein.

Several tests are available for measuring the amount of total and antigen-specific IgE. Measurement of antigen-specific IgE by the RAST (radioallergosorbent test) or FAST (fluorescent allergosorbent test) (see below) is now becoming an important adjunct to skin testing in selected instances; and, as these tests become better standardized and less expensive, they may overtake skin testing as the method of choice for evaluating specific hypersensitivity in instances where large numbers of samples are tested. Both of these tests and their clinical usefulness are discussed in this chapter. Another method of gauging responsiveness to a specific allergen is measurement of release of histamine from whole blood or leukocytes.

The techniques involved in histamine release are an *in vitro* counterpart of the skin tests but are approximately one-hundred-fold more precise. The correlation between results obtained by skin tests and histamine release is excellent although not complete. The histamine release technique can be used to measure patient sensitivity, to characterize and standardize antigens, and for the measurement of blocking antibodies (IgG, IgG4).

Direct antigen challenge, either by the oral or inhaled route, is advocated by some investigators as the only truly reliable method of objectively testing patients' reactivity or sensitivity to an antigen, particularly for assessing gastrointestinal or bronchial reactions. Unfortunately, these challenge procedures are also more likely to induce unpleasant or potentially dangerous reactions than the other methods described. They must be rigorously controlled and performed by a physician with resuscitation equipment readily available. The procedure for inhalation challenge is presented elsewhere.

STANDARDIZATION OF ALLERGENS

Manufacturing methods for allergenic extracts have changed very little during the last 50 years since allergy has been a medical specialty. The industry has applied much better controls over manufacturing, testing, and storage. Although manufacturing facilities have become very elegant with state-of-the-art environmental controls and analytical instrumentation, the basic method of making an allergenic extract has seen little improvement. The standard practice for many years has been to soak the allergen in an aqueous solution containing buffers, sodium chloride, glycerine, and/or phenol followed by sterilization by filtration. With few exceptions there are no reference preparations against which the potency or composition of the extract can be compared, nor any real measures applied to the finished product to determine potency or composition. Allergy has been the only area of medicine to employ injectable substances that do not have guaranteed potency or authoritative dosage recommendations based on controlled clinical studies.

Several companies saw the need for better allergenic extracts and sought to achieve this through the application of the better commercial technology available. The first step was to define the ideal extract, which would be:

1. free from extraneous, non-allergenic material
2. potent
3. stable
4. standardized
5. efficacious

The next step was to address each of these characteristics:

Free From Extraneous Material

The ultimate extract would contain only purified allergens, but at this point in time it is not commercially feasible. Some companies decided to remove components of the extract with molecular weights above 100,000 and below 1,000. This decision was based on the following assumptions:

1. Known allergens have molecular weights between 100,000 and 1,000 and would be retained.

2. Material over 100,000 M.W. and under 1,000 M.W. is extraneous material and would be eliminated.
3. Viruses are larger than 100,000 M.W. and would be removed. This is of particular importance in epidermal extracts.
4. Endotoxins from gram-negative bacilli are larger than 100,000 M.W. and would be removed.
5. Mycotoxins are smaller than 1,000 M.W. and would be removed. This is particularly important in mold and housedust extracts.

Potency

1. The process would allow adjustment of potency during manufacturing.
2. Potency would be established by skin testing.

Stable

Recently the effects of time, temperature, and diluent on stability by isoelectric focusing (IEF), RAST inhibition, crossed immunoelectrophoresis (CIE), crossed radioimmunoelectrophoresis (CRIE) and dye-binding protein assay were studied. It was found that:

1. The higher the storage temperature above refrigerator temperature, the more rapid the decrease in potency.
2. Extracts in 50 percent glycerine were more stable than nonglycerinated aqueous extracts.
3. Proteins in extracts disappeared at different rates indicating not only a decrease in potency but a change in specificity.

Extracts should be freeze-dried providing the best stability up to the time of reconstitution. The amount per vial should be small enough to be used rather quickly, but large enough so that the user would not be required to reconstitute too frequently. Five ml per vial is optimal.

Standardized.

The FDA Office of Biologics recently published guidelines by which a manufacturer can establish reference preparations.

1. Pollen Extracts: For pollen extracts a manufacturer must assure lot-to-lot potency by RAST inhibition and isoelectric focusing (IEF). Other assays such as radial immunodiffusion (RID) can be used where applicable. Antigen E and R_a5 content of Short Ragweed are assayed this way.
2. Non-Pollen Extracts: Non-pollen extracts are evaluated on an individual basis. Where an assay for a specific antigen such as the RID for Cat Allergen-I is available, it may be used to assure lot-to-lot uniformity.

3. Clinical Data: Prior to approval, some puncture and intradermal skin testing data must be provided to demonstrate the range of reactivity of the extract.

4. Labeling: Once standardized, an extract will be labeled in Allergy Units (AU). Extracts that are statistically equivalent to the reference will be labeled 100,000 AU. Thus, the potency of a standardized extract is established by skin testing and the lot-to-lot uniformity is maintained by RAST inhibition, RID, IEF, or some other appropriate laboratory technique. Extracts should be manufactured and tested in accordance with these guidelines.

An inhibition assay using IgE FAST™ (fluorescent allergosorbent test) microtitration plate technology was recently developed as an alternative to the 3-day RAST inhibition procedure for the comparison of potencies of allergenic extracts. The test procedure utilizes microtitration wells as a solid-phase support for the coating of specific allergens. Binding of allergen-specific IgE to the coated wells is inhibited in a dose dependent manner by allergenic extracts. An objective fluorometer is used for the measurement of the relative fluorescence signal emitted from each test well.

The relative potencies of ten pairs of allergenic extracts were determined using the FAST inhibition method. The results correlated well with those obtained by RAST inhibition. Because the FAST inhibition procedure is completed within one day, it is especially useful for in-process testing during the manufacturing of standardized allergenic extracts.

Efficacy

Efficacy cannot be properly evaluated until a uniform standard of potency has been established. Determination of potency by skin testing in humans is a necessary prerequisite to efficacy studies of allergenic extracts. Controlled clinical trials by skin testing to determine the potency of the extract are a significant part of the development of Standardized Allergenic Extracts.

IN-VIVO EVALUATION OF IMMEDIATE HYPERSENSITIVITY

Skin Testing

Direct reproduction of an immediate allergic reaction by introducing a small amount of extract of suspected allergen into the skin is ingrained in the practice of medicine as a diagnostic aid. A large number of tests can be done in a short time, the results appear in a matter of minutes, and the result, when positive, is striking both to the patient and to the physician. The early work of Prausnitz and Kustner showed that wheal and erythema reactions in the skin were the result of serum antibodies specific for the allergen being tested. The presence of IgE antibodies on mast cells and basophils sensitizes them so that a repeat contact with the allergen results in rapid (15–20 min) secretion of histamine and other mediators, which show their characteristic activity in the skin by the development of a wheal, a sharply circumscribed localized area of edema, surrounded by a flare, a less exactly defined area of erythema surrounding the wheal. It was early recognized that a positive skin test simply reproduced to a minor degree, in the skin, the disease that was causing the patient's problem in other tissues. As the procedure was usually safe, it caught on rapidly in diagnosis and has been used much more frequently than direct challenges to tissues.

Skin tests, however, do not always elicit a reaction when a challenge by another route will. This is seen most frequently in drug allergy.

INDICATIONS

The indications for skin testing are to confirm suspicion that an individual's symptoms are allergic in origin. This is based on a review of the character of the symptoms, along with time and place of occurrence. Suspicion of allergy, however, should not be an excuse to perform skin tests to all possible allergens. Skin tests should only be performed with those allergens that, from the history, have some likelihood of causing the patient's symptoms.

PROCEDURE

Although testing may be carried out by a nurse or technician, a physician should always be within immediate calling distance, as generalized allergic reactions are rare but distinctly possible occurrences. A rubber tourniquet to place above the skin test site on an extremity and 1:1,000 aqueous epinephrine should be on hand as the first measure employed in treating a generalized reaction. The prick and intradermal tests provide the most consistent and interpretable results in skin testing. Each is described here, and the two are then compared. Histamine controls should always be placed to judge the quality of both techniques. For the prick test, a 1 percent histamine solution (1 mg/ml) is employed. This concentration gave a 6.4 mm mean diameter flare with a standard deviation of 2.1 mm in a control series. For the intradermal test, 0.01 per cent histamine base solution is employed (0.275 mg of histamine phosphate per ml of diluent, Eli Lilly & Co.). Failure to react to histamine can result from improper technique, prior use of antihistamines and drugs or systemic illness resulting in certain forms of immune paralysis. A diluent control utilizing 0.4 percent phenol should also be employed. Dermatographic individuals may give wheal and flare reactions to the trauma involved in placing the test, so that all tests appear positive. These patients should be tested by an alternative method, (i.e. *in vitro*).

Prick tests may be performed either on the volar surface of the lower or upper arm, or on the back. If large numbers of tests are to be performed, the back is preferable so that the tests can be properly spaced. The skin is cleaned with isopropyl alcohol or 70 percent ethyl alcohol. The testing sites are marked with an appropriate code. Sites should be at least 5 cm apart to prevent overlap. A single drop of test solution is applied to each test site from containers with rubber bulk droppers. A sterile testing needle is passed through the drop and inserted into the skin. The needle is then withdrawn with a slight lifting of the skin. The solution is wiped away approximately 1 minute later, and the prick lesion should be superficial enough not to cause bleeding. Either a 26-gauge × 0.5 inch needle or a special testing needle provided by the antigen manufacturer may be used, and a new needle is used for each test. When fully developed, lesions are read with a millimeter rule. The wheal and erythema is smaller by this method than by the intradermal method, so the same grading system does not apply and grading is not always done. The means obtained by measuring the widest and narrowest borders are recorded for induration and erythema. End-point titrations are possible with prick tests by utilizing varied antigen concentrations. The prick test requires approximately 1000-fold higher concentration of antigen than an intradermal test for a positive reaction of the same size in the same patient or in patients with equivalent sensitivities. Recently, disposable standardized devices have been available (Stallerpoint) allowing time saving and less painful large series of prick tests.

INTRADERMAL SKIN TESTS

The arm is the usual preferred site for intradermal testing. This method provides increased sensitivity, and a tourniquet may be employed in an adverse reaction. As a rule, fewer tests are required with this method, because many practitioners choose to screen for exquisite sensitivity with the prick technique and eliminate the significant reactants from intradermal testing. Skin tests sites are cleansed and marked as described above. Sterile disposable plastic 1-ml tuberculin syringes with 26-gauge × 3/8 inch needles are filled with approximately 0.05 ml of the test solution; all bubbles must be carefully expelled, as these, when injected into the skin, produce induration reactions that reduce testing precision. When the arm is used, the skin should be stretched by grasping from behind. The syringe is placed at an angle of 45° to the arm, with the bevel of the needle facing down. The point of the needle is inserted in a forward lifting motion, as if to pick up the skin with the tip of the needle. As the tip enters the skin, the pick-up motion is gradually converted to a forward and downward pressure, while the barrel is lowered to eliminate the angle it previously formed with the surface. The bevel should penetrate the skin with the tip between the layers of the skin. With the index finger, fluid is forced into the skin, producing a small wheal. About 0.02 ml of fluid will give a wheal approximately 3 mm in diameter. Some practitioners prefer to introduce 0.05 ml as an amount easier to measure on the syringe, although the amount does not influence the size of the eventual reaction as much as the allergen concentration. If no wheal is formed or an air bubble enters the skin, an alternate site should be chosen.

A series of tests are placed and then inspected after 15 minutes. Occasional patients will take longer to develop a mature reaction; when no reaction or only a small reaction occurs at 15 minutes, the sites should be reinspected at 20–30 minutes. When the reactions have fully developed, they are measured with a millimeter rule. The greatest and smallest diameter of the wheal and erythema are measured. Reactions are often irregular in shape; thus, the diameters measured are not necessarily at right angles. Both diameters are measured, added, and then halved and recorded. Grading systems vary greatly from one center to another. Appropriate standardization will probably not occur until antigens become standardized.

Reactions read at 15 minutes should be reinspected at 30 minutes; if these are significantly larger, the reactions should be reread and the original readings disregarded. A late reaction (4–6 hours) is seen in some patients, and may be IgE mediated.

REAGENTS

In most instances, a concentrated commercial allergen extract is purchased, and serial dilutions are made by the practitioner for testing. The diluting fluid may be purchased in ready-made vials containing either 4.5 or 9.0 ml of solution. A ten-fold dilution series is then made by adding either 0.5 or 1.0 ml, respectively, to a vial, mixing thoroughly, withdrawing the same amount, and adding to the next vial, and so on. A fresh syringe should be employed each time the mixed fluid is withdrawn, as enough material may remain in the syringe from a more concentrated material to alter the concentrations considerably after serial dilutions. The diluting fluid usually is a phosphate-buffered physiologic saline at pH 7.4 with 0.4 percent phenol added to inhibit bacterial growth. Studies indicate that this fluid may allow a significant adsorption of protein to glass, resulting in a loss of up to 90 percent of biologic activity in the high dilutions required for intradermal testing. Addition of human serum albumin (0.03 percent) or Tween 80 (0.005 percent) prevents adsorption to glass.

END POINT TITRATION

Until improved methods for standardization of allergen extracts are in more general use, the physician or laboratory must approach each new batch of allergenic extract with the suspicion that it may be either considerably more or less potent than the previous lot. Each new lot should be compared with the old one by simultaneous end point testing in a few reactive patients to determine whether the potencies of the lots are similar.

Although a single concentration of an allergen may be selected for testing and the reaction graded for positivity, additional information may be obtained with a threshold dilution titration of skin tests performed employing a ten-fold dilution series. In this method, a low concentration (unlikely to produce a large reaction) is tested first. If no reaction is produced, 10-fold and 100-fold higher concentrations are then placed. If positive, these reactions are graded; if negative, higher concentrations are placed until either a positive reaction is elicited or the highest concentration available shows no reaction. Alternatively, if the original test is 3+ or greater positive, lesser concentrations are tested until a concentration is reached that gives either a trace or negative reaction. The lowest dilution required for a 1+ or 2+ reaction is considered the end point. When this end point falls between two dilutions, (i.e., the stronger gives a 3+ or 4+ reaction and the weaker gives a trace or negative reaction), the end point is considered to be intermediate between the two dilutions.

INTERPRETATION

As with the indications for skin tests, interpretation of results is complex. Skin tests do not always correlate with challenge by direct routes. For example, in respiratory allergy, skin tests are often positive when attempts at bronchial challenge fail to reproduce measurable bronchospasm. In contrast, in some patients bronchial challenge is positive when skin tests are negative. Careful attempts to demonstrate this phenomenon with the well-characterized allergen, ragweed, however, have shown reasonable agreement between skin tests and respiratory challenge, so that some of the discrepancies between the two methods may result from differences in technique.

Currently, two alternatives are available to skin testing for demonstrating the presence or absence of IgE-mediated reactions. These are direct estimation of serum IgE antigen-specific antibodies by the radioallergosorbent test (RAST) or the FAST, and histamine release from peripheral blood leukocytes. RAST and FAST offer a quantitative level of antigen-specific IgE, but give no information with respect to threshold for clinical sensitivity. Histamine release depends on the amount of IgE fixed to the basophils and is also subject to influences of intracellular events leading to histamine secretion. Skin tests are subject to variability from the patient's responsiveness to mediators, anatomic skin sites, drug use, hormonal state, etc. When skin tests, histamine release and RAST (or FAST) are compared, the demonstrable differences are small, with similar information obtained from each method. Whatever the technique employed, the potency and stability of the allergens employed is as important to control as the technique used in performing the tests. The choice of techniques for assaying a patient's sensitivity, therefore, often depends on such practical matters as cost and convenience rather than the superiority of one of these methods over another. The ease and simplicity of skin testing make it the procedure of choice in regular diagnostic usage, despite the extra discomfort to the patient compared with a single venipuncture. Under certain circumstances, however, there may be advantages to each method (see below).

Not every positive skin test can be correlated with symptoms actually induced by that allergen; however, when threshold dilution testing is employed, the higher the dilution required for a positive test, the greater the likelihood of clinical significance. Tests may also be falsely negative when a patient is truly clinically sensitive. This can be due to the variability of potency and stability of allergenic extracts, but there may also be a few patients who have only local sensitivity and, therefore, respond only to a direct provocative test. The level of sensitivity in a dilution series required to indicate clinical significance may vary considerably from one allergen to another. In general, pollen and animal dander extracts are highly potent, whereas mold and dust extracts give positive tests only when a large amount of protein is introduced. Further identification of allergens and development of more accurate methods of standardization offer a hope of making skin test reactions to extracts a more reproducible phenomenon.

IN-VITRO EVALUATION OF IMMEDIATE HYPERSENSITIVITY

Measurement of Total Serum Immunoglobulin E

IgE represents a distinct immunoglobulin class. Through sensitization and subsequent contact with an allergen, (with resulting mast cell release of vasoactive substances), it is responsible for induction of immediate hypersensitivity reactions. Like other immunoglobulins, IgE is composed of two light and two heavy chains, with a molecular weight of 190,000. Its concentration in serum is very low compared to the major circulating immunoglobulins. The serum pool, however, may only reflect absorbed spillover from locally produced sources or reflect traffic patterns, as the major reservoir is in the tissues in areas of high antigen contact. Total serum immunoglobulin E (IgE) is present in normal adults in nanogram per milliliter quantities.

Methods that reproducibly detect less than 100 ng of IgE protein per ml are divided into two groups: solid-phase radioimmunoassays and radioimmunoprecipitation (double-antibody) assays. The solid-phase methods have in common the insolubilization of anti-IgE antibody. This insoluble antibody has been employed in a competitive binding assay using radiolabeled IgE with standards of known IgE content, or it can be used to bind serum IgE in a noncompetitive fashion, with the amount bound determined by subsequent incubation with a radio- or enzyme-labeled anti-IgE. The competitive binding assay, called the radioimmunosorbent test (RIST), is commercially available in kit form, as are the individual reagents (Pharmacia Laboratories, Piscataway, New Jersey). The advantages of the method include completion in a single day, lack of need of precipitating antisera, and the commercial availability of all required reagents. It can be used in clinical settings to distinguish normal from clearly elevated levels of serum IgE in adult patients. However, when low levels of serum IgE must be measured accurately or when serial studies are required, radioimmunoprecipitation is preferred.

The radioimmunoprecipitation (double antibody) assay for serum IgE protein is unsurpassed in precision and reproducibility and is the method of choice for clinical purposes. Unlike solid-phase radioimmunoassays, it requires the addition of a second antibody after completion of the competitive binding incubation in order to separate bound from free antigen, (i.e., IgE). This precipitating antiserum must be available in large quantities (often at considerable cost) and the assay generally requires two days to complete. Its other disadvantage is that inherent in all competitive binding assays–namely, nonspecific interference by serum factors at high concentrations.

Radioimmunoassays (RIA) making use of ^{125}iodine labeled antibodies are subject to strict regulations and a federal license of the U.S. Nuclear Regulatory Commission (NCR); decay, inherent to radionuclides, prevents long shelf life and puts a strain on final cost. Monoclonal anti-IgE antibody technology allows a reduction of background, with a "cleaner" assay. Alkaline phosphatase and betagalactosidase enzyme immunoassays are more flexible than immunoperoxidase assays. Microtiter plate or microtitration wells assays allow rapid determination with computerized data reduction. Emission of fluorescence signals allows more precise determinations than absorption of light in a spectrophotometer. All these considerations should be kept in mind before selecting a system, and will ultimately influence volume and cost.

INDICATIONS

Clinical situations in which a total serum IgE level may be diagnostically useful are listed in Table 16-1.

Serial tests on patients with allergic disorders may be used to confirm the seasonal elevations in serum total IgE level regularly seen after high-level exposure to allergens to which the patient is sensitive. In pathologic conditions associated with high serum IgE levels, (e.g., parasitism) serial assays may be useful in documenting therapeutic effectiveness. Serum IgE levels may also be useful in providing supportive evidence of the differential diagnosis of allergic disease in difficult cases. The clinician, however, must be

Table 16-1

Differential Utility of Total Serum IgE in Allergic Disease

Syndrome	Total serum IgE [IU/ml]	Interpretation
Rhinitis	>200	Favors allergic component
	<50	Favors nonallergic component
Asthma	>200	Consistent with atopic component
	<50	Suggests intrinsic (nonatopic) disease or minor atopic component
Atopic Dermatitis	>400	Consistent with atopic dermatitis in absence of other explanations
	<50	Atopic dermatitis unlikely
Allergic bronchopulmonary aspergillosis	>500	Supports diagnosis
	<300	Virtually excludes diagnosis in untreated patient
Urticaria	>200	Possible allergic mechanism
	<50	IgE mechanism unlikely but not impossible.
Unexplained eosinophilia	>2000	Suggests parasitism
	450–2000	Compatible with parasitic infections
	200–450	Nonspecific

aware that the use of the total serum IgE level can neither definitively rule in or out an allergic diagnosis. That is, although allergy and elevated serum IgE are related, some patients with elevated serum IgE levels have no allergic symptoms, while others with unequivocal allergic problems clinically have normal or low total serum IgE levels.

INTERPRETATION

Serum IgE values are expressed in international units per milliliter. One IU is equivalent to approximately 2.4 ng of IgE protein. As with the other Ig classes, serum IgE levels are age-dependent. The IgE level of cord sera is very low–probably less than 2 IU/ml–and IgE does not cross the placental barrier in significant amounts. Mean serum IgE levels progressively increase with age until about 12 years of age, after which there is a gradual decline to adult levels. After the age of 12 years, serum IgE greater than 333 IU/ml (800 ng/ml) is generally considered abnormally high. The great majority of patients with elevated serum IgE levels have atopic disorders such as allergic rhinitis, "extrinsic" asthma and atopic dermatitis. There is, however, considerable overlap between nonatopic and atopic populations. For example, the mean serum IgE level in one study of adults with allergic asthma was 1589 ng/ml (range, 55 to 12,750 ng/ml); however, only about one half of these asthmatic patients had IgE levels above 800 ng/ml, the upper limit of normal for the nonatopic population. Atopic dermatitis is associated with extremely high serum IgE levels, with only about 20 per cent of these patients having serum IgE levels within the normal range. Allergic urticaria and anaphylactic reactions are also commonly associated with elevated serum IgE levels.

Serum IgE levels vary with levels of exposure to allergens. Patients with pollen allergies increase their basal serum IgE levels several-fold during their relevant pollen seasons. Immunotherapy with allergenic extracts also elevates IgE levels during the early phase of treatment, sometimes elevating the total serum IgE. Alternatively, total IgE levels may drop below baseline with blunted seasonal rises after successful immunotherapy.

Basal levels of serum IgE appear to be under genetic control, with high IgE levels inherited as a simple Mendelian recessive trait. Additionally, numerous pathologic conditions, particularly parasitism, boost basal IgE production. T lymphocytes probably play an important role in the regulation of IgE and other immunoglobulin synthesis. Elevated serum IgE levels are seen in patients with T cell malignancies such as Hodgkin's disease, whereas chronic lymphocytic leukemia and multiple myeloma are associated with low levels of IgE. Rare examples of IgE myeloma have been documented, however. It must be kept in mind that IgE production is but one variable in most allergic disorders. Total serum IgE levels can only be interpreted properly with respect to other pertinent clinical information, including the personal and family history of allergic disorders known to be associated with elevated IgE levels.

RADIOALLERGOSORBENT TEST (RAST) AND FLUORESCENT ALLERGOSORBENT TEST (FAST) FOR ANTIGEN-SPECIFIC SERUM IMMUNOGLOBULIN E

The radioallergosorbent test (RAST), a solid-phase radioimmunoassay, and FAST, an enzyme immunoassay with fluorescence emission are the current methods of choice for serologic determination of antigen-specific IgE antibody.

The other *in vitro* test for specific serum IgE is radioimmuno-diffusion, a time-consuming, cumbersome and semiquantitative test that has largely been abandoned in favor of RAST and FAST. The basic principle of the RAST is simple. Allergen-coated particles are incubated in the study serum, during which time specific antibody of all immunoglobulin classes is bound. The particles are then washed, and a second incubation is undertaken with a radiolabeled, high specific anti-IgE antibody. The radioactivity bound is directly related to the antigen specific IgE antibody content of the test serum. Results are then compared with a standard reference serum. The assay requires 24–48 hours to complete. Unfortunately, the RAST has been subjected to numerous technical variations. These have generally involved the use of different polymers for allergen insolubilization. The commercial supplier of RAST kits (Pharmacia, Piscataway, New Jersey) has settled upon the use of allergen-coated paper disks because of the ease of washing and manipulation. For most clinical diagnostic purposes, the use of paper disks is satisfactory.

Several investigators have found that the absorption of antibodies to plastic surfaces produced immobilized antibody preparations equally effective for enzyme immunoassays. The advantages of this kind of immobilization are its simplicity, its ease of handling, and the fact that it requires only small quantities of antibody.

Plastic solid phases have also been criticized. Theoretically, only a small quantity of material is fixed; due to hydrophobicity, denaturation of the adsorbed macromolecules may take place with time, and sometimes desorption of the immobilized antibody or allergen can occur. Through a proprietary process these problems have been controlled in FAST. Covalent coupling of antibody to cellulose produces stable immobilized antibody preparations that give reproducible results in enzyme immunoassays. Cellulose discs have been criticized for not binding all relevant allergen molecules, for increased nonspecific binding of IgE in serum samples with elevated IgE (>500 IU/ml), for competition for allergen of nonspecific and/or blocking factors and antibody.

Independent studies have demonstrated that ELISA may measure antibodies to different component(s) of the allergen extract, which may bind preferentially to the plastic surface of the well; nonspecific and/or blocking factors or antibody do not compete in ELISA, and this ELISA may detect a population of high affinity IgE antibodies; nonspecific IgE interference was a factor of class differences in RAST but not in IgE FAST.

The enzymes most often used in ELISA are horseradish peroxidase, *Aspergillus niger* glucose oxidase, *Escherichia coli* and veal intestinal alkaline phosphatase and *E. coli* β-galactosidase. In a comparative study, although the four enzymes detected equally small quantities of IgE, the dose–response curves of alkaline phosphatase and β-galactosidase were superior to those of glucose oxidase and peroxidase. With alkaline phosphatase, a linear plot was obtained for quantities of human IgE ranging from 1 to 1,000 IU. The sensitivities of the measurements in this case were equal to that achieved with RIA.

The relative instability of the various substrates used to measure oxidoreductases like peroxidase and glucose oxidase can be a serious drawback in the use of oxidoreductase in enzyme immunoassays requiring a long incubation time. Using fluorescent techniques, procedures have been developed that can measure extremely small quantities of enzyme. Such procedures allow measurement of very small quantities of antigen or antibody. Amounts of human IgE as low as 0.05 IU/ml have been measured.

In 1981, a new fluorescence enzyme immunoassay for IgE quantitation was developed. This test differs from other *in vitro* tests in that it uses a monoclonal antibody to determine the allergen-specific and total IgE in human serum. This immunoassay makes use of a high-speed fluorometer with built-in data reduction capability and microtitration wells as solid-phase support for immobilization of specific allergen or anti-IgE antibody. The allergen-specific IgE test (IgE FAST) can be completed in less than 6 hours.

INTERPRETATION OF TEST RESULTS

In the allergen-specific IgE assay, results are expressed in international units of IgE per milliliter of serum (IU/ml). Each international unit is approximately equivalent to 2.4 ng. Human serum IgE, which is obtained from the National Institutes of Health in Bethesda, Maryland, is used as the primary references. In this test, a serum IgE level of greater than 0.03 IU/ml correlates with a clinical history and symptoms of allergy. The sensitivity of the test is 0.02 IU/ml. The monoclonal antihuman IgE antibody used in this test system was found to have no cross reactivity to other human immunoglobulins and serum albumin.

INDICATIONS

There is some controversy regarding the appropriate use of RAST or FAST for clinical diagnosis. It is generally agreed, however, that RAST and FAST provides information similar to that obtained by direct intradermal skin testing, using the measured wheal and flare response at 15–20 minutes as the criterion.

False-positive RAST or FAST tests rarely occur except with complex allergen mixtures like dust extracts, which may nonspecifically bind IgE. Alternatively, when low-sensitivity RAST systems are employed, the skin test may be positive when the RAST test is negative. The clinical significance of these false-negative RAST tests is unresolved. Economically, in small numbers, skin testing is less expensive than RAST assays and has the advantage of immediate results.

There are, however, some clinical situations in which RAST and FAST assays may offer advantages over direct skin testing. In young children or apprehensive adult patients, a single venipuncture may be better tolerated by both patient and physician than skin testing with multiple allergens. In some patients, dermatographism or severe dermatitis (particularly eczema) may interfere with proper interpretation of the skin test, and FAST or RAST offer an acceptable alternative. RAST or FAST can be employed in patients whose skin test results may be altered by medication such as antihistamines (which often cannot be withdrawn). Further, RAST and FAST assays may be useful in a few selected patients with suggestive clinical histories but negative skin tests, principally to provide independent confirmation of the lack of IgE antibodies. Similarly, FAST or RAST may also prove useful in the future (after appropriate standardizations) for evaluating food allergy, where skin tests correlate poorly with clinically reproducible reactions, and oral challenge is at best cumbersome and, at times, relatively contraindicated owing to the extreme nature of the reaction (history of anaphylaxis with laryngoedema or shock). RAST or FAST may be useful in differentiating shocklike reactions mediated by direct vasoactive amine release (such as ASA or iodinated contrast media reactions) from truly IgE-mediated anaphylactic reactions. Additionally, RAST or FAST may be employed any time the nature of the reaction in question is so severe that the physician wishes not to subject the patient to the possible risk of reaction from skin testing with the offending antigen (e.g., Hymenoptera venom sensitivity).

Currently, the major disadvantage of RAST for clinical use is the difficulty of transforming RAST or FAST results into levels of clinical sensitivity. The correlation between RAST assay and intradermal skin testing is very good when carefully performed with the use of the same allergen extract for skin testing and for RAST or FAST assay. None of the commercially available RAST kits has been standardized with respect to clinical symptomatology or direct skin testing. The clinical laboratory desiring to provide RAST or FAST assay results should make an effort to provide physicians with some basis for interpretation. This is not easily accomplished, as such data had to be gathered independently for each allergen. Currently, research attempts relating circulating IgE levels to clinical status are under way. Large-volume FAST or RAST testing allows significant reduction in cost. In the future, these advances may result in the FAST or RAST becoming the method of choice for evaluation of IgE-mediated disorders.

INTERPRETATION

Commercial RAST kits, available from Pharmacia Laboratories, utilize a single birch pollen reference serum and sorbent as a standard for all of their RAST assays. Results are expressed as negative or 1+ to 4+ (or protein nitrogen units), depending on binding relative to an arbitrary division of the standard curve. This grading system may be easily misinterpreted by the clinician to imply corresponding severity of clinical disease. Such inference is not justified, since in some allergen systems the most sensitive individuals do not exceed 2+ on the birch pollen standard curve. Ideally, each RAST sorbent system should have its own specific reference serum drawn from the most highly sensitive patients available.

Currently, each laboratory must determine the clinical correlations necessary to provide useful interpretations of the RAST assay results. Standardization of RAST data in units of absolute antibody content will help solve this problem. Precise clinical interpretation of specific antibody content, however, will have to await clinical correlation data, which are not yet available.

HISTAMINE RELEASE

Allergic reactions depend not only on circulating IgE but also on a number of other factors, including the balance between blocking antibodies and IgE on the target cells, and the ability of basophils or mast cells to release other mediators. Histamine release from the leukocytes of allergic individuals is an excellent *in-vitro* correlate of immediate hypersensitivity. This reaction is initiated by the addition of antigen to which the individual is allergic, and is due to the presence of antibody fixed to the basophil membrane. Histamine is released from the basophil, the only circulating cell that contains histamine. The addition of serum or plasma usually is not essential for the release of histamine from human basophils. However, normal serum will enhance the release when reaction conditions are suboptimal (i.e. with limited antigen concentrations). The serum of allergic individuals also contains blocking antibodies (IgG antibodies) that compete for antigen and possibly (a controversial point) prevent it from reaching IgE-sensitized basophils; the concentration of these antibodies increases as a result of hyposensitization therapy.

For several reasons histamine release has had only limited clinical application: (1) the histamine extraction and the fluorometric assay are cumbersome and time-consuming procedures; (2) large amounts of blood are required; (3) the method is technically complicated. Several recent technical advances, however, have made possible the routine use of histamine release from leukocytes as an *in-vitro* technique for the diagnosis and study of allergy. The extraction and assay of histamine by the fluorometric technique is an accurate and sensitive method for determination of this biologically active molecule. The method is based on the coupling of histamine with ophthalaldehyde at a highly alkaline pH to form a fluorescent product. The fluorescence of the histamine-o-phthalaldehyde complex is more intense and more stable at an acid pH. To remove histidine and other interfering compounds, the histamine is extracted prior to the condensation step. Protein is removed from the sample to be analyzed by perchloric acid precipitation; the histamine is extracted into n-butanol from the alkalinized salt-saturated solution. Histamine is recovered in an aqueous solution of dilute HCl by adding heptane. This dilute HCl solution is then used for the condensation of histamine with o-phthalaldehyde. Moreover, recently a completely automated, sensitive histamine analysis system has been developed. The system can be used with a broad range of histamine concentrations, and at the highest sensitivity is capable of analyzing samples that contain 0.05–5 ng of histamine (in 0.5 ml).

This procedure can be utilized to evaluate histamine release from washed leukocytes and whole blood. The whole blood system should be used as a general survey method to give information on the allergic status of patients. The washed leukocyte system is used for experimental studies on the release of mediators, the effect of pharmacologic agents on the release mechanism, the effect of immunotherapy on cell sensitivity and for measurement of blocking antibody.

INDICATIONS

In ragweed-allergic individuals, there is a good correlation between the severity of clinical symptoms and *in vitro* histamine release. In these patients, there is excellent correlation of histamine release with skin test, symptom scores, and the level of serum IgE specific for antigen E (a well characterized antigenic component of ragweed). Both the antigen concentration at which histamine is released and the magnitude of histamine release are good correlates of the clinical severity of disease. Patients with high concentration of ragweed-specific IgE release histamine with low concentrations of antigen E. There is good correlation in ragweed-and grass-allergic individuals between the concentration of antigen required to release 50 percent histamine and the skin sensitivity as determined by intradermal tests. Histamine release can, therefore, be used as a quantitative measure of the clinical sensitivity of a patient. The histamine release method also allows quantitation of the level of blocking antibody and measurements of the effect of hyposensitization on this antibody.

Passive sensitization of normal leukocytes allows quantitation of the relative amount of specific IgE antibody. The radioallergosorbent test (RAST) gives similar information and has the further advantage that it can be more easily standardized. The RAST assay, however, requires more antigen than do histamine release studies.

Purification of an antigen can be followed by determination of its ability to release histamine. Similarly, the system is very useful for studying the effect of allergen modification on its ability to release histamine. There are a number of potential advantages to the use of the histamine release reaction as an alternative to skin testing. The *in-vitro* test completely avoids the possibility of an anaphylactic reaction, an important consideration for some allergens. There is also no danger of sensitizing a patient or boosting a previous immune response, as might occur during repeated skin tests. The test is also useful in the rare patient who cannot be skin tested because of dermatologic conditions and in children. *In vitro* tests also permit the use of antigens that have not been purified or that cannot be used clinically.

INTERPRETATION

Immunotherapy of patients results in several changes in histamine release results: there is often an increase in the level of blocking antibody, a decrease in cell sensitivity and reactivity, and a progressive but slow decrease in the serum antigen-specific IgE levels. The changes in cell sensitivity and reactivity, with some cells releasing no histamine, are most often seen in pediatric cases. Increase in the level of blocking antibody correlates with effectiveness of immunotherapy. Cellular sensitivity may fall prior to seasonal exposure, and there is a post-seasonal rise that appears to be less in patients on immunotherapy.

It should be emphasized that the skin test for immediate hypersensitivity using a number of common allergens and a dilution of 2 + end point is currently the simplest method of assessing the presence or absence of allergy. The *in-vitro* histamine methods are useful complements to the clinical evaluation of patients and supply quantitative data on the degree of sensitivity of a patient. The automated histamine analysis system makes the assay more sensitive and far simpler to apply to routine use; undoubtedly these factors will make this test more useful in the future.

Allergic reactions depend on a number of factors, including the presence of specific IgE, the concentration of blocking antibodies and the ability of basophils or mast cells to release mediators. The amount of histamine released when an allergen is added to whole blood *in vitro* is due to the interaction of all these factors. This test, therefore, more closely simulates the allergic reaction occurring *in vivo* than do measurements of the concentration of allergen-specific IgE. Histamine release from whole blood correlates closely with a patient's skin sensitivity. Over 90 percent of patients who have skin tests greater than or equal to 3 + at 100 PNU or less release significant histamine when antigen is added to whole blood. In contrast, the test is positive in less than 2 percent of skin test-negative patients.

In most clinical studies a very close correlation has been found between the results of skin tests with ragweed pollen, antigen E or grass pollen, and histamine release (e.g., the correlation coefficient between cell sensitivity and skin test sensitivity is approximately 0.8). There is also a highly significant correlation between the cell sensitivity and how symptomatic the patient is during the pollen season. There are, however, some patients with very little histamine release (less than 15 percent) at any concentrations who are very sensitive by skin tests. The meaning of this is not clear. Finally, there is also good correlation between the level of specific ragweed IgE antibody in the serum and the cell sensitivity; however, patients with the same level of anti-ragweed serum IgE might vary in cell sensitivity by 100- to 1000-fold. Therefore, cell sensitivity also measures the effectiveness of the histamine release mechanism. These correlations do not necessarily hold for patients on immunotherapy.

THE EOSINOPHIL IN ALLERGIC DISORDERS

Eosinophils are granule-laden, intensely eosin staining, specialized polymorphonuclear leukocyte seen circulating in increasing numbers or accumulated in local infiltrates primarily in allergic or parasitic disorders. Indeed, it has long been speculated that the entire system of hypersensitivity reactions is related to defense against such parasitic infestation, with allergic reactions being an unpleasant (and at times life-threatening) result of improper regulation of this system. The eosinophil's integral participation within this system has been utilized as evidence of the presence of hypersensitivity type reactions when eosinophils are encountered in high concentrations in the circulation or in tissue accumulations. As with other cellular elements of the hematopoietic system, the formation, migration, kinetics, and functional involvement in the immune inflammatory processes of the eosinophil are extremely complex, and the reader is directed to reference sources for further details. Likewise, it is increasingly apparent that the eosinophil participates in many disorders, apart from the well-recognized allergic and parasitic processes, such as inflammatory, neoplastic and immunodeficiency diseases (Table 16-2), and the clinician is cautioned against automatically and exclusively thinking of the former disorders when elevated levels are encountered.

Eosinophils originate from precursor myeloid cells in the bone marrow and pass through the circulation to reside in tissues–the gastrointestinal tract, skin, and lungs being the most heavily infiltrated. Disorders with increased utilization of eosinophils demonstrate enhanced marrow proliferation, more effective mobilization, and selective redistribution.

PERIPHERAL BLOOD EOSINOPHILIA

Circulating eosinophils are normally seen in low numbers in the blood of healthy individuals. The normal range of blood eosinophilia in adults (cells per cubic millimeter) is about 0 to 500. Norms for children are somewhat higher (mean of 240 cells/mm^3, with 95 percent confidence limits of 0 to 740) and show a moderate degree of sex and age dependence, with higher values exhibited by boys and with peaks in the age range of 4–8 years. Other sources of variations in assessing blood eosinophil levels have also been identified. Exercise can be responsible for transient elevations, whereas emotional stress, physical abuse, β-adrenergic agents (e.g., epinephrine) and hormonal influences of the menstrual cycle serve as lowering influences. Diurnal variations in blood eosinophil numbers have been described, with peak values occurring late at night and minimal values in the morning—the opposite of the diurnally varying levels of circulating adrenal corticosteroids, agents known for eosinopenic effects.

Since eosinophils are present in relatively low numbers in the blood compared to other cellular elements, accurate quantitation is difficult. By counting a total of 100 white blood cells (WBC) in a differential study, a small sampling error of one or two cells may have a relatively large effect on the total level of a blood element normally present as only 1–3 percent of the total white cell pool. In an effort to minimize such potential sampling errors, larger cell numbers should be counted in WBC differentials (e.g., 500 to 1000 total cells), or larger volumes of blood (1 mm^3) may be processed by techniques designed to obscure other WBC and to specifically stain eosinophils.

Despite these difficulties, sampling of blood remains the best available method for assessing host responses characterized by eosinophilia. The eosinophil is not primarily a blood element and it is found concentrated several hundredfold in the marrow and tissues. Thus, circulating cells reflect only those that are trafficking between sites of production and function. There are pathologic situations, especially in certain chronic conditions, in which tissue eosinophilia is prominent but peripheral blood eosinophilia is minimal or absent. Thus, although the quantitative assessment of peripheral blood eosinophilia can be important diagnostically, results must be interpreted with an understanding of the kinetics of the eosinophil and an appreciation of the technical limitations and potential sampling variations involved.

TISSUE EOSINOPHILIA

Eosinophils produced in the marrow traffic only briefly through the circulation before finally reaching the tissues, where they presumably carry out their still incompletely understood functions. However, because of the inaccessibility of some involved sites and technical difficulties in sampling and studying tissue-localized cells, information about the tissue eosinophil, especially in humans, is limited. Although eosinophils are distributed intravascularly throughout the body in the normal animal, extravascularly they appear to localize preferentially in certain tissues. Characteristically the densest infiltrations of eosinophils outside the bone marrow occur in the gastrointestinal tract (especially the small bowel and stomach) and the lungs (primarily the perivascular and peribronchial regions). The density of eosinophils is much less in the skin than in the gut or lungs, but the great mass of the skin makes it the chief reservoir of eosinophils among tissues. Eosinophils migrate to areas of inflammation and specific antigenic challenge under the influence of a number of tissue, mast cell, lymphocytic, and leukocytic mediators. Although phagocytic properties are known, their quantity and bactericidal power are less than those of neutrophils. Eosinophils play a major modulatory role in immediate and delayed inflammatory reactions.

A number of studies demonstrate a strong link between the eosinophil and the lymphoid immune system. In certain parasitic infections (e.g., trichinosis and schistosomiasis), the development of eosinophilia has been shown to be absolutely dependent on the presence of a functional T cell immune system. Close association between eosinophils and macrophages observed

Table 16-2

Commonly Occurring Causes of Eosinophilia*

Disorder	Tissue	Blood
Respiratory Tract		
Loeffler's syndrome	+++	+++
Eosinophilic pneumonia	+++	++
Allergic asthma	++	++
Intrinsic asthma	++	++
Tropical eosinophilia	+++	+++
Bronchopulmonary aspergillosis	++	++
Allergic rhinitis	++	+
Chronic sinusitis/polyposis	++	++
Gastrointestinal Tract		
Eosinophilic gastroenteritis	+++	++
Skin		
Atopic dermatitis	++	++
Urticaria	++	++
Exfoliative dermatitis		
Scabies	+	+
Toxic epidermal necrolysis	++	+
Erythema neonatorum	+	+
Dermatitis herpetiformis	++	++
Pemphigus	+	+
Impetigo	+	+
Urinary Tract		
Interstitial nephritis	++	++
Interstitial cystitis	++	+
Granulomatous prostatitis	++	0
Adrenal		
Addison's disease	0	++
Liver		
Cholestatic hepatotoxicity (drug-induced)	+++	++
Lymphoproliferative		
Hodgkin's disease	++	++
Mycosis fungoides	+	+
Angioblastic lymphoid hyperplasia	++	++
Eosinophilic granuloma	+++	0

* (+++, ++, +) indicate degrees of eosinophilia.

Table 16-2

Continued

Disorder	Tissue	Blood
Eye		
Allergic conjunctivitis	+ +	+
Vernal conjunctivitis	+ +	+
Rheumatic		
Eosinophilic fasciitis	+ + +	+ + +
Hypersensitivity angiitis	+ + +	+ + +
Allergic granulomatosis	+ +	+ +
Serous myopericarditis	+ + +	+ + +
Immunodeficiency		
Wiscott-Aldrich syndrome	+ +	+ +
Buckley syndrome	+	+ +
IgA deficiency with allergy	+ +	+ +
Neoplasia		
Tumors with inflammation	+ +	+
Carcinoma of the lung	+ +	+
Carcinoma of the ovary	+ +	+ +
Carcinoma of the stomach	+ +	+
Hematologic Disorders		
Eosinophilic leukemia	+ + +	+ + +
Hypereosinophilic syndrome	+ + +	+ + +
Cyclic neutropenia	0	+ +
Drugs		
Mast cell degranulators	+	+
Aspirin intolerance	+ + +	+ + +
Infection		
Bacterial—Scarlet fever	0	+
Parasitic—Helminths;	+ + +	+ + +
Pneumocystis carinii	+ +	+ +

From Stewart SR, Gershwin ME: Allergic disease and the evaluation of immediate hypersensitivity reactions, in Halstedt JA and Halstedt CH (eds): The Laboratory in Clinical Medicine. Interpretation and Applications. Philadelphia, PA, W.B. Saunders, 1981, pp 612–633. Used with permission.

morphologically has led to speculation that the eosinophil may play a role in the afferent limb of the immune response by helping to process certain kinds of antigens or even to generate some types of antibodies.

CLINICAL ASSESSMENT

Eosinophils normally complete their cycles in the loose, submucous connective tissue of the respiratory, gastrointestinal, genital tracts, and skin; thus, the presence of small numbers of these cells in histologic sections of nasal, bronchial, stomach, appendiceal, prostatic, and uterine tissue can be a normal finding. The presence of a few eosinophils in nasal secretions, sputum, stool, urine, and urethral discharge may represent a wash-out phenomenon. Furthermore, since the spleen may serve as a reservoir for eosinophils, the finding of small collections of these cells among other cellular elements should be considered normal.

With proper attention to materials and techniques, the total eosinophil count can be a reliable indication of absolute numbers of cells. Normal cyclic fluctuations, however, can result in hourly inconsistencies. Consistent eosinophil elevations, regardless of the time of day the blood is sampled, give added significance to the finding. Coincident factors of stress, infection, drug intake, and hormonal and menstrual influences can also account for day-to-day variations. The monitoring of peripheral blood eosinophil counts, although frequently more feasible, is usually less profitable than direct examination of tissue biopsies and secretions, as progression or resolution of local eosinophilic lesions can occur without corresponding reflection on cell numbers in the peripheral blood. Identification of eosinophil leukocytes within nasal and brochial mucosa and corresponding eosinophilia of the nasal secretion and sputum are commonplace findings in atopic populations. There is no arbitrary figure, however, that can give significance to eosinophil percentages in secretions, exudates, blister contents, or body fluids. Atopic diseases, however, IgE-mediated disorders and related allergic processes are associated with eosinophil differential determinations of 25–100 percent at the involved serous surfaces or within fluid secretions.

Circulating blood eosinophils normally localize temporarily in respiratory tract tissue awaiting extrusion, although the exact mechanism whereby the lung serves as a filtering bed is not clear. It is conceivable that accumulations of trafficking eosinophils may account for transient circumscribed shadows on chest x-ray films in situations in which such findings are associated with high peripheral blood eosinophilia in the absence of other primary pulmonary disorders. In contrast, and by definition, Loeffler's syndrome is an asymptomatic or minimally symptomatic self limited condition with peripheral blood eosinophilia and transient migratory pulmonary infiltrates visualized radiographically. The infiltrates, which may be unilateral or bilateral, have a patchy distribution, but are predominantly found at the pleural surfaces and most often in the upper lung fields. Typically, Loeffler's syndrome resolves within four weeks and is generally agreed to represent an allergic response to a variety of agents. When pulmonary eosinophilic infiltrates reflected by radiographic shadows persist for periods of longer than three to four weeks and are accompanied by definite symptoms, such variants of eosinophilic pneumonia likely have initiating factors that differ from those of the benign Loeffler's syndrome. Localized parasitic, fungal or bacterial infections, hypersensitivity pneumonitides and drug allergy comprise a heterogenous group that may account for prolonged pulmonary eosinophilic syndromes. Histopathologic findings of varied mixtures of multiple cell types and different pathologic types of involvement, including granulomas and angiitis, suggest that immunopathologic and eosinotactic effector mechanisms are involved. Tropical eosinophilia is one condition of this nature in which diffuse miliary mottlings with consolidation visualized on chest x-ray films accompany both bronchial and constitutional symptoms. The finding of microfilaria within pulmonary nodules suggest the host's ability to sequester and contain parasites within the lung parenchyma, possibly as a result of the extremely vigorous antibody responses generated, especially IgE.

Although the IgE-related immunopathogenesis of allergic asthma certainly provides potential mechanisms for generating eosinophilia, it is seldom accompanied by evidence of radiographic pulmonary infiltrates in the absence of complicating factors. There are two noteworthy exceptions to the absence of parenchymal eosinophilic collections in asthma: bronchopulmonary aspergillosis in which fungal allergens greater than 4μ in size gain access to the peripheral airways; and situations that allow for the escape of inhaled allergens out of the bronchi, for example, into bronchiectactic cavities.

Mechanisms of eosinophilia in nonatopic asthma, rhinitis, and sinusitis are incompletely understood. The small degrees of eosinophilia found in the nasal secretions of vasomotor rhinitis could reflect nonspecific effects of physical, hormonal, or endocrine factors on a mast cell rich nasal mucous membrane. However, the degree of eosinophilia in tissue, secretion and peripheral blood in hyperplastic sinusitis, nasal polyps, and in asthma not associated with other evidence of allergy (i.e., aspirin intolerance triad) may exceed those of allergic disorders. The cause of this observation is unknown.

INFLUENCE OF DRUGS

Pharmacologic influences can affect eosinophil development and regulation at different levels of the cells' life cycle. As a result, eosinophilia or eosinopenia occurs during administration of certain drugs. Normal and elevated levels of circulating eosinophils and neutrophils may fall rapidly when leukocyte precursors in the bone marrow are inhibited by cytotoxic and immunosuppressive agents. However, selective changes limited to the eosinophil may be seen in the temporary eosinopenia induced by β-adrenergic agonists, such as isoproterenol and epinephrine. Conversely, a β-adrenergic blocking agent such as propranolol reverses the eosinopenic effect of epinephrine and may actually raise the number of circulating eosinophils.

Depending on dose, route, and duration of administration, certain drugs may elicit variable degrees of local tissue eosinophilic infiltration and/or circulating blood eosinophilia as a function of their chemical actions in effecting mast cell degranulation, apart from any postulated immunologic relationships. Included in this category are codeine, morphine, dextran, polymyxin, protamine, stilbamidine, viomycin, and D-tubocurarine. Like isoproterenol and epinephrine, drugs of the theophylline series should also favor reductions in eosinophil numbers by enhancing intracellular levels of cyclic AMP and inhibiting discharge of mast cell inflammatory mediators.

The finding of eosinophilia among other manifestations of adverse effects of drugs is extremely variable. When present, eosinophilia should only serve as a lead in considering diagnostic possibilities among hypersensitivity versus nonimmunologic causes. Eosinophilia with drug reactions is likely to occur in those syndromes involving skin (e.g., exfoliative dermatitis, urticaria, erythema nodosum, erythema multiforme), the respiratory tract (eosinophilic pneumonitis) or connective tissues of the vasculature (angiitis). Also, the eosinophilias accompanying drug reactions associated with IgE responses are of greater prominence than those occurring with IgG antibody-mediated serum sickness reactions.

Discontinuation of a drug upon appearance of an adverse allergic drug reaction would appear appropriate. Considerable judgement is often required, however, when asymptomatic eosinophilia is discovered in a patient receiving a therapeutic agent. Drugs that are most frequently associated with the development of eosinophilia include ampicillin, penicillin, streptomycin, paraminosalicyclic acid, diphenylhydantoin, arsenicals, gold, phenothiazines, sulfonamides, and nitrofurantoin. They are also the agents most frequently incriminated in severe allergic reactions associated with eosinophilia. Persistently high or progressively rising eosinophil cell counts should, therefore, give reason for caution when dealing with these drugs. Generally, the drug should be discontinued, since eosinophilia in this setting implies presumptive evidence for appearance of sensitizing IgE antibodies.

The mechanism of eosinophilia associated with the acetylsalicylic acid (aspirin)-intolerant patient is unknown. The nature of clinical manifestations of the asthma-nasal polyposis-hyperplastic sinusitis syndrome with which intense eosinophilia is occasionally associated has suggested to some that its development may be on the basis of β-adrenergic blockade. The finding that aspirin induced asthma is related to the inhibition of prostaglandin synthesis may be important in the suggested role of eosinophil prostaglandins in mast cell modulation.

ACKNOWLEDGEMENTS

The authors appreciate the contributions granted by Walter G. Peter, III, Director, Publications Department, American Society for Microbiology on behalf of/and of Lawrence M. Lichtenstein, M.D., Ph.D., Philip S. Norman, M.D., N. Franklin Adkinson, Jr., M.D., and Reuben P. Siraganian, M.D., Ph.D. for their respective chapters in the "Manual of Clinical Immunology", pp. 775–821, 1980). They also thank Francisque Leynadier, M.D., Hopital Rothschild, Paris, France and Irene B. Haydik, M.D., Clinical Director, Allergy Division, NMS Pharmaceuticals Inc., Newport Beach, California for their important and original work. The secretarial assistance of Nikki Rojo was excellent.

REFERENCES

Avrameas S: Heterogeneous enzyme immunoassays, in A Voller, et al (eds): Immunoassays for the '80's. Lancaster, England, M.T.P. Press, Ltd, 1981

Benveniste J: The human basophil degranulation test as an *in vitro* method for the diagnosis of allergies. Clin Allergy 11:1, 1981

Bruce CA, et al: Diagnostic tests in ragweed allergic asthma. J Allergy Clin Immunol 53:230, 1974

Bryant DA, Burns MW, Lazarus L: The correlation between skin tests, bronchial provocation tests and the serum level of IgE specific for common allergens in patients with asthma. Clin Allergy 5:145, 1975

Coca AF: Studies in specific hypersensitiveness. V. The preparation of fluid extracts and solutions for use in the diagnosis and treatment of the allergies with notes on the collection of pollens. J Immunol 7:163, 1922

Conroy MC, Orange RP, Lichtenstein LM: Release of the slow reacting substance of anaphylaxis (SRS-A) from human leukocytes by the calcium ionophore A23187. J Immunol 116:1677, 1976

Coombs RRA, Gell PGH: Classification of Allergic Reactions, in PGH Gell, RRA Coombs (eds): Clinical Aspects of Immunology, 2nd ed., Oxford, England Blackwell Scientific Publications, 1968

Douglas WW: Histamine and antihistamines; 5-hydroxytryptamine and antagonists, in: LS Goodman, A Gilman (eds): The Pharmacological Basis of Therapeutics, 5th ed, New York, Macmillan, 1975

Dry J, Leynadier F, Luce H: Human basophil degranulation in dermatophagoides allergies. Ann Allergy 44:308, 1980

Friesen GL, Jones RM: Standardized and partially purified allergenic extracts: concept and clinical evaluation of potency. Immunol Allergy Practice 6:163, 1984

Gleich GJ, Yunginger JW, Stobo JD: Laboratory methods for studies of allergy. Principles and interpretation, in: E Middleton Jr, CE Reed, EE Ellis (eds): Allergy: Principles and Practice. St. Louis, C.V. Mosby, 2nd edition, 1983

Goetzl EJ, Austen KF: Purification and synthesis of eosinophilotactic tetrapeptides of human lung tissue: identification as eosinophil chemotactic factor of anaphylaxis. Proc Natl Acad Sci (USA) 72:4123, 1975

Golbert TM: A review of controversial diagnostic and therapeutic techniques employed in allergy. J Allergy Clin Immunol 56:170, 1975

Greaves MW, Yamamoto S, Fairley VM: New in-vitro test for IgE-mediated hypersensitivity in man. Br Med J 2:623, 1972

Halpern GM: Serological markers of human allergic disease. I. Immunoglobulin E Immunol Allergy Pract 6:197, 1984

Ishizaka K: Biology of Immunoglobulin E, in: P Kallos, BH Waksman, A de Weck (eds): Progress in Allergy, Vol. 19, Basel, Switzerland, S Karger, AG, 1975, p. 60

Knauer KA, Adkinson Jr NF: Clinical significance of IgE, In: E. Middleton, Jr., C.E. Reed, E.E. Ellis (eds): Allergy: Principles and practice. St Louis, CV Mosby, 2nd edition, 1983

Lichtenstein LM, Margolis S: Histamine release in vitro: inhibition by catecholamines and methylxanthines. Science 161:902, 1968

Lichtenstein LM, Norman PS, Winkenwerder WL, et al: In vitro studies of human ragweed allergy: changes in cellular and humoral activity associated with specific desensitization. J Clin Invest 45:1126, 1966

Lichtenstein LM, Ishizaka K, Norman PS, et al: IgE antibody measurements in ragweed hay fever: relationship to clinical severity and the results of immunotherapy. J Clin Invest 52:472, 1973

Lichtenstein LM, Osler AG: Studies on the mechanisms of hypersensitivity phenomena. IX. Histamine release from human leukocytes by ragweed pollen antigen. J Exp Med 120:507, 1964

May CD, Lyman M, Alberto R, et al: Procedures for immunochemical studies of histamine release from leukocytes with small volume of blood. J Allergy 46:12, 1970

Mayer M: The complement system. Sci Am 229:54, 1973

Norman PS: In vivo methods of study of allergy: skin and mucosal tests, techniques, and interpretation, in: E Middleton, Jr, CE Reed, EE Ellis (eds): Allergy: Principles and Practice. St. Louis, CV Mosby, 2nd edition, 1983

Parish WE: Detection of reaginic and short-term sensitizing anaphylactic or anaphylactoid antibodies to milk in sera of allergic and normal persons. Clin Allergy 1:369, 1971

Patterson R, et al: Immunotherapy, in: E Middleton, Jr, CE Reed, EE Ellis (eds): Allergy: Principles and Practice. St. Louis, C.V. Mosby, 2nd edition, 1983

Samter M, Beers RF, Jr: Intolerance to aspirin: clinical studies and consideration of its pathogenesis. Ann Intern Med 68:975, 1968

Solley GO, Gleich GF, Gordon RE, et al: The late phase of the immediate wheal and flare skin reaction. J Clin Invest 58:408, 1976

Siraganian RP, Hook WA: Complement-induced histamine release from human basophils. II. Mechanism of the histamine release from human basophils. II. Mechanism of the histamine release reaction. J Immunol 116:639, 1976

Stewart SR, Gershwin ME: Allergic diseases and the evaluation of immediate hypersensitivity reactions, in Halstedt JA and Halstedt CH (eds): The Laboratory in Clinical Medicine. Interpretation and Applications. Philadelphia, PA, W.B. Saunders, 1981, pp 612–633.

Tsay YG, Halpern GM: IgE fluoroallergosorbent (IgE FAST™) test: concept and clinical applications. Immunol Allergy Practice 6:169, 1984

Wasserman SI, Goetzl EJ, Austen KF: Inactivation of slow-reacting substance of anaphylaxis by human eosinophil arylsulfatase. J Immunol 114:645, 1975

Yunginger JW, Gleich GJ: Seasonal changes in IgE-antibodies and their relationship to IgG-antibodies during immunotherapy for ragweed hay fever. J Clin Invest 52:1268, 1973

Yunginger JW, Jones RT, Gleich GJ: Studies on Alternaria allergens. II. Measurement of the relative potency of commercial Alternaria extracts by the direct RAST and by RAST inhibiton. J Allergy Clin Immunol 58:408, 1976

Roger W. Fox
Richard F. Lockey

17

Role of Immunotherapy in Asthma

Immunotherapy is used to treat allergic respiratory disorders, in particular, allergic rhinitis (hayfever) and allergic asthma. Over forty clinical immunotherapy studies, 18 in asthma, have been done. Fifteen of these 18 studies of allergic asthma have demonstrated some measure of benefit from immunotherapy, and three have not. The role of immunotherapy in the management of asthma, however, remains controversial, because it is extremely difficult to determine efficacy of a nonbronchodilator treatment modality, such as immunotherapy.

Much of our knowledge about immunotherapy is derived from the allergic rhinitis studies. Mast cells and basophils in nasal and bronchial secretions and mucosal surfaces of allergic subjects appear to respond similarly to inhalant allergens. The benefits observed to occur from the immunologic changes in allergic rhinitis subjects on immunotherapy, therefore, should theoretically also benefit subjects with allergic asthma.

HISTORY

The recognition that allergic disease can be treated immunologically was noted as early as 1903 when Dunbar of Hamburg, Germany, attempted to passively immunize grass-sensitive hayfever subjects by applying animal-(horse and geese) derived grass pollen antisera to the subjects' nasal mucosa. Several years later, Leonard Noon suggested that active immunization with

BRONCHIAL ASTHMA, Second Edition
ISBN 0-8089-1814-1

grass pollen vaccine should be attempted in allergic subjects. He had been working in Almroth Wright's laboratory where the successful prophylactic immunization against typhoid fever had been discovered, and his idea was a natural follow-up to this work. With the assistance of his botanist sister, Dorothy Noon, who devised methods for collecting grass pollens, he began an active immunization program for grass sensitive allergic rhinitis subjects. Soon after Noon's work appeared, John Freeman published data suggesting decreased symptomatology in subjects with allergic rhinitis treated with grass extract injections. Cooke, in 1915, formally introduced immunotherapy into the United States by reporting the treatment by pollen immunization of 114 subjects with hayfever and asthma. This procedure, first referred to as desensitization, was modified in many ways over the next half century and became an accepted method of treating allergic diseases.

In modern terminology, "desensitization" is more appropriately used when referring to the rapid, temporary depletion of IgE and/or chemical mediators of anaphylaxis by repeated sublethal doses of antigen, such as penicillin. The terms immunotherapy and hyposensitization are currently used most commonly. Immunotherapy is the preferred term used by most authors and found in most modern textbooks and articles, since it implies immunologic manipulation of the allergic responses to an allergen resulting in a therapeutic effect. Hyposensitization refers to the decreased sensitivity to allergens with observed clinical improvement and demonstration of alterations in various immunologic and allergic parameters from the administration of allergenic extracts.

CLINICAL TRIALS

Clinical trials to study a nonbronchodilator treatment modality, such as immunotherapy, are difficult to perform for many reasons, some of which include the following: first, asthma has a variable course; second, numerous factors in addition to IgE-mediated reactions contribute to the clinical manifestations; third, single allergen sensitivity is uncommon; fourth, it is difficult to match asthmatic subjects with similar demographics, comparable severity and similar allergen sensitivity; fifth, spirometry and/or peak flow determinations may not be adequate to measure the response to immunotherapy.

Over 40 controlled clinical trials have been done with a variety of allergens in subjects with seasonal allergic rhinitis and/or asthma. The best studies that demonstrate efficacy in allergic rhinitis have used a species of ragweed or antigen E, various grasses, mountain cedar, or birch pollen extracts, and those demonstrating benefit in asthma have used a species of ragweed, various grasses, *Alternaria,* house dust, house dust mite, cat pelt, and cat allergen 1 extracts. Mixtures of pollens and molds to treat allergic respiratory disorders have also been used in some clinical trials. Collective analysis of these studies is difficult due to the variation in study design and methods, although the majority demonstrated between 60 and 90 percent partial or complete improvement after immunotherapy. In many studies, daily symptom scores and the physicians' clinical assessments were used to determine efficacy with or without regard to the amount of allergen extract administered. In other studies, immunologic parameters such as blocking antibody (IgG), specific IgE, basophil histamine release, and lymphocyte blast transformation were measured before and after treatment. Changes in bronchial sensitivity have also been assessed by allergen bronchoprovocation testing. Several investigations have adequately studied the effect of immunotherapy on both the early phase and late phase pulmonary response to allergen challenge. The late phase asthmatic response is very important, since it seems to more closely reflect the clinical disease of asthma.

Essential features of a controlled study of immunotherapy should include: (1) selection of appropriate allergic subjects, (2) random assignment of subjects to treatment and placebo groups, (3) high dose immunotherapy with a standardized extract or extracts, (4) double-blind assessment, (5) incorporation of a sensitive index to measure response, e.g. symptom scores, concomitant medications used, peak flow determinations, spirometric studies, response to bronchoprovocation challenge (both early and late responses) and/or changes in immunologic parameters [specific IgE, basophil histamine release, blocking antibody (IgG and IgA), T-suppressor cell function and lymphocyte blast transformation to allergen], and (6) statistical analysis of data.

Although 18 of the immunotherapy studies in allergic asthma contain some of the above features, very few contain all of them, a difficult feat (Table 17-1). Fifteen of these studies reported beneficial results, three did not. The improvement, for the most part, was directly related to the total dose of extract administered and the duration of therapy, (i.e. the higher the cumulative dose, the better the response).

With few exceptions, interpretation of the data is difficult, because the clinical criteria for including study subjects have not been well defined, and most studies used nonstandardized extracts. Even when objective measurements are done to determine response, such as tolerance to allergen bronchoprovocation, it is difficult to measure or correlate these findings with a clinical response.

The first double-blind controlled study was done by Bruun, who treated 100 adult chronic asthmatic subjects with dust extract. The criteria for dust sensitivity was not defined except on clinical terms. Perennial immunotherapy was used, although the amount of extract received by each subject was not reported. After 2 years of treatment, 74 of 95 improved whereas 28 of 82 improved on placebo.

Frankland and Augustin did the first double-blind controlled study with

Table 17-1
Clinical Studies of Immunotherapy in the Treatment of Asthma

Author Date	Age	Allergen	Duration	Treated Subjects	Control Subjects	Evaluation	Significant Difference
Brunn, 1949	Adults	Dust	2 yr, perennial	95	82	Symptoms	Yes (vs placebo)
Frankland, Augustin, 1954	Adults and chldren	Grass (timothy, cocksfoot)	1 yr, preseasonal	31	26	Symptoms	Yes (vs placebo)
Johnstone, 1957	Children	Ragweed	1 yr, perennial	22	13	Symptoms	Yes (high vs low dose and placebo
Citron, et al., 1958	Adults	Grass (timothy, cocksfoot)	1 yr, preseasonal	13	5	Symptoms, broncho-provocation	Yes (vs placebo)
Johnstone, Crump, 1961	Children	Multiple	4 yr, perennial	131	42	Symptoms	Yes (high vs low dose and placebo)
McAllen, 1967	Adults	Grass mix (mineral oil emulsion)	4 yr, preseasonal (1 to 3 inj)	31	—	Symptoms, broncho-provocation	Yes (before vs after)
Johnstone, Dutton, 1968	Children (under age 16)	Multiple	14 yr, perennial	130	210	Symptoms	Yes (high vs low dose and placebo)
Forgacs, Swan, 1968	Over 7 yr of age	Dust, low dose	1 yr (15 inj)	33	37	Symptoms, peak flow	No (vs placebo)

Study	Population	Allergen	Duration			Measure	Result
Aas, 1971	Children	House dust	2.5 to 3 yr, perennial	52	28	Symptoms, broncho-provocation	Yes (vs placebo)
Smith, 1971	11 to 48 yr	Mite	16 wk	11	11	Symptoms	Yes (vs placebo)
Tuchinda, Chai, 1973	Children	Multiple	5 to 12 mo	10	5	Broncho-provocation	Yes (high vs low dose)
Bruce, et al., 1977	Adults	Ragweed (low dose)	1 yr, perennial	13	17	Symptoms, broncho-provocation	No (vs placebo)
Warner, et al., 1978	Children	Mite	1 to 2 yr, perennial	27	24	Symptoms, broncho-provocation	Yes (late phase reaction)
Taylor, et al., 1978	Adults	Cat Pelt	1 yr	5	5	Broncho-provocation	Yes (vs placebo)
Davis, et al., 1979	Adults	Mite	4 mo and cross over to placebo; 18 mo, perennial	19	10	Symptoms	No (high and low dose vs placebo)
Metzger, et al., 1983	Adults	Alternaria	1 yr, perennial	10	6	Broncho-provocation	Yes (late phase)
Ortolani, et al., 1984	15 to 45 yr	Grass mixture	1 yr, perennial	8	7	Symptoms	Yes (vs placebo)
Ohman, et al., 1984	Adults	Cat allergen 1	4 mo	9	8	Symptoms, broncho-provocation, cat exposure	Yes (vs placebo)

timothy and cocksfoot grass extract. A total of 20,000 Noon units (equivalent to 1.0 ml of a 1:50 w/v pollen extract) were administered. Fifty-seven asthmatic subjects, with or without rhinitis, were included in the 200 studied, and the remainder had only allergic rhinitis. Ninety-four percent of the subjects treated with commercial extracts or extracts made by the investigators attained moderate or more improvement as measured by clinical assessment. This compared to 30 percent of those who received placebo. Johnstone reported similar results with ragweed extract administered to four groups of allergic asthmatics. The best results were associated with the high dose therapy compared to low dose therapy or placebo.

Citron, et al., in another study, measured bronchial sensitivity to timothy and cocksfoot grass pollen extracts by inhalational testing before and after immunotherapy with these extracts and compared responses to untreated controls. Reduction of bronchial sensitivity to antigen challenge, as measured by the mean fall in FEV_1 in 12 of 13 treated subjects, correlated with improvement of symptoms of asthma in all 13 during the subsequent pollen season.

Johnstone and Crump studied asthmatic children with different degrees of sensitivity to various inhalant allergens including pollens, danders, molds, house dust, and bacterial vaccines (bacterial vaccines are ineffective and no longer used) and randomly assigned them to high dose or low dose immunotherapy or to placebo. Once maintenance was achieved, injections were given monthly for 4 years. High dose therapy was more effective than low dose or placebo therapy as measured by the number of asthma attacks and days of wheezing.

McAllen, et al., in a controlled study, demonstrated an incremental increase in bronchoprovocation challenge tolerance and improved symptom scores before and after the grass pollen season for 4 subsequent years in subjects treated preseasonally each of those years with a mixture of 12 grass pollens in a mineral oil emulsion (mineral oil containing extracts are no longer used because of the high incidence of local complications such as sterile abscesses). There was general correlation between challenge tolerance and symptomatic improvement during the grass seasons. Johnstone and Dutton, over 14 years, studied high and low dose immunotherapy with a variety of allergens compared to placebo in children up to age 16 years. They reported significant improvement in the treatment group versus placebo, but also indicated that high dose immunotherapy was more effective than low dose therapy.

In 1971, Aas studied house dust sensitive asthmatic children who had positive bronchoprovocation with house dust extracts. These subjects were exclusively house dust sensitive with or without rhinitis and were prick skin test positive at 1:10,000 w/v. Bronchial reactivity to house dust was less in the two groups treated with house dust extracts than in the placebo group. Smith found a significant difference in symptom scores and medication usage between asthmatic subjects treated for 16 weeks on immunotherapy with house dust mite (*Dermatophagoides pteronyssinus*) versus placebo.

Tuchinda and Chai, using various allergens, in a 5 to 12 month double-blind study of 15 childhood asthmatics, found that the high dose treatment group had less bronchial sensitivity by inhalational challenge than did the low dose treatment group. There were no differences in clinical symptoms between the two groups despite decreased bronchoprovocation sensitivity.

Warner, et al., studied children ages 5 through 14 years who were sensitive to *D. pteronyssinus* by skin tests and bronchial challenge tests. In this 1 to 2 year study of perennial immunotherapy with dust mite or placebo, improvement as measured by symptom scores and pulmonary function tests, occurred in both groups, but drug scores were less only in the actively treated group. The most interesting finding was the reduced or absence of the previously observed delayed or late phase bronchial response in 10 of 22 treated subjects. A reduced late asthmatic response was observed in 1 of 24 placebo treated subjects. Only 4 of 27 treated subjects had a reduced immediate response to dust mite allergen.

Metzger, et al., studied 10 seasonal allergic asthmatics before and after high dose, *Alternaria*, perennial immunotherapy. These subjects had positive methacholine and *Alternaria* bronchoprovocation tests. Eight of nine showed a reduction in the late asthmatic response, averaging 60.8 percent less following immunotherapy. The late asthmatic response was totally ablated in one subject and nearly so in another. Before therapy, five subjects had a late asthmatic response that required several days to subside. After immunotherapy, all late asthmatic responses had resolved by the morning after challenge. Three subjects required a 1.2 – 33-fold increase in allergen dose to produce an early asthmatic response. Methacholine PD_{20} was increased from 28 to 158 breath units (p value < 0.04) in the treated group compared to six untreated *Alternaria* sensitive asthmatics who retained their dual asthmatic responses to *Alternaria* and in whom methacholine sensitivity was unchanged. The authors concluded that immunotherapy may preferentially reduce the severity of the late asthmatic response over that of the early asthmatic response and may concurrently reduce bronchial airway hyperresponsiveness.

Ortolani, et al., in a year long double-blind controlled study of immunotherapy with a mixed grass pollen extract of equal parts timothy, sweet vernal, and velvet grasses, concluded that grass pollen-induced asthma was reduced symptomatically (Fig. 17-1) and was associated with a rise in timothy-specific IgG, the only grass specific IgG measured. No significant differences in the early asthmatic response were noted in bronchoprovocation sensitivity to the grass extract mixture or in the amount of timothy-specific IgE, the only one measured, in serum or nasal secretions.

A model to study immunotherapy is domestic cat-induced asthma, because the causative agent can be easily identified by history, and the

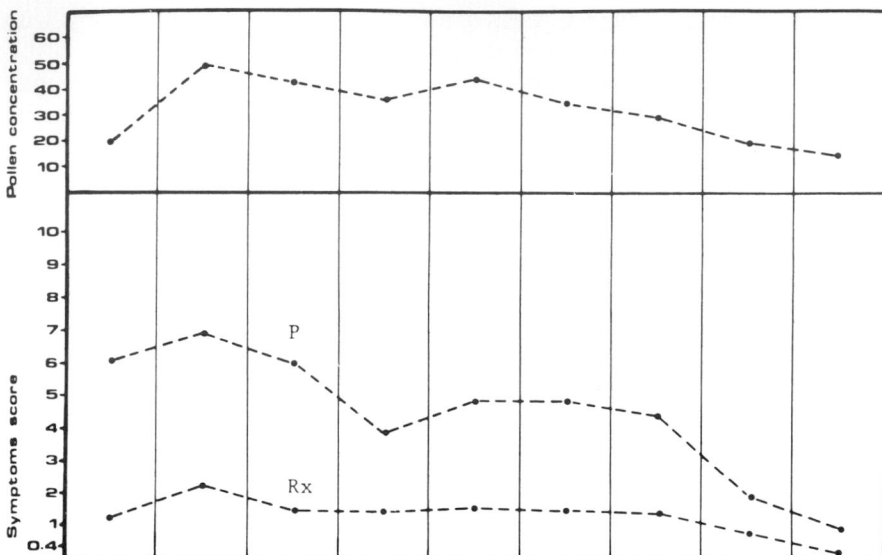

Fig. 17-1. Comparison of weekly average pollen count (ordinate, upper section) versus weekly average symptom scores (lower section) in placebo (P) and actively treated (Rx) subjects during the May to June grass pollen season (weeks marked on abscissa). For both the actively treated group and the group treated with placebo, there was a correlation between pollen exposure and symptoms ($r = 0.71$, $p < 0.05$ and $r = 0.88$, $p < 0.05$, respectively). (From Ortolani C, Pastorello E, Moss R, et al: Grass pollen immunotherapy: a single year double-blind, placebo-controlled study in patients with grass pollen-induced asthma and rhinitis. J Allergy Clin Immunol 73:286, 1984. Used with permission.)

clinical symptoms of bronchial asthma can be reproduced by intentional exposure to cats. Twenty to 30 percent of asthmatic subjects have documented sensitivity to cat allergens as reported in studies from different parts of the world. Immunotherapy studies by Taylor, et al., demonstrated decreased bronchial sensitivity in subjects treated with cat pelt extract as compared to placebo-treated controls. The isolation and purification of cat allergen 1 permitted the administration of a standardized allergen to cat-sensitive asthmatics in another study. Nine subjects were treated with cat allergen 1 and 8 with placebo in this second double-blind study. The cat 1 allergen-treated subjects had diminished skin tests (Fig. 17-2) as compared to placebo-treated subjects, increased tolerance to bronchoprovocation (Fig. 17-3) and decreased symptoms following cat exposure. IgG to both cat allergen 1 (Fig. 17-4) and cat albumin increased significantly in the treated group. There was no significant change in basophil sensitivity to cat allergen 1 and no demonstrable change in methacholine challenge sensitivity. The 4 months of immunotherapy with cat allergen 1 resulted in a significant reduction of

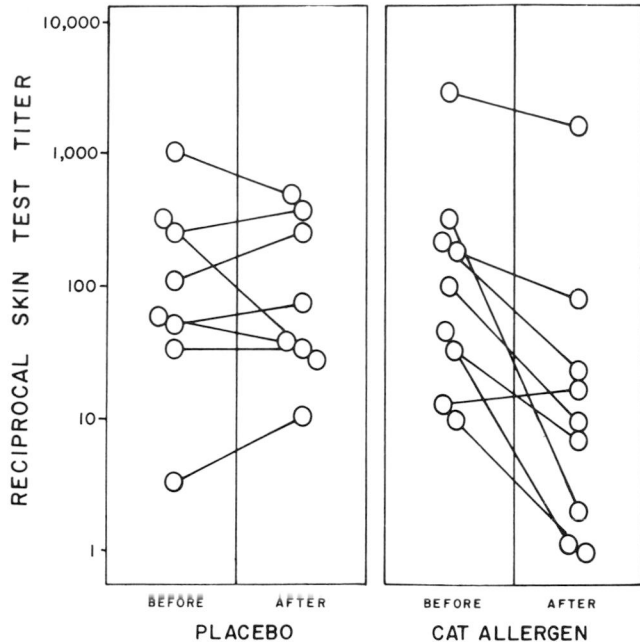

Fig. 17-2. Skin test responses. The geometric mean of reciprocal prick test titer changed from 82 to 76 in the placebo-treatment group (NS) and from 94 to 9.8 in the active treatment group (p < 0.01). A comparison of change from baseline between the placebo- and active-treatment groups revealed a highly significant difference (< 0.01). (From Ohman JL, Findlay SR, Leiterman KM, et al: Immunotherapy in cat-induced asthma. Double-blind trial with evaluation of in vivo and in vitro response. J Allergy Clin Immunol 74:234, 1984. Used with permission.)

cutaneous and bronchial sensitivity to cat allergen 1 as well as a decrease and delay in onset of asthmatic and ocular symptoms upon exposure to an environment in which cats had been housed (Fig. 17-5).

Three negative studies of immunotherapy in asthma have been completed. The first, done in 1968 by the Committee of the British Tuberculosis Association, was a study in which mild perennial asthmatic subjects with positive skin tests to dust extract were treated either with house dust extract or placebo by 14 physicians in their offices. The treatment groups were given house dust extract in a series of weekly injections. Efficacy was based upon the treated subject's daily assessment of symptoms, medications used and respiratory flow rates determined monthly by the investigators. There were no statistical differences in measured parameters between the treated and placebo groups. A major flaw in this study is that low dose dust immunotherapy was used. Bruce, et al., administered either placebo or low dose ragweed extract, a mean dose of 11 micrograms in a double-blind controlled study of

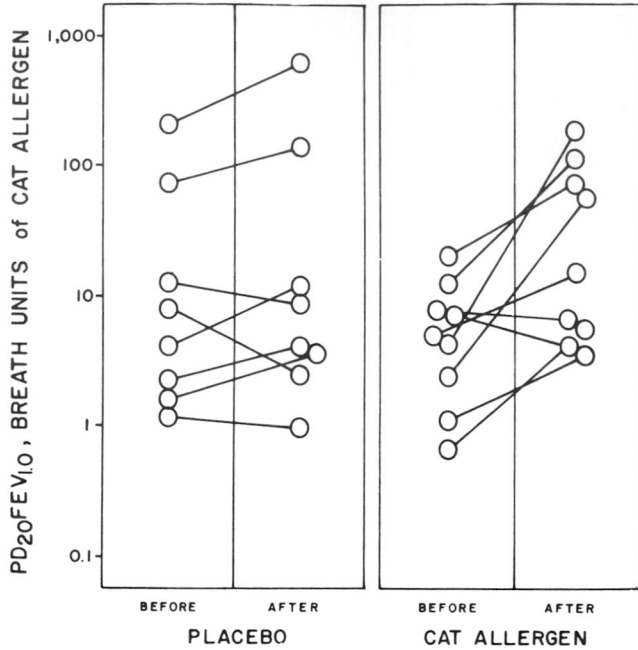

Fig. 17-3. Bronchial provocation with cat allergen. The geometric mean cumulative provocation dose of cat allergen in BU was defined as one inhalation (containing 0.05cc) of a 1.0 mg/ml solution for methacholine or one inhalation of a 1:100 dilution (0.04 units of cat allergen 1 per ml) from cat allergen. BU that resulted in a 20% drop in the $FEV_{1.0}$ ($PD_{20}FEV_{1.0}$ allergen) changed from 8.8 to 12.3 BU in the placebo-treatment group (NS) and from 4.27 to 20.7 BU in the active-treatment group (p < 0.05). A comparison of change from baseline between the placebo- and active-treatment groups revealed no significant difference. (From Ohman JL, Findlay SR, Leiterman KM, et al: Immunotherapy in cat-induced asthma. Double-blind trial with evaluation of in vivo and in vitro response. J Allergy Clin Immunol 74:234, 1984. Used with permission.)

autumnal asthma. There were no differences between placebo and treated groups, although the authors indicated that sensitivity to other allergens, such as *Alternaria* and other molds, may have accounted, in part, for the lack of immunotherapy efficacy. A British Thoracic Society double-blind collaborative study on immunotherapy with high dose mite (*D. pteronyssinus*) extract, 1 ml of 0.3 percent versus placebo, in mite sensitive subjects, demonstrated a slight clinical improvement only in the nonglucocorticosteroid dependent asthmatics and deterioration of symptom scores in some of the glucocorticosteroid dependent asthmatics. The committee of physicians assessing the results felt that only marginal benefits were derived and did not consider allergic immunotherapy warranted.

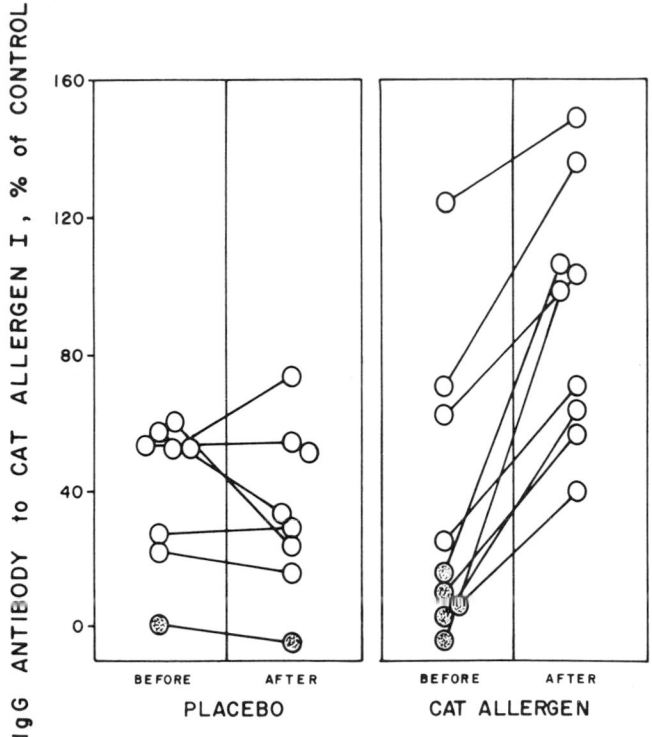

Fig. 17-4. IgG-antibody response to cat allergen 1. Mean IgG-antibody levels to cat allergen 1 changed from 41% to 35% of standard in the placebo-treatment group (NS) and from 35% to 91% in the active-treatment group (p < 0.001). A comparison of change from baseline between the placebo- and active-treatment groups revealed a highly significant difference (p < 0.001). Shaded circles represent values that fall within the 95% confidence interval of repetitive measurements of the normal control serum. (From Ohman JL, Findlay SR, Leiterman KM, et al: Immunotherapy in cat-induced asthma. Double-blind trial with evaluation of in vivo and in vitro response. J Allergy Clin Immunol 74:237, 1984. Used with permission.)

INDICATIONS

A suitable method to decide which subject is a potential candidate for immunotherapy is to separate them into three categories. First, those subjects should be treated with allergic diseases who cannot be sufficiently controlled by environmental changes and/or by therapeutic regimens and in whom the disease has caused significant morbidity. The second group consists of subjects with some, but not all, of the above criteria. A trial of immunotherapy may be justified. The third group are those in whom injection therapy is unwarranted because the disease is not atopic in etiology, not progressive,

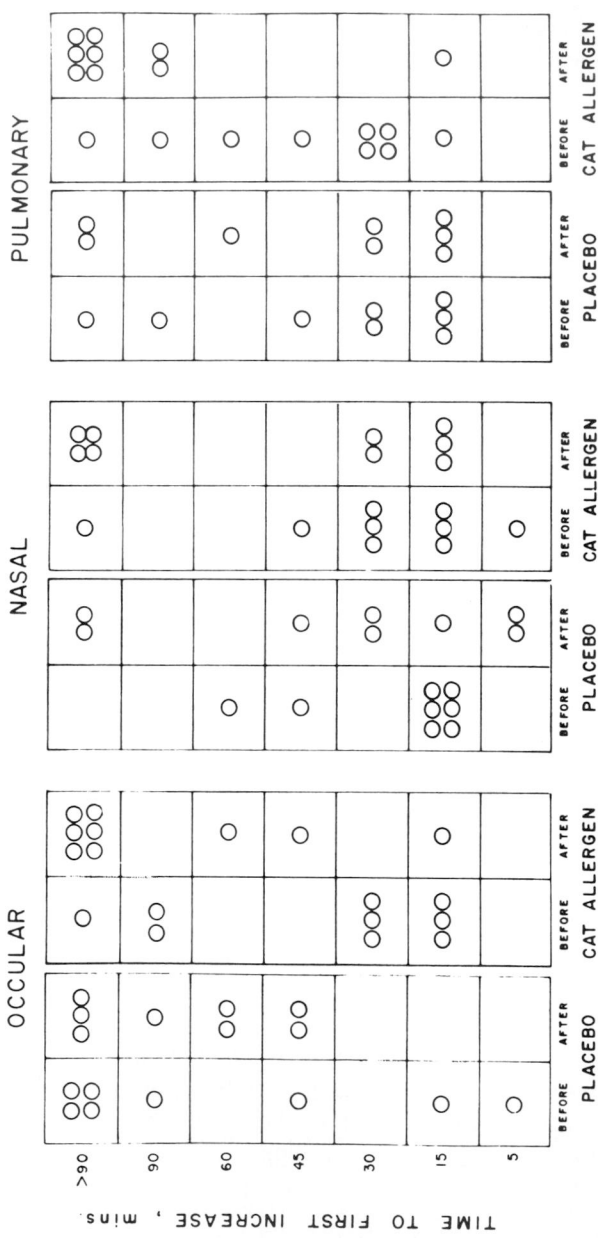

Fig. 17-5. Time to first increase in symptoms on exposure to cats. Subjects were requested to record a symptom score after 15-minute time intervals after entering a room with cats. The time to a first increase in symptoms was recorded for each patient before and after treatment. For ocular symptoms (left panel) there was a significant delay in the appearance of symptoms only with active treatment (p < 0.05). A comparison of change scores from baseline in the placebo- and active-treatment groups revealed no significant difference. There was no significant difference in time to a first increase in nasal symptoms before and after treatment in either the placebo- or active-treatment groups (middle panel). A highly significant delay in pulmonary symptoms occurred only with active treatment (p < 0.05) (right panel). In addition, a comparison of change scores from baseline in the placebo- and active-treatment groups revealed a significant difference (p < 0.05). (From Ohman JL, Findlay SR, Leiterman KM, et al: Immunotherapy in cat-induced asthma. Double-blind trial with evaluation of in vivo and in vitro response. J Allergy Clin Immunol 74:235, 1984. Used with permission.)

has not resulted in morbidity, and/or is easily controlled by environment manipulation or with medications.

In any event, the final decision regarding initiation of immunotherapy should be made by the trained specialist familiar with the complexities of this form of therapy. The treated subject must also be informed of the type of response to expect, time necessary to receive treatment, expense involved and the potential risks, since deaths have occurred (see below).

INHALANT ALLERGEN EXTRACTS USED

Aqueous pollen, dust mite, and mold extracts are primarily used in immunotherapy to treat allergic respiratory diseases. Extracts of animal epithelia are usually used only to treat subjects whose livelihood depends on close association with animals, such as veterinarians. Although a variety of allergenic extracts, including foods and bacterial vaccines, have been used in the past, they have not been proven effective and are no longer used.

Most present day allergen extracts are poorly standardized. Extraneous materials found in some extracts include proteins (such as enzymes), carbohydrates, pigments, mycotoxins, and endotoxins. Various manufacturers employ a variety of methods to produce identically labelled allergen extracts. Source materials used to prepare extracts may vary from manufacturer to manufacturer. Such factors have caused significant lot-to-lot and manufacturer-to-manufacturer variations in biological potency of these extracts. Even though the labels of different extracts may be identical in terms of weight/volume (w/v) (ragweed extract, 1:10 w/v, is prepared by extracting one gram of ragweed pollen in 10 ml of buffer) or protein nitrogen units (PNU) per ml (an inexact method of precipitating nitrogen-containing substances in an extract by using phosphotungstic acid), neither designation indicates true biologic potency of the extract. The Food and Drug Administration (FDA), World Health Organization International Laboratory for Biological Standards, pharmaceutical firms which produce these extracts, and professional organizations such as the American Academy of Allergy and Immunology and the American College of Allergists are currently working to standardize all allergen extracts. Some of these are already available in the United States and on the international markets (see below).

Most allergen extracts in the United States are prepared with aqueous buffers and a bacteriostatic agent such as phenol, 0.4 percent. Other extracts may be marketed in glycerine, 50 percent, with or without phenol. Lypholyzed extracts are freeze-dried powders and must be reconstituted in aqueous solutions prior to use. Glycerinated and lypholyzed extracts are more stable during storage than are aqueous extracts, however, glycerinated extracts may cause pain at injection sites. Allergens are also marketed as alum-precipitated extracts. Some of the alum-precipitated extracts are prepared using a pyridine extraction and others are not. Such extracts are absorbed more slowly, permit an increase in the total quantity of allergen delivered, produce fewer systemic reactions during therapy, and require fewer injections to reach a maintenance dose. In the case of ragweed, the antigenicity of the alum-precipitated extract was substantially altered by pyridine extraction. More data on efficacy of alum-precipitated extracts are necessary.

SELECTION OF ANTIGENS

The selection of antigens included in the extracts is based on the knowledge of aeroallergen surveys, clinical history, appropriately performed and interpreted skin tests, and/or radioallergosorbent test (RAST) results. Allergens that elicit positive skin tests are correlated with the seasonal and/or exposure related symptoms, for example, oak pollen skin reactivity and asthma, which occurs in the spring, or dust mite skin sensitivity and wheezing associated with house cleaning.

Most allergic subjects have a significant allergic history and skin test reactivity to more than one allergen. Many allergens are present in the atmosphere simultaneously. For example, a variety of tree pollens and mold spores are present during the spring as are various weed pollens and mold spores in the fall. Therefore, mixtures of allergens are necessary when symptoms occur during a particular season and both pollen and mold sensitivity exists. In such instances, it is important to limit the contents of the extract to the most relevant and important allergens. A vial containing a single allergen extract is appropriate in some cases when the treated subject is very sensitive to the identified allergen or when only one aeroallergen, such as short ragweed, is considered important.

A second approach is to treat severely allergic subjects who have a spectrum of sensitivities by using mixtures of specific botanical groups (e.g., trees, weeds, and grasses) appropriate for the region. The concentration and the amount of the individual extract constituent can be varied dependent on the relative importance of each.

The clinical efficacy of immunotherapy has been demonstrated with a selected number of allergens derived from certain species of ragweed, grasses, and trees; *Alternaria*; house dust; a species of dust mite; and cat allergen 1 and cat pelt. Immunotherapy with other allergens, such as other molds, grasses, trees, and weeds, is standard practice even though controlled studies have not been done. The assumption and clinical experience are that these other allergen extracts are also beneficial, often in combination with the studied extracts. Efficacy and immunologic studies using mixtures of allergens are lacking.

Methods of Administration

Perennial immunotherapy is the most widely used and accepted form and is associated with the best clinical response. Injections are administered year round to achieve a higher cumulative dose of allergen. High dose immunotherapy has been shown to result in a longer and more significant clinical response and is associated with more pronounced immunologic changes than other forms of immunotherapy, such as coseasonal and preseasonal immunotherapy, which are not commonly used. Injections are initially administered either once or twice weekly beginning with a weak dilution of extract and increasing the amount and concentration to a maintenance dose or the highest tolerated dose. Once this is achieved, depending on the clinical response, the injection interval may be prolonged gradually by weekly increments to every 4–6 weeks.

Preseasonal immunotherapy is similar in methodology, except that therapy is started several months prior to the season and discontinued during the season. It is then resumed in a similar fashion the following year. Coseasonal immunotherapy is a method used by some physicians to treat allergic symptoms during the pollen season. Intradermal or subcutaneous injections of low dose aqueous extract are given at frequent intervals; however, proper studies have not been carried out to prove efficacy.

Several other forms of therapy, which are very controversial and have not been proven to be efficacious in controlled studies, include skin-test endpoint titration to determine optimal dosage for immunotherapy, intracutaneous and subcutaneous provocation and neutralization, and sublingual provocation and neutralization.

Dosage and Techniques

The dilution of extract, which can be safely administered for the initial injection, is dependent on several factors. The most important include the degree of skin test sensitivity and severity of clinical symptoms. If marked sensitivity exists to an offending allergen, the initial dose for immunotherapy should be small, such as 0.05 ml of 1:100,000 w/v or 1:1,000,000 w/v. Moderate skin sensitivity to high concentrations of intradermal testing extracts usually means relative safety in beginning with higher concentrations of extracts such as 0.05 ml of 1:10,000 w/v. Another factor to be considered is the biological activity of the allergen. Ragweed, grass, tree, and animal derived allergens appear to be more likely to cause systemic reactions than are mold and dust allergens; therefore, with these former antigens, a weaker dilution is the usual rule for initial injections.

The risk of severe systemic reaction is always present when allergen extracts are being administered. Therefore, extreme caution is mandatory by those responsible. Because of this risk, the injected subject should be advised to receive injections in a medical facility in which a physician is present. The extract is usually given by a nurse familiar with the technique of immunotherapy as long as a physician is available to treat a systemic reaction.

The proper vial should be selected and the label checked several times prior to the injection. A 1.0 ml tuberculin syringe with a 3/8-inch 26- or 27-gauge needle is ideal for this purpose. Using customary sterile technique, the proper amount of extract is withdrawn into the syringe. The needle can then be wiped with an alcohol sponge to remove allergens, thereby reducing the likelihood of a local reaction. After wiping the skin with alcohol, the tissue of the arm is held taut with one hand while the needle is thrust into the subcutaneous tissue at a 45° angle on the posterolateral aspect of the lower portion of the arm. By aspirating, one decreases the likelihood of injecting into adjacent vessels thereby decreasing the chance of rapid absorption or direct intravascular injection of antigen. If blood does appear, a second site should be chosen for the injection. The extract is injected at a moderate rate with occasional aspirations of the plunger to be sure intravascular injection is not occurring. The needle is then withdrawn, and a cotton swab is held over the site for several minutes.

The treated subject is required to wait in the physician's office for 20–30 minutes after an injection. Usually severe reactions will occur in this allotted time and can be instantly treated. Strenuous exercise should be avoided for several hours after an injection to decrease the likelihood of rapid absorption associated with vasodilation and increased circulation. Careful records are necessary, and the treated subject must be questioned prior to the administration of a subsequent injection to determine whether local or systemic symptoms appeared following the previous injection.

Duration

The length of time for which immunotherapy is continued is determined by several factors, including response to therapy, the nature and severity of the disease being treated, and the desire to continue therapy in view of the clinical response obtained. Immunotherapy for respiratory allergies is usually continued for a minimum of 3–5 years. Once complete or substantial amelioration of symptoms is observed and this response maintained with the injection therapy for a year or two, discontinuation may be attempted. If immunotherapy is discontinued and symptoms recur, it can be resumed following an appropriate clinical evaluation. Immunotherapy may be continued until the treated subject is asymptomatic or greatly improved for at least a year before therapy is again stopped. Cessation of immunotherapy is recommended for those who have not benefited clinically after a year of uninterrupted maintenance immunotherapy. Although most treated subjects experience clinical benefit within the first months of immunotherapy, others may take a year or two to achieve maximum effect.

Immunologic Changes

A variety of immunologic changes have been demonstrated associated with immunotherapy that may, in part, be responsible for the relief of allergic symptoms. Among these changes are: (1) a blunting of the usual seasonal rise in the IgE following allergen exposure and a slow decline over several years in the level of specific IgE; (2) a rise in serum IgG (blocking antibody) which blocks the allergen from reacting with the IgE bound to mast cells; (3) increase in blocking IgA and IgG in mucosal secretions; (4) reduced basophil reactivity and sensitivity to allergens as determined by in vitro leukocyte histamine release; (5) reduced in vitro lymphocyte blast transformation to allergen; and (6) generation of allergen specific suppressor T cells.

Each of these changes do not usually occur in every subject, and those that are important in ameliorating symptoms are not well defined. One change, however, that correlates to some extent with clinical results has been the serum titer of specific IgG. Studies show that when high dose immunotherapy is reached, IgG levels plateau and usually do not increase despite additional allergen extract administered. No immunologic test adequately predicts the clinical response, although those who fail to make specific IgG do not usually improve symptomatically. The observed immunologic changes are, for the most part, highly specific for the allergens administered which reemphasizes the importance of accurately identifying relevant allergens before beginning such therapy.

Treatment Failure

Lack of clinical response to immunotherapy is usually secondary to one of the following. First, the treated subject does not have IgE mediated disease and is being inappropriately treated. Second, appropriate allergens are not being utilized. For example, exacerbations in the fall may be due to mold and weed sensitivity, whereas the treated subject is only receiving weed extract. Third, proper environmental controls have not been instituted. Fourth, the treated subject has not received maximal tolerated doses of allergen extract. Fifth, the allergen extract is not sufficiently potent and is not standardized. Sixth, new sensitivities have developed that have not been recognized and/or treated. Seventh, aggravation of symptoms from concomitant drugs is occurring, (e.g., reserpine, propranolol, and/or sympathomimetic nasal sprays). Eighth, coexisting medical and/or surgical diseases exist, such as hypothyroidism, nasal polyposis, sinusitis, nasal septal deviation, or bronchiectasis. Finally, there is unrealistic patient expectation of treatment. Immunotherapy does not eliminate symptoms in most cases, it ameliorates symptoms.

Reactions

Local swelling and/or redness frequently develop at the injection site. It is thought that this may predispose an impending systemic reaction with subsequent injections if this swelling is severe and/or is gradually increasing with each injection. Therefore, if swelling is severe, the dose of extract is reduced, followed by repeated attempts to increase the amount and concentration to the highest tolerated dose or a predetermined maximum dose.

Systemic reactions to immunotherapy occur with varying frequency. The incidence is low, and the most common systemic allergic reactions are mild in nature. The systemic reaction rate to immunotherapy probably is related to the potency and allergenicity of the administered extract and the degree of clinical sensitivity of those subjects receiving immunotherapy. For example, in a survey conducted by the American Academy of Allergy and Immunology, of 1,430 patients administered Hymenoptera venom extract, 178 (12.5 percent) had 336 reactions, 8 of which were severe and 48 of which were of moderate severity.

Lamson reported the first anaphylaxis fatality from immunotherapy in 1929. Six other fatalities from immunotherapy injections have been reported in the literature up to 1980. In 1985, 13 additional fatalities were reported based on a retrospective survey (1973–1984) of the members of the American Academy of Allergy and Immunology. Although clinical errors accounted for several of these deaths in which details were reported, the majority of subjects died even though immunotherapy and treatment of the systemic reactions appeared, for the most part, to be optimal.

The most common systemic reaction associated with immunotherapy is mild and consists of generalized urticaria and/or angioedema. More severe systemic reactions, which manifest clinically as rhinoconjunctivitis, laryngoedema, bronchospasm, nausea, vomiting, and hypotension, also occur.

Proper emergency equipment and treatment should be immediately available in an office or medical facility in which allergen extracts are administered. A physician should be present to treat systemic reactions, first, with epinephrine as early as possible to prevent more serious reactions from occurring. β-adrenergic blocking agents may exacerbate asthma and seem to potentiate anaphylactic reactions and, therefore, are not recommended for general use in these subjects.

Immunotherapy has not been associated with other side effects, and although immune complex mediated disease is theoretically possible and has been reported, a cause and effect is unlikely. Pregnant subjects, in general, are not started on immunotherapy until after delivery to avoid a possible systemic reaction requiring treatment, although those already on maintenance therapy can be continued. There have been no reported fatalities and/or fetal abnormalities associated with this form of therapy used during pregnancy.

A patient consent form is advisable because of the reported fatalities associated with immunotherapy. For those patients receiving immunotherapy outside the allergists' offices, detailed immunotherapy instructions are necessary from the prescribing allergist to the physician and staff administering the injections.

PROGRESS IN RESEARCH

Allergen extracts are marketed by many pharmaceutical firms. Standardization of allergen extracts in the future will be based on actual measurements of biologic activity as compared to allergen extract standards. These standards can be obtained from the Laboratory of Allergenic Products, Office of Biologic Research and Review, Center for Drugs and Biologics, Food and Drug Administration, Bethesda, Maryland 20205, and from the WHO International Laboratory for Biological Standards at NIBSC, Holly Hill, Hampstead, London, NW36RB, United Kingdom. They are labeled in universally recognized units *Allergy Units* (AU) in the United States and *International Units* (IU) outside the United States. This process of standardization will be superior to standardization by techniques not based on biological activity such as w/v or PNU. For example, short ragweed standardized extract is assigned a value of 100,000 AU/ml for convenience and lot-to-lot consistency when the vial is reconstituted with the proper amount of sterile diluent. Physicians and investigators will be able to communicate more accurately about degrees of sensitivity. A statement that a positive skin test produced by a specific number of AUs or IUs should communicate the sensitivity to others in mutually understood terms. Investigators can also describe the sensitivity of a group under study in terms that allow comparison with other groups. Doses used will also be quantitative so physicians can accurately describe the dose an individual has received, and investigators can communicate what they believe is the optimum dose in terms that can be confirmed in other research centers. This is not to say that there will be perfect transferability of information about extracts from different sources simply because they are labeled in AUs or IUs. The variability and biological measurements based on different groups of subjects make some variation in extract standards at different times or places inevitable. For this reason, despite similar labelling, physicians will still have to be cautious while transferring treated subjects from extracts made by one company to extracts made by another.

Formaldehyde or glutaraldehyde modified allergens are also being developed but are not yet approved by the FDA for general use. Chemically modified extracts, because of their decreased allergenicity, should not as readily induce allergic reactions, yet should retain their immunogenicity. The potential advantages of these preparations, with reduced allergenicity, are to permit larger initial amounts of extract and higher maintenance therapy plus decrease the number of injections needed for effective therapy. This would decrease the cost and inconvenience of receiving injections. For example, polymerized ragweed extract (glutaraldehyde treated) has been proven efficacious, safe, and cost-effective in several clinical trials. A 15 week injection course with this extract gave good clinical results in hayfever sufferers, and the benefits persisted several years without supplemental immunotherapy. The IgG blocking antibody increased 11 fold. Allergoids, produced by formaldehyde modification, also appear to be safe and effective. No major side effects have been noted in over seven years of study using various allergens including ragweed, oak, and plantain pollen allergoids. These studies demonstrate that this therapy should be equally or more effective than aqueous immunotherapy and have a lower incidence of systemic reactions. Ten visits are required to achieve maintenance, and booster injections are necessary every three months.

CONCLUSION

Many factors, including allergic ones, trigger asthma. Immunotherapy offers the allergic patient a form of therapy that alters his/her hypersensitivity to specific environmental allergens. It thereby reduces the asthmatic symptoms caused by those allergens and may decrease nonspecific bronchial hyperreactivity. In some cases, immunotherapy has been shown to affect both the early and late phases of the asthmatic reactions to allergens, although the late asthmatic reaction appears to be more affected than the early phase. Further studies are necessary to more clearly define the optimal methods of immunotherapy to treat asthmatic subjects.

ACKNOWLEDGMENTS

We thank Peggy L. Hales and Pat A. Walsh for their secretarial assistance and Samuel C. Bukantz, M.D. for his editorial advice.

REFERENCES

Aas K: Hyposensitization in house dust allergy asthma. Acta Paediatr Scand 60:264–268, 1971

Bruce CA, Norman PS, Rosenthal RR, et al: The role of ragweed pollen in autumnal asthma. J Allergy Clin Immunol 59:449–459, 1977

Bruun E: Control examination of the specificity of specific desensitization in asthma. Acta Allergol 2:122–128, 1949

Citron KM, Frankland AW, Sinclair JD: Inhalation tests of bronchial hypersensitivity in pollen asthma. Thorax 13:229–232, 1958

Davis D (Chairman): A trial of house dust mite extract on bronchial asthma. Mite Allergy Subcommittee of the Research Committee of the British Thoracic Association. Br J Dis Chest 73:260–270, 1979

Forgacs P, Swan AV: Treatment of house dust allergy. A report from the Research Committee of the British Tuberculosis Association. Br Med J 3:774–777, 1968

Frankland AW, Augustin R: Prophylaxis of summer hayfever and asthma: controlled trial comparing crude grass pollen extracts with isolated main protein component. Lancet 1:1055–1057, 1954

Franklin W: Controlled studies of immunotherapy in asthma. New Engl and Regional Allergy Proceedings 4:208–211, 1983

Johnstone DE: Study of the role of antigen dosage in the treatment of pollenosis and pollen asthma. J Dis Child 94:1–5, 1957

Grammar LC, Shaghnessy MA, Suszko IM, et al: Persistence of efficacy after a brief course polymerized ragweed allergen: a controlled study. J Allergy Clin Immunol 73:484–489, 1984

Johnstone DE, Crump L: Value of hyposensitization therapy for perennial bronchial asthma in children. Pediatrics 27:39–44, 1961

Johnstone DE, Dutton A: The value of hyposensitization therapy for bronchial asthma in children—a 14-year-old study. Pediatrics 42:793–802, 1968

Lockey RF, Bukantz SC: Diagnostic tests and hyposensitization therapy in asthma, in Weiss EB, Siegel MS (eds), Bronchial Asthma, Mechanisms and Therapeutics. Boston, Little, Brown and Company, 1976, pp 613–637

Lockey RF, Fox RW: Allergic emergencies. Hospital Medicine 15:64–78, 1979

Lockey R, Peppe B, Baird I, et al: Hymenoptera venom study, treatment result. J Allergy Clin Immunol (Supplement) 71–120, 1983

Lockey R, Benedict L, Turkeltaub P: Fatalities from immunotherapy and skin testing. J Allergy Clin Immunol (Supplement) 75:166, 1985

McAllen MK, Heaf PJD, McInroy P, et al: Depot grass pollen injection in asthma: effect of repeated treatment on clinical response and measured bronchial reactivity. Br Med J 1:22–25, 1967

Metzger WJ, Donnelly BA, Richardson HB: Modification of late asthmatic response (LAR) during immunotherapy for Alternia-induced asthma. J Allergy Clin Immunol (Supplement) (Abstract 121) 71:119, 1983

Mosbeck H: House dust mite allergy. Allergy 40:81–91, 1985

Norman PS: Immunotherapy. Prog Allergy 32:318–346, 1982

Norman PS, Lichtenstein LM, Kagey-Sobotka A, et al: Controlled evaluation of

Allergoid in the immunotherapy of ragweed hayfever. J Allergy Clin Immunol 70:248–260, 1982

Ohman JL, Findlay SR, Leiterman KM: Immunotherapy in cat-induced asthma. Double-blind trial with evaluation of in vivo and in vitro response. J Allergy Clin Immunol 74:230–239, 1984

Ortolani C, Pastorello E, Moss R, et al: Grass pollen immunotherapy: a single year double-blind, placebo-controlled study in patients with grass pollen-induced asthma and rhinitis. J Allergy Clin Immunol 73:283–290, 1984

Patterson R: Clinical efficacy of allergen immunotherapy. J Allergy Clin Immunol 64:155–158, 1979

Reed CE, Swanson MC, Agarwal MK, et al: Allergens that cause asthma. Identification and quantitation. Chest 83 (Supplement) 40s–44s, 1985

Rocklin RE: Clinical and immunologic aspects of allergen-specific immunotherapy in patients with seasonal allergic rhinitis and/or allergic asthma. J Allergy Clin Immunol 72:323–334, 1984

Smith AP: Hyposensitization with *Dermatophagoides pteronyssinus* antigen. Trial in asthma induced by house dust. Br Med J 4:204–206, 1971

Taylor WW, Ohman JL, Lowell FC: Immunotherapy in cat induced asthma. A double-blind trial with evaluation of bronchial response to cat allergen and histamine. J Allergy Clin Immunol 61:283–289, 1978

Tuchinda M, Chai H: Effect of immunotherapy in chronic asthmatic children. J Allergy Clin Immunol 51:131–138, 1973

Warner JO, Sothill JF, Price JF, et al: Controlled trial of hyposensitization to *Dermatophagoides pteronyssinus* in children with asthma. Lancet 2:912–915, 1978

Zieger RS, Schatz M: Immunotherapy of atopic disorders. Present state of the art and future perspectives. Med Clin of N America 65:987–1012, 1981

R. Michael Sly

18

Treatment of Asthma in Children

Asthma is a chronic pulmonary disease characterized by hyperirritability of the airways manifested by recurrent episodes of generalized airway obstruction that is usually reversible either spontaneously or following appropriate treatment. Allergy is not the only cause of asthma, but medical histories and the results of allergy skin testing have implicated allergy as a cause of asthma in the great majority of asthmatic patients from 5 to 45 years of age. Allergy is a somewhat less frequent cause of asthma in children less than 5 years old and a much less frequent cause in those less than 2 years old. Other causes of asthma include viral respiratory infections, exercise, inhalation of cold air, changes in weather, air pollution, and emotional stress.

When allergy causes asthma interaction between allergen and a specific IgE antibody, bridging adjacent IgE molecules attached to the surfaces of mast cells, causes interaction between IgE receptors, transmethylation of membrane phospholipids, and movement of calcium ions into the cell. Simultaneously the combination of allergen with antibody activates adenylate cyclase to stimulate formation of cyclic adenosine monophosphate (cAMP) from adenosine triphosphate. The increased intracellular concentration of cAMP initiates a series of biochemical events that causes movement of mast cell granules to the surface of the cell in the presence of calcium ions. Solubilization of the contents of the granules occurs. Granules fuse with each other and then with the cell membrane, releasing stored mediators. These mediators include histamine, a kallikrein, eosinophil chemotactic factors, neutrophil chemotactic factors, and other mediators.

BRONCHIAL ASTHMA, Second Edition
ISBN 0-8089-1814-1

393

Either specific or nonspecific perturbation of cell membranes can liberate arachidonic acid from membrane phospholipids directly by the action of phospholipase A_2 or indirectly by sequential actions of phospholipase C and diglyceride lipase after activation of the phospholipases. Metabolism of arachidonic acid by the cyclo-oxygenase pathway causes formation of the various prostaglandins, while metabolism by the lipoxygenase pathway leads to formation of the leukotrienes. Leukotrienes C, D, and E comprise slow reacting substance.

The actions of these mediators released from mast cell granules or generated in response to the antigen-antibody combination cause the signs and symptoms of asthma. Histamine, bradykinin, leukotrienes C, D, and E, PGD_2, $PGF_{2\alpha}$, and thromboxane A_2 can all cause bronchoconstriction. Histamine, bradykinin, PGE, and leukotrienes C, D, and E can cause increased capillary permeability and consequently mucosal edema. Histamine can cause secretion of mucus in the airways both directly through action on H2 receptors and indirectly by acting on irritant receptors to cause reflex parasympathetic stimulation of submucosal glands. Several products of arachidonic acid metabolism are even more potent than histamine in stimulating secretion of mucus (leukotrienes C and D, HETEs, $PGF_{2\alpha}$, PGD_2, PGI_2, and PGE_1).

Airway obstruction with hyperinflation results from the bronchoconstriction, mucosal edema, and increased production of secretions. Lack of uniform ventilation and mismatching of ventilation and perfusion contribute to alveolar hypoventilation with consequent hypercapnia and hypoxemia. Both respiratory acidosis and metabolic acidosis can occur.

Inhalation of allergen can cause immediate bronchoconstriction that remits within 1–2 hours, but in as many as half of allergic asthmatics bronchoconstriction may recur 4–6 hours after exposure to allergen. This late phase reaction may persist 2–5 hours or longer. In rare asthmatics inhalation of allergen may elicit a late bronchoconstrictive response without immediate bronchoconstriction. Increased bronchial irritability, identified by the dose of inhaled, nebulized methacholine, or histamine necessary to cause significant airway obstruction, occurs after late bronchoconstrictive responses and may persist as long as one week after the challenge with allergen. Bronchial hyperreactivity, characteristic of both allergic and nonallergic asthma, also follows viral respiratory infections. There is a general correlation between bronchial reactivity and the severity of asthma as measured by the frequency of need for bronchodilators and adrenal corticosteroids.

Modification of Release of Mediators

One can prevent or interrupt the chain of events that follows interaction of allergen with the IgE antibody by elimination of allergens, pharmacologic prevention or modification of release of mediators, inhibition of the actions of mediators, or reversal of their actions. Cromolyn prevents movement of calcium ions into the cell, inhibiting both immediate and late phase asthmatic responses to inhaled allergen at least partly through this action. Cromolyn can also reduce bronchial hyperreactivity, possibly partly because of its inhibition of late phase responses. Cholinergic agents such as acetylcholine or methacholine cause bronchconstriction by direct action on smooth muscle, but cholinergic stimulation also increases formation of cyclic guanosine monophosphate from guanosine triphosphate and enhances antigen-induced mediator release. Accordingly an anticholinergic agent such as atropine or ipratropium bromide can cause both bronchodilation and inhibition of mediator release.

β-adrenergic stimulation with an agent such as isoproterenol causes an increase in the formation of cyclic adenosine monophosphate from adenosine triphosphate through interaction with adenylate cyclase. Such an increase in the concentration of cAMP that precedes challenge of the mast cell with allergen inhibits release of mediators. In smooth muscle increased concentrations of cyclic AMP cause bronchodilation by augmenting sequestration of calcium.

The mechanism of the beneficial effect of theophylline in asthma is unknown. Theophylline enhances contractility of fatigued diaphragm, increases phrenic nerve activity, and inhibits bronchoconstriction induced by inhaled adenosine, which is released by allergenic challenge. Its chief mode of action is not inhibition of the phosphodiesterase responsible for degradation of cAMP because therapeutic doses of theophylline cause only a 10 percent inhibition of phosphodiesterase. Furthermore some phosphodiesterase inhibitors are not bronchodilators.

Adrenal corticosteroids can have several beneficial effects. One of the most important is induction of plasma proteins, macrocortin or lipomodulin, that inhibit activation of phospholipase A_2 and thus inhibit liberation of arachidonic acid from membrane phospholipids. Corticosteroids can also prevent or reverse tolerance to β-adrenergic drugs by preventing or reversing β-adrenergic receptor uncoupling from the adenylate cyclase system. Steroids also inhibit resynthesis of histamine, decrease vascular permeability, and inhibit the late asthmatic response to inhaled allergen.

ELIMINATION OF ALLERGENS AND IRRITANTS

Elimination of exposure to the offending allergen is the most effective treatment for any allergic condition. Medical histories and testing implicate allergenic components of house dust mites and house dust most frequently of all possible allergens. Precautions that minimize exposure to these allergens

Table 18-1
Preparation of a dust-free bedroom

1. Remove all carpet and rugs, leaving a plain, wooden floor or tile. Small, cotton throw rugs may be acceptable if washed at least weekly in a washing machine.

2. Remove curtains and venetian blinds. Shades are acceptable. Use curtains only if they can be laundered weekly.

3. Clean the room and closet thoroughly and wax the floor.

4. Close and seal hot air vents unless there is a central HEPA filter or a central electronic air filter. As an alternative fiber glass or cheesecloth filters may be placed over air vents, but do not place flammable material in contact with metal that may become hot.

5. Encase all mattresses, box springs, and pillows in air tight, dustproof covers, sealing with adhesive tape where the zipper ends. Durable covers are available from Allergen-Proof Encasings, Inc., 1450 East 363rd St., Eastlake, Ohio 44094 and Allergy Control Products, 28 High Ridge Avenue, Ridgefield, Ct. 06877.

6. Any comforters, quilts, mattress pads, and pillows should be filled only with dacron or polyester. Replace pillows each year unless encased in allergen-proof covers. Launder blankets and bedspreads at least monthly.

7. Any stuffed toys must be filled only with polyester or another synthetic stuffing.

8. Eliminate upholstered furniture and minimize other furniture.

9. Eliminate bookshelves with books.

10. Dust the room daily and clean thoroughly at least weekly, including window sills, tops of window frames, and tops of doors. Vacuum the covered mattress at least weekly.

11. Air the room thoroughly during and after cleaning; otherwise keep doors and windows closed. The allergic patient should avoid the room for at least 1 hour after vacuuming or cleaning.

12. Keep only clothing in current use in the closet. Keep the closet door closed.

Reprinted by permission of Elsevier Science Publishing Co., Inc., modified from Sly RM: Textbook of Pediatric Allergy,p 307. New Hyde Park, NY, copyright 1985 by Medical Examination Publishing Co., Inc.

are of established benefit in the control of allergic asthma in such patients (Table 18-1). Upholstered furniture, carpet, and mattresses are the richest sources of mites in homes. Mites are most prolific at 25°C and 80 percent relative humidity and are rarely found at relative humidity less than 50 percent. They are rarely found at altitudes greater than 1600 meters, probably because of low humidity. Accordingly air conditioning to reduce humidity can reduce proliferation of mites. Monthly treatment of carpet and upholstered furniture with an acaricide, primiphos methyl, available in the United Kingdom, is effective in reducing contamination with mite allergen.

Minimizing exposure to sources of dust and mites in the bedroom often affords adequate control of exposure for a child, who often spends more time in his bedroom than in any other room of the house. When outdoors or at school there is usually no exposure to house dust. Mechanical, high efficiency particulate air (HEPA) filters are effective in removing dust, mold, and pollen from the air. Placing such a unit on the bedside table can assure inhalation of clean air while the youngster sleeps. Central units are also available. Electronic air filters are equally effective but produce ozone, which may have adverse pulmonary effects.

Exposure to allergenic fungi can occur both indoors and outdoors. Complete avoidance is impossible, but substantial reduction in exposure is often feasible at least indoors. Scrupulous cleaning of bathrooms, kitchens, and laundry rooms is necessary with special attention to shower stalls and curtains, sinks, refrigerator drip trays, and garbage pails. Use of a dehumidifier may be necessary to prevent growth of fungi in damp basements. Outdoors avoidance of dead leaves, mulch, hay, and ensilage is appropriate.

Cats and dogs are sources of potent allergens. Their complete elimination from the home of the allergic patient is necessary for optimal control of exposure. Neither confinement of the animal to a single room nor confinement of the patient to a single room is a satisfactory solution because of inevitable dissemination of allergen by activity of occupants of the house if not by a forced air heating and cooling system. Allergy to other fur-bearing household pets can also occur. Exposure to allergen can continue for several months after elimination of an animal from the house, and resultant continued symptoms may raise doubts over the wisdom of what has usually been a distasteful decision to eliminate an animal that may have become as much a part of the family as the child. The result of a trial visit to the home of a relative who has no animals or a vacation at a hotel where no animals are permitted may be sufficiently convincing to provide guidance for an appropriate decision regarding the pet. Animals never permitted indoors are much less likely to be problematic and less likely to be covert sources of exposure to allergen. Symptoms that occur only with exposure to an animal outdoors obviously indicate allergy to the animal.

Elimination of a feather pillow can cause dramatic relief of symptoms due to allergy to feathers. A kapok-filled sofa pillow is not a satisfactory substitute because sensitization to kapok can also occur. Pillows filled with polyester or dacron are safe.

Irritants can cause airway obstruction in both allergic and nonallergic asthmatic subjects. Cigarette smoke is still the most common irritant to which patients are exposed, and either active or passive smoking can cause airway obstruction. Maternal smoking increases both the frequency and the severity of asthma in children. Accordingly cigarette, cigar, and pipe smoking should be prohibited in the home of the asthmatic subject. Avoidance of public facilities where smoking is permitted is best for all asthmatic patients and may be essential for patients with severe asthma. Travelers can seek accommodations in hotels or rooms where smoking is proscribed.

Other sources of inhaled irritants include wood-burning stoves, gas ranges, kerosene heaters, and fireplaces. Proper venting and adjustment are essential when complete avoidance is impossible. Use of an exhaust fan during cooking reduces exposure to irritating cooking fumes.

Industrial and motor vehicular air pollution can also cause airway obstruction in asthmatic subjects. Avoidance of strenuous exercise is wise during periods of intense air pollution, and the patient should remain indoors, breathing filtered air when possible.

Treatment of food allergy depends upon dietary elimination of the offending food. Supplying suggested menus and recipes as well as lists of dietary sources of the allergen facilitates compliance with diets that eliminate common allergens with many sources in the diet such as egg, milk, and wheat. Recipes and lists are available in textbooks of allergy and from manufacturers and the American Dietetic Association (620 N. Michigan Ave., Chicago, Illinois 60611).

Highly restrictive diets should not be imposed for more than brief periods without detailed evaluation of their ability to meet nutritional needs. Supplemental B and D vitamins are necessary when milk and cereals are eliminated completely. Elimination of citrus fruits requires supplementation with vitamin C. Prolonged dietary elimination of milk necessitates supplementation with calcium unless the child is receiving adequate volumes of a substituted formula that contains calcium.

Patients with sensitivity to sulfites must avoid ingestion of sulfites, which are often added to or sprayed onto fresh fruits and vegetables, shellfish, beer, and wine. They must avoid acidic soft drinks, which contain sulfur dioxide. Because of the likelihood of inadvertent exposure it is prudent for such patients to carry loaded epinephrine syringes for use in emergencies.

It is imperative that patients with sensitivity to aspirin avoid aspirin, other nonsteroidal antiinflammatory agents, and the numerous medications that contain aspirin and are available without prescription.

PHARMACOLOGIC TREATMENT

Pharmacologic treatment is essential to optimal management of acute airway obstruction due to asthma and can be effective in preventing recurrent asthma and maintaining normal pulmonary function. Drugs of established value include β-adrenergic agonists, theophylline, cromolyn, adrenal corticosteroids, and anticholinergic agents.

BETA-ADRENERGIC AGONISTS

β-adrenergic agonists can cause bronchodilation and inhibition of release of mediators from mast cells. Accordingly one would expect a drug such as isoproterenol to be one of the most effective drugs for the treatment of asthma, and it remains the standard against which other β-adrenergic agonists are usually compared. Nevertheless it suffers from several serious limitations. It is metabolized rapidly by catechol-o-methyltransferase, causing a short duration of action of only 1–2 hours. It is metabolized to 3-methoxyisoproterenol, a weak β-adrenergic blocking agent, which although produced in only small amounts, blocks to some extent the very actions for which the isoproterenol has been administered. Inactivation by intestinal and hepatic sulfatases prevents effectiveness after oral administration; accordingly inhalation is the optimal method of administration.

Inhalation of isoproterenol sometimes elicits a decrease in arterial PO_2 despite lessening of airway obstruction, probably because of reversal of compensatory pulmonary vasoconstriction, aggravating further the ventilation-perfusion imbalance typical of acute asthma. These decreases have rarely exceeded a few torr, and the greatest decreases of as much as 25 torr have occurred in patients with relatively high baseline PO_2 who could best tolerate some decrease. Similar changes in arterial PO_2 can follow subcutaneous injection of epinephrine or intravenous administration of aminophylline. This adverse effect can be prevented by simultaneous administration of supplemental oxygen.

Inhalation of isoproterenol has aggravated airway obstruction in a few patients in whom temporary improvement has been followed by increased airway obstruction within one hour. Discontinuation of treatment with isoproterenol has elicited clinical improvement in some patients who previously had been using metered dose inhalers more frequently than recommended.

Inhalation of isoproterenol at usually recommended doses causes little or no cardiac stimulation in asthmatic subjects, but inhalation of 520 μg from a metered dose inhaler may increase heart rate by 20 percent. Intravenous administration has been associated with myocardial ischemia and fatal myocardial necrosis.

Isoproterenol's rapid onset of action and short duration of action encourage overuse. Efforts to develop safer drugs with longer durations of action have led to the introduction of metaproterenol, terbutaline, albuterol, fenoterol, and bitolterol mesylate, which elicit longer lasting bronchodilation than isoproterenol (5–6 hours or more after inhalation of terbutaline, albuterol, and fenoterol; 6–8 hours after bitolterol). Most of these are effective after oral administration, but inhalation is the route of choice because of rapid onset of bronchodilation following very small doses that cause minimal side effects at recommended doses (Table 18-2). Cardiac stimulation can follow oral or intravenous administration.

In general metaproterenol has been studied more extensively in children than have the newer β-adrenergic agonists, but albuterol administered by inhalation at doses recommended for adults also seems safe for children as young as three years of age. Onset of action, time to peak bronchodilation, and duration of bronchodilation after doses equivalent for peak brochodilation are similar to metaproterenol, terbutaline, albuterol, and fenoterol, but 2 inhalations (180 μg) of albuterol causes more bronchodilation than 2 inhalations (1.3 mg) of metaproterenol. Bitolterol is hydrolyzed by pulmonary esterases to the active catecholamine, colterol. More extensive accumulation and hydrolysis of bitolterol in the lungs than in the heart may minimize potential cardiac effects. Measurement of pulmonary function after treatment is not the most accurate index of duration of pharmacologic effect because apparent bronchodilation may be due partly to failure of bronchoconstriction to recur after it has been relieved. The chief advantage of inhaled albuterol over inhaled metaproterenol is the longer duration of inhibition of exercise induced asthma of up to 6 hours after inhalation of albuterol. Inhaled metaproterenol inhibits exercise induced asthma in most subjects no longer than 30 minutes after treatment. Fenoterol prevents exercise induced asthma as long as 4 hours after inhalation. Inhaled terbutaline causes inhibition for as long as 1 hour; bitolterol, 45 minutes; but neither has been studied longer after inhalation.

Inhalation of a β-adrenergic agonist from a metered dose inhaler usually elicits as much bronchodilation as inhalation from a powered nebulizer, which may require 6–8 times as much drug for equivalent bronchodilation. During severe airway obstruction, use of a powered nebulizer may be more effective. Optimal technique for use of a metered dose inhaler requires a slow inhalation from functional residual capacity to total lung capacity held for 10 seconds. Intervals of several minutes between 2 or 3 inhalations enhance response. Use of a spacer tube or cone can increase pulmonary deposition of aerosol by permitting evaporation of the large propellant particle that surrounds each bronchodilator particle, reducing the particle size to one that can reach the lower airway before deposition. The spacer also permits a decrease in the speed at which the particles are traveling before reaching the orophar-

Table 18-2
Beta Adrenergic Agonist Drugs

Drug	Route	Dose
Albuterol	Inh	180 μg q 4–6 h (MDI)
	Oral	0.1 mg/kg tid or 2–4 mg tid-qid (>2 years old)
Bitolterol mesylate	Inh	740–1110 μg q 8 h (MDI)
Ephedrine	Oral	0.5–1 mg/kg q 4–6 h (max 50 mg q 4 h)
Epinephrine, 1:1,000, aqueous	SC	0.01 ml/kg (max 0.3 ml) q 20 min × 3 if necessary. May repeat in 4 h.
Epinephrine, 1:200, aqueous suspension (Sus-Phrine)	SC	0.005 ml/kg (max 0.3 ml). May repeat in 8 h.
Ethylnorepinephrine (Bronkephrine)	SC	0.01–0.02 ml/kg (max 0.5 ml). May repeat in 20 min.
Fenoterol	Inh	160–320 μg q 4–6 h (MDI)
Metaproterenol	Inh	0.1–0.3 ml q 4–6 h (inhalant solution, 5%, diluted in 3 ml saline and nebulized)
	Inh	1.0–2.5 ml q 4–6 h (inhalant solution, unit dose, 0.6%, nebulized)
	Inh	1.3–1.95 mg q 4–6 h (MDI)
	Oral	0.5 mg/kg q 6–8 h (max 20 mg qid)
Terbutaline	Inh	0.1 mg/kg q 4–6 h (max 6 mg, nebulized)
	Inh	400 μg q 4–6 h (MDI)
	SC	0.01 mg/kg (max 0.25 mg). May repeat in 20 min (max 0.5 mg in 4 h).
	Oral	0.075 mg/kg or 2.5 mg q 6 h tid (max 5 mg q 6 h tid).

Inh = by inhalation
SC = by subcutaneous injection
MDI = metered dose inhaler
max = maximum

ynx, minimizing deposition by impaction in the pharynx. Use of a chamber such as the Inhal-Aid or Aerochamber obviates the need for synchronization of inhalation with actuation of the inhaler, enabling children as young as 3 years of age to receive effective treatment with metered dose inhalers.

Continual treatment with either inhaled or oral β-adrenergic agonist drugs can cause tolerance manifested by some decrease in the peak and duration of bronchodilation that follow each dose. Regular treatment with terbutaline, albuterol, or fenoterol for 12–13 weeks may reduce peak improvement in FEV_1 and duration of bronchodilation by 30–60 percent. Tolerance usually becomes maximal within the first 2 weeks of treatment when it occurs and may extend to all β-adrenergic drugs, not only the drug that induced tolerance. Adrenal corticosteroids administered by intravenous injection can restore responsiveness to β-adrenergic agonists within one hour in such patients, however, and concurrent treatment with inhaled or oral corticosteroids can minimize tolerance induced by a β-adrenergic agonist. Continual treatment can induce tolerance to tachycardia and tremor as well as to bronchodilation.

Concurrent administration of bronchodilators by both inhaled and systemic routes may enhance bronchodilation, and treatment with a β-adrenergic agonist and theophylline together can have an additive effect on bronchodilation. Consequently combined therapy can minimize adverse side effects by reducing the dose of each drug required for the same bronchodilating effect that would otherwise require a larger dose of a single drug.

Simultaneous treatment with an oral beta agonist and theophylline has caused chest pain with electrocardiographic changes in a few asthmatic children in whom both the chest pain and the electrocardiographic abnormalities resolved after discontinuation of the beta agonist. Chest pain and electrocardiographic changes have followed inhalation of beta agonists in rare asthmatic adults who also have had cardiovascular disease. Oral beta agonists can cause premature ventricular contractions in susceptible adults with chronic obstructive pulmonary disease. Generally beta agonists seem quite safe at recommended doses, however. The chief potential hazard to the use of an inhaled beta agonist may be overdependence by a patient who may use larger and larger doses at shorter and shorter intervals, not recognizing the loss of effectiveness of the drug and the need for other therapy. This loss of responsiveness may be due to tolerance, inflammation, or both. Loss of responsiveness is less likely to remain unrecognized with the more recent drugs than with isoproterenol because of their longer durations of action. When loss of responsiveness to the beta agonist occurs, however, the patient must know how to contact a physician for adjunctive therapy. Completely unsupervised use of these drugs may be dangerous.

THEOPHYLLINE

The major mode of action that accounts for the beneficial effect of theophylline in asthma remains unknown, but extensive investigation has established a sound basis for safe, effective treatment with theophylline.

There is a logarithmic linear relationship between bronchodilation and serum theophylline concentration over the range of 5–20 μg/ml. Accordingly a doubling of the serum concentration of 5 to 10 μg/ml causes a proportionately greater improvement in FEV_1 than doubling the concentration from 10 to 20 μg/ml. Most children require serum concentrations of at least 10 μg/ml to approach optimal bronchodilation, and most experience adverse side effects at concentrations that exceed 20 μg/ml. The threshold for side effects varies from patient to patient, however, and many children have nausea or vomiting at serum concentrations of 15 μg/ml or even less, especially if they have not been receiving prolonged treatment with theophylline.

Signs and symptoms of theophylline toxicity include restlessness, nausea, vomiting, irritability, headache, abdominal pain, hematemesis, twitching, convulsions, pallor, fever, diarrhea, insomnia, tachycardia, premature ventricular contractions, and coma. Irreversible brain damage or death can occur. Serious adverse effects usually occur at excessive serum theophylline concentrations; convulsions are rare at concentrations less than 30 μg/ml.

Serum theophylline concentrations are not predictable from the dose alone, however, because of substantial variations in rates of metabolism and elimination of the drug from patient to patient. Serum half lives range from 1–10 hours in different patients. Serum half life in a healthy, young adult can vary by as much as 55 percent within 3–4 days, although serum half lives in individual asthmatic children usually remain relatively stable over periods of several months.

Ninety percent of absorbed or infused theophylline is usually eliminated after metabolism in the liver by cytochrome P450 enzymes. As a result liver disease reduces clearance of the drug substantially, increasing serum concentrations. Many other factors can also decrease clearance of theophylline (Table 18-3). Viral respiratory infections with influenza A and adenovirus causing fever and seroconversion can cause prolongation of the serum theophylline half life, and administration of influenza vaccine can increase the serum half life in some patients for as long as 21 days after immunization.

Renal failure has a negligible effect on clearance of theophylline because only 10–15 percent of the drug is excreted without prior hepatic biotransformation into relatively inactive metabolites after the neonatal period. Renal clearance of theophylline is dependent upon the rate of urine flow. Consequently clearance is elevated at high serum theophylline concentrations after

Table 18-3
Factors That Can Decrease Theophylline Clearance and
Magnitude of Effect

Factor	Percentage Decrease in Clearance
Heart failure	60
Liver disease (cirrhosis, acute hepatitis)	30–75
Viral respiratory disease	Increase in serum half life of 70%
Renal failure	10–15
High carbohydrate, low protein diet	20
Dietary xanthines	Modest
Troleandomycin	50
Erythromycin	25
Cimetidine	40 (23–100)
Oral contraceptives	34
Allopurinol	25
Propranolol	40 in smokers; 20 in nonsmokers
Influenza trivalent vaccine	Increase of 145% in serum half life

single doses because of the diuretic effect of theophylline. Less diuresis follows multiple dosing, and consequently there is less effect on renal clearance.

Concurrent treatment with erythromycin can decrease theophylline clearance sufficiently in some patients that a decrease of at least 25 percent in theophylline dosage is warranted, especially in patients with serum theophylline concentrations that have ranged from 15–20 μg/ml at the dose of theophylline they have been receiving. In patients with serum theophylline concentrations, less than 10 μg/ml there may be relatively little risk from the doubling of the serum concentration that may occur with treatment with erythromycin.

Cimetidine can have an even more profound effect on theophylline clearance than erythromycin. Fortunately ranitidine, another H_2 receptor antagonist, does not affect theophylline clearance.

Oral contraceptives, large doses of allopurinol, and treatment with propranolol can also decrease theophylline clearance, but use of propranolol is contraindicated in patients with asthma.

Smoking either tobacco or marijuana can increase theophylline clearance probably because of induction of hepatic microsomal enzymes by polycyclic hydrocarbons (Table 18-4). The effect of ingestion of charcoal-broiled beef is ascribed to the same mechanism.

High protein, low carbohydrate diets can also increase theophylline clearance, whereas high carbohydrate, low protein diets or dietary xanthines such as caffeine or theobromine can have an opposite effect. Dietary changes

Table 18-4
Factors That Can Increase Theophylline
Clearance and Magnitude of Effect

Factor	Percentage Increase in Clearance
Smoking	
Tobacco	50
Marijuana	50
Tobacco and Marijuana	90–100
High protein, low carbohydrate diet	55
Charcoal-broiled beef	30
Phenobarbital	33
Phenytoin	80
Isoproterenol (intravenous infusion)	20

are likely to have a clinically relevant effect on theophylline clearance, only when they are major changes continued for more than several days, however.

Treatment with therapeutic doses of phenobarbital daily for 4 weeks can increase theophylline clearance, but treatment for 2 weeks may have no effect on clearance. Phenytoin causes a much more substantial increase in theophylline clearance that may require an increase in theophylline dosage within 10 days. Theophylline inhibits absorption of phenytoin, on the other hand. Accordingly it is best to avoid use of these two drugs together if possible. Carbamazepine may also increase clearance of theophylline.

Administration of isoproterenol by intravenous infusion may increase theophylline clearance by 6–42 percent and may require an increase in theophylline infusion rate to maintain optimal serum concentrations.

Rates of clearance of theophylline also vary with age. Average dose requirements beyond the neonatal period are indicated in Table 18-5, but because of individual variations in rates of clearance and susceptibility to adverse effects one should initiate therapy at 1/2–2/3 the average dose and later increase dosage gradually if necessary. Signs or symptoms of toxicity may necessitate reductions in dosage. Obesity does not affect the recommended loading dose, but requires determination of maintenance dosage by ideal body weight and clinical response.

Serum theophylline concentrations that follow administration of an oral preparation are determined by absorption as well as variables that affect metabolism and excretion. Absorption from liquid preparations is rapid and complete, eliciting peak serum theophylline concentrations at 1/2–1 1/2 hours. Peak concentrations usually occur 1 1/2–2 1/2 hours after administration of a plain uncoated tablet or capsule containing theophylline for rapid absorption. Wide peak to trough fluctuations in serum concentrations inevitable with

Table 18-5
Average Theophylline Dosage
Requirements by Age

Age (years)	Dose (mg/kg/24 hours)
< 1	8 + 0.3 × age (weeks)
1–9	24
9–12	20
12–16	16–18
> 16	12–13

Initial dosage ½–⅔ average for age

such preparations and the inconvenience of frequent administration at intervals of 6 hours or less to maintain adequate serum concentrations and adequate control of symptoms led to the development of sustained release preparations. These are available as tablets or bead-filled capsules. Sustained release tablets should be broken only where scored, but the beads from capsules are suitable for sprinkling on a teaspoonful of applesauce for swallowing by young children unable to swallow tablets. The youngster must not chew the beads before swallowing, however. The contents of capsules cannot be divided accurately for administration of a smaller dose because some beads contain no theophylline. The increase in intervals between doses possible with use of a sustained release preparation enhances compliance with recommended drug regimens.

Peak serum theophylline concentrations usually follow administration of most sustained release preparations by 4–8 hours and usually occur 6–10 hours after administration of TheoDur, Sustaire, or Uniphyl. Absorption of sustained release preparations is delayed at night, however, possibly because of the recumbent position, and peak concentrations may not be reached until time for the next dose in the morning in patients receiving the drug at intervals of 12 hours. Administration of TheoDur tablets, Slobid Gyrocaps, or Somophyllin CRT capsules with a meal usually delays attainment of the peak concentration by 1–2 hours without affecting bioavailability. Administration of Theolair SR with a meal can cause a much more extreme delay in attainment of the peak concentration to as long as 20 hours after administration of a dose with breakfast. This product dissolves much more rapidly in alkaline solutions than in acid solutions. The combination of its pH-dependent dissolution and nocturnal delays in gastric emptying may cause inadequate serum concentrations during the evening and early night and excessive concentrations the following morning without the precaution of administration before meals. Administration of TheoDur Sprinkle with meals not only delays reaching peak concentration, but also reduces bioavailability by as much as 50 percent or more, depending on the type of meal. Accordingly TheoDur Sprinkle should be administered 1 hour before or 2 hours after meals.

Selection of a suitable product often permits effective control of asthma in children as young as 2 years of age with administration of the sustained release preparation at intervals of 12 hours, but some young children require administration at intervals no longer than 8 hours. Few data are available to indicate safety or efficacy of administration of ultrasustained release preparations to children at intervals of 24 hours. Because of the shorter gastrointestinal transit time typical of most children administration of a preparation such as Uniphyl once daily is probably more appropriate for adults than children.

Because of the numerous variables that can affect absorption and elimination of theophylline determination of serum theophylline concentrations is often necessary to assure optimal therapy. Determination of peak concentrations is of greatest value for indicating when the dose can be increased safely or when possible side effects are likely to be due to theophylline toxicity. Trough concentrations are of value in evaluating the need for increasing the dose when symptoms occur or shortening the interval between doses. Serum concentrations are of greatest value at steady state after 5 half lives of the drug have elapsed following initiation of regular dosing. Recommendations for adjustment of dosage for various peak concentrations at steady state when control of symptoms is inadequate or dosage is excessive are designed to achieve concentrations of 10–20 μg/ml. Changes in dosage when near this range should be cautious because relatively small changes in dosage may elicit larger changes in serum concentration than anticipated (Table 18-6).

There are several rapid, accurate, sensitive, specific methods for deter-

Table 18-6

Theophylline Dosage Adjustments Recommended for Various Peak Serum Concentrations.

Concentration (μg/ml)	Adjustment in Total Daily Dosage
<5	100% increase in 2–4 equal increments at intervals of 2 days
5–7.5	50% increase in 2 equal increments at intervals of 2 days
8–10	20% increase
11–13	10% increase if necessary for control of symptoms
14–20	10% decrease if side effects present
21–25	10% decrease
26–30	25% decrease after omitting next dose
31–35	33% decrease after omitting next dose
>35	50% decrease or more after omitting next 2 doses

From Hendeles L, Weinberger M, Wyatt R, et al: Guide to oral theophylline therapy for the treatment of chronic asthma. Am J Dis Chil 132:876, 1978. Used with permission.

mination of serum theophylline concentrations that require less than 1 ml of blood. These include the enzyme multiplied immunoassay (EMIT), radioimmunoassay, fluorescence immunoassay, and high performance liquid chromatography. With appropriate calibration the Ames Seralyzer permits reasonably accurate determination of serum or plasma concentrations that are less than 20 μg/ml within 30 minutes (15 minutes for plasma).

Treatment of serious toxicity from oral administration of theophylline includes induction of vomiting or gastric lavage followed by administration of a slurry of 30 gm activated charcoal. Administration of the charcoal should be delayed until after vomiting if ipecac has been given to induce emesis because activated charcoal absorbs ipecac as well as theophylline. Administration of charcoal several times at intervals of 2 hours or less is helpful, especially after ingestion of a sustained release theophylline preparation. The charcoal can remove theophylline that has already been absorbed as well as theophylline that remains in the gastrointestinal tract. A saline cathartic is also indicated. Serum concentrations of 60 μg/ml or more 4 hours after ingestion may indicate a need for consideration of hemoperfusion with resin or activated charcoal cartridges. Some have recommended consideration of hemoperfusion at serum theophylline concentrations of 40–60 μg/ml when associated with unusually slow clearance or symptoms of toxicity, but administration of activated charcoal by mouth or nasogastric tube may also be effective in such patients.

CROMOLYN

The primary mode of action of cromolyn is probably prevention of movement of calcium ions into mast cells with consequent inhibition of release of mediators from mast cells, possibly by inducing phosphorylation of a certain protein. Phosphorylation of this protein also occurs 30–60 seconds after stimulation of rat peritoneal mast cells with anti-IgE or with compound 48/80, and may therefore, constitute a natural mechanism for termination of the secretory response. Cromolyn does not inhibit release of mediators from basophils.

Pretreatment with cromolyn can prevent both immediate and late asthmatic responses to inhaled allergen or to exercise. It can prevent bronchoconstriction induced by inhalation of cold air or inhalation of ultrasonically nebulized distilled water. It can prevent the decrease in tracheal mucus velocity induced by challenge with allergen in asthmatics. It can also inhibit bronchoconstriction induced by toluene diisocyanate, sulfur dioxide, and in some patients, inhaled methacholine or histamine aerosols. Its inhibition of bronchoconstriction unrelated to mediator release requires another mode of action, possibly inhibition of neural transmission by afferent C fibers.

Cromolyn can prevent seasonal increases in bronchial reactivity and may reduce bronchial reactivity within 8 weeks of treatment.

Cromolyn can elicit improvement in 60–89 percent of asthmatic subjects with adequate trials. Although improvement usually occurs within the first 2 weeks of treatment, therapy for as long as 3 months may be necessary to elicit the maximal improvement possible and therefore to identify all patients with a potential for improvement with the drug. After improvement has followed initial treatment with 20 mg qid the dose can usually be reduced to 20 mg tid without loss of control of asthma. When response is inadequate, a larger dose of 40 mg tid or qid may be effective. Sufficient bronchodilation to assure satisfactory delivery of the inhaled cromolyn to the lower airways is necessary to assure an adequate trial of the drug, and this may require an initial increase in use of bronchodilators or brief treatment with adrenal corticosteroids.

Children less than 5 years old can rarely inhale cromolyn effectively from the Spinhaler, but the cromolyn nebulizer solution permits treatment of these young children and the few older children in whom inhalation of cromolyn powder triggers coughing or wheezing. Inhalation of a β-adrenergic agonist shortly before inhalation of cromolyn usually prevents the coughing or wheezing that may follow deposition of cromolyn on highly irritable airways. An air compressor such as the DeVilbiss #561 compressor with a nebulizer delivers cromolyn solution effectively for inhalation even by infants. The cromolyn solution is compatible with both metaproterenol inhalant solution and terbutaline solution. Both cromolyn and the bronchodilators are stable in such solutions for at least one hour. Accordingly cromolyn and the bronchodilator can be nebulized simultaneously for patients who need both.

Significant adverse reactions including maculopapular eruptions, urticaria, and angioedema occur in only 1–2 percent of patients treated with cromolyn. Nasal congestion or pulmonary infiltrates with eosinophilia have been rare side effects. A few swallows of water after each treatment prevents the most common minor side effect, throat irritation due to deposition of cromolyn powder.

Indications for treatment with cromolyn include unavoidable exposure to an offending allergen such as a dog or cat, seasonal or perennial asthma that requires frequent or continual use of bronchodilators or adrenal corticosteroids, and prevention of exercise induced asthma, especially when protection is required for little more than 1 hour. Some clinicians prefer a trial with cromolyn to continual treatment with bronchodilators because of the lesser frequency of side effects with cromolyn.

It is prudent to discontinue treatment with cromolyn powder temporarily during acute asthma or status asthmaticus, when its delivery to the lower airways is impaired and when it is more likely to trigger further airway obstruction, but continued treatment with nebulized cromolyn rarely aggravates airway obstruction.

ADRENAL CORTICOSTEROIDS

Although adrenal corticosteroids are quite effective in the treatment of asthma, their use is limited by numerous possible adverse side effects (Table 18-7). The most common side effect, suppression of the hypothalamic-pituitary-adrenal axis, depends upon dose, duration of treatment, and the

Table 18-7
Possible Complications of Therapy with Adrenal Corticosteroids

Acceptable Complications	
Excessive weight gain	Insomnia
Edema	Headache
Polyphagia	Euphoria
Facial mooning	Fatigue
Development of "buffalo hump"	Increased urinary frequency and
Acne	nocturia
Ecchymoses	Leg cramps
Striae	Abdominal pain
Hypertrichosis	Leukocytosis

Serious Complications	
Endocrine	Hematopoietic
Hypothalamic-pituitary-adrenal	Agranulocytosis
suppression	Musculoskeletal
Diabetes mellitus	Growth suppression
Central nervous system	Myopathy
Psychosis	Tendon rupture
Pseudotumor cerebri	Osteoporosis
Convulsions	Aseptic necrosis
Neuritis	Ocular
Cardiovascular	Posterior subcapsular cataracts
Hypertension	Glaucoma
Thromboembolism	Exophthalmos
Arteritis	Serum electrolytes
Congestive heart failure	Hypokalemia
Gastrointestinal	Cutaneous
Peptic ulcer	Erythema nodosum
Pancreatitis	Dermatitis
Adverse effects on infection	Subcutaneous
Enhancement of virulence	Panniculitis
Masking of signs and symptoms	Fetal
Activation of latent infections	Adrenal insufficiency
Allergic	

corticosteroid selected. Some adrenal suppression can follow a single dose of hydrocortisone, and as little as 2.5 mg daily of prednisone can maintain adrenal suppression.

Adrenal function usually returns to normal within 9 months after discontinuation of treatment with exogenous corticosteroids, and plasma cortisol (hydrocortisone) concentrations may become normal within 2 weeks after discontinuation of daily treatment with prednisone in children. Adrenal insufficiency may persist longer than usual after discontinuation of treatment with steroids in rare patients, however, and fatal adrenal insufficiency has occurred as long as 24 months after discontinuation of treatment with steroids. Accordingly children at risk for adrenal insufficiency should receive supplemental parenteral corticosteroids when faced with stress such as the stress of status asthmaticus.

Suppression of linear growth may occur when the corticosteroid dosage is more than twice the normal daily secretion rate of cortisol of 12 mg/M^2. Severe asthma can also suppress growth, however, and a growth spurt may occur when severe asthma is brought under control with corticosteroids.

Use of the smallest dose necessary for adequate control of symptoms and administration for the shortest time possible minimizes adverse effects of corticosteroids. Administration of prednisone, prednisolone, or methylprednisolone at a dose of 2 mg/kg/day divided into 3 or 4 equal doses (total daily dose 20–80 mg) usually controls asthma within 3 days, but treatment for more than 3 days is necessary occasionally. After treatment for only a few days the corticosteroid can be discontinued or the dosage can be decreased gradually over several days and then discontinued. Dosage should be large enough to control symptoms.

When prolonged treatment with a corticosteroid is necessary for adequate control of asthma, inhaled beclomethasone, triamcinolone acetonide, or flunisolide is least likely to cause adverse effects (Table 18-8). Inhaled beclomethasone probably induces adrenal suppression only at doses that

Table 18-8
Recommended Doses of Inhaled Adrenal Corticosteroids

Corticosteroid	Children's Dose	Adult Dose
Beclomethasone dipropionate	42–84 μg tid-qid (max 420 μ/day)	84 μg tid-qid (max 840 μg/day)
Flunisolide	500 μg bid	500–1,000 μg bid
Triamcinolone acetonide	100–200 μg tid-qid (max 1,200 μg/d)	200 μg tid-qid (max 1,600 μg/d)

max = maximum dose
d = day
Beclomethasone and triamcinolone are usually equally effective when administered bid rather than tid or qid.

exceed 14 μg/kg/day. Even doses that exceed this cause other side effects of treatment with steroids less frequently than oral corticosteroids.

Dysphonia may occur as a side effect of treatment with inhaled corticosteroids in as many as 30 percent of adults treated with recommended doses and 50 percent of those treated with doses as high as 1600 μg/day of beclomethasone. The dysphonia is usually intermittent, but occasionally severe and persistent. It is often associated with vocal abuse. It may be due to a bilateral adductor vocal cord deformity, possible a manifestation of local steroid myopathy. Improvement often follows avoidance of vocal stress without discontinuation of treatment. The condition is reversible with discontinuation of treatment with inhaled corticosteroids, but it may persist 8–12 weeks after stopping treatment. Rarely as long as one year may be necessary for complete recovery.

Clinical oropharyngeal candidiasis occurs less frequently as a complication of treatment with inhaled corticosteroids, and its frequency is also related to the dose. It is usually mild and may remit spontaneously or responds rapidly to treatment with nystatin. It rarely necessitates discontinuation of the inhaled steroid. Rinsing the mouth after each treatment or use of a spacer tube or chamber for delivery of the inhaled corticosteroid minimizes the frequency of oropharyngeal candidiasis and may possibly also reduce the frequency of dysphonia.

Tracheobronchial and pulmonary biopsies of patients treated with inhaled beclomethasone for more than 1 year have disclosed no adverse effects.

Inhaled beclomethasone at recommended doses can maintain adrenal suppression previously induced by oral corticosteroids. Fatal adrenal insufficiency has occurred in such children during acute asthma because of underestimation of the severity of the airway obstruction and inadequate supplemental oral corticosteroids.

If continual treatment with an oral corticosteroid becomes necessary, administration of prednisone, prednisolone, or methylprednisolone as a single morning dose on alternate days reduces the risk of adrenal suppression and other side effects likely with daily oral steroids. Dexamethasone is not a suitable choice for treatment on alternate days because of its longer biologic half life.

ANTICHOLINERGIC DRUGS

Beneficial effects of anticholinergic drugs in asthmatic subjects include abolition of resting smooth muscle tone, inhibition of reflex bronchoconstriction, a decrease in the volume of tracheobronchial secretions, and inhibition of release of mediators from mast cells. Inhalation of nebulized atropine sulfate delivered by a dosimeter at doses of 0.05–0.1 mg/kg causes prompt bronchodilation that peaks within 1 hour and is sustained for 5 hours in asthmatic children. These doses may cause unacceptable side effects of tachycardia, dryness of the mouth, and blurring of the vision in adults, for whom a maximal dose of 0.025 mg/kg may be more appropriate. Atropine can elicit further bronchodilation even in asthmatic adults already treated with inhaled beta agonists, intravenous theophylline, and systemic corticosteroids for acute asthma.

Because of unpredictable systemic absorption of atropine sulfate adverse, side effects can occur at recommended doses and these can include mental confusion. Quaternary derivatives of atropine that are highly polar and lipid-insoluble are poorly absorbed across biologic membranes and do not cross the blood-brain barrier. Accordingly minimal systemic effects follow inhalation. Ipratropium bromide, one of these derivatives, is an effective bronchodilator in infants and children with airway obstruction. Bronchoconstriction that has followed inhalation of nebulized ipratropium bromide in occasional patients is not entirely accounted for by hypotonicity of the solution in which it has usually been administered.

Ipratropium affords protection against methacholine-induced bronchoconstriction but not histamine-induced or allergen-induced bronchoconstriction.

The combination of an anticholinergic drug and conventional doses of beta agonists can cause significantly more bronchodilation than either drug alone in some asthmatic patients.

EXPECTORANTS

Medications marketed as expectorants are not of established value in the treatment of asthma. Iodides can cause numerous side effects, including hypothyroidism and goiter, and therefore should be avoided. The value of water itself may be limited to prevention of dehydration and consequent inspissation of tracheobronchial secretions. Overhydration should also be avoided during treatment of status asthmaticus, and this requires frequent clinical assessment of the state of hydration.

IMMUNOTHERAPY

At least 15 published, placebo-controlled studies indicate beneficial effects of immunotherapy in patients with allergic asthma due to allergy to inhalant allergens including ragweed pollen, grass pollen, mountain cedar pollen, cat allergen, house dust, and *Dermatophagoides pteronyssinus*. Immunotherapy can induce specific, IgG blocking antibody. It can suppress the usual seasonal increase in specific, IgE antibody, and with treatment over

several years it can reduce specific IgE concentrations in the serum. Immunotherapy can reduce basophil reactivity and sensitivity to allergen, and it can
induce increases in specific IgG and IgA antibodies in secretions. It can
reduce lymphocyte responses to allergen in vitro. Immunotherapy can also
inhibit late phase asthmatic responses to inhaled allergen.

Response to immunotherapy is specific for allergens included in the
allergy extract and dependent upon the doses administered, requiring relatively large doses for efficacy. Although small doses are ineffective, treatment must begin with small doses to avoid systemic reactions to the
injections of extract. Therapy usually continues until the patient has been free
of significant symptoms or substantially improved for 1–1½ years. Improvement usually occurs in 80–90 percent of patients appropriately treated for
allergy to unavoidable inhalant allergens such as pollens or mites. Improvement usually occurs during the first year of treatment, but some who do not
improve during the first year improve during the second year.

Treatment extracts should contain only allergens to which the patient has
demonstrable allergy because immunotherapy can induce hypersensitivity
where previously there was none. Results of allergy skin testing should
correlate with the clinical history.

Controlled studies have failed to verify a beneficial effect of immunotherapy with bacterial vaccines.

Immunotherapy is indicated for most patients with allergic asthma due to
allergy to unavoidable inhalant allergens, but is not appropriate for those who
have recently failed to respond to an adequate trial of immunotherapy with
large doses of potent allergenic extracts that have included all relevant allergens.

INTERMITTENT ASTHMA

Patients who experience mild or moderate airway obstruction due to
asthma less frequently than 6 times each year require drug therapy that will
afford rapid relief of symptoms. An inhaled β-adrenergic agonist is the most
rapidly effective form of therapy suitable for administration at home. The
best choice is albuterol or fenoterol because of sustained bronchodilation for
5–6 hours and long lasting inhibition of exercise induced asthma for 6 hours
after albuterol and 4 hours after fenoterol. Dosages are indicated in Table 2.
An Inhal-Aid or Aerochamber permits effective delivery of the drug from the
metered dose inhaler for children 3–6 years old and for older children who
may be unable to coordinate actuation of the canister with inhalation. Children who are younger than 3 years old and older children who may be unable
to inhale the drug effectively from the chamber during moderately severe
airway obstruction require nebulization of the β-adrenergic agonist by an air

compressor such as the DeVilbiss #561 compressor with nebulizer. Either metaproterenol inhalant solution or terbutaline solution can be nebulized.

The patient should receive continual treatment with a brochodilator for 4–5 days after coughing and wheezing remit because some airway obstruction is likely to persist for several days after relief of symptoms. A sustained release theophylline preparation is most convenient for this purpose because of the possibility of dosing at intervals of 8 or 12 hours, and convenience correlates with compliance. Theo-Dur tablets, Slo-Bid Gyrocaps, and Somophyllin-CRT capsules are suitable sustained release preparations with bioavailability unaffected by meals. Sprinkling beads from the capsule on a teaspoonful of applesauce permits even children unable to swallow tablets or capsules to enjoy the benefits of a sustained release preparation, but the child must not chew the beads before swallowing them.

Both the inhaled beta agonist and the sustained release theophylline preparation are started at the first indication of symptoms. The inhaled beta agonist is continued only as required for relief of symptoms, but the theophylline is continued for 4–5 days after symptoms have resolved.

Infants and toddlers who cannot swallow sustained release beads require administration of a liquid theophylline preparation or metaproterenol syrup at intervals of 6 hours.

Asthma of whatever frequency requires inquiry into the possible cause and its elimination when possible. Consideration of immunotherapy may be appropriate depending on the frequency and severity of symptoms and signs.

FREQUENT OR CONTINUAL ASTHMA

Patients with symptoms of airway obstruction several times each month or somewhat less frequently if symptoms have been severe require continual drug therapy when avoidance of allergens is impossible or affords inadequate control of symptoms. It is warranted when abnormal peak expiratory flow rate or FEV_1 persists even without symptoms and may be justified by persistent abnormalities of more sensitive parameters of pulmonary function such as maximal midexpiratory flow rate.

Use of a sustained release theophylline preparation is most practical because of the long dosing interval and the bronchodilating effect. Some prefer a trial of prophylaxis with cromolyn because of the remarkable paucity of side effects of cromolyn. Whichever drug is used requires supplemental therapy with an inhaled beta agonist for relief of acute asthma that may occur despite the prophylactic therapy.

When continual treatment with theophylline at optimal doses fails to afford adequate control of symptoms and restoration of pulmonary function to normal a trial of cromolyn is indicated.

When the combination of bronchodilators and cromolyn fail to provide sufficient control a trial with an inhaled corticosteroid (beclomethasone, flunisolide, or triamcinolone) is appropriate. Cromolyn and inhaled corticosteroids are effective only after adequate delivery to the lower airways. Accordingly initiation of therapy with either requires control of airway obstruction if necessary with oral corticosteroids. Continued treatment with prednisone, prednisolone, or methylprednisolone as single doses in the morning on alternate days may be necessary if attempts to discontinue the oral corticosteroid are unsuccessful.

EXERCISE-INDUCED ASTHMA

Nasal breathing or a scarf wrapped around the nose and mouth or a cold weather mask that forms a reservoir where the last exhalation warms and humidifies air before inhalation can minimize the airway obstruction induced by strenuous exercise in asthmatics. When these measures are inadequate pretreatment with inhaled albuterol or fenoterol can inhibit exercise induced asthma for 4–6 hours. Cromolyn is less effective in inhibiting exercise induced asthma beyond the first hour after treatment, although it has some effect for as long as four hours. A sustained release theophylline preparation may be most convenient for inhibition of exercise induced asthma in a youngster who may be exercising unpredictably throughout the day, but optimal effectiveness would require continual treatment or administration of an unusually large dose to maintain the serum theophylline concentration at 15–20 μg/ml if tolerated. When a single drug does not afford adequate protection, combinations of an inhaled beta agonist with cromolyn or theophylline or all three drugs may be more effective.

A warm-up period before strenuous exercise may help minimize exercise induced asthma whether by induction of a refractory period that may persist 60–90 minutes or by some other mechanism.

Appropriate pretreatment with medication enables most children with asthma to exercise normally, but for the rare asthmatic in whom these measures are not protective activities that require only brief, intermittent exercise are likely to be more tolerable than those that require sustained strenuous exercise. Swimming is usually tolerated especially well.

PROPHYLAXIS FOR ALLERGEN EXPOSURE

Pretreatment with cromolyn is the method of choice for prevention of asthma due to predictable, unavoidable exposure to inhaled allergens. Inhalation of 20 or 40 mg is most effective during the first hour after treatment but may provide some protection for a few hours. Fortunately the drug's safety permits repeated treatment at frequent intervals if necessary.

ACUTE ASTHMA

When moderately severe airway obstruction due to acute asthma fails to improve within 15 minutes after adequate inhalation of a β-adrenergic agonist or within 30–60 minutes after oral administration of a bronchodilator the patient should seek additional immediate treatment at a physician's office or an emergency room. Patients should recognize progressive decreases in duration of bronchodilation after regular administration of an inhaled beta agonist as another indication of need for further medical intervention. Regular monitoring of pulmonary function at home with a portable instrument such as the Mini-Wright Peak Flow Meter or Pulmonary Monitor facilitates recognition of a need for additional therapy in those patients unable otherwise to recognize dangerous increases in airway obstruction.

Factors that contribute to poor responsiveness of airway obstruction to bronchodilators include inadequate dosage or inadequate inhalation technique, mucosal edema, inspissated tracheobronchial secretions, superimposed infection, acidosis, and induction of tolerance to β-adrenergic agonists. Inhaled beta agonists themselves may cause airway obstruction in rare patients. Patients are at special risk for dangerous airway obstruction during the week after discharge from the hospital after hospitalization for treatment of status asthmaticus.

Administration of 1–3 doses of 1:1,000 aqueous epinephrine by subcutaneous injection is the most commonly employed treatment for acute asthma requiring emergency treatment in the United States (Table 18-2). After satisfactory improvement injection of epinephrine suspension provides more sustained relief. Administration of terbutaline by subcutaneous injection is at least as effective and requires fewer injections because of its longer inherent duration of action. Inhalation of a β-adrenergic agonist is usually at least as effective as subcutaneous injection of epinephrine or terbutaline and is much less likely to cause adverse side effects such as tachycardia, vomiting, and muscle tremor. Inhalation therapy may be less effective than subcutaneous injection with very severe airway obstruction that may restrict delivery of the inhaled drug to some airways. The inhaled beta agonist should be delivered by simple nebulization with supplemental oxygen to prevent worsening of hypoxemia and to help correct hypoxemia already likely to be present. Intermittent positive pressure is neither necessary nor advisable because it can aggravate airway obstruction and can increase the risk of pneumothorax. Treatment with one of the more recently introduced beta agonists by inhalation may necessitate a somewhat longer period of observation to assure airway obstruction does not recur than with subcutaneous injection of epinephrine. Inhalation therapy is safer but more time consuming than injection therapy; parenteral therapy may be more effective for patients with the most severe airway obstruction.

Failure of adequate response to appropriate doses of a beta agonist establishes the diagnosis of status asthmaticus, which is discussed elsewhere in this volume.

ALLERGIC RHINITIS

Effective treatment of allergic rhinitis to facilitate filtration, warming, and humidification of inspired air is essential to optimal management of asthma in patients who have both asthma and allergic rhinitis. Avoidance of allergens and irritants such as smoke is often helpful, but drug therapy is often necessary. Treatment with H_1 antihistamines is more effective in controlling nasal discharge, sneezing, and nasal itching than in relieving nasal congestion. Preliminary data suggest treatment with an H_1 and an H_2 antihistamine in combination may help alleviate nasal congestion. Treatment with an H_1 antihistamine can cause bronchoconstriction in a small proportion of patients with asthma, however, and H_1 antihistamines are generally considered contraindicated in status asthmaticus.

Systemic decongestants often cause side effects that include tachycardia, hypertension, insomnia, nervousness, irritability, headache, nausea, vomiting, and abdominal pain. Topical decongestants spare the patient these side effects, but use for more than a few days in succession can cause rhinitis medicamentosa with increased nasal congestion.

Topical cromolyn rarely causes significant side effects and often elicits dramatic relief of symptoms of allergic rhinitis. It is most effective when treatment has been initiated before exposure to the allergen. One spray (5.2 mg) of a 4 percent solution to each nostril 4–6 times each day is usually necessary for optimal protection. Associated sneezing, nasal irritation, sore throat, or headache has necessitated discontinuation of its use in rare patients.

Intranasal beclomethasone dipropionate aerosol, 42 μg to each nostril bid-qid, or flunisolide nasal solution, 25 μg to each nostril tid or 50 μg to each nostril bid (50 μg to each nostril bid–50 μg to each nostril tid for adults), usually controls symptoms of allergic rhinitis. Mild sneezing, a transient burning sensation, and occasional epistaxis have rarely necessitated discontinuation of topical beclomethasone or flunisolide. Adrenal suppression apparently does not occur at recommended doses even in patients who are also receiving recommended doses of inhaled beclomethasone for control of asthma. Nasal biopsies of patients with allergic rhinitis treated as long as 3$^{1}/_{2}$

years with intranasal beclomethasone have disclosed no adverse effects of therapy. Septal perforation has followed prolonged treatment in two patients who had regularly directed the steroid spray toward the nasal septum.

Improvement may occur within a few days after initiation of treatment with either intranasal cromolyn or intranasal beclomethasone or flunisolide, but maximal benefit may not occur until after 1–2 weeks of treatment. Neither topical cromolyn nor topical corticosteroid is likely to be effective if adequate access to the nasal mucosa is impaired by severe nasal obstruction. Instillation of a topical decongestant a few minutes before treatment with cromolyn or the steroid may be necessary during the first few days of therapy to assure adequate treatment when substantial nasal congestant is present.

UNLABELED USE OF APPROVED DRUGS

Many of the drugs that are safest and most effective for the treatment of asthma and allergic rhinitis are not labeled for use in children. The United States Food and Drug Administration regulates industry rather than physicians, however. Lack of approval of a drug should be guided by all information available regarding safety and effectiveness in children rather than the package insert alone. Use of a drug not labeled for use in children, however, must be distinguished from use of a drug contraindicated in children because investigation has shown it to be unsafe or ineffective in children.

REFERENCES

Berman BA, Ross RN: Cromolyn. Clin Rev All 1:105–121, 1983
Brown LA, and Sly RM: Comparison of Mini-Wright and standard Wright peak flow meters. Ann All 45:72–74, 1980
Casale TB, Kaliner M: The pathophysiology of asthma. Clin Proceedings 39:200–209, 1983
Cavanaugh MJ, Cooper DM: Inhaled atropine sulfate: dose response characteristics. Am Rev Respir Dis 114:517–524, 1976
Ellis EF: Theophylline. Clin Rev All 1:73–85, 1983
Fairshter RD, Habib MP, Wilson AF: Inhaled atropine sulfate in acute asthma. Resp 42:263–272, 1981
Hendeles L, Weinberger M: Theophylline. Pharmacother 3:2–44, 1983
Ishizaka T: Analysis of triggering events in mast cells for immunoglobulin E-mediated histamine release. J All Clin Immunol 67:90–96, 1981
Mitchell EB, Wilkins S, McCallum Deighton J, et al: Reduction of house dust mite allergen levels in the home: use of the acaricide, pirimiphos methyl. Clin All 15:235–240, 1985
Orgel HA, Kemp JP, Tinkelman DG, et al: Bitolterol and albuterol metered-dose

aerosols: comparison of two long-acting beta$_2$-adrenergic bronchodilators for treatment of asthma. J All Clin Immunol 75:55–62, 1985

Rohatgi N, Sly RM: Comparison of pulmonary monitor and Wright peak flow meter. J Asthma Res 17:149–152, 1980

Schwartz AL, Lipton JM, Warburton D, et al: Management of acute asthma in childhood. Am J Dis Child 134:474–478, 1980

Siegel SC: Adrenal corticosteroids in the treatment of asthma. Clin Rev All 1:123–146, 1983

Sly RM: Current theories of the pathophysiology of asthma. J Asthma 20:419–427, 1983

Sly RM: Unlabeled use of approved drugs. J All Clin Immunol 71:515–517, 1983

Sly RM: *Textbook of Pediatric Allergy*. New Hyde Park, New York, Medical Examination Publishing Co., 1985, pp 12–187

Sly RM, Anderson JA, Bierman CW, et al: Adverse effects and complications of treatment with beta-adrenergic agonist drugs. J All Clin Immunol 75:443–449, 1985

Suschitzky JL, Sheard P: The search for antiallergic drugs for the treatment of asthma—Problems in finding a successor to sodium cromoglycate. Prog in Med Chem 21:1–61, 1984

Toogood JH, Jennings B, Greenway RW, et al: Candidiasis and dysphonia complicating beclomethasone treatment of asthma. J All Clin Immunol 65:145–153, 1980

Williams AJ, Baghat MS, Stableforth DE, et al: Dyphonia caused by inhaled steroids: recognition of a characteristic laryngeal abnormality. Thorax 38:813–821, 1983

Geoffrey Kurland
Albin B. Leong

19

The Management of Status Asthmaticus in Childhood

Asthma affects up to 10–12.5 percent of the pediatric population, and acute exacerbations of asthma are a common problem. A severe exacerbation, status asthmaticus is potentially life-threatening. Young children in particular may develop respiratory failure and acidosis secondary to severe asthma with frightening speed. For this reason, it is imperative that the clinician treat such patients vigorously, before the development of respiratory failure.

DEFINITION

The term *status asthmaticus* is difficult to define to the satisfaction of all clinicians. For the purpose of this review, we shall refer to status asthmaticus as a clinical condition characterized by acute severe wheezing, which is refractory to the administration of β-adrenergic agents by subcutaneous injection or aerosol. Although this is a broad definition, it suggests that status asthmaticus is seen in those patients who have failed to adequately improve after accepted emergency treatment of asthma.

PATHOPHYSIOLOGY

It is beyond the scope of this chapter to discuss the pathophysiology of asthma in great detail, and the reader is referred to Chapters 2, 3, and 4 and review articles by Kurland and Leong, Downes, and Boushey and co-workers for a full discussion of this topic.

Several aspects of the pathophysiology of asthma are of especial importance to the clinician dealing with the acutely ill asthmatic child, and will be briefly discussed at this time. Figure 19-1 depicts the pathophysiology of status asthmaticus. Acute asthma results in airway obstruction, a reduction in lung compliance, and hyperinflation of the thorax. Because of the relatively

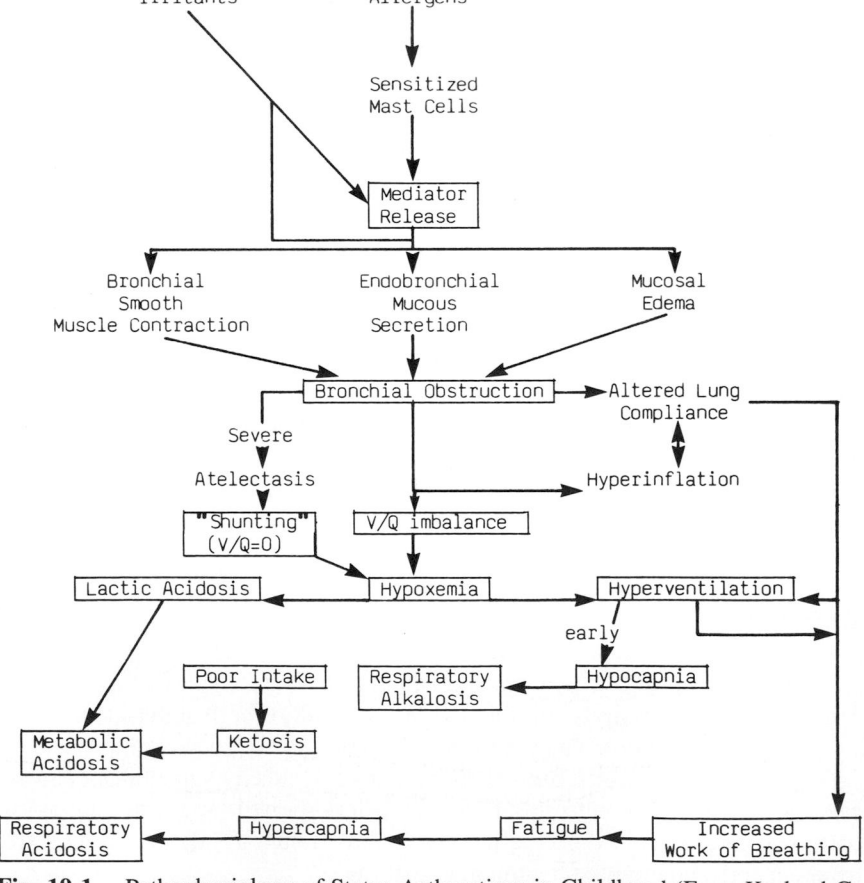

Fig. 19-1. Pathophysiology of Status Asthmaticus in Childhood (From Kurland G, Leong AB: The management of status asthmaticus in infants and children. Clin Rev Allergy 3:37, 1985. Used with permission.)

more horizontal placement of ribs in children, as well as a lower diaphragmatic position in childhood, the mechanical forces involved in respiration are less efficient. There are fewer fatigue-resistant fibers in the infant diaphragm, increasing the likelihood of fatigue in young acutely ill asthmatics. Obstruction of airways leads to ventilation/perfusion inequality and a widened alveolar-arterial gradient for oxygen. The majority of severely ill asthmatic children, therefore, will have some degree of hypoxemia. The small size of peripheral airways in infants increases airway resistance, and mucous production secondary to asthma will aggravate this condition. Further, the paucity of collateral channels of ventilation (pores of Kohn and Lambert's Canals), heightens the possibility of atelectasis secondary to this mucous production. An initially rapid respiratory rate and adequate or supranormal alveolar ventilation commonly lead to a respiratory alkalosis. A decreased oral intake of fluids and an increased respiratory rate with insensible fluid losses contribute to ketosis. With severe hypoxemia, lactic acidosis may be seen. All of these physiological changes may depress respiratory muscle and myocardial contractility, both of which can result in respiratory failure, cardiac arrhythmias, hypoperfusion, hypoxemia, and a combined respiratory and metabolic acidosis with potentially fatal consequences.

INITIAL ASSESSMENT OF THE ACUTELY ILL ASTHMATIC CHILD

We will discuss the history, physical and laboratory examinations, and therapeutics separately. In many cases, it is possible to obtain most of the history, carry out the physical examination, and initiate appropriate therapy for the asthmatic child simultaneously. Because of the potentially life threatening nature of severe asthma in childhood, we recommend that this be done whenever possible. A detailed history usually can await the initiation of treatment and clinical improvement.

History

A directed, rapid, and focused history is essential. The circumstances of the acute exacerbation, recent medication history, and complicating features such as fever or emesis should be ascertained. A limited knowledge of past hospitalizations, use of corticosteroids, and pattern of previous asthmatic episodes is important, but the clinician should obtain this information rapidly.

Physical Examination

Like the history, the physical examination of the acutely ill asthmatic child should be rapid, with attention paid to specific areas. Vital signs must include the patient's weight, temperature, respiratory rate, cardiac rate and rhythm, and blood pressure. The pulsus paradoxus, the accentuation of the normal variation in cardiac output with the respiratory cycle, is often increased in acute asthma and is related to the degree of hyperinflation. In children, there is some evidence that the degree of pulsus paradoxus present is indicative of the severity of asthma and the likelihood of success in outpatient management.

Although the chest, lungs, and heart are often examined first, the rapid assessment of the ears (to rule out otitis media), nose and sinuses (to rule out sinusitis and flaring of the alae nasi), and throat should be carried out. The neck should be palpated to assess tracheal location and to rule out the presence of subcutaneous emphysema secondary to pneumomediastinum.

A complete, yet rapid examination of the chest and lungs are central in the assessment of the acutely ill asthmatic child. The configuration of the chest, including the antero-posterior diameter, symmetry of expansion, and presence of any pectus deformity should be noted. The use of accessory muscles of respiration will alert the physician to the severity of the episode, as they are an indication of airway obstruction. The chest wall should be quickly percussed to assess both for areas of dullness suggesting atelectasis or consolidation and as an indication of the degree of hyperinflation. Auscultation of the chest, preferably with a differential stethoscope, should be done with attention to the degree of wheezing, unequal areas of air exchange, the prolongation of the expiratory phase, the presence of adventitious sounds, and the adequacy of air exchange.

The cardiac examination should include the palpation of the chest in addition to auscultation. The presence of a right ventricular heave and a loud pulmonic component of the second heart sound may indicate cor pulmonale (rare in childhood asthma). A palpable liver edge is a further indication of hyperinflation. The extremities should be assessed for nail bed cyanosis. Clubbing, if present, should suggest a diagnosis other than asthma such as cystic fibrosis. The neurologic examination should concentrate on the mental status of the child. Confusion, restlessness, irritability, and coma are all signs of impending respiratory failure.

Laboratory Evaluation

While laboratory tests are helpful in the management of children with severe asthma, therapy must not await their completion. A chest x-ray may document atelectasis, consolidation, pneumothorax, or pneumomediastinum, any of which may require specific actions related to therapy. In most instances, however, the chest x-ray will not reveal pathology that will require alterations in therapy. Further, radiology facilities are often not immediately available to the clinician. To await an x-ray while deferring therapy or to send

Table 19-1
Clinical asthma score used by Downes (Downes and Heiser, 1981)

Score	Cyanosis (or PaO$_2$ in torr)	Inspiratory breath sounds	Use of accessory muscles	Expiratory wheezes	CNS Function
0	None (70–100)	Normal	None	None	Normal
1	In air ($\leq$ 70 in air)	Unequal	Moderate	Moderate	Depressed or agitated
2	In 40% 0$_2$ ($\leq$ 70 in 40% oxygen)	Decreased or absent	Maximal	Marked	Coma

Impending Respiratory Failure: Score $\geq$ 5 or PaCO$_2$ = 55 torr or rising between 45 and 55 torr.
Respiratory Failure: Score $\geq$ 7 or PaCO$_2$ $\geq$ 65 torr.

a child with impending respiratory failure to a radiology facility are unwarranted.

Because most infectious triggers of childhood asthma are viral rather than bacterial, sputum cultures are generally not indicated in acute asthma. Complete blood counts and differential counts are not helpful, especially if the patient has received subcutaneous epinephrine as part of the initial therapy. Serum electrolytes, blood urea nitrogen determination, and urinalysis are helpful to assess hydration. A blood theophylline level is mandatory in patients who have recently received this medication. Arterial blood gases are useful in specific settings and these will be discussed in the section on therapy.

Physical findings and laboratory data are useful in clinically scoring patients. Several scoring systems have been devised, but one of the most widely used is that of Downes and his coworkers. This scoring system, shown in Table 19-1, is helpful *prognostically,* to help delineate those patients who require hospitalization or are at increased risk of developing respiratory failure, and *directive,* to establish the subset of patients requiring specific intervention such as intravenous isoproterenol or mechanical ventilation.

GENERAL MANAGEMENT

Nursing Care

Severely ill asthmatic children, particularly those in impending respiratory failure, should be cared for in an intensive care setting, preferably one with pediatric expertise. Skilled pediatric nursing is essential in the management of children with status asthmaticus. In addition to monitoring objective data such as vital signs and urine output, an experienced pediatric nurse can help alleviate anxiety and establish rapport with an acutely ill child. This will better allow for the use of equipment such as oxygen masks or nasal prongs, the inhalation of β-adrenergic agents, and the placement of intravenous lines and drawing of blood. The astute nurse can, furthermore, provide the physician with early warning of deterioration of the patient.

Oxygen

As previously mentioned, children with status asthmaticus are almost uniformly hypoxemic. In one study, the average PaO_2 in children with acute asthma was reduced to 60 torr. Because a reduction in PaO_2 below this level may lead to desaturation of hemoglobin and decreased oxygen content of the arterial blood, the use of oxygen is essential in the therapy of status asthmaticus. Most children will have a normalization of their PaO_2 by an inspired oxygen concentration of 30–50 percent. The use of Venturi mask, nasal prongs, or head hood oxygen must be individualized to the size of the patient, his cooperation, and availability of equipment. A parent holding an oxygen tubing blowing on the face of an acutely ill uncooperative infant is often better for the nursing staff, physician, and (most importantly) the patient and parent, than the option of restraining the infant so that he will stay confined in a Plexiglass head hood with a known amount of oxygen.

The theoretical possibilities of respiratory depression, creation of atelectasis, or other detriments of relatively short term administration of oxygen to the acutely ill childhood asthmatic are undetermined, but felt to be insignificant risks. Further, because the cardiac toxicities of methylxanthines and β-adrenergic agents are potentiated by hypoxemia, oxygen therapy may decrease the likelihood of myocardial dysrhythmias.

Hydration

Tachypnea, fever, a decreased intake secondary to respiratory distress, and emesis are all potential causes of an increased insensible water loss or decreased intake in children with status asthmaticus. It is not uncommon for such patients to be relatively dehydrated. Indeed, severe hypovolemia and shock requiring intravenous volume expanders has been reported in some adults with severe asthma.

Although commonly accepted, the rapid infusion of large volumes of intravenous fluids to children with status asthmaticus has the potential of leading to pulmonary edema. Further, there is little evidence that intravenous fluids will result in less viscous sputum in these patients. It is therefore recommended that patients with status asthmaticus have their urine specific gravity and BUN concentration determined. If necessary, rehydration at a rate of 1.25–1.5 times maintenance rate is suggested. The infusion rate can be slowed to a maintenance rate when the BUN and urine specific gravity are normal and the urine output is 1–2 ml/kg/hour. There is no advantage to any specific rehydrating solution. The authors commonly use 5 percent dextrose in 0.2 percent saline with added potassium chloride.

Recent studies have suggested that an increased antidiuretic hormone secretion is common in children with status asthmaticus. This should be considered in patients with hyponatremia or especially concentrated urine. When indicated, simultaneous determination of serum and urine electrolytes and osmolalities will help establish the diagnosis. The treatment for this syndrome is fluid restriction rather than the marked increase in fluids described previously.

Sodium Bicarbonate

Although metabolic acidosis and ketosis may be seen in severe status asthmaticus, the administration of sodium bicarbonate ($NaHCO_3$) in this situation is controversial. If alveolar ventilation is already compromised, the increased CO_2 following $NaHCO_3$ administration may worsen the respiratory component of the acidosis. On the other hand, severe acidosis is associated with a decrease in the responsiveness of bronchial smooth muscle to bronchodilators such as theophylline and β-adrenergic agents. Adults with status asthmaticus who require mechanical ventilation may maintain a satisfactory pH while allowing for an elevated $PaCO_2$ if $NaHCO_3$ is administered. This may potentially lessen the risk of barotrauma in such patients.

The authors recommend that $NaHCO_3$ be administered only in the presence of a low pH (<7.2) preferably secondary to both respiratory and metabolic acidosis. The dosage used is:

$$NaHCO_3 \text{ (meq)} = \text{(Base Deficit)} \times \text{Body Weight (Kg.)} \times 0.3$$

THE PHARMACOLOGIC MANAGEMENT OF STATUS ASTHMATICUS

With the improved understanding of the cellular mechanisms responsible for both allergic disease and the maintenance of normal bronchomotor tone and airway caliber, improved pharmacologic agents are available to treat acute asthma. More selective β-agents, the use of pharmacokinetic data in theophylline administration, and the aggressive use of corticosteroids have all had their effect on the management of asthma. Newer agents such as anticholinergics may soon gain an important role in the treatment of status asthmaticus. Several of the available medications act in an additive or synergistic fashion. The authors recommend their joint use for this reason. Table 19-2

Table 19-2
Summary of the Basic Management of Status Asthmaticus in Childhood

Directed history and physical examination

Laboratory Evaluation (as indicated)
  Theophylline level (see Fig. 19-2)
  Arterial blood gas
  Serum electrolytes with BUN
  Complete blood count
  Urinalysis with specific gravity
  Chest x-ray
  Pulmonary function tests (FEV$_1$, FVC, PEFR)
  Bacterial cultures

Initial treatment:
  Humidified oxygen, 30–50%
  Intravenous fluids, based on state of hydration, serum chemistries, and ability to
    take oral fluids.
  Intravenous theophylline (Fig. 19-2 and Table 19-3)
  Intravenous corticosteroid options:
    Methyl prednisolone sodium succinate: 1–2 mg/kg bolus, then 1 mg/kg every
      4–6 hr, or 2 mg/kg/24 hr continuously; OR
    Hydrocortisone sodium succinate: 5–7 mg/kg every 4–6 hr, or 2 mg/kg/hr for 12
      hr then 1 mg/kg/hr, or 2 mg/kg bolus then 0.5 mg/kg/hr; OR
    Dexamethasome phosphate: 0.25 mg/kg every 8–12 hr, or 0.25 mg/kg bolus
      then 0.3 mg/kg/24 hr.
  Aerosolized β-adrenergic agent and suggested dosage options
    Metaproterenol 5% solution: 0.1–0.3 cc (based on patient age and size) diluted in
      2–3 cc saline, up to every 30 min. for 2 hr, then every hr for 4 hr, then every 2–4
      hr; OR
    Isoetharine, 1% solution: 0.25–0.5 cc (based on patient age and size), diluted in
      2–3 cc saline, every 1–4 hr; OR
    Isoproterenol, 1:200 solution: 0.1–0.3 cc (based on patient age and size) diluted in
      2–3 cc saline, every 1–4 hr.

outlines the initial medical management of children with status asthmaticus.
A more detailed pharmacologic discussion of each of these agents may be
found in Chapter 18.

Adrenergic Agonists*

Although epinephrine (adrenaline) has been the standard therapeutic
agent for the treatment of acute asthma since the early part of this century, the

---

* See also Chapter 22.

improved understanding of the pharmacology of agents related to epinephrine has greatly improved the medical armamentarium in the recent past. The elucidation of the α- and β-adrenergic systems and the further subdivision of the beta into the more selective β_1 and β_2 receptors has permitted the development of the β_2-selective agents with greater bronchodilatory effect relative to their effect on cardiac rate and contractility.

The delivery of β-adrenergic agents by inhalation to infants and children with status asthmaticus remains somewhat controversial. Certainly, there is good evidence that this method of delivery is effective in children who can co-operate with the technique. There is controversy over the ability of the airway of the young infant (less than 20 months of age) to respond with bronchodilatation after the administration of a β-adrenergic agent. Further, the very young infant, acutely ill with asthma, is often uncooperative with attempts at the administration of such agents. The concomitant use of oral and inhaled β-adrenergic agents is advocated by some investigators, on the grounds that the sites of action of oral and inhaled medications may be additive.

The dosage, choice, and exact mode and frequency of administration of β-adrenergic agents are all difficult to state as absolutes. Although *in vitro* data may show major differences in potency of various agents, *in vivo* studies are much more difficult to carry out and interpret. Isoproterenol, the former mainstay of inhaled adrenergics, has both β_1 and β_2 effects and is a potent bronchodilator. The more selective β_2 agents such as isoetharine, metaproterenol, terbutaline, fenoterol, albuterol, and carbuterol, have fewer undesirable β_1 effects, but are not more potent bronchodilators on a molar basis when compared with isoproterenol. However, the newer agents, with the exception of isoetharine, have the advantage of a longer duration of action.

The authors currently administer inhaled β_2-adrenergic agents to all children with status asthmaticus except those receiving intravenous isoproterenol. We have utilized metaproterenol, 0.01 ml/kg/dose of a 5 percent solution diluted in 2.5–3.0 ml of normal saline, by aerosol administration up to every 30 minutes for 2 hours, then hourly for 4 hours without noting deleterious side effects. Less frequent administration of metaproterenol, however, is often adequate adrenergic therapy for many children with status asthmaticus.

METHYLXANTHINES.†

Methylxanthines have a long and controversial history in the treatment of acute asthma. Theophylline remains the most important of these agents and will, therefore, be the subject of this discussion. Structurally related to caf-

---

†See also Chapter 18.

feine, theophylline is completely and rapidly absorbed from the gastrointestinal tract, but its intravenous use is particularly important in the treatment of status asthmaticus. Dilute solutions of theophylline in 5 percent dextrose, ready for intravenous use, are now available.

The therapeutic index of theophylline is narrow, and side effects include life-threatening cardiac arrhythmias and seizures. The availability of rapid and accurate assays for blood levels of theophylline enables clinicians to use this medication more safely. The understanding of the pharmacokinetics of theophylline is one of the most important developments in the treatment of patients with status asthmaticus.

The administration of theophylline as the ethylenediamine *salt* (aminophylline) intravenously in periodic infusions has been supplanted by the use of pure theophylline in dilute solution as a continuous intravenous infusion. This allows for a stable serum theophylline level, which can minimize side effects and allow for more uniform bronchodilatation. The prerequisite for the safe administration of theophylline in any form is the ability to rapidly measure blood theophylline levels.

Because the bronchodilatation secondary to theophylline is related to the blood concentration, it is necessary to establish a therapeutic blood level as soon as possible in the acutely ill patient. The initiation of a theophylline infusion with a *loading* dose, or bolus, to establish this level is important, as the achievement of a therapeutic level with only a slow continuous infusion would be prohibitively delayed. Multiple factors must be taken into account before deciding on both the correct loading dose and the infusion rate for each patient. These include the age of the patient, any recent theophylline administration, the presence of a febrile viral illness, and the use of other medications such as macrolide antibiotics (e.g. erythromycin) which may interfere with theophylline clearance. Several schedules and computer-assisted methods for the safe administration of theophylline by continuous infusion have been devised. Our suggested treatment schedule for theophylline is outlined in Table 19-3 and Figure 19-2.

If no theophylline preparation has been recently taken, the patient is given a loading dose of 4–6 mg/kg lean body weight over 30 minutes. If oral theophylline has been taken, a blood theophylline level is drawn and sent *stat* and the loading dose is decreased.

The infusion solution is either 0.8 mg/ml or 1.6 mg/ml of theophylline in 5 percent dextrose. This solution is *piggy backed* into the intravenous rehydration solution. The loading dose is administered over 30 minutes and the rate then immediately decreased to provide the continuous infusion. The previously obtained prebolus level can be used to make readjustments in the infusion. If the level is very low and the clinician has given a low bolus infusion, then an additional bolus may be administered. If signs of theophylline toxicity appear, or if the prebolus level already suggests the potential

Table 19-3
Theophylline: suggested initial dosage for
maintenance intravenous infusion. (See also,
Figure 19-2. The initial infusion dosage
should be modified and/or levels followed
more closely in the presence of factors
affecting clearance.)

Patient Age	Theophylline Infusion Rate (mg/kg/hr)
Infants: 6–52 weeks	(Age in weeks $\times$ 0.008) + 0.21
1–9 years	0.8
9–12 years	0.7
12–16 years (non-smoker)	0.7
12–16 years (smoker)	0.5

Notes: (1) Theophylline (mg) = Aminophylline (mg) $\times$ 0.8; (2) In obese
patients, use lean body weight to calculate theophylline dosage; (3) Total
initial dosage in older patients who have not previously received theophylline should not exceed 900 mg/24 hr; (4) Serum theophylline levels must
be followed in all patients receiving theophylline by continuous intravenous infusion.

danger of a toxic level with the bolus infusion, the infusion can be interrupted, the theophylline level determined, and the infusion rate then adjusted.

After approximately 6 hours of uninterrupted infusion of theophylline,
the blood theophylline level should be determined and the projected steady-
state level calculated. If the 6 hour and the projected level are both in the
therapeutic range, the infusion is continued and the true level obtained in 12–
24 hours. The infusion can be further modified if any of the levels are out of
the therapeutic range.

Of major importance is the need for clinical judgement. If symptoms
suggestive of theophylline toxicity appear, or if the patient deteriorates and a
subtherapeutic theophylline level is suspected, then a blood theophylline
level is mandatory. The ability of the laboratory to provide rapid determination of blood theophylline levels is paramount in enabling the clinician to use
this medication effectively and safely.

CORTICOSTEROIDS.‡

For over 30 years, corticosteroids have been a mainstay in the pharmacologic management of allergic disease, including asthma. Despite this, the
evidence documenting the beneficial effects of corticosteroids in status
asthmaticus is not absolutely conclusive. There have been relatively few
rigorous, double-blind, well controlled studies of the effects of cortico-

---

‡ See also Chapter 18.

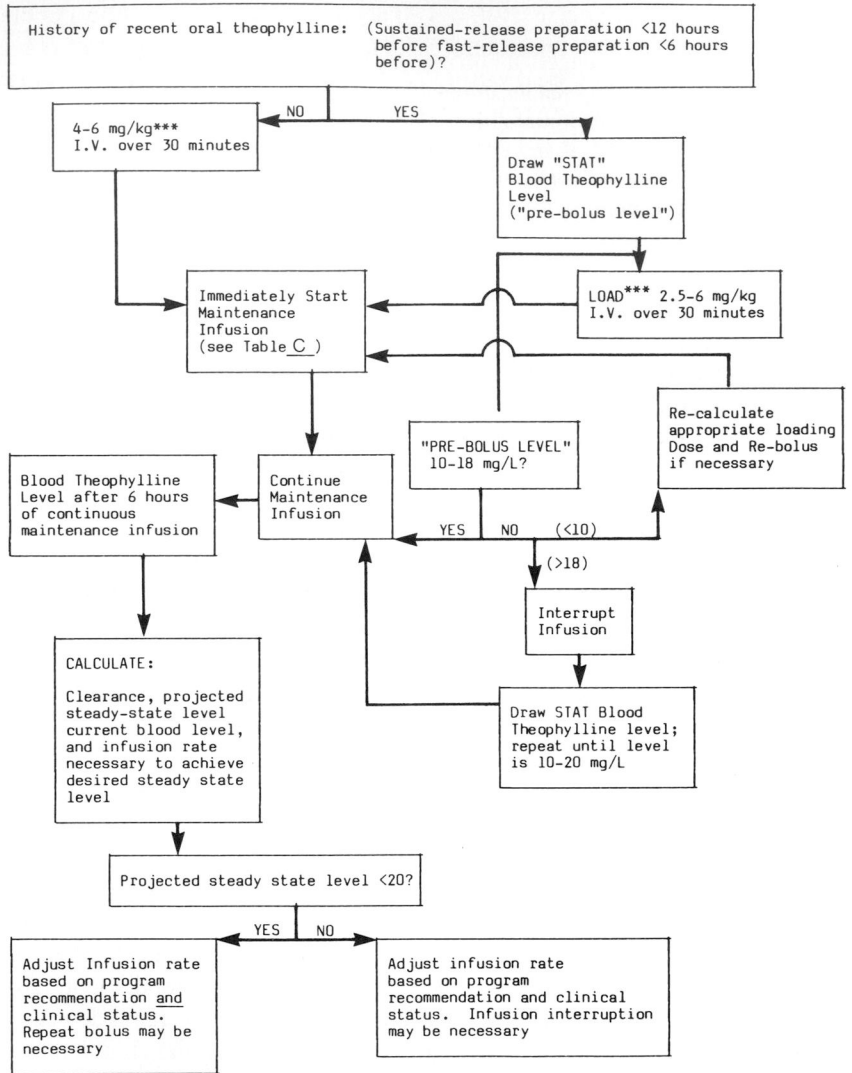

Theophylline*: Decision Making** During Treatment of Status Asthmaticus

History of recent oral theophylline: (Sustained-release preparation <12 hours before fast-release preparation <6 hours before)?

NO → 4-6 mg/kg*** I.V. over 30 minutes

YES → Draw "STAT" Blood Theophylline Level ("pre-bolus level")

LOAD*** 2.5-6 mg/kg I.V. over 30 minutes

Immediately Start Maintenance Infusion (see Table C)

Re-calculate appropriate loading Dose and Re-bolus if necessary

"PRE-BOLUS LEVEL" 10-18 mg/L?

Blood Theophylline Level after 6 hours of continuous maintenance infusion

Continue Maintenance Infusion

YES   NO   (<10)

(>18)

Interrupt Infusion

CALCULATE:

Clearance, projected steady-state level current blood level, and infusion rate necessary to achieve desired steady state level

Draw STAT Blood Theophylline level; repeat until level is 10-20 mg/L

Projected steady state level <20?

YES   NO

Adjust Infusion rate based on program recommendation and clinical status. Repeat bolus may be necessary

Adjust infusion rate based on program recommendation and clinical status. Infusion interruption may be necessary

*All doses are given as Theophylline. Theophylline (mg) = Aminophylline (mg) x 0.8.

**Decision making utilizes projected values from programmable calculator.(94) Clinical judgment of need for blood theophylline levels, based on patients condition should always take precedence.

***Use lean body weight for calculating loading dose.

****Adjustment of loading dose when there is a history of recent theophylline dose is based on the history of recent dosage(s) and preparation(s), compliance, and previous theophylline levels, if available.

Fig. 19-2. Theophylline: Decision Making During Treatment of Status Asthmaticus (From Kurland G, Leong AB: The management of status asthmaticus in infants and children. Clin Rev Allergy 3:37, 1985. Used with permission.)

432

steroids on acute asthma in children. The weight of the literature coupled with a large amount of anectdotal evidenced strongly supports the use of corticosteroids in this clinical setting. A further important point is that there are few, if any, side effects from a relatively brief course of corticosteroids, as long as the total dose is not excessive. In most instances, the need for high doses of corticosteroids in children with status asthmaticus is less than 5 days. With improvement, the dosage is reduced to a more reasonable, single daily dose.

While there is agreement that corticosteroids should be used in acute asthma of childhood, there is little agreement on the corticosteroid preparation, dosage, or dosing interval that is optimal in this setting. The Section on Allergy and Immunology of the American Academy of Pediatrics recently recommended that children with status asthmaticus be treated with an intravenous loading dose of hydrocortisone hemisuccinate, dexamethasone phosphate, or betamethasone phosphate equivalent to 1–2 mg/kg of prednisone, followed by the administration of the equivalent dosage over the following 24 hours, either by continuous infusion or in divided doses. There are no studies to specifically support this recommendation. Currently, the authors use intravenous methylprednisolone in a dose of 1 mg/kg every 6 hours. This dosage has the advantage of being easy to remember, and it is the equivalent of a high dose of prednisone with few side effects.

Because corticosteroids are not rapidly acting, with 6–8 hours being required before a clinical effect is seen, it is imperative that they be used early. Observing a child who has severe asthma and witholding corticosteroids while hoping that theophylline and β-adrenergic agents will provide satisfactory relief of the bronchospasm is assuming a risk that probably exceeds the small risk of the corticosteroids.

The clinician often is faced with an acutely ill asthmatic patient who has received corticosteroids within the past year. If the dosage received could potentially result in the suppression of the hypothalamic-pituitary-adrenal axis in the patient, corticosteroids should be administered to prevent adrenal insufficiency as well as to treat the acute asthmatic episode.

Isoproterenol by Continuous Intravenous Infusion

Several authors have suggested that the continuous intravenous infusion of isoproterenol (CIIS) is an alternative to mechanical ventilation in children with severe asthma who develop impending respiratory failure. The strongest proponent of this technique is Downes, who, with his coworkers, has a large experience with this technique. There are specific advantages of intravenous isoproterenol, which include its rapidity of onset, potency, and rapid metabolism. The authors agree with Downes that CIIS be used in children with status asthmaticus and impending respiratory failure despite therapy with intravenous theophylline, corticosteroids and inhaled β-adrenergic agents. The criteria for the use of CIIS includes a clinical score (Downes) $\geq$ 5, or $PaCO_2 \geq$ 55 torr or rapidly rising between 45 and 55 torr. In patients with severe acidosis and a markedly elevated $PaCO_2$, however, mechanical ventilation may be more prudent.

Major complications of CIIS include cardiac arrhythmias, especially ventricular tachycardia, and bronchorrhea. These complications generally respond to discontinuing or interrupting the infusion. Because one of the metabolites of isoproterenol, 3-0-methylisoproterenol, is a weak beta-blocker with a prolonged half-life, β-adrenergic blockade is a theoretical risk. For this reason, CIIS should be tapered slowly to prevent rebound bronchospasm from β-adrenergic blockade. Myocardial ischemia and/or necrosis are also potential complications of CIIS, and both of these have been documented in patients receiving CIIS.

A summary of a technique for delivering CIIS is outlined in Table 19-4. While Downes advocates discontinuing theophylline during CIIS, the authors and others continue this medication. It must be pointed out that theophylline clearance may be increased during the administration of isoproterenol. Further as both theophylline and isoproterenol are potentially cardiotoxic, the theophylline level, blood gases, and isoproterenol infusion must be carefully monitored.

Intravenous access for isoproterenol must be secured with a well functioning intravenous line reserved for this medication only. Arterial blood gases must be monitored using an indwelling arterial catheter. Delivery of isoproterenol by an infusion pump assures control over the infusion rate. Isoproterenol is diluted in 5 percent dextrose and initially infused at a rate of 0.05 mcg/kg/minute. If neither clinical response nor adverse effects are seen after 15–20 minutes, the infusion is doubled to administer 0.1 mcg/kg/minute. Arterial blood gases are obtained at least 10 minutes after every alteration of the infusion rate. The dose is doubled every 15–20 minutes until a rate of 0.8 mcg/kg/minute is achieved or until improvement is noted. If a clinical response is not achieved, the rate is increased by 0.2–0.4 mcg/kg/minute increments until a clinical response is seen or toxicity is noted. The maximum recommended dosage is 6.0 mcg/kg/minute, although the average dosage required to see initial improvement is usually far less (0.3 mcg/kg/minute in Downes' series).

A clinical response to CIIS is defined as a decrease in the $PaCO_2$ to less than 55 torr or a reduction of $PaCO_2$ by 10 percent from the preinfusion value. If tachycardia (180–200/min) supervenes, or if a cardiac dysrhythmia is noted, the infusion must be promptly decreased or terminated. Usually, patients who respond to CIIS have a nearly simultaneous improvement in their respiratory status with a decrease in $PaCO_2$ and an increase in heart rate to greater than 140–150 bpm.

After clinical improvement is noted, the infusion rate must usually be

Table 19-4
Intravenous isoproterenol in childhood status asthmaticus with
impending respiratory failure. (See text for details.)

Preparation
    Arterial catheter placement
    Separate indwelling intravenous access for isoproterenol
    Continuous EKG monitoring
    Discontinue aerosolized beta-adrenergic agents
    Notify arterial blood gas laboratory of need for frequent determinations
    Baseline laboratory: Arterial blood gas, EKG, theophylline level, cardiac enzymes

Isoproterenol Infusion
    Initial isoproterenol dilution for intravenous use:
        Use standard ampule: 0.2 mg/ml
        Dilution: Patient's weight (kg) $\times$ 0.15 = mg of isoproterenol added to 100 ml of
          5% dextrose

    Example: 20 kg patient: 20 $\times$ 0.15 = 3.0 mg added to 100 ml of 5% dextrose

    Initial dose: 0.05 mcg/kg/min = 2 ml/hr of above dilution

    Measure arterial blood gases 15–20 min after initiation and after each dosage
      change

    Increase isoproterenol by a factor of 2 every 15–20 min up to a level of 0.8
      mcg/kg/min. Increments thereafter are by 0.2–0.4 mcg/kg/min.

Increase isoproterenol until one of the following:
    $PaCO_2$ decreases to < 55 torr *or* decreases by at least 10% of preinfusion $PaCO_2$.
    Further increase may be required to achieve or maintain normocapnia.

    Tachycardia > 200 bpm: decrease infusion rate.
    Cardiac dysrhythmia: discontinue infusion.
    Maximum isoproterenol dosage is unknown. Downes suggests a maximum of
      6 mcg/kg/min.

Measure cardiac enzymes and theophylline every 12–24 hr, EKG every 24 hr.

After $PaCO_2$ improves, *continue* isoiproterenol infusion at least, 12–24 hr, then
    slowly taper over 24–36 hr.
    Average duration of infusion required is 2 days.
    Stop infusion if patient stable on rate of 0.1 mcg/kg/min.

increased to achieve normocapnia. The infusion rate is continued for at least 12 hours and then gradually tapered over at least 24 hours, while the child is closely monitored. Rebound bronchospasm necessitating a transient increase in the infusion rate during tapering has been described. When the tapered dosage is 0.1 mcg/kg/minute, the infusion is discontinued.

When a patient is treated with CIIS, the blood theophylline level, serum cardiac enzymes, and EKG must be closely monitored along with arterial blood gases.

MECHANICAL VENTILATION

Mechanical ventilation was the sole treatment of impending respiratory failure in severe asthma prior to the description of CIIS, and it is still required in some severe cases. The technique is not without morbidity or mortality, however. Complications may include barotrauma, oxygen toxicity, mechanical failure of the ventilator equipment, occlusion of the endotracheal tube, intubation of the esophagus or of a mainstem bronchus, and postextubation subglottic stenosis.

In children requiring mechanical ventilation for respiratory failure, intravenous access should be established as rapidly as possible. Intubation should be carried out by the most skilled available individual, preferably an anesthesiologist with pediatric experience. A nasogastric tube should be passed to evacuate stomach contents and minimize the risk of aspiration. Premedication to facilitate intubation usually includes intravenous atropine (10–20 mcg/kg), ketamine (2 mg/kg) and succinylcholine (4 mg/kg). Orotracheal intubation is the most rapid method to establish a controlled airway. If prolonged intubation is likely, then elective nasotracheal intubation can be carried out under controlled circumstances. Because high airway pressures are often required to mechanically ventilate children with severe asthma, a large bore endotracheal tube should be used. This will minimize the need for high flow rates and will also decrease the overall resistance encountered during mechanical ventilation. For patients under the age of 8–10 years, an uncuffed endotracheal tube is generally used; older patients will require an endotracheal tube with a low-pressure high-volume inflatable cuff.

Following intubation, a chest x-ray to document endotracheal tube position and to detect pneumomediastinum, pneumothorax, or atelectasis is mandatory. If a pneumothorax is present, closed chest thoracostomy tube drainage is usually necessary. Continuous monitoring of the cardiac rate and rhythm and the placement of an indwelling arterial catheter for blood pressure and blood gas determinations are essential. A bladder catheter to document urine flow is also recommended.

A volume-preset ventilator is most useful in treating the acutely ill asthmatic child with respiratory failure. A delivered tidal volume of 15–20 ml/

kg, after allowing for internal compliance of the ventilator and the tubing is a reasonable starting point. Positive end-expiratory pressure (PEEP) is not recommended, as it adds to expiratory obstruction. A prolonged expiratory phase (inspiratory:expiratory ratio of 1:1.5 or greater) allows for improved ventilation. A slow rate of ventilation will provide adequate inspiratory and expiratory times as well as minimizing turbulent flow which increase resistance. At the start of mechanical ventilation, 100 percent oxygen should be delivered, while arterial blood gases are used to direct changes in ventilator settings. When possible, PaO_2 should be maintained between 80 and 100 torr. The $PaCO_2$ may be allowed to rise to a level somewhat above the physiologic range, as long as the pH is not less than 7.30. In some instances, it may be necessary to administer $NaHCO_3$ to correct the arterial pH even though alveolar ventilation, as reflected by the $PaCO_2$, is still inadequate.

Neuromuscular blockade with intravenous pancuronium bromide in a dose of 0.1 mg/kg every hour or by continuous infusion allows for coordination of the patient with the ventilator and reduces the risk of barotrauma. Intravenous diazepam may be given at a dose to provide sedation (0.2–0.3 mg/kg) every 1–3 hours. Morphine sulfate is also effective for sedation, although it theoretically may result in nonspecific histamine release from tissue mast cells.

Because of the increased risk of atelectasis in the paralyzed mechanically ventilated child with severe asthma, close attention to pulmonary toilet and clearance of thick secretions from the airways is important. The use of a side port valve to allow for continued ventilation during suctioning will reduce the risk of hypoxemia. If significant atelectasis is present and is unresponsive to routine suctioning and chest physiotherapy in the ventilated patient, flexible fiberoptic bronchoscopy is suggested.

Generally, mechanical ventilation of children with severe asthma and respiratory failure is required for 12–24 hours. CIIS may be given during mechanical ventilation, although the same complications of CIIS may be seen and the same technique for delivery of CIIS is utilized.

Although occasional children will tolerate a tapering IMV rate while breathing spontaneously, this technique of weaning from the ventilator is not advised. Before attempting to discontinue mechanical ventilation, Downes states that the following criteria should be met by the patient:

1. There should be a sustained bronchomotor response to intravenous isoproterenol or subcutaneous epinephrine, characterized by a decrease in either wheezing or peak airway pressure for at least 1 hour.
2. The chest x-ray should demonstrate a decrease in hyperaeration, no significant atelectasis, and no air leak (e.g., pneumothorax).
3. The $PaCO_2$ should be less than 45 torr, and the minute ventilation should be less than 150 percent of the predicted normal for age, sex, and height.
4. The PaO_2 should be greater than 200 torr in 50 percent oxygen.

When these criteria are met, the patient is usually ready for extubation. Chest physiotherapy and tracheobronchial suctioning are carried out in preparation for extubation. The patient is given intravenous atropine (20 mcg/kg) and neostigmine (70 mcg/kg), which should lead to spontaneous respirations. Once the patient demonstrates vigorous spontaneous respirations, he should be allowed to ventilate through a *T-piece* adaptor while breathing an increased oxygen concentration. Arterial blood gases should be followed to ensure adequate PaO_2 and $PaCO_2$ levels. If the patient is thus clinically stable for several hours, without evidence of deterioration, atelectasis, or respiratory acidosis, the endotracheal tube can be removed. After extubation, oxygen should be delivered by mask, other medications for the treatment of asthma should be continued, and the patient should be observed closely for signs of deterioration.

COMPLICATIONS

Children with status asthmaticus may suffer from complications of the illness as well as those related to therapy. Most of the important complications secondary to therapy have been already discussed.

It is estimated that up to 25 percent of children requiring hospitalization for acute asthma have abnormalities on chest radiographs. Of these findings, the most frequent was the presence of perihilar infiltrates, although atelectasis and pneumomediastinum are fairly common (5–20 percent). Pneumothorax in children with acute asthma is rare. The chest radiograph is more useful in patients with findings such as decreased breath sounds or localized rales, but only rarely does the x-ray lead to a major change in therapy.

Mucous plugging, leading to atelectasis or airway obstruction is occasionally noted in children and adults with severe asthma. This complication can lead to worsening hypoxemia in the patient affected; further, severe atelectasis may compromise gas exchange and perfusion in the unaffected lung. There are several reports of the efficacy of bronchopulmonary lavage using the flexible bronchoscope in adults with severe atelectasis.

As mentioned earlier, fluid therapy must be carefully administered in children with acute asthma because of the potential for pulmonary edema or the syndrome of inappropriate antidiuretic hormone secretion (SIADH). Recent data suggests that ADH levels are elevated in many children with acute asthma. These findings support the cautious use of fluids in such patients.

Electrocardiographic evidence of cor pulmonale has been noted in some adults with acute severe asthma ($PaCO_2 \geq 45$ torr, pH ≤ 7.39). Studies to document clinically significant cor pulmonale in children with status asthmaticus are not available, although it is not felt to be a major problem. If present, it is probably secondary to the combination of the markedly negative pleural pressures and an increase in the right heart transmural pressure.

A rare poliomyelitis-like illness resulting in permanent residual weakness which occurred during the recovery from an acute exacerbation of asthma has been described by Hopkins and Shield. In this syndrome, isolated lower motor neuron paralysis without evidence of sensory loss occurs usually in one extremity. Appearing from 4–11 days after the onset of acute asthma, this syndrome has a rapid progression and may present with meningeal signs, muscle pain or tenderness. A cerebrospinal lymphocytic pleocytosis with an elevated protein are sometimes seen. The etiology is unclear, and no specific viral agent has been implicated.

PROJECTIONS FOR THE FUTURE

The treatment of status asthmaticus has improved in the past several decades. With an improved knowledge of the current pharmocologic management of asthma, safer drugs will become available. With an increased understanding of the cellular basis for acute asthma, unique and more specific medications will no doubt follow.

Newer β-adrenergic agents with an improved β_2 specificity and a longer half-life are currently under intense development. Albuterol (salbutamol) is one such agent, which has recently been released in this country for oral and hand-held pressurized aerosol usage. It is widely used in Europe and may eventually supplant aerosolized metaproterenol and intravenous isoproterenol in this country. Fenoterol is another β_2-adrenergic agent with a long duration of action that should become available in the near future. Terbutaline, already used as an oral and injectable preparation in adults, has undergone study in children. A subcutaneous injection of 12 mcg/kg of terbutaline has bronchodilatation approximately equal to 10 mcg/kg of epinephrine, with fewer side effects. Bitolterol has been recently released as a hand-held metered dose inhaler, but is limited to use in adults. There are other β_2-adrenergic agents being developed, including pirbuterol, carbuterol, and clenbuterol.

A major advancement in the understanding of the pathophysiology of asthma is the delineation of the role of the parasympathetic nervous system. It has been recognized for centuries that parasympatholytic medications were effective in the treatment of asthma. Aerosolized atropine is an effective bronchodilator, but is limited by side effects such as dry mouth, blurred vision, tachycardia, and urinary retention. Ipatroprium bromide, a quaternary ammonium derivation of atropine, has received widespread interest because of its greater bronchomotor selectivity without the degree of side effects seen with atropine. It is an effective bronchodilator in children and has an additive effect with albuterol in adults. A second promising preparation is glycopyrollate, which has had preliminary trials in childhood asthmatic subjects and is especially noteworthy because of its duration of action, which approaches 12 hours. The development of both of these new agents should spur the further investigation and development of new antimuscarinic agents for childhood asthma.

Because of the postulated roles played by calcium in the maintenance of bronchomotor tone, the release of mast cell mediators, and the production and secretion of mucous in the airway, calcium channel blocking agents are potential additions to the pharmacologic armamentarium. At present, the use of any of these agents is experimental, although there is preliminary evidence that nifedipine is a mildly effective bronchodilator.

The search for other medications to treat acute asthma has included α-adrenergic antagonists, inhaled antihistamines, and inhibitors of the lipoxygenase pathway of arachidonaic acid metabolism. The latter avenue of research is based on the recent identification of certain leukotrienes as being the potent bronchoconstrictors known as the slow reacting substance of anaphylaxis (SRS-A). Thus far, the available substances are not well enough studied to justify speculation on their ultimate clinical usefulness. It is likely, however, that continued research to develop both more specific bronchodilators and medications to interrupt the pathogenic mechanisms of asthma at the cellular level will be successful.

ROLE OF PREVENTION

It should be stressed that status asthmaticus is a life-threatening event within the course of a complex disease. As such, the prevention of the acute exacerbations of asthma must remain a foremost priority of the clinician, the patient, and the patient's family.

An especially sobering observation is that of the childhood asthmatic who has sudden death before he or she can receive medical assistance. Kravis and her coworkers have noted several characteristics of children with chronic asthma that place them at an increased risk for sudden death. These include: (1) medication related factors, such as inappropriate use of corticosteroids, excessive usage of adrenergic aerosols, and noncompliance; (2) unsuspected pulmonary pathology; (3) serious psychosocial maladaption; (4) early, severe onset of wheezing, particularly in the first year of life; and (5) prediliction for abrupt airway narrowing. Other studies have also underscored the importance of early intervention, including systemic corticosteroids and maximal bronchodilator therapy. This is especially true in patients at known increased risk for severe bronchospasm upon exposure to a significant *trigger*. Further, the need for family and patient education as well as close medical follow up are essential to these patients. Through prevention, it is hoped that the life-threatening exacerbations of asthma can be kept to a minimum. Meanwhile, it is necessary that physicians treating asthmatic children recognize the potential severity of their asthma. By maintaining the expertise to care for the acutely ill asthmatic child, the physician can minimize the morbidity and mortality of this disease.

REFERENCES

American Academy of Pediatrics, Section on Allergy and Immunology: Management of asthma. Pediatrics 68:874, 1981.

Bohn D, Kalloghlian A, Jenkins J, et al: Intravenous salbutamol in the treatment of status asthmaticus in children. Crit Care Med 12:892, 1984

Boushey HA, Holtzman MJ, Sheller JR, et al: Bronchial hyperreactivity. Am Rev Respir Dis 121:389, 1980

Cavanaugh MJ, Cooper DM: Inhaled atropine sulfate: dose response characteristics. Am Rev Respir Dis 114:517, 1975

Cohen RM: A pharmacokinetic approach to the use of theophylline in status asthmaticus. Ann Allergy 54:1, 1985

Downes JJ, Heiser MS: Status asthmaticus in children, in Gregory GA (ed) *Respiratory Failure in the Child.* New York, Churchill Livingstone, 1981, pp 107–133

Downes JJ, Wood DW, Harwood I, et al: Intravenous isoproterenol infusion in children with severe hypercapnia due to status asthmaticus. Crit Care Med 1:63, 1973

Downes JJ, Wood DW, Striker TW, et al: Arterial blood gas and acid base disorders in infants and children with status asthmaticus. Pediatrics 42:238, 1968

Garra B, Shapiro GG, Dorsett CS, et al: A double-blind evaluation of the use of nebulized metaproterenol and isoproterenol in hospitalized asthmatic children and adolescents. J Allergy Clin Immunol 60:63, 1977

Gross NJ, Skorodin MS: Anticholinergic, antimuscarinic bronchodilators. Am Rev Resp Dis 129(5):857, 1984

Hendeles L, Weinberger M: Theophylline: A "state of the art" review. Pharmacotherapy 3:2, 1983

Herman JJ, Noah ZL, Moody RR: Use of intravenous isoproterenol for status asthmasticus in children. Crit Care Med 11:716, 1983

Johnson BE, Suratt PM, Gal TJ, et al: Effect of inhaled glycopyrrolate and atropine in asthma. Chest 85:325, 1984

Kattan M, Gurwitz D, Levison H: Corticosteroids in status asthmaticus. J Pediatr 96:596, 1980

Kravis LP, Kolski GB: Unexpected death in childhood asthma. Am J Dis Child 139:558, 1985

Kurland G, Leong AB: The management of status asthmaticus in infants and children. Clin Rev Allergy 3:37, 1985

Lawford P, Jones BJM, Milledge A: Comparison of intravenous and nebulized salbutamol in initial treatment of severe asthma. Br Med J 1:84, 1978

Gibbe H. Parsons

20

Treatment of Asthma in Adults

The wheezing patient usually arrives in the physician's office with the diagnosis already made. Often family members also have had asthma and the symptoms of the disease are easily recognized, (i.e., episodic chest tightness, cough with little sputum, wheezing, and shortness of breath). Less commonly, such symptoms are not recognized as asthma and patients believe they suffer from frequent *colds* or, in older patients, heart failure or exacerbations of chronic bronchitis.

Once the diagnosis of asthma is confirmed, the physician must address the type of medical management to be used. Individual physicians who treat asthmatics have a different set of background experiences in managing cases of different etiologies and severities and have witnessed both dramatic successes as well as chronic failures. There is no specific drug regimen appropriate for all patients, and in any given case there may be widely divergent views between physicians regarding the specifics of treatment. Nonetheless, the general goals of therapy can usually be agreed upon, despite different approaches to management. All regimens of therapy should have a major goal to keep the patient functional and able to live and work with minimal interference from disease symptoms or drug side effects. Indeed, frequent emergency room visits or hospital admissions represent a failure of adequate outpatient management.

The success in management can often be measured by the degree of independence the patient has from the physician. If patients receive adequate education so that they understand the nature of the disease, the early symp-

BRONCHIAL ASTHMA, Second Edition
ISBN 0-8089-1814-1

toms of an asthmatic attack, the basic pharmacology of the drugs available for treating asthma, and how to take the drugs, they may not only avoid the necessity for emergency room visits and hospital admissions, but may significantly reduce dependence upon the physician. Indeed, there are many mild asthmatics who are able to control symptoms adequately with over-the-counter preparations such as aerosolized epinephrine, and remain independent from physicians. Nonetheless, the majority of asthmatics will eventually develop intermittent episodes of more severe bronchospasm, leading to a physician evaluation. This chapter deals with the approach to these patients including selected aspects of diagnosis, therapeutics, a few special problems, and unifying concepts for patients education.

DEFINING THE PATIENT'S DISEASE

The patient's history is important, not only in establishing the diagnosis of asthma, but also for defining those factors that trigger or exacerbate attacks. Indeed, the diagnosis of asthma (Table 20-1) is aided by a history of episodic dyspnea, cough, chest tightness, and wheezing, a history of allergic rhinitis or atopic dermatitis, or a family history of asthma, hay fever, or atopic dermatitis. Reduced expiratory flow rates that improve significantly after bronchodilator inhalation define the functional abnormality of the disease and an increased blood eosinophil count and eosinophils in sputum are common (some would say invariable) findings in asthma. Moreover, when sputum is produced and can be examined, inspissated mucus casts of small airways known as Curschmann's spirals may be seen. In addition, elongated octahedral bodies, easily visible on unstained wet mounts, and known as Charcot-Leyden crystals, may be present and are thought to be formed from

Table 20-1
Aids in the Diagnosis of Asthma

History
    Episodes of chest tightness, cough, wheezing, dyspnea
    Atopic dermatitis, allergic rhinitis
    Family history of same
Laboratory findings
    Reduced expiratory flow rates improved by bronchodilators
    Increased quantitative blood eosinophil count
Sputum examination
    Eosinophils
    Curschmann's spirals
    Charcot-Leyden crystals
    Shed respiratory epithelial cells or Creola bodies.

the granule material from degenerated eosinophils. Finally, sputum examination may reveal shed respiratory epithelial cells, identifiable by their cilia. When found in clumps, the latter are known as Creola bodies. Eosinophils and polymorphonuclear neutrophils may also be noted.

The initial evaluation of every asthmatic should include a search for factors that may precipitate and perpetuate an asthmatic attack (Table 20-2). Frequently, the patient will be able to identify allergens that are associated with attacks of asthma. For example, exposure to cats, house dust, plants, feathers, or other inhalants may predictably cause wheezing. Foods or drugs may also be associated by the patient with asthma attacks.

Upper respiratory tract infections frequently precipitate or aggravate symptoms. Although the mechanism is unclear, damage to the respiratory epithelium may expose irritant receptor nerve endings in bronchial mucosa to a host of nonspecific irritants that provoke bronchospasm. Normal (non-asthmatic) individuals have been shown to have increased bronchial reactivity to irritant inhalation during an upper respiratory infection. Other occult infections, particularly sinusitis, should be searched for. Sinus films are frequently abnormal in asthmatic adults. Where sinusitis is discovered appropriate treatment may markedly improve asthmatic symptoms. This important treatable cause of asthma should not be overlooked.

Aspirin sensitivity may be present in up to 28 percent of asthmatics. Because wheezing may follow the ingestion of aspirin by several hours, the patient may not associate the two events as being related. A well described syndrome of aspirin induced asthma, nasal polyps, and usually perennial asthma has been called the ASA triad. Other nonsteroidal antiinflammatory agents also usually induce asthma in these patients, suggesting that the mechanism may involve inhibition of cyclooxygenase, (the enzyme responsible for conversion of arachadonic acid to prostaglandins) possibly with an increase in formation of the leukotriene bronchoconstrictors via the lipoxygenase pathway. Curiously, a small group of asthmatics appear to get relief rather than bronchospasm from aspirin. In general, asthmatics should be advised to avoid the use of aspirin.

Table 20-2
Factors That Can Precipitate
an Asthma Attack

Specific allergens—inhaled or ingested
Infections (URI, sinusitis)
Aspirin intolerance (ASA triad)
Isoproterenol abuse
Nonspecific irritant inhalation
Exercise
Emotional upset

Excessive use of isoproterenol inhalers can induce airway narrowing. The proposed mechanisms include formation of a metabolic breakdown product of isoproterenol that is a weak β-adrenergic receptor blocking agent, and that smooth muscle in the airway, acting to structurally support an open airway, is relaxed, allowing airway collapse on expiration. Regardless of the mechanism, if flow rates can be shown to decrease with isoproterenol or symptoms are noticeably worsened with drug use (or overuse), isoproterenol should be discontinued.

Finally, as noted elsewhere in this text, nonspecific irritants, exercise, and emotion may also be important historic events in the evaluation of asthma.

Most asthmatics will have attacks triggered by more than one of the above factors and developing a known set of precipitating factors for each patient is a part of "defining the disease" that not only helps the patient understand his disease but points toward methods of effective management.

Although bronchial asthma is classically described as being comprised of intrinsic and extrinsic groups, this distinction is often difficult. The extrinsic (atopic) asthmatic is said to wheeze on exposure to an extrinsic allergen, to have seasonal symptoms in many instances, and to manifest elevated serum IgE levels and positive allergy skin tests. The intrinsic (nonatopic) asthmatic, by contrast, is said to have perennial wheezing triggered by nonspecific physical factors and upper respiratory infections, to have normal serum IgE levels, and negative allergy skin tests. This division, which is somewhat imprecise due to *overlap* in certain cases, serves little useful purpose in terms of predicting the severity of disease, and aids in planning strategies of management only insofar as the patient with clear-cut atopic asthma is more likely to respond to environmental manipulation, desensitization, or cromolyn sodium inhalations.

CLINICAL PATTERNS OF BRONCHIAL ASTHMA

Clinically, asthma may present in many ways, from infrequent, mild, short-lived episodes of wheezing to perennial intractable symptoms with periodic exacerbations of status asthmaticus (Table 20-3). Effective management requires an appreciation of these patterns, a few of which will be mentioned.

Cough as the sole manifestation of asthma is probably uncommon, although cough is a frequent prelude to the dyspnea and wheezing that is soon to follow. Chronic cough without wheezing may be seen in asthmatics with primarily large airway bronchoconstriction responsive to smooth muscle relaxing drugs such as isoproterenol. Such patients have hyperreactive airways when challenged with inhaled methacholine, and usually do not produce sputum.

Table 20-3
Some Clinical Patterns in Asthma

Cough as a sole manifestation
Exertional dyspnea only
Prolonged recovery from acute attack
Asthma in the elderly
Chronic asthmatic bronchitis
The "brittle" asthmatic
The "morning dipper"
The "irreversible" asthmatic

Exertional dyspnea may also be the sole or predominant symptom of an asthmatic attack. Studies in patients with this symptom suggest that exertional dyspnea is caused by mucosal edema or mucus secretions in peripheral airways. Cessation of exertion or production of sputum often relieves the symptom. The exertional dyspnea may last for hours to days, and may represent either a prodrome of a more severe attack or a residual airways obstruction during resolution of an asthmatic attack. Either cough or exertional dyspnea can occur in the absence of wheezing.

The prolonged duration of recovery from an acute attack has not been adequately emphasized, particularly in the emergency room setting. When appropriate bronchodilator therapy is given for an acute attack of moderate severity, and the patient no longer has subjective complaints, wheezing is usually audible by auscultation and airway resistance is still markedly increased. When wheezes can no longer be heard and the patient is considered "well" by the physician, significant abnormalities in expiratory flow rates may still persist. Several weeks of adequate outpatient therapy may be required before spirometric and lung volume values return to normal. This residual airway obstruction present on leaving the emergency room may serve as a base upon which subsequent attacks can form. It is thought that large airways constriction has a more rapid reversibility than the peripheral *silent zone*. It should be noted that bronchial smooth muscle constriction affects large airways, whereas slowly reversible edema and mucus plugging plays a more prominent role in the peripheral airways.

Asthma in the elderly may be difficult to diagnose because the symptoms may mimic those of congestive heart failure or angina, and because the fact that asthma may have its onset at any age is frequently overlooked. Elderly patients who develop asthma often have chronic bronchitis, but also note the sudden onset of increased breathlessness, wheezing, and paroxysmal nocturnal dyspnea. A history of familial atopy, elevated blood eosinophils, or the presence of sputum eosinophils should lead to a trial of bronchodilators.

Chronic asthmatic bronchitis is a term used to describe chronic bronchitis with sputum production in which episodic or perennial bronchoconstriction and wheezing occur. Such cases are occasionally difficult to diagnose because spirometric values do not normalize with bronchodilator aerosols and symptoms are incorrectly attributed to the bronchitis alone. The frequency of bronchial infections in these patients may make their exacerbations of asthma more frequent and severe.

The *brittle asthmatic* is a patient who has intractable asthma but with extreme variability. Indeed, the severity of bronchospasm may change quickly. A rapid response may be seen with β-adrenergic stimulators, but no regimen of drug therapy is successful in stabilizing these individuals. Such patients are often accused of malingering or having *emotional* asthma because of the rapid changes in asthma symptoms.

The *morning dipper* has dips in peak expiratory flow rates in the early hours of the morning, often around 2–4 A.M. The symptom of increased wheezing at night may be the clinical manifestation in some asthmatics. The cause of early morning or nocturnal worsening of symptoms is unclear, but does not appear due to variation in endogenous steroid level as it is not obliterated by infusions of hydrocortisone. Additionally, it is not related to the supine position, allergens, or night time per se. In fact, a day-shift worker who changers to night shift will still experience symptoms towards the end of the sleeping hours.

The *irreversible asthmatic* is one whose peak expiratory flow rates never normalize but demonstrate fluctuations spontaneously and occasionally in response to steroids. These individuals do not have evidence of chronic bronchitis or emphysema, but can be confused with these two diseases because they never have normal flow rates. Some of these individuals have a very slow response to steroids, requiring 1–2 weeks for improvement to be seen.

DRUG THERAPY OF ASTHMA

The pharmacologic treatment of asthma can be simplified by defining the five major classes of drugs that are available for use: sympathomimetics or epinephrine-like agents, methylxanthines, cromolyn, steroids, and anticholinergic agents. The great majority of asthmatics can be adequately managed by the appropriate use of these five groups, and an orderly addition of drugs from one category at a time is the usual approach. There are, of course, several other types of drugs that may be helpful in selected cases and these will be briefly mentioned.

SYMPATHOMIMETICS

As has been discussed elsewhere in this text cyclic 3'5'-adenosine monophosphate (cyclic AMP) causes bronchial smooth muscle relaxation and bronchodilation. The β-adrenergic agents cause bronchodilation by stimulating the enzyme adenyl cyclase, resulting in the conversion of adenosine triphosphate (ATP) into cylic AMP.

Although sympathomimetics have been available for decades the concept of β_1 and β_2 receptors is relatively new. In the 1960s Lands compared sympathomimetics for lipolytic, cardiac stimulation, bronchodilation, and vasoactive effects. Those drugs that were lipolytic also caused cardiac stimulation. Those that caused bronchodilation also caused vasodilation (and glycogenolysis and skeletal muscle stimulation). Thus the concept of β_1 (cardiac stimulation) and β_2 (bronchodilation) receptors was developed. More recently it has been recognized that β_2 specificity is more apparent when drugs are given as aerosols. Sympathomimetics given as tablets or subcutaneously lose much of their selective action on the β_2 receptor. Some patients will respond better to one sympathomimetic than another; thus some experimentation among the various agents is always indicated if the first drug is ineffective or causes excessive side effects (see Fig. 20-1).

When given as an aerosol or subcutaneously, sympathomimetics may cause a transient fall in arterial oxygen tension in the range 5–10 mm Hg. Because pulmonary vessels may be dilated before bronchial dilation occurs,

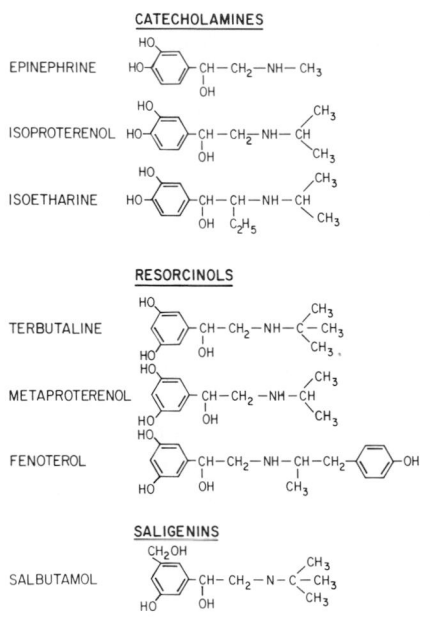

Fig. 20-1. Structure of various sympathomimetic agents used in the treatment of asthma.

shunting of poorly oxygenated blood into the left atrium may increase transiently. Supplemental oxygen is, therefore, advisable in hypoxemic asthmatics before bronchodilator administration.

The proper method of inhaling aerosol drug from a metered dose inhaler (MDI) deserves mention because it is so frequently performed incorrectly. The aerosol is released as fairly large droplets with a high velocity. As the propellant rapidly vaporizes, droplets become smaller, allowing more distal penetration on inhalation. If inhalation is very rapid, particles will impact on the posterior wall of the pharynx or at airway branch points due to the velocity of the particles. Thus a *slow* deep inhalation from a cloud of aerosol generated at the open mouth is optimal.

A breath hold will allow maximal distal airway deposition of drug. Waiting for a minute or more before the next inhalation will allow some bronchodilation to occur so the next inhalation will result in deeper penetration of the aerosol. To assure that the patient is performing this maneuver correctly, watch carefully as the patient shakes the inhaler to produce proper mixing of the drug and propellant, exhales fully, holds the canister upright, places the mouthpiece near the open lips, fires the inhaler while inhaling slowly and deeply, holds the breath for about 10 seconds, and then waits for one minute before the next inhalation. Washing the mouth out with water may remove excess drug from buccal mucosa, reduce absorption and thereby reduce systemic side effects.

Patients that cannot coordinate a slow inhalation with actuating the MDI are not uncommon. These patients may benefit from use of a spacer or other chamber into which the aerosol is released before inhalation. The aerosol then stabilizes and is slowly inhaled from the chamber without the need for coordinating the activation of the MDI. Spacers are now being built into a number of MDI systems.

Epinephrine

Epinephrine is a potent sympathomimetic agent with α, β_1, and β_2 activity (Table 20-4) that was first used in the early 1900s both subcutaneously and as an aerosol. Like other catecholamines (Fig. 20-1) epinephrine is rapidly metabolized by methylation of a hydroxy group by catechol-O-methyl transferase (COMT) or by sulfatization. This limited duration of action may result in a common clinical event. An asthmatic patient in the emergency room gets rapid relief from subcutaneous epinephrine and is discharged only to return in 3–4 hours with a return of symptoms. Subcutaneous epinephrine 0.1–0.5 mg is extremely valuable in treating rapidly progressive bronchospasm but should never be the sole treatment. An aqueous solution plus a crystalline suspension of the drug, (e.g., SusPhrine, has a more prolonged effect lasting 8–10 hours). Epinephrine in oil is available for intramuscular use with a

Table 20-4
Sympathomimetic Effects

Stimulation	Tissue	Effect
α-receptor	Bronchial muscle	Weak contraction
	Bronchial blood vessels	Constriction
	Cardiac muscle	Excitation
β_1-receptor	Cardiac muscle	Stimulation
	Fatty tissue	Lipolysis
β_2-receptor	Bronchial muscle	Relaxation
	Bronchial blood vessel	Dilation
	Skeletal muscle	Tremor
	Liver and muscle	Glycogenolysis

duration of action up to 16 hours, but sterile abscesses at the site of injection limit the usefulness of this preparation. The racemic mixture of D- and L-epinephrine in a 2.25 percent solution is used for aerosol treatments. One possible advantage of this drug over pure beta agents is that the α-adrenergic effects may constrict bronchial mucosal vessels and shrink swollen membranes. This action has led to its use in croup in children and in laryngotracheobronchitis. In wheezing caused by propranolol or β-blockade the alpha effects of epinephrine may worsen the condition. The cardiac stimulation effects of epinephrine probably make more selective β_2 agents preferable.

Ephedrine

Ephedrine has been used in the United States since the early 1920s and was the only oral sympathomimetic agent available for several generations. Until metaproterenol became available in 1961 ephedrine was and is widely

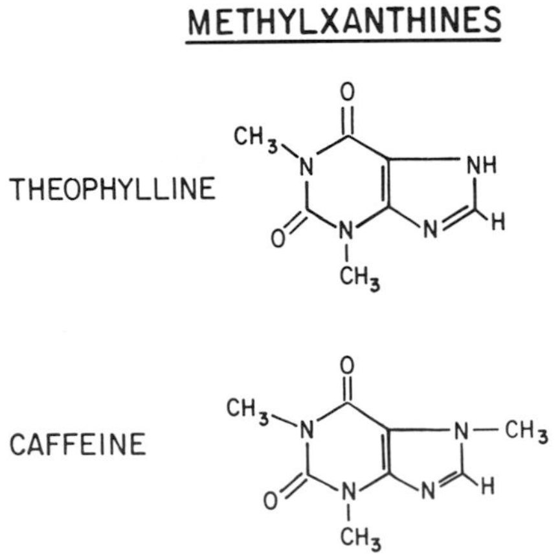

METHYLXANTHINES

THEOPHYLLINE

CAFFEINE

Fig. 20-2. Comparison of the structures of theophylline and caffeine. The side effects of the two drugs are similar.

used today in fixed combination preparations such as Tedral (theophylline, ephedrine, phenobarbital) and Marax (theophylline, ephedrine, hydroxyzine). Ephedrine acts by both direct β_2 stimulation and release of stored catecholamines. The latter mechanism probably accounts for the tachyphylaxis that develops with large doses or prolonged use of the drug. The usual dosage of ephedrine is 15–50 mg with a duration of action of about 4 hours. As excess central nervous system stimulation is a major side effect of the drug, sedatives such as phenobarbital or hydroxyzine are often given concurrently. Moreover, urinary retention in males, hypertension, insomnia, and potentiation of the effects of monoamine-oxidase-inhibitor drugs are other major side effects. In adults there is little reason to recommend ephedrine over more recently developed β_2-specific oral bronchodilators. Its major indication may well be in a patient who has taken ephedrine for years and is reluctant to switch to another preparation. During an acute severe attack, ephedrine is not the drug of choice.

Isoproterenol

Available since 1941, isoproterenol has been widely used as a very potent pure β-adrenergic stimulator. As it has both β_1 and β_2 activity, one can predict that its use will often result in cardiac stimulation as well as the desired bronchodilation. Like the catecholamines, epinephrine and isoetharine, isoproterenol is rapidly metabolized by COMT and has a duration of action of 1–2 hours. The methylated compound, 3-methoxy-isoproterenol, is a weak β_2 blocker, but this rarely results in bronchoconstriction.

The onset of action with inhaled isoproterenol is often within 1 minute. Hand-held metered aerosols are in common use and differ to some degree in the administered dose per inhalation. A patient may find Isuprel Mistometer better that Medihaler-Iso. The difference between the two preparations is mainly in delivered dose: 125 μg versus 75 μg per puff. Reports of isoproterenol-aerosol-related deaths in Great Britain in the past may have been related to much higher drug doses per puff in those metered aerosol systems. Both isoproterenol and Freon propellant overdose may have caused fatal arrhythmias, but this complication is not commonly noted with current preparations. The usual metered aerosol dose is 1–4 inhalations 4 times a day; the frequency may be increased to every 4 hours in mild-to-moderate attacks.

Isoproterenol 1:200 solution is frequently used in IPPB and other types of nebulizers. 0.5–1 ml of the drug is added to 2 ml of water or saline so that continuous nebulization will occur over 5–15 minutes. Undiluted drug in the same dose may be used in equally effective but much less expensive handheld or compressor-driven nebulizers. Because cardiac arrhythmias may occur with isoproterenol, monitoring of heart rate and blood pressure is advisable during initial aerosol delivery.

Isoetharine

Isoetharine has been available since 1950 as a metered aerosol and as a solution for nebulization. Although isoetharine is a weaker bronchodilator than isoproterenol, it is more β_2 specific. The duration of action, due to the ring structure, is 1–3 hours. Bronkometer delivers 340 μg per puff and is used as 1–4 puffs every 4 hours. The 1-percent solution Bronkosol is used in doses of 0.5 ml in water or saline in IPPB devices, hand-held or compressor-driven nebulizers. Isoetharine has been very popular as the only bronchodilator in mild asthmatics or as supplemental therapy in asthmatics on other drugs. This largely β_2 specific drug causes fewer cardiac side effects than isoproterenol or epinephrine.

Bitolterol

Bitolterol mesylate, available in 1985, is a "pro drug" that is hydrolyzed by an esterase, which has its highest concentration in the lungs, to the active catecholamine colterol. Therefore it is not active immediately, a disadvantage compared to other β-adrenergic agents. Colterol is structurally similar to Isoproterenol but has a greater β_2 specificity. The bitolterol structure protects against metabolism by COMT thus the duration of action is prolonged to 6–8 hours, similar to albuterol. As with all aerosol sympathomimetics, the duration of action appears shorter in patients on steroids, presumably the group with more severe disease.

Metaproterenol

Metaproterenol, available since 1961, resembles isoproterenol except that the hydroxy groups are rearranged on the benzene ring. This structural alteration renders COMT ineffective as a metabolizing enzyme. Thus metaproterenol, as well as terbutaline and fenoterol, termed resorcinols, all have a longer duration of action than the catecholamines.

Metaproterenol is available as tablets (10 or 20 mg), syrup (10 mg/tsp), solution for aerosol (50 mg/ml), or metered dose inhaler 650 μg/puff, and its duration of action is about 3–5 hours. The drug is a relatively selective β_2 agent although, like all the sympathomimetic drugs, this β_2 selectivity is less apparent when the drug is given orally. The syrup may be given to children over 6 years of age. Tachycardia and tremor are two common side effects. Skeletal muscle stimulation, a β_2 effect, results in hand tremors that usually diminish after the drug is taken for a week or two. The usual aerosol dose for adults is 15 mg (0.3 ml) with 2 ml water or saline in a compressor-driven nebulizer. When cost has been compared, this sympathomimetic has often been less expensive than other β_2 specific agents. The longer duration of action compared to isoproterenol or isoetharine and the relative β_2 specificity have made this a popular aerosol agent.

Terbutaline

Terbutaline has been available since 1974 in both a subcutaneous injection and a tablet form and is now available as an aerosol as well. A resorcinol, terbutaline is longer acting than epinephrine or isoproterenol, lasting 3–5 hours. The aerosol metered dose inhaler (200 μg/puff) commonly given as 2 puffs four times daily is more β_2 selective than oral or subcutaneous forms of administration of the drug. Tolerance to the aerosol does not appear to develop with continued use over several months. When given subcutaneously terbutaline and epinephrine appear to differ mainly in duration of action. It can be argued that epinephrine is preferable as a subcutaneous agent because if excess dosage causes unwanted side effects, the duration would be shorter with epinephrine than terbutaline.

Fenoterol

Fenoterol, a resorcinol, differs from metaproterenol and terbutaline primarily by a longer duration of action. This relatively β_2 specific aerosol has a duration of action of 6–8 hours in some studies. As has been noted with other sympathomimetic aerosols, fenoterol is very effective in preventing exercise induced asthma, but this protection is shorter than the bronchodilator duration of action. Thus, either 2 or 4 200 μg puffs inhibited exercise induced asthma for less than 4 hours. The β_2 selectivity and long duration of action of fenoterol may make it an aerosol of choice.

Albuterol

Albuterol, or salbutamol, is a saligenin and is resistant to degradation by COMT, resulting in a prolonged duration of action up to 6–8 hours. In addition it is relatively β_2 specific, especially, as an aerosol. Albuterol is available as 2 mg or 4 mg tablets and as the more popular aerosol metered dose inhaler that delivers 90 μg/puff. The usual dose is 2 puffs every 4–6 hours. As with all sympathomimetics the β_2 specificity is greater with the aerosol delivery of a smaller total dose to the airways than a larger dose orally. In addition there is no rationale to use more than a single oral sympathomimetic at any one time as the side effects are additive, and it is prudent when possible to use the aerosol agent alone without adding a tablet sympathomimetic.

METHYLXANTHINES

Although the bronchodilator properties of theophylline were known in 1921, clinical studies and general use of the drug did not occur until the late

1930s. The theophylline bronchodilators are now in common use for the treatment of asthma and form a cornerstone of therapy. Theophylline is a methylated xanthine structurally resembling caffeine (Fig. 20-2) with side effects resembling those of too much coffee; this is an analogy many patients understand. Parenthetically, an occasional asthmatic patient will report that bronchospasm is relieved by drinking coffee or warm tea.

Concepts about the mechanism of action of the theophyllines have changed over the last several years. Although theophyllines do inhibit phosphodiesterase, the enzyme responsible for degradation of cyclic AMP, this does not appear to be the mechanism of action for the methylxanthines. Phosphodiesterase is not inhibited by the low concentrations of theophylline that result in bronchodilation. In addition other phosphodiesterase inhibitors are not bronchodilators. A currently popular proposed mechanism of action is that methylxanthines inhibit adenosine, an agent that induces bronchospasm in asthmatic patients. Adenosine and theophylline are structurally similar and theophylline competitively inhibits adenosine receptors. Elucidation of the true mechanism of this bronchodilator awaits further studies.

Theophylline is well absorbed from the gastrointestinal tract as are salts of the drug, oxtriphylline (the choline salt), aminophylline (the ethylenediamine salt) and others (Table 20-5). Aminophylline, however, because of greater water solubility, is the theophylline commonly used intravenously.

Therapeutic bronchodilation occurs at serum levels above 5 μg/ml with greater effect at higher levels. Side effects, however, are common above 20 μg/ml. Therefore, the general therapeutic goal is to maintain serum levels between 10 and 20 μg/ml. Achieving this level is somewhat complicated by the variation in drug half life between individuals. The average half life is 8 hours with a range of 3–9 hours. In general children, adult smokers, and 25 percent of adult non smokers eliminate theophylline rapidly whereas theophylline is metabolized slowly in patients with heart failure, liver disease, pneumonia, COPD, or old age. Thus no single daily dose results in a therapeutic drug level is all patients.

The goal of therapy is to have a constant therapeutic theophylline level around the clock. Fluctuations in serum theophylline levels can be reduced by decreasing the rate of drug elimination (a patient variable over which we have no control), shortening the dosing interval (a prescribing variable), or slowing the rate of drug absorption (a product variable). Increasing dosing frequency is often impractical. However, a growing selection of sustained release theophylline products have become available (Table 20-5). The ideal slow release product would mimic a continuous intravenous infusion (e.g., release the same mg of drug each hour) (zero order kinetics) as opposed to release of the same percentage of the remaining drug each hour (first order kinetics). However, when there is very slow drug release with first order kinetics the difference from zero order kinetics is indistinguishable.

Table 20-5
Oral Theophylline Preparations

Trade Name	Percent Anhydrous	Contents
Aminophylline	85	Aminophylline
Choledyl	64	Oxtriphylline
Theolair	100	Anhydrous theophylline
Elixophylline	100	Anhydrous theophylline
Lufylline	70	Dyphylline 200 mg
Tedral tablets	100	Theophylline 130 mg
		Ephedrine 25 mg
		Phenobarbital 8 mg
Marax	100	Theophylline 130 mg
		Ephedrine 25 mg
		Hydroxyzine 10 mg
Bronchotabs	100	Theophylline 100 mg
		Ephedrine 24 mg
		Phenobarbital 8 mg
		Glyceryl guaiacolate 100 mg
Theodur*	100	Anhydrous Theophylline
Respbib*	100	Anhydrous theophylline
Constant T*	100	Anhydrous theophylline
Somophyllin-CRT†	100	Anhydrous theophylline
Slo-Phyllin Gyrocaps†	100	Anhydrous theophylline
Uniphyl‡	100	Anhydrous theophylline
Theo-24‡	100	Anhydrous theophylline

* Slow release preparations as tablets
† Slow release preparations as bead filled capsules
‡ Very slow release preparations as tablets.

The slow release products may allow twice daily (BID) or even daily, (QD) dosing if the patient is not a rapid metabolizer. The trough level of theophylline may be subtherapeutic in the rapid metabolizer requiring shorter dosing intervals (e.g., Q8H or Q6H despite the slow release of the drug). Thus, children, smoking adults, and about 25 percent of nonsmoking adults may require Q8H dosing intervals for most slow release products.

Theophylline dosage should be carefully reviewed at the time each prescription is written. The percent theophylline by weight varies with the preparation. For example elixophylline is 100 percent anhydrous theophylline but aminophylline is 83 percent theophylline and choledyl is 64 percent theophylline. Most of the newer preparations are 100 percent theophylline.

In the acute asthmatic attack intravenous aminophylline is commonly used. A loading dose of 5.6 mg/kg is given *slowly* by over 20 minutes (to prevent cardiac arrhythmias) followed by a continuous infusion of 0.5 mg/kg/hour with subsequent adjustments based on serum levels. When increasing theophylline dosage it is important to be aware that the percentage increase in subsequent serum level is usually greater than the percentage increase in dose, thus gradual increases in dosage are best.

In the less severe chronic asthmatic, oral theophylline is indicated without the need for a loading dose. The average theophylline dose requirement is 13 mg/kg/day not exceeding 900 mg/day in divided dose. The daily dose should be half this in patients with hepatic or cardiac dysfunction including cor pulmonale. Serum levels should be measured as peak levels, 3–7 hours after most slow release preparations. This should be drawn at steady state after at least 48 hours of drug when no doses have been missed and no other medications affecting drug metabolism have been started or stopped. Some of the current methods of measuring serum theophylline (e.g., the EMIT assay) are so specific that dyphylline is not detected, a major reason to avoid using this methylxanthine product.

The side effects of theophylline (Table 20-6) resemble those of excessive caffeine. Central nervous system stimulation and gastrointestinal distress are frequently seen at serum levels over 15–20 μg/ml. Tremor is much less commonly seen with theophyllines than with β_2 sympathomimetics. Rarely, generalized grand mal seizures present as the first sign of theophylline toxicity and seizures have occurred at serum levels as low as 25 μg/ml. In one study the mean serum level of 8 patients with theophylline-induced seizures was 53 μg/ml with a range of 25–70 μg/ml, but diarrhea, melena, and hematemesis are primarily reported in massive overdoses, often in children. The nausea is related mainly to blood level. Thus, improvement of nausea by switching from aminophylline to oxtriphylline probably reflects the reduced theophylline in the latter drug. Tachycardia, arrhythmias, and blood pressure

Table 20-6
Theophylline Side Effects

Gastrointestinal Irritation	Cardiovascular
Nausea	Tachycardia
Vomiting	Arrhythmias
Diarrhea	Hypotension
Hematemesis	Hypertension
Melena	Renal
CNS Stimulation	Diuresis
Restlessness	Other
Insomnia	Flushing
Irritability	Fever
Headache	
Tremor	
Twitching	
Seizures	

changes are seen mainly, but not solely, with intravenous drug administration. Finally, diuresis commonly occurs and cutaneous flushing and low-grade fever are occasionally seen with toxic serum drug levels. When initiating therapy with theophylline compounds it is imperative that the patient learn the side effects and be able to recognize them early so that corrective action can be taken. Rectal suppositories provide an alternate route of administration but unpredictable absorption (i.e., often rapid with resultant high serum levels) makes this a less desirable method of giving the drug.

Fixed combinations of theophylline, ephedrine, and often a tranquilizer or expectorant are in common use (Table 20-5). When a patient does well on such a combination and wishes to continue, no alterations in therapy are required. These fixed combinations are not entirely rational, however, and the patient might do as well on only the theophylline or the β_2 agent. These combination products should not be initial therapy in a newly diagnosed asthmatic.

ADRENOCORTICAL STEROIDS

Following the discovery by Hench in 1949 that cortisone was effective in treating rheumatoid arthritis, this class of drugs has found wide application in many diseases. Despite many potential side effects, steroids are of great use in severe cases of asthma. The corticosteroids, all synthetic analogues of hydrocortisone, are similar in most metabolic effects, but differ in sodium-retaining properties, equivalent dosage, and biologic half-life (Table 20-7). Oral corticosteroids are well absorbed. However, because steroids are poorly soluble in water they are ofter conjugated with phosphate or succinate for intravenous or intramuscular use.

The mechanism of improvement of asthma with steroids is unclear. They may prevent the release of chemical mediators of bronchoconstriction, or alternatively enhance the effect of sympathomimetics on the β_2 receptors. The beneficial effects do not occur immediately. Depending upon the severity

Table 20-7
Corticosteroids

Preparation	Equivalent Dose (mg)	Biologic Half-life (hrs)
Hydrocortisone	20	8–12
Cortisone	25	8–12
Prednisone	5	12–36
Prednisolone	5	12–36
Methylprednisolone	4	12–36
Dexamethasone	0.75	36–54

of the attack, steroid benefit may be inapparent for 3–6 hours or longer. In some cases of severe chronic asthma, steroid effect may not be seen for days.

The decision to initiate steroid use can be difficult. In general, any asthmatic severe enough to require hospitalization should be given steroids. Corticosteroids may be lifesaving if the disease is progressing and may shorten the course of the illness regardless of its status. The general rule is to use high doses initially in an attempt to control the disease and then to taper the drug rapidly within 5–7 days to avoid side effects. The initial dose of steroids for severe asthma should be 50–100 mg of methylprednisolone IV (or prednisone orally) initially and then about half that dose every 4–6 hours until the desired effect is obtained. The dose is then rapidly reduced by about 50 percent each day, watching for exacerbations, in an attempt to have the patient back to the baseline steroid dose in a short time (Table 20-8). Although side effects of acute psychosis, edema formation, and hypokalemic alkalosis can occur, the severity of disease usually warrants the risk. Prednisone or methylprednisolone with less salt-retaining properties are preferable to hydrocortisone in this setting.

Maintenance steroids for outpatients are associated with greater potential for side effects. In general, steroids are only given when other measures fail. Only when adequate doses of methylxanthines plus β-adrenergic agents and cromolyn have been given without adequate control of symptoms is chronic oral prednisone considered. It is clear that higher doses of steroid are required to initiate a remission from a severe attack than are required to maintain control subsequently. Prednisone should be given as a single A.M. dose so that serum levels are highest when endogenous cortisone levels are highest. This timing of administration appears to reduce the suppression of the

Table 20-8
Guidelines for Steroid Therapy

Start with high doses for exacerbations (e.g., prednisone 40–80 mg/day)
After control of symptoms, taper rapidly (within 5–7 days) to baseline steroid dose
For "chronic" steroid use, try to keep daily dose of prednisone below 10 mg/day
Give daily dose in the A.M.
Attempt alternate-day steroids if more than 7.5 prednisone/day is required
Use 2–3 times daily dose for "on" days initially
Use beclomethasone dipropionate aerosol or other inhaled steroids to avoid need for, or reduce dose of, oral prednisone.

hypothalamic-pituitary-adrenal axis. The lowest possible dose should be used, hopefully 5–10 mg/day. Side effects of chronic steroid use are multiple (Table 20-9) and serious. Osteoporosis and posterior subcapsular cataracts are irreversible when they occur, but other adverse effects improve with dose reduction. It is known that tuberculosis can reactivate when steroids are given for long periods. Considering the number of asthmatics on steroids, reactivation tuberculosis is surprisingly infrequent. If the patient requiring steroids has a positive PPD, has evidence of old tuberculosis, and has never been treated or been given a year of prophylaxis, isoniazid administration should be strongly considered.

The frequency of steroid side effects reduced by using short-acting steroids (prednisone, prednisolone, or methylprednisolone), small daily doses, and more recently, alternate-day steroids. The rationale for using steroids only every 48 hours is that the therapeutic effects may last longer than the metabolic effects responsible for most of the complications of long-term therapy. Alternate-day steroid administration appears to cause much less hypothalamic-pituitary-adrenal axis suppression, less hyperglycemia, and less Cushingoid change than daily steroid use. If the patient requires more than 7.5 mg prednisone per day, alternate-day steroids should be tried. The usual method of switching from daily to alternate-day steroids is to give 2–4 times the usual daily dose on alternate days. Someone requiring 10 mg prednisone per day, for example, may require 20–40 mg on alternate days. The alternate-day dose is then gradually reduced. On the day without prednisone the unwanted effects of steroids are reduced and often the asthma is still controlled. During exacerbations, however, steroids will have to be increased to daily doses, often using increased dosage.

Withdrawal from steroids after even short periods of daily use may be associated with a host of symptoms–depression and arthralgias being fairly

Table 20-9
Adverse Effects of Corticosteroids

Cushingoid appearance
Hyperglycemia
Psychosis, mood changes
Acne, purpura, hirsutism
Muscle wasting
Osteoporosis,* vertebral collapse
Suppression of hypothalamic-pituitary-adrenal axis
Posterior subcapsular cataracts*
Sodium retention, edema, hypertension
Hypokalemic metabolic alkalosis
May reactivate tuberculosis

* Irreversible.

common (Table 20-10). The physician can alleviate patient anxiety if these symptoms are discussed in advance of a withdrawal regimen.

INHALED STEROIDS

Inhaled corticosteroids have been widely used in the management of moderate to severe asthma. These topically active steroids are absorbed but are rapidly inactivated, thus providing local airway antiinflammatory effect without systemic side effects. Beclomethasone dipropionate has been available in the U.S. since 1976 but triamcinolone acetate, budesonide, flunisolide, and others are either currently available or being studied. Beclomethasone dipropionate, is usually used at 2 inhalations 4 times a day (400 μg/day) with a maximum recommended dose of 1000 μg/day. Some authors recommend doses exceeding this level when systemic steroid intake can successfully be reduced by use of the inhaled agent. The maximum dose of beclomethasone is probably equivalent to 5–15 mg or oral prednisone per day without the systemic side effects. Untoward effects of all the inhaled steroids include sore throat, oral candidiasis (treated by stopping the drug, reducing the dose, or giving mystatin drops), and the emergence of allergic symptoms such as atopic dermatitis or allergic rhinitis as the oral steroid is tapered. Washing the mouth out after each use may reduce the incidence of oral candidiasis. Inhaled steroids have no role in treating acute severe asthma. By contrast they are very useful in chronic asthma ofter allowing a reduction in systemic steroid dose. The use of a spacer on the inhaler may reduce oral and laryngeal deposition of the drug thereby reducing side effects.

Cromolyn Sodium

Cromolyn sodium (also known as disodium cromoglycate in England) was approved for use in the United States in 1973. This drug has no intrinsic bronchodilator, or antiinflammatory activity. Nor does it inhibit the mediators

Table 20-10
Symptoms of Steroid Withdrawal

Malaise, headache
Depression
Arthralgias, myalgias
Abdominal pain
Anorexia, nausea, vomiting
Orthostatic hypotension, dizziness
Exacerbation of asthma or other allergic symptoms

of immediate hypersensitivity. It appears to act in part by preventing the release of mediators of bronchoconstriction from the mast cell, probably by blocking calcium entry into the cell. There is some evidence that cromolyn inhibits reflex bronchoconstriction as well. Finally there is evidence that cromolyn may reduce bronchial reactivity or level of *twitchiness* in response to histamine, antigen, and cold air. A patient, thus, treated during a pollen season with cromolyn may have less frequent and milder asthma attacks with the use of this drug.

Because of its mechanism of action, cromolyn is for prophylactic use only and has no role in an acute asthma attack. The drug comes in several forms, a white powder inhaled from a 20 mg capsule via a turbo-inhaler device, the Spinhaler, and as a liquid in 20 mg, 2 ml vials to be used with a compressor driven nebulizer. The duration of action is at least 5 hours and probably longer, and the usual dose by either route is 20 mg 4 times a day. Also a metered dose inhaler is now available. When cromolyn is beneficial, the effectiveness appears unchanged even with prolonged use.

Cromolyn sodium is not effective in all asthmatics. The presumed mechanism of action suggests that it should be of greatest usefulness in allergen-induced bronchospasm, especially if given immediately before allergen inhalation. Clinical studies suggest that up to 50 percent of adults will have a decreased frequency or severity of asthma attacks when using cromolyn. Our experience is that considerably less than 50 percent of adult asthmatics experience relief when using this drug. The success rate may be higher in children. Surprisingly, many perennial asthmatics without definable allergens will also respond. In addition, exercise-induced asthma can often be prevented by cromolyn use, although sympathomimetics are equally effective and cheaper. Finally, some patients with aspirin-induced asthma also respond to cromolyn prophylaxis. The usefulness of this drug thus appears to extend beyond pure allergen-induced asthmatics. A summary of characteristics is given in Table 20-11.

Improvement with cromolyn use is often seen after several days of drug inhalation, but many cases require 2–4 weeks before a response is noted. If no effect is apparent after 1 month, little is to be gained by continuing the drug. Perhaps the greatest single value of cromolyn is to allow the steroid dose to be reduced or avoided entirely, particularly in children. As cromolyn is prophylactic only, it has no role in the treatment of an acute attack. In fact, the irritation to the airways caused by inhaling the dry powder may exacerbate the bronchospasm.

There are few side effects of cromolyn except for the mechanical effects of causing throat and airway irritation, dry mouth, cough, and perhaps reactive bronchospasm. The use of a bronchodilator aerosol immediately before cromolyn powder inhalation may prevent cough and perhaps reactive bronchospasm. These side effects are not a problem with the liquid form of the

Table 20-11
Consensus on Cromolyn

Prophylactic only
Best results in "seasonal" allergic asthma
Some improvement in perennial asthmatics
Most patients should have a trial
Inhibits exercise—induced asthma
May reduce bronchial reactivity
May reduce steroid requirement
No apparent loss of effectiveness with time
Two to four weeks required to assess effect
Minor local side effects are common—dry mouth, irritation of
    airways, cough, bronchospasm
Major side effects are rare

drug. Rare cases of skin rashes, eosinophilic pneumonia, and allergic granulomatosis have occurred, but in general cromolyn is a remarkably benign
drug. Finally, careful coaching of the patient in the proper use of the Spinhaler is important. For example, if one exhales into the device so that the
powder gets damp, the pierced holes in the capsule may become clogged so
the powder cannot be dispersed.

The availability of liquid cromolyn has been a major benefit to many
asthmatics. A hand held bulb nebulizer cannot easily be used to deliver the
volume of 2 ml of cromolyn so we have found that compressor driven
nebulizers for home use are necessary. These devices can then be used as
well to deliver sympathomimetic liquids in aerosol form. Many patients
experience major improvement in symptoms when they take their aerosol
medications via this route as it allows ready titration of dosage, and does not
require the hand-breath coordination needed for use of metered dose inhalers.

ANTICHOLINERGIC AGENTS

Anticholinergic agents in the form of stramonium cigarettes were used
for the treatment of asthma in the early 1800s. More recently atropine and
newer anticholinergics with limited systemic effects have been used in
Europe. Atropine sulfate as an aerosol (0.025 mg/kg) causes bronchodilation
in asthmatics and bronchitis-emphysema patients by blocking vagal parasympathetic acetylcholine-mediated bronchoconstriction. Atropine, however, is
readily absorbed and results in dry mouth, tachycardia, meiosis, skin flushing, mental changes, and urinary retention. In addition atropine may reduce
mucus secretion, ciliary activity, and transport rates of mucus. Nonetheless

the drug is useful in some acute asthma episodes because it produces some bronchodilation beyond that obtained by sympathomimetics alone.

The newer atropine-like quarternary ammonium compounds of atropine methonitrate, ipratropium bromide (Atrovent, Sch 1000), and glycopyrrolate methylbromide are topically active, are not well absorbed, and therefore, produce the desired bronchodilation without the atropine-like side effects either systemically or on the mucociliary function. They have been shown to be effective in exercise-induced asthma, antigen and irritant induced wheezing, and particularly in asthma due to β-adrenergic receptor blockade.

The anticholinergic agents appear to be more efficacious in the airway obstruction of bronchitis and emphysema than in asthma. The reverse is true for the sympathomimetics. Therefore the atropine-like drugs may be most rational where chronic bronchitis or emphysema is accompanied by asthma. As the quarternary ammonium compounds become approved by the FDA for use in asthma, a broader experience may clarify their exact indications.

OTHER DRUG THERAPY

The calcium channel blocking agents nifedipine and verapamil have been extensively used to treat angina and supraventricular arrhythmias respectively. Recently nifedipine (20 mg sublingual) has been shown to provide some protection against exercise-, histamine-, and antigen-, induced bronchospasm. Verapamil has been less effective. It seems unlikely that these agents will become first line drugs in the treatment of asthma. However, in an asthmatic patient needing treatment for angina, the use of nifedipine rather than a beta blocker (that might cause bronchoconstriction) would be very rational.

Tranquilizers and sedatives have in the past enjoyed some popularity in the treatment of asthma because the dyspneic patient is, indeed, anxious. Anxiety is the natural response to the increased work of breathing, the feeling of suffocation, and the concern of family members. However, verbal reassurance and relief of bronchospasm using bronchodilators is the treatment of choice for anxiety. The hazards of dangerous depression of the respiratory drive usually outweigh any possible benefit from treatment of the symptom of anxiety.

Mucolytic agents seem rational in light of the tenacious sputum characteristic of asthma, but aerosolized acetylcysteine or Mucomyst is a potent airway irritant due in part to its alkaline pH. Cough and bronchospasm can be aggravated in asthmatic patients by the use of this drug. There appears to be little role for these agents in the treatment of asthma, except in occasional patients. Concomitant use of a bronchodilator aerosol is imperative.

NONDRUG THERAPY OF ASTHMA

Immunotherapy for asthma, using graded injections of an extract of the allergen to which the patient is sensitive, is intended to decrease the patient's symptoms upon reexposure. This form of therapy is more efficacious for hay fever than for asthma, and is most likely to be helpful in seasonal asthmatics, a group usually quite responsive to sympathomimetics and methylxanthine. The benefit to adult perennial asthmatics is usually disappointing. In patients with moderate to severe asthma, however, a screening for a specific unsuspected allergen for which immunotherapy might be helpful is appropriate.

General measures such as adequate physical and emotional rest, proper diet, and adequate fluid intake are important in asthma therapy. If specific allergens consistently provoke attacks, these should, of course, be avoided. Patient education as to the nature of the disease and treatment modalities is perhaps the single most important nondrug treatment.

PATTERNS OF MANAGEMENT

The choice of medications for management of asthma depends on the severity of the symptoms. The patient with mild and intermittent wheezing should be given a β_2 specific sympathomimetic in a metered dose inhaler with careful (and repeated) instructions on its use. Inhalations should be used as needed and before exposure to stimuli known to produce symptoms (e.g., exercise).

When the asthma is of moderate severity with frequent exacerbations, perhaps superimposed on chronic wheezing, the aerosol β_2 sympathomimetic is to be used regularly (interval depends on duration of action) and methylxanthines are added. Care is used to titrate a stable continuous therapeutic serum theophylline level usually using the slow release preparations. If this combination does not control symptoms the addition of cromolyn is appropriate. At this point a compressor driven nebulizer is often prescribed for home use. Liquid cromolyn is used at home as is a liquid beta sympathomimetic. Away from home the powdered cromolyn can be used. The nebulizer allows upward titration of the sympathomimetic dose without depending on the hand-breath coordination and often improves symptom control dramatically.

When the asthma is severe with very frequent exacerbations ofter superimposed on chronic wheezing, the use of steroids is added to the above regimen. Preferably steroids are added only after maximal sympathomimetic, methylxanthine, and cromolyn therapy has been achieved. Then inhaled steroids are added and increased to maximally recommended doses in an attempt to control wheezing. Finally daily oral corticosteroids, usually prednisone, are instituted and titrated to control symptoms with a single A.M. dose being used. Attempts to move to alternate day dosing should be made. Every effort should be made to allow symptom control without long term systemic steroids. The use of oral sympathomimetics on top of maximal doses of aerosol beta agonists (that have fewer side effects) is not entirely rational but should be tried. Aerosolized atropine or a topically active anticholinergic aerosol should be tested. A search for allergens that could be treated with immunotherapy (or avoidance) and a search for occult infection (e.g., sinusitis) should be carried out. During an acute exacerbation, higher doses of systemic steroids temporarily are entirely appropriate. The care of more severe cases is discussed in the chapter on status asthmaticus.

SPECIAL PROBLEMS

There are several special problems involved in the care of asthmatics that should be emphasized. Cough fractures of ribs may occur in asthmatics, causing pain and splinting. It is important to document such events not only to exclude more serious causes of the pain, but also to prove to the patient that the pain is not "imagined." Symptoms of rib fracture are relieved by splinting with a simple chest binder, although intercostal nerve blocks or potent analgesics are occasionally necessary. The rib ends usually stabilize and become painless within 2 weeks. Pneumomediastinum or pneumothorax that may occur spontaneously during an asthma attack also present with chest pain and/or increased shortness of breath. Presumably due to high alveolar pressures with rupture of alveolar walls and retrograde air dissection toward the mediastinum, pneumomediastinum requires no treatment other than reassurance. Pneumothorax, unless miniscule in degree, usually requires closed intercostal drainage. Asthma attacks accompanied by fleeting pulmonary infiltrates and expectoration of brown mucus plugs should alert the physician to the possibility of allergic bronchopulmonary aspergillosis. This important but uncommon complication of asthma is reviewed elsewhere in this text. Severe asthmatics or those prone to severe exacerbations should probable be considered for influenza vaccinations, and perhaps pneumococcal vaccination as well, in hopes of preventing infections that may aggravate symptoms. Finally, patient education continues to be of paramount importance for adequacy of symptom control, proper drug and nondrug therapy, and development of a treatment program that will result in the most functional state. Using this approach the successful treatment of asthma can be a rewarding experience for both the patient and the physician.

REFERENCES

Berman BA: Cromolyn: past present, and future. Ped Clin North Amer 30:915–930, 1983

Bukowsky M, Nakatsu K, Munt PW: Theophylline reassessed. Ann Intern Med 101:63–73, 1984

Busse WW: The precipitation of asthma by upper respiratory infections. Chest 87:44S–48S, 1985

Gross NJ, Skorodin MS: Anticholinergic, antimuscarinic bronchodilators. Amer Rev Resp Dis 129:856–870, 1984

Heel RC, Brogden RN, Speight TM, et al: Fenoterol: a review of its pharmacological properties and therapeutic efficacy in asthma. Drugs 15:3–32, 1978

Hendeles L, Weinberger M: Theophylline, a "state of the art" review. Pharmacotherapy 3:2–44, 1983

Kemp JP, Chervinsky P, Orgel HA, et al: Concomitant bitolterol mesylate aerosol and theophylline for asthma therapy, with 24 hr electrocardiographic monitoring. J Allergy Clin Immunol 73:32–43, 1984

Mathison DA, Stevenson DD, Tan EM, et al: Clinical profiles of bronchial asthma. JAMA 224:1134–1139, 1973

Mathison DA, Stevenson DD, Simon RA: Precipitating factors in asthma. Aspirin, sulfites, and other drugs and chemicals. Chest 87:50S–54S,1985

McFadden ER Jr: Exertional dyspnea and cough as preludes to acute attacks of bronchial asthma. New Engl J Med 292:555–559, 1975

McFadden ER Jr, Kiser R, DeGroot WJ: Acute bronchial asthma, relations between clinical and physiologic manifestations. New Engl J Med 288:221–225, 1973

Morris HG: Mechanisms of action and therapeutic role of corticosteroids in asthma. J Allergy Clin Immunol 75:1–13, 1985

Newman SP, Clarke SW: The proper use of metered dose inhalers. Chest 86:342–344, 1984

Orgel HA, Kemp JP, Tinkelman DG, et al: Bitolterol and albuterol metered-dose aerosols: comparison of two long acting beta$_2$-adrenergic bronchodilators for treatment of asthma. J Allergy Clin Immunol 75:55–62, 1985

Russi EW, Ahmed T: Calcium and calcium antagonists in airway disease. A review: Chest 86 :475–482, 1984

Slepian IK, Mathews KP, McLean JA: Aspirin-sensitive asthma. Chest 87:386–391, 1985

Spector SL: The use of corticosteroids in the treatment of asthma. Chest 87:73S–79S, 1985

Stevenson DD, Mathison DA, Tan EM, et al: Provoking factors in bronchial asthma. Arch Intern Med 135:777–783, 1975

Turner-Warwick M: On observing patterns of airflow obstruction in chronic asthma. Br J Dis Chest 71:73–86, 1977

Zwillich CW, Sutton FD Jr, Neff TA, et al: Theophylline-induced seizures in adults. Ann Intern Med 82:784–787, 1975

Hillary Don

21

Management of Status Asthmaticus in Adults

Status asthmaticus is a severe, life-threatening exacerbation of bronchial asthma that fails to improve with conventional treatment. Conventional treatment should include three subcutaneous injections of epinephrine at 15-minute intervals. Status asthmaticus brings with it the possibility of the need for mechanical ventilation unless prompt and vigorous treatment is instituted. The use of the term "status asthmaticus" has the disadvantage of drawing attention away from other aspects of severe asthma, such as that patients die at home, and in some cases within minutes of the onset of an attack, before "conventional treatment" can be instituted. In some ways, therefore, it is better to describe "severe acute asthma" rather than status asthmaticus.

Reported mortalities are shown in Table 21-1, and have a mean of 1.23 percent of patients hospitalized for status asthmaticus. Mean mortality for children (1.2 percent) is similar for that of adults (1.3 percent). Asthma remains a potentially lethal disease, and its mortality has not declined significantly over the last 20 years. The causes of death are shown in Table 21-2. Progressive disease is commonly associated with obstruction due to plugging of small airways with thick tenacious mucus; mucosal edema with eosinophilic cellular infiltrate, and hypertrophy and spasm of the bronchial smooth muscle may be only secondary findings. Therapy may be inappropriate in that, for example, systemic steroids may be utilized too late or in too small a quantity, or overdosage with theophylline may occur, with seizures and hypoxemia. The use of sedative drugs has been associated with deaths in status asthmaticus due to depression of the respiratory center. Tension

BRONCHIAL ASTHMA, Second Edition
ISBN 0-8089-1814-1

Table 21-1
Variations in Published Mortality
of Severe Acute Asthma
Between 1963 and 1976

Period	Age	Number	Mortality %
1963–1965	Children	31	0
1965–1967	Children	91	4.3
1966–1968	Adults	80	2.8
1972	Children	324	0.3
	Adults	237	1.7
1970–1974	Children	356	0.3
1974	Adults	127	0.8
1968–1975	Both	2933	0.9
1967–1975	Adults	811	1.0
1974–1976	Adults	1345	0.2

pneumothorax or pneumomediastinum are not infrequent companions of status asthmaticus, whether or not positive-pressure breathing treatment is used. Mechanical failure of the ventilator was the sole cause of death in one study of patients in status asthmaticus. Hemodynamic instability may be created by hypovolemia due to poor fluid intake. Pulmonary edema has been reported, produced by hypervolemia. Finally, sudden death may occur, with no obvious antecedent warning or precipitating factor. This occurs predominantly between the hours of midnight and 6 A.M. and correlates with excessive diurnal variation in peak expiratory flow rate (PEFR).

Table 21-2
Causes of Mortality in Severe Acute Asthma

Progressive asthma not responding to therapy
Failure by physician to appreciate the severity of disease
Inappropriate therapy
    too little, e.g., corticosteroids
    too much, e.g., isoproterenol, aminophylline
Sedative or narcotic drug administration
Associated pulmonary problems
    infection
    pneumothorax
    aspiration of gastric contents
Malfunction or accident with mechanical ventilation
Hemodynamic problem
    hypovolemia, shock
    pulmonary edema, hypervolemia, negative pleural pressure
Sudden cardiac arrest

CLINICAL PICTURE OF STATUS ASTHMATICUS

Respiratory System

The patient with severe acute asthma usually complains of dyspnea, wheezing, and fatigue. The history of the patient's respiratory disease is important in helping to assess both the etiology and severity of disease, and the following should be noted:

1. The history of previous attacks of severe asthma, the length of time the episode persisted, treatments instituted, and whether mechanical ventilation had been required.
2. Whether the patient has recently had, or been in contact with an upper respiratory tract infection; this may be a clue to the precipitating cause. Fifty percent of episodes of acute asthma have been related to prior upper respiratory tract infections, although a viral rather than bacterial organism is usual.
3. The duration of the present episode is important, as more persistent obstruction is likely due to mucus impaction rather than simple spasm of smooth muscle.
4. The patient's usual medication regimen, and whether there have been any recent changes.
5. Drugs the patient is taking that may have precipitated or caused the attack of asthma. Drugs incriminated include the beta-blocking agents propranolol, acebutalol and nadolol, and nonsteroidal anti-inflammatory drugs such as aspirin, naproxen, indomethacin, and zomepirac.
6. Environmental exposure to airway irritants such as ammonia, nickel, dusts, and fumes should be sought. Many forms of occupational asthma can be prevented by appropriate changes in the environment. There may also be a history of exposure to an allergen that provokes bronchospasm.

Physical examination of the patient almost invariably reveals expiratory rhonchi. Breath sounds may be distant and difficult to hear. With increasing severity, the intensity of the expiratory rhonchi may diminish as air entry fails. The respiratory rate is frequently increased to 24–30 breaths per minute in more severe attacks. Tidal volume usually diminishes. The chest wall may appear hyperinflated, and ventilatory movement may be difficult to detect. The use of accessory muscles, particularly the sternomastoid, is usually evident and correlates well with the severity of disease. When this sign is present in adults, the 1-second forced expiratory volume ($FEV_{1.0}$) is usually less than 1 liter, maximum midexpiratory flow is below 40 liter/minute, and specific conductance is less than 0.05 liter/second per cm of water per liter. The disappearance of this sign also corresponds well with improvement in mechanical impairment. The relief of dyspnea and subjective wheezing with recovery is still associated with significant disease—mean airway resistance 200 percent of predicted, and mean residual volume 230 percent of predicted value. Even with the complete absence of abnormal physical findings, considerable impairment of static and dynamic lung volumes remain.

Pulmonary function tests are the most reliable objective assessment of the severity of acute asthma, and usually show:

1. An increase in airway resistance and a decrease in specific conductance.
2. Hyperinflation of the lungs, with total lung capacity (TLC) 130 percent of predicted. This alteration is thought due to trapping of gas in the lung in combination with loss of lung recoil, increased outward recoil of the chest wall, and increased strength of contraction of the inspiratory muscles.
3. Functional residual capacity (FRC) may be increased twofold.
4. Residual volume (RV) may be increased up to 400 percent of predicted values.
5. Narrowing of the large airways is detected by measurement of maximum expiratory flow rate (MEFR) and airway resistance (R_{aw}), which may be 20 percent and 500 percent of predicted normal values, respectively.
6. Combined large and small airway function is assessed by the $FEV_{1.0}$ and the maximum expired flow rate at 50 percent vital capacity. Mean values in acute asthma for $FEV_{1.0}$ of 30 percent of predicted have been shown, but values as low as zero have been recorded because of the inability of patients to cooperate for the test in extreme cases.
7. A reduction of the oxygen partial pressure in arterial blood (PaO_2) is almost invariable when breathing room air, and correlates with a reduction of $FEV_{1.0}$. The alveolar-arterial oxygen tension gradient ($P(A-a)O_2$) is increased to 40 Torr from a normal value of 5 Torr. Calculated venous admixture is 7.9 percent as compared to a normal value of two percent.
8. Variable effects on arterial carbon dioxide ($PaCO_2$) are found. Initially, hyperventilation with hypocapnia is the rule. With mild obstruction, mean values for the $PaCO_2$ of 25 Torr, at pH 7.44 have been described. With worsening disease the $PaCO_2$ increases as the $FEV_{1.0}$ declines below 20 percent predicted. The dead-space fraction of tidal volume (V_D/V_T) is increased to 0.45 from normal values of 0.3. Capillary determinations of PaO_2, $PaCO_2$, and pH have shown similar changes during acute asthma, and correlate with arterial values.
9. The ventilation response in asthmatic patients to hypoxia is described as normal or reduced. The response to hypercapnia and obstruction to airflow is normal or supernormal.
10. Roentgenograms of the chest customarily show clear, hyperlucent lung

fields with hyperinflation, even when upper respiratory infection is a predisposing factor. Pneumomediastinum, subcutaneous air, or pneumothorax may be visible. Pneumoperitoneum may be found occasionally.

Cardiovascular System

The heart rate is commonly increased; a rate above 114 beats per minute is indicative of severe airways obstruction. Systolic and diastolic systemic pressures are often increased. Frequently, systemic systolic pressure diminishes more than the usual amount during spontaneous inhalation; pulsus paradoxus is defined as existing when this fall in systolic pressure exceeds 10 Torr, and its presence correlates well with both outcome and severity of asthma in adults and children. Pulsus paradoxus is present in patients when $FEV_{1.0}$ is less than 20 percent of their best $FEV_{1.0}$ during recovery. However, pulsus paradoxus may be present in mild, and absent in severe, airways obstruction.

The electrocardiogram (EKG) is frequently abnormal in status asthmaticus. The most common finding is P pulmonale, which is a P wave with an amplitude greater than 2.5 mV. This finding is indicative of hypercapnia ($PaCO_2$ >44 Torr) and more severe obstruction. ST-segment and T-wave abnormalities are found in approximately 10 percent of patients, suggesting myocardial ischemia.

Pulmonary artery systolic and diastolic pressures related to atmospheric pressure in patients with severe acute asthma have been shown to be normal. However, mean pleural pressure becomes markedly negative during acute asthma, and consequently pulmonary artery and right ventricular transmural pressures are increased. Right ventricular afterload is also increased.

Radioisotope lung scans frequently show clear-cut focal perfusion abnormalities during an acute attack of asthma. The mechanism for these alterations in perfusion is not known, but focal hypoxia or air trapping has been postulated.

ABNORMALITIES ASSOCIATED WITH STATUS ASTHMATICUS

Intravascular Volume

Hypovolemia, with blood volume reduced by 10 percent, is common in patients in status asthmaticus. This is accompanied by an increase in hematocrit and plasma protein concentration. The reason for this apparent loss of plasma is not obvious. The deficiency of intravascular volume may predispose to circulatory collapse.

Hypervolemia has also been described and an increase in antidiuretic hormone is found in some patients with acute asthma. Water intoxication and hyponatremia may therefore occur, and should be considered as a possible cause of an altered state of consciousness.

Pulmonary Edema

An increase in lung water will further increase small airways obstruction in status asthmaticus, and impair gas exchange. In addition to hypervolemia, the mechanics of breathing may cause pulmonary edema. The tendency for small airways to close elevates the FRC and increases the distending pressure. Mean pleural pressure is therefore more negative throughout tidal breathing, and becomes slightly positive during exhalation only during severe obstruction. Mean pleural pressure in one study during tidal breathing in children with status asthmaticus ranged from $^-7.7$ to $^-25.5$ cm H_2O, compared to the normal of $^-5$ cm H_2O. The decrease in pressure will lower lung interstitial pressure, favoring the filtration of edema fluid into the lung.

Adrenal Failure

All asthmatic patients who have previously received steroids must be treated with systemic steroids during an acute attack of asthma, as their adrenal response to stress may be diminished or absent.

Central Nervous System

As the acute episode of asthma progresses, patients frequently become irrational and confused. They may become obtunded and finally comatose. The causes of these changes are not clear. Hypoxemia or hypercapnia may be factors. Fatigue, the effects of medications, and possibly water intoxication may also contribute. A decrease in the level of consciousness is a grave sign, not only of increased disease but also of the loss of the patient's ability to cooperate with proposed therapies.

Metabolic Studies

Metabolic acidosis is common during severe acute asthma, with an increase in lactic and pyruvic acids. Increased glycolysis and anaerobic respiratory muscle glycolysis during extreme airways obstruction may be the cause of the changes.

In patients with acute asthma, serum glutamic oxaloacetic transaminase, lactic dehydrogenase, and creatinine phosphokinase activities are significantly increased. Serum sodium and potassium are normal. The mean serum value for the 2,3-diphosphoglycerate concentration is elevated to 17.5 μmol/g of hemoglobin, as compared with the normal upper limit of 16 μmol/g hemoglobin; this is presumably a compensatory mechanism to enhance oxygen delivery at the tissues.

Lung Disruption

Lung disruption, with air found in the mediastinum, subcutaneous tissue, pleural space, or peritoneal cavity, is surprisingly rare in severe acute asthma. In two studies, chest radiographs of patients with acute asthma failed to reveal a single example of lung disruption. Other studies have suggested that pneumomediastinum or pneumothorax occurs in about two percent of patients with acute asthma.

Differential Diagnosis

The patients' complaints of dyspnea and wheezing, together with the physical findings of expiratory rhonchi and retractions, make the diagnosis of an acute attack of asthma so obvious that they unfortunately obscure the need to seek alternative explanations.

Upper Airway Obstruction

Intrathoracic tracheal obstruction predominantly will cause expiratory rhonchi that are indistinguishable from bronchospasm. Such tracheal obstruction can be caused by tracheal stenosis, an aberrant pulmonary artery, or a foreign body. Diagnosis is helped by the pattern of onset of the respiratory distress, but may only be confirmed by bronchoscopy.

Although extrathoracic tracheal or laryngeal obstruction produces primarily inspiratory obstruction, it can mimic asthma. Spastic adduction of the vocal cords can present as asthma. We have seen airway obstruction caused by the administration to an elderly patient of a large therapeutic tablet, which adhered to the back of the tongue, being mistaken for acute asthma, and being unsuccessfully treated with intravenous aminophylline.

Pulmonary Embolism

Dyspnea and expiratory rhonchi are presenting symptoms in some patients with pulmonary embolism. Diagnosis may be difficult, as both asthma and acute pulmonary embolism may show focal filling defects on perfusion scan of the lungs. If the usual clinical differentiating features are not clear, a pulmonary angiogram may be necessary.

Pulmonary Edema

Pulmonary edema is often associated with peribronchial cuffing and expiratory rhonchi. The edema may be associated with high left-ventricular filling pressure, and diagnosis may require a pulmonary-artery balloon flotation catheter. Pulmonary edema with normal filling pressures is difficult to diagnose, but may be suspected in the clinical setting.

Pulmonary Infection

Acute bronchitis or bronchiolitis may mimic asthma. Examination of the sputum by Gram stain may be helpful. Elevation of the white blood cell count is not a distinguishing feature, as it is often elevated in acute asthma without infection.

Lung Disruption

Air in the interstitium of the lung or in the mediastinum may compress airways, mimicking airway smooth muscle spasm. The patient with pneumothorax may also present with expiratory rhonchi.

Aspiration of Gastric Contents

Dyspnea and expiratory rhonchi may be produced following aspiration of gastric contents. Usually, the chest radiograph will be abnormal after aspiration. Sometimes, however, the diagnosis of aspiration pneumonia is one of exclusion.

Drugs

A clinical picture identical to that of acute asthma may be produced by a hypersensitivity reaction or a direct effect of drugs.

Factitious Asthma

The characteristic findings of acute asthma can be readily mimicked by a patient. A history of asthma can be provided, respirations can be labored, the accessory muscles used, and wheezes made audible. Symptomatic relief with therapy can be simulated. More objective signs of asthma will usually uncover this form of factitious illness. These include absence of hypoxemia and a normal alveolar-to-arterial oxygen tension gradient, lack of hyperinflation on chest radiograph, and normal small airway function soon after resolution of symptoms. Bronchial reactivity is absent.

DRUG THERAPY IN STATUS ASTHMATICUS

The mainstay of treatment of status asthmaticus is pharmacologic in nature. The routes of choice for administration of drugs are subcutaneous, intravenous, or inhalation. Oral and rectal administration do not have a place in the treatment of severely ill patients because of the lesser predictability of the length and extent of action.

Subcutaneous Injection of Medications

Epinephrine is the drug of choice in the initial treatment of severe asthma. This agent stimulates α, β_1, and β_2 adrenergic receptors and in addition to its effects on airway resistance, has been shown to cause in normal people:

1. an increase in heart rate
2. an increase in cardiac output
3. an increase in systemic systolic blood pressure
4. a fall in systemic diastolic pressure
5. a decrease in vascular resistance

In adult patients with acute asthma, the subcutaneous injection of epinephrine (0.25 mg) has the following effects:

1. onset with 15 minutes
2. maximum effect at 45 minutes
3. duration of approximately 2.5 hours
4. a 20-percent increase in PEFR
5. no change in heart rate
6. a slight fall in systemic and diastolic pressures

The injection of epinephrine (0.5 mg) has similar effects to 0.25 mg except for the following:

1. the duration of effect increases to more than 3 hours
2. PEFR increases 40 percent
3. pulse rate decreases slightly

In children, epinephrine 0.01 mg/kg (with a maximum dose of 0.3 mg) has no effect on heart rate and systemic systolic pressure, but decreases diastolic pressure. Repeating the dosage in 30 minutes has the same effect, or lack of effect, on these hemodynamic variables.

Terbutaline, a drug with more selective β_2-adrenergic activity, has been introduced with the expectation of equivalent bronchodilation to epinephrine, but with less marked effect on hemodynamics. In a comparison of these two agents in the normal human, terbutaline (0.25 mg) increases heart rate and cardiac output to the same degree as 0.5 mg epinephrine.

In adult patients with acute asthma 0.25 mg terbutaline produces an increase in pulmonary function similar to 0.5 mg epinephrine, except that (1) the duration is less (2 hours as compared with 3 hours), and (2) the heart rate increases slightly.

In children the subcutaneous injection of terbutaline 0.01 mg per kg of body weight (up to a maximum of 0.3 mg) during an acute attack of asthma, when compared to the identical dose of epinephrine, has the following effects:

1. terbutaline has twice the effect on the $FEV_{1.0}$—an increase of 40 percent as compared with 23 percent with epinephrine.
2. the improvements in the clinical index (a composite score utilizing the extent of wheezing, retractions of the chest wall and nasal flaring) are similar.
3. the respiratory rate decreases similarly after either drug.
4. heart rate increases slightly with terbutaline, but is unchanged with epinephrine.
5. systemic systolic pressure is not significantly altered by either drug.
6. systemic diastolic pressure is reduced approximately 4 Torr by either drug.

Terbutaline (0.01–0.02 mg/kg body weight) has also been shown to reduce the $PaCO_2$ and increase the PaO_2 in patients with status asthmaticus.

In summary, subcutaneous injection of epinephrine remains the route and drug of choice for initial treatment of patients in status asthmaticus. For adult patients, a dose of 0.3–0.5 mg of a 1:1,000 solution should be used. This can be repeated as necessary every 20 minutes. No maximum dose is described, but it should probably not be repeated more than three times. In children, the dose of epinephrine (1:1,000) is 0.01 mg/kg, to a maximum of 0.3 mg and no increase in heart rate should be expected. A small decrease in systemic systolic and diastolic pressure will usually occur. No clear advantage of subcutaneous terbutaline has been demonstrated.

Intravenous Aminophylline (Theophylline Ethylenediamine)

Aminophylline plays a central role in the therapy of reversible bronchoconstriction. Traditionally, aminophylline is considered to work through inhibition of phosphodiesterase and increasing intracellular cyclic AMP. This in turn mediates smooth muscle relaxation and inhibits the release of histamine by mast cells. It may also act as a prostaglandin antagonist. The mechanism producing bronchodilatation, and even the hypothesis that bronchodilatation is the major benefit produced by aminophylline, has been challenged, however. Other facets of the pharmacologic properties of aminophylline that might contribute to improvement of the patient's status are the diuretic effect, the central stimulation of ventilation, and the increased contractility of the diaphragm caused by the drug. Aminophylline also increases right and left ventricular ejection fractions in patients with chronic obstructive pulmonary disease, whether or not ventricular function is depressed in the control state. Heart rate and systemic blood pressure increase slightly.

When aminophylline is administered intravenously there is considerable variation in plasma theophylline levels produced among patients, and in the same patient at different times and in different disease states. The effect of theophylline on airways increases with increasing plasma concentrations. The effect on $FEV_{1.0}$ increases from 30 to 80 percent as plasma levels increase from 5 to 20 $\mu g/ml$. However, nausea and vomiting are observed at approximately 15 $\mu g/ml$, cardiac arrhythmias at 40 $\mu g/ml$, and convulsion when 50 $\mu g/ml$ is exceeded. The therapeutic range of plasma concentration of theophylline, therefore, lies between 10 and 20 $\mu g/ml$.

Theophylline is eliminated by biotransformation in the liver and excretion of the breakdown products in the urine. The mean plasma half-life of theophylline in normal adults is 4.5 hours. The half-life varies with the age of the patient, the severity of the airways obstruction, the presence of pneumonia, congestive heart failure, liver disease, with a history of cigarette smoking, and in the presence of various drugs.

Clearance is increased in the presence of acidemia, such that at pH 7.3, twice the dose of aminophylline would be required to increase the plasma theophylline concentration by 10 $\mu g/ml$ when compared to that required at pH 7.5. Ideal or lean body weight or PaO_2 do not alter theophylline clearance.

The dosage of intravenous aminophylline should be modified with these factors in mind. A suggested dosage schedule to produce a plasma theophylline level of approximately 10 $\mu g/ml$ is (1) a loading infusion of 6 mg/kg over 20 minutes (this should be reduced if the patient has already received theophylline); and (2) a standard maintenance infusion of 0.5 mg/kg hour, modified as follows:

1. children (under age of 19 years), increase to 0.6 mg/kg per hour
2. cigarette smokers, increase to 0.8 mg/kg per hour
3. congestive heart failure reduce to 0.2 mg/kg per hour
4. liver disease, reduce to 0.2 mg/kg per hour
5. pneumonia, reduce to 0.2 mg/kg per hour

6. patients receiving cimetidine, erythromycin, or troleandomycin,
    reduce to 0.3 mg/kg per hour

Further regulation should be by measurement of plasma theophylline
concentration, because the above dosage schedule may still provide either
subtherapeutic or toxic levels.

In summary, failure of the patient with acute asthma to improve following the subcutaneous injection of epinephrine necessitates the administration
of intravenous aminophylline. Aminophylline and catecholamines in vitro
work synergistically, although this additive effect has not been demonstrated
in acute asthma.

Inhaled Sympathomimetic Agents

Isoproterenol is a potent sympathomimetic agonist that has both β_1 and
β_2 effects in man. Administered by inhalation, it has relatively little effect on
heart rate or blood pressure as compared with similar bronchodilation produced by parenteral use.

In adult patients with stable asthma the inhalation of 0.3 mg isoproterenol by Freon inhaler produces the following effects:

1. a 20-percent increase in $FEV_{1.0}$
2. a decrease of 45 percent in airway resistance
3. a fall in FRC of 20 percent
4. a 50-percent increase in maximum flow at 25 percent of vital capac-
    ity
5. a time of onset that varies with the specific test but ranges from 30
    seconds to 10 minutes
6. peak effect is found in 15 minutes
7. duration of significant effect is 1–2 hours
8. infrequently, a mild increase in heart rate
9. neither systolic nor diastolic blood pressure is affected

Palpitations may be noted in a small percentage of people.

In approximately one-half of adult asthmatic patients inhaling nebulized
isoproterenol, the PaO_2 decreases by 7 Torr and the $P(A-a)O_2$ increases 12
Torr when breathing air. The alveolar-arterial oxygen tension when breathing
pure oxygen is not altered.

The dose of inhaled isoproterenol is an arbitrary decision because variable amounts, as low as 10 percent, of the administered dose may be retained
in the lung. In adults, 2.5 mg of isoproterenol (0.5 percent) added to saline
(1.5 ml) is administered by nebulizer and can be repeated every 30 minutes,
depending upon clinical response. Alternatively, 0.25–0.5 mg can be inhaled
from a Freon dry aerosol.

For children, 2.5 mg of isoproterenol should be diluted to 2 ml with saline and the child given 10–15 breaths. This can be repeated at 30-minute intervals, as long as pulse rate stays below 180 beats/min.

The administration of more specific β_2-agonists by inhalation has the advantage of longer duration of action. The effects of terbutaline in stable asthmatics are as follows:

1. An inhaled dose of 1.5 mg increases the $FEV_{1.0}$ by 45 percent, the maximum flow at 25 percent of vital capacity by 80 percent, and specific airway conductance by 140 percent.
2. Significant effect is detected within 5 minutes. Maximum effect is found at 1 hour. The response persists at least 6 hours.
3. The percentage change in pulmonary function tests following 0.5 mg is approximately half the effect of 1.5 mg. The duration of action is still at least 6 hours, however.
4. There are no significant alterations in heart rate, nor in systemic blood pressure.
5. Hypoxemia is not usual after administration of inhaled terbutaline.

In summary, inhalation of a beta agonist should be commenced when the effect of repeat subcutaneous epinephrine has been assessed and the priming dose of intravenous aminophylline is infused. The drug most commonly used in the past was isoproterenol. The drug of choice is probably a more specific β_2- agonist (metaproterenol, terbutaline, salbutamol, or fenoterol), which has a more prolonged effect, and perhaps causes less hemodynamic alterations. There is not, however, documented significant clinical advantage of these agents over isoproterenol.

Corticosteroids

Corticosteroids have been used in the management of status asthmaticus for at least 25 years. Double-blind controlled studies have shown an improvement in $FEV_{1.0}$ when intravenous corticosteroids were added to the management of patients with acute asthma who had been documented to be refractory to 8 hours of conventional treatment. The benefit of the steroids became apparent after approximately 10 hours of therapy. The dose and type of corticosteroid best used is not known.

The mode of action of corticosteroids in relieving status asthmaticus is not known, and is probably multiple. The adverse effects of using corticosteroids for short durations (2 or 3 days) are insignificant. Weighed against their proven advantages in status asthmaticus, they should be started as soon as the diagnosis is made.

The dosage and type of corticosteroids are arbitrary: (1) hydrocortisone 7 mg/kg as a loading dose, followed by 7 mg/kg every 8 hours, or (2) dexamethasone, 0.3 mg/kg as a loading dose, followed by 0.3 mg/kg every 24 hours. Corticosteroids should be continued at this dosage for 48 hours and then tapered over 2 days.

Antimuscarinic Agents

Although atropine has been used for several hundred years in the treatment of asthma, the role of inhaled antimuscarinic agents in the treatment of severe asthma is uncertain.

In adult patients with acute asthma, aerosolized atropine methonitrate (1.5 mg) causes an increase of 44 percent in the $FEV_{1.0}$ and inhaled salbutamol (200 μg) a 50-percent increase. The effect of atropine lasts 4 hours, and that of salbutamol lasts 2 hours. The dosages of drugs used has been shown to produce a maximum response, but the combination of salbutamol (200 μg) and atropine (1.5 mg) causes a 75-percent increase in the $FEV_{1.0}$.

Ipratropium bromide is a longer acting antimuscarinic agent than atropine, and has fewer side effects. In an inhaled dosage of 1 mg it was shown to be as effective a bronchodilating agent as inhaled salbutamol (5 mg) in patients with acute asthma.

The role of the antimuscarinic drugs in acute asthma is not established. The customary therapeutic sequence at present is to initially administer a subcutaneous adrenergic agent such as epinephrine. This is repeated, and if improvement in the patient's status is not evident, an intravenous loading dose of aminophylline, followed by a continuous infusion, is commenced. Inhaled beta receptor agonists are also administered. Corticosteroids are added. Should the patient fail to improve, or even deteriorate, inhaled atropine or ipratropium should be given.

INTERMITTENT POSITIVE-PRESSURE BREATHING (IPPB)

Although accepted by custom, the use of intermittent positive-pressure breathing is not well established in proven utility. Delivery of bronchodilating agents by IPPB has been shown to have no advantage over hand nebulizers in adults and children, although marginal benefit from IPPB has been claimed by some workers.

It should be noted that studies of the effect of IPPB during acute asthma have regulated peak inspiratory airway pressure to values between 10 and 20 cm H_2O. These pressures are low when treating a patient with airways obstruction. Without ensuring that the delivered volume is greater than the patient's voluntary inspiratory effort, IPPB would not be expected to be of value. IPPB in severe acute asthma is used mainly in patients who are not responding to other forms of therapy. It also has a place in the management of patients who are familiar with IPPB and believe that it is of value. Although part of its value may be psychological support, that aspect of care is of particular importance in the management of patients with severe asthma.

CHEST PHYSIOTHERAPY

Although the value of chest physiotherapy has not been proven, breathing exercises and assisted coughing are probably beneficial. In addition, the psychological component may be therapeutic.

ADDED INSPIRED OXYGEN

Hypoxemia is frequent in patients with severe acute asthma while the patient is breathing air, and augmented inspired oxygen is always necessary. Arterial oxygen tension should be maintained above 60 Torr by means of nasal prongs or a face mask. Arterial carbon dioxide tension may rarely be elevated by increasing PaO_2, but the hazard of hypoxemia is greater than the potential fall in pH.

HUMIDITY

A predominant pathologic finding in patients with status asthmaticus is obstruction of airways due to tenacious mucus. The administration of added humidity to the inspired gas is probably of benefit to loosen secretions and allow productive coughing. Humidity is produced either by nebulized particles or by heated vapor. Either method may, in some patients, provoke bronchospasm. Nebulized normal saline has been claimed to have no associated bronchospasm. Monitoring the effect is therefore essential. Correction of systemic dehydration with intravenous fluid therapy is also important.

SODIUM BICARBONATE

Correction of metabolic acidosis and partial compensation for respiratory acidosis has been recommended in patients with status asthmaticus. Although correction of the underlying deficit is imperative, persistent metabolic acidosis should be corrected by administration of small amounts of sodium bicarbonate, using the equation

administered $NaHCO_3$ (mEq) = base deficit (mEq) $\times$ 0.3 body weight in kg

Dangers of bicarbonate administration include the possibility of cerebral acidosis, due to the relative impermeability of the blood-brain barrier to bicarbonate compared to the ease of movement of carbon dioxide. In addition, ventilatory drive may be blunted, hypokalemia is frequent, and the severity of the asthmatic attack may be disguised.

ANTIBIOTICS

The use of broad-spectrum antibiotics is not warranted unless there is evidence of bacterial infection. Although upper respiratory infections have been frequently incriminated as the trigger for status asthmaticus, these infections are usually viral.

Criteria for the presence of infection are (1) otitis media, (2) purulent pharyngitis, and (3) lobular infiltrate on chest roentgenogram. The leukocyte count is deceptive, being frequently raised to $10,000-20,000/mm^3$ in patients with acute asthma.

INTRAVENOUS FLUID THERAPY

The infusion of intravenous fluids is governed by the same general principles as in any severely ill patient. The initial deficit should be replaced, as hypovolemia is common. Generous replacement has been advocated, with the purpose of promoting the hydration of pulmonary secretions. There is, however, no evidence that intravenous fluid therapy aids lung clearance. In view of the possible development of pulmonary edema due to predominantly negative pleural pressures, the aim should be to maintain satisfactory intravascular volume without producing hypervolemia.

Potassium should be added to the intravenous fluids, as hypokalemia is common in status asthmaticus, particularly when treated with corticosteroids.

PROGRESSIVE AIRWAYS OBSTRUCTION

Clinical recovery from status asthmaticus usually occurs within minutes or hours of the institution of the therapies outlined in the preceding sections. Hypercapnia, pulsus paradoxus, and changes in the electrocardiogram disappear first, within hours. The $FEV_{1.0}$ and PEFR normalize more slowly, and may take more than 7 days. The patient's symptoms may become normal when $FEV_{1.0}$ is still reduced to 30 percent predicted. Functional residual capacity and RV remain elevated even when TLC is normal.

A percentage of patients, however, do not respond to the therapies already outlined. The differential diagnosis must be reexamined to ensure that a discrete identifiable factor has not been overlooked, such as tracheal stricture. Potentiating factors must also be sought: pulmonary embolism or edema, pneumomediastinum, pneumothorax, aspiration of gastric contents, or pneumonia.

Careful observation of the patient must be maintained, as sudden death, particularly in the early hours of the morning, is not uncommon. Danger signals in the patient's progress include:

1. altered mental state, with developing coma
2. increase in pulsus paradoxus above 20 Torr
3. tachycardia in the adult above 120 and in children above 180 beats/minute
4. $PaCO_2$ increasing to levels above 65 Torr
5. progressive hypoxemia as inspired oxygen is increased
6. increased use of accessory muscles
7. inspiratory breath sounds diminished or absent
8. increased hyperinflation on chest roentgenogram
9. PEFR below 100 liters/minute or a $FEV_{1.0}$ less than 0.5 liters, and failure to improve with bronchodilators

Continued deterioration can be halted by the use of a continuous intravenous infusion of isoproterenol, or by the institution of mechanical ventilation.

Intravenous Sympathomimetic Agents

The use of an intravenous infusion of a beta receptor agonist such as isoproterenol has been recommended in patients who have failed to improve in spite of the treatments already described. The initial infusion of isoproterenol 0.1 μg/kg per minute is increased in steps of 0.1 μg/kg per minute every 15 minutes if the patient does not respond. The usual maximum dose is approximately 0.5 μg/kg per minute. However, inhalation of the beta receptor agonists is as effective as the intravenous route, with less systemic toxicity.

Endotracheal Intubation and Mechanical Ventilation

Mechanical ventilation is instituted when the severity of the disease continues to increase in the face of maximum drug therapy. The benefits from mechanical ventilation are:

1. Minute ventilation is augmented or provided entirely by the ventilator. This spares the work of breathing by the patient, and maintains a normal $PaCO_2$ and pH.

2. PaO_2 is maintained because the larger tidal volumes provided by the machine will help reverse atelectasis or pulmonary edema.
3. The patient will be able to be given either narcotics or sedatives, and will be able to rest.
4. The presence of an endotracheal tube will allow improved pulmonary toilet in a patient who is unable to cough effectively.

Endotracheal Intubation

The indications for performing endotracheal intubation and beginning mechanical ventilation are not clearly defined or rigid. The following is a list of factors that guide the decision:

1. Possibly the most important factor is alteration in the patient's mental state. The onset of drowsiness, confusion, irritability, or coma is ominous because of its cause—possible cerebral hypoxia—and its consequence—lack of ability to cooperate with needed therapies.
2. Persistent hypoxemia (PaO_2 less then 60 Torr) in the presence of maximum inspired oxygen fraction.
3. Increasing $PaCO_2$ (above 65 Torr) with decreased pH (less than 7.25).
4. Persistent and increasing metabolic acidosis.
5. Increasing fatigue, with marked retraction of the accessory muscles of breathing and intercostal indrawing.
6. Diminished or absent inspiratory breath sounds as tidal volume diminishes, with either increased or decreased expiratory rhonchi.

Endotracheal intubation can be performed by either the nasal or oral route. The initial route of tracheal intubation in the adult patient is via the nose. The advantages of this route compared with the oral are that the tube can usually be inserted during maintained spontaneous breathing using only topical anesthesia, it is more easily secured once inserted, and it is more comfortably maintained for the patient. The disadvantages of the nasal route are the occurrence of nasal hemorrhage, obstruction of the tube by pressure from the walls of the nasal passage, and maxillary sinusitis. The oral route allows the passage of a shorter, wider endotracheal tube.

The procedure of nasotracheal intubation must be carefully planned and prepared. The patient is informed of the procedure and is connected to a cardiac monitor. The nasal mucosa is sprayed with cocaine (4 percent) to produce topical anesthesia and local vasoconstriction. The lubricated endotracheal tube is inserted into the nostril and advanced slowly and firmly. Through a feeding tube inserted to the distal end of the endotracheal tube, 1 percent lidocaine (maximum 10 ml) is injected in front of the tube. The tube is advanced, using audible or visible (by water condensation) guides, through the larynx. The tube is secured and its position relative to the nares is noted.

Auscultation of the chest checks the position of the tube. A chest roentgenogram is mandatory, however, as auscultation is an unreliable guide.

Should the nasal route not be possible, tracheal intubation is accomplished through the mouth. Although intubation through this route can be achieved with topical anesthesia alone, it is probably easier and safer to perform oral intubation after the patient has been sedated with diazepam and paralyzed with succinylcholine. The oral route is probably safer in children.

An endotracheal tube with an internal diameter of at least 8 mm should be used in adult patients, to facilitate endotracheal suctioning and allow fiberoptic bronchoscopy should this be needed for diagnostic or therapeutic reasons. The endotracheal tube should be constructed from clear plastic material certified for tissue compatibility by animal implantation tests. The material must not irritate mucous membranes, and should be smooth and sufficiently flexible to conform to the patient's anatomy. The tube should not kink at small radius nor flatten due to the pressure of the cuff or the walls of the upper airway. A radiographic marker must be present at the distal end of the tube. The cuff should have a high residual volume with high compliance when inflated.

The complications of endotracheal intubation include the following:

1. At the time of insertion, hypoxemia, reflex cardiac arrhythmia, and vomiting with possible aspiration may occur. Trauma to the mucosa and hemorrhage may be caused by the nasal route.
2. The endotracheal tube breaks the continuity of the patient's natural lung clearance mechanisms, and may introduce infection.
3. The tube may be incorrectly placed into the esophagus or a mainstem bronchus.
4. The endotracheal tube may become obstructed by kinking, by an overinflated cuff compressing the tube or evaginating over the end of the tube, or by materials such as blood clots or secretions within the lumen.
5. Erosion of the trachea may occur, with development of a tracheo-mediastinal or tracheo-esophageal fistula.
6. Following removal of a tube, laryngeal problems such as airway obstruction or hoarseness may occur for a variable length of time. Stenosis of the trachea may also be found.

Management of Mechanical Ventilation

After insertion of the endotracheal tube, the patient's spontaneous breathing is gently assisted by means of a hand ventilating device. Sedative or narcotic drugs are carefully administered intravenously. The drugs of choice are:

1. Morphine sulfate by intravenous injection. Increments of 2–4 mg may be given. Although releasing histamine and theoretically increasing airway resistance, it is commonly used in this situation.
2. Diazepam, 2–4 mg IV can be added, or used alone.
3. Ketamine hydrochloride has been advocated for use in patients with acute asthma. The drug has been shown to reduce airway resistance and increase compliance in patients with preexisting airways obstruction.
4. If severe bronchospasm persists, inhalation of halothane can be used. Halothane results in bronchial dilatation and has been used effectively in patients with severe asthma.

Frequently in children but only occasionally in adults, the administration of drugs that block the neuromuscular junction is necessary. The drug of choice is pancuronium, a nondepolarizing agent that rarely causes hypotension, but may frequently produce tachycardia. Intravenous titration of 0.05 mg/kg dosages should be carried out in either adult or pediatric patients.

For adult patients, mechanical ventilation that is time or volume cycled is then started. Pressure cycled ventilators have the major disadvantage of delivering decreased tidal volumes when airway resistance increases or lung or chest wall compliance decreases. On the other hand, with children who have uncuffed endotracheal tubes in place, and therefore a variable leak around the tube, a pressure cycled ventilator may provide a more constant tidal volume. A parallel breathing circuit should also be used, allowing spontaneous breathing of the same inspired oxygen fraction as is used for the mechanical breath.

A tidal volume between 8 and 12 ml/kg of body weight is delivered. This is approximately 20 percent less than the size of the tidal volume selected for most patients being mechanically ventilated for other causes of acute lung disease. The reason for this reduction is to minimize gas trapping and hyperinflation, reducing the harmful effect of positive intrathoracic pressure on hemodynamics and reducing the risk of lung disruption. It has been recommended that peak inspiratory pressure be kept at or below 50 cm H_2O to reduce the possibility of barotrauma. Moderate hypercapnia is then tolerated in some patients. Titration of intravenous sodium bicarbonate can be used to maintain near normal pH.

The frequency of ventilation is adjusted while considering the following factors:

1. The expiratory phase must allow near complete emptying of the lungs. This can be judged by watching the patient's chest wall or the filling of an expiratory spirometer if in place.
2. The minute ventilation should not produce marked hyperventilation. Sudden hypocapnia in combination with preexisting compensatory meta-

bolic alkalosis can cause seizures and cardiac arrhythmias. The $PaCO_2$ should be adjusted to produce mild alkalemia (pH 7.45).

3. The frequency will usually be between 8 and 16 per minute in adults, but higher rates—up to 30 per minute—may be necessary in children.

The inspiratory flow rate is adjusted with the ventilatory rate to maintain 1:2 inspiratory-to-expiratory ratio, and the inspired oxygen fraction (F_1O_2) is set at 1.0 and the PaO_2, $PaCO_2$, and pH are determined. The F_1O_2 is then adjusted to maintain the PaO_2 at approximately 100 Torr.

Mechanical ventilation is continued, together with sedation with morphine or diazepam. Endotracheal suctioning is carried out every 1–2 hours. Instillation of up to 50 ml of normal saline prior to suctioning may facilitate removal of secretions. The bronchodilator therapy instituted prior to endotracheal intubation is maintained. A greater percentage of any drug nebulized through the endotracheal tube will be delivered to the airways and lung compared to through a face mask or oral airway, so a reduction in dosage may be necessary.

Care of the patient includes

1. Monitoring the function of the ventilator and endotracheal tube by setting appropriate alarms and careful observation.
2. Daily chest radiograph.
3. Daily Gram stain of sputum.
4. Measurement of forced vital capacity at appropriate intervals.
5. Monitoring PaO_2, $PaCO_2$, and pH at intervals not greater than every 6 hours; an indwelling arterial line is therefore advisable.
6. Positive end-expiratory pressure (PEEP) can be applied if oxygenation needs to be improved or inspired oxygen reduced. The risk of further hyperinflation and lung disruption would seem considerable in a patient who already has hyperinflated lungs. It has been suggested, however, that PEEP may treat severe bronchospasm, reducing gas trapping and peak airway pressure during mechanical ventilation of patients with acute severe asthma.
7. The placement of a nasogastric tube and the administration of antacids.
8. Nutrition should be started as soon as practicable, either by the intravenous or alimentary route.

Failure of the Patient to Improve During Mechanical Ventilation

The patient may fail to improve during mechanical ventilation, despite continuation of the therapies already instituted. Additional treatments can be used and assessed.

PULMONARY LAVAGE

Instillation of large volumes of fluid into the airway may be therapeutic. Solutions containing normal saline, acetyl-cysteine, a beta agonist, and a corticosteroid have been found effective.

INHALED ANESTHETIC AGENTS

Inhalalation of halothane has been used to reduce airway resistance and peak respiratory airway pressure. Anesthesia has been maintained for 4–5 days in this way.

PLASMAPHERESIS

Apparent benefit has been reported in a patient with severe chronic asthma. Plasmapheresis, if proven effective in this setting, is probably too slow in the onset of its benefit to be of value in severe acute asthma.

EXTRACORPOREAL MEMBRANE OXYGENATION

Support by extracorporeal membrane oxygenation can prevent immediate death, although it does not improve ultimate survival of patients with the adult respiratory distress syndrome. Its successful use in severe acute asthma has been reported in the management of a patient who was moribund in the face of maximal treatment. Extracorporeal support restored the patient's hemodynamic status, and allowed pulmonary lavage. The presumed eventual reversibility of the severe acute asthmatic attack makes the patient in some ways an ideal candidate for extracorporeal support.

Hazards of Mechanical Ventilation

The complications of mechanical ventilation in status asthmaticus seem to be more frequent than when ventilation is maintained for other causes of acute lung disease. Common problems are

1. Mechanical problems with the ventilator and its circuitry are possibly the greatest hazard. They have been reported to occur in 20 percent of patients.
2. Depression of cardiac output. During inflation, positive-pressure ventilation creates increasingly less negative pleural pressure, and in fact the pressure may become positive. This increases intrathoracic venous pressure, which in turn may reduce venous return, with consequent depression of cardiac output. Pulmonary vascular resistance is also increased. The rise in venous pressure may also elevate the back pressure in the hepatic and renal circulations. Although cardiac filling may be decreased due to the more positive pleural pressure, it is possible that left ventricular function is aided as the positive pressure tends to reduce afterload.

3. Lung disruption is not frequent. Air can track from the bronchovascular bundle to almost any part of the body. Mediastinal air, subcutaneous emphysema, and pneumothorax are each reported to occur in approximately 20 percent of patients. Pneumoperitoneum is more rare, and occurs in less than 5 percent of patients.
4. Hyperinflation, either of both lungs or of discrete areas in the lungs, may occur. This is presumably due to a ball-valve effect aggravated by limited expiratory time.
5. Fluid retention is described as a consequence of positive-pressure ventilation. Increases in both antidiuretic hormone and aldosterone have been attributed to this mode of ventilation.

Mortality in Patients Mechanically Ventilated for Status Asthmaticus

Mean mortality for patients mechanically ventilated for severe acute asthma is approximately 12 percent, and does not seem to have declined over the past 20 years. The latter finding is surprising in view of the advances in respiratory care, but it may represent selection of more sick patients for mechanical ventilation. The causes of death in this group of patients include hypoxic brain damage in about one third of patients, pneumothorax, mechanical ventilator failure, sepsis, cardiac arrhythmias, and inexorable deterioration in the patient's condition due to the underlying disease.

Discontinuing Mechanical Ventilation

Although the criteria for discontinuing mechanical ventilation have received considerable attention in the literature, no combination of factors has been shown to cover all aspects of the problem. The management of weaning must therefore be tailored to the individual patient. Some guidelines are

1. The mechanics of breathing are the major focus, and recovery of vital capacity is the most important variable. Vital capacity should exceed approximately 10 ml/kg body weight.
2. Expiratory rhonchi should be lessened, and may be absent when extubation is finally accomplished.
3. The patient is awake and cooperative.
4. A period of spontaneous ventilation is tolerated for at least 45 minutes, with $PaCO_2$ less than 50 Torr.

The period of mechanical ventilation in patients with severe acute asthma is usually brief, averaging about 60 hours. Following extubation, humidified oxygen is administered. The patient's medications are then tapered and discontinued or changed to the oral route as appropriate over the next 2–3 days. The patient should be reassured that the necessity for use of mechanical ventilation for support during the acute episode of severe asthma does not imply that the disease will in the future involve more frequent or more severe attacks. Many patients have demonstrated improved pulmonary function in the years following an episode of acute asthma that required tracheal intubation and mechanical ventilation.

REFERENCES

Don H: Status asthmaticus in adults. Clin Rev Allergy 3:69–93, 1985

Don H: Wheezing, in Don H (ed): Decision Making in Critical Care. Toronto, BC Decker, 1985, p. 70–71

Don H: Acute asthma, in Don, H (ed): Decision Making in Critical Care. Toronto, BC Decker, 1985, p. 76–77

Fanta CH, Rossing TH, McFadden ER, Jr: Emergency room treatment of asthma. Relationships between therapeutic combinations, severity of obstruction and time course of response. Am J Med 72:416–422, 1982

Fanta CH, Rossing TH, McFadden ER, Jr: Glucocorticoids in acute asthma. A critical controlled trial. Am Rev Respir Dis 125:94(S), 1982

MacDonnell KF, Moon HS, Sekar TS, et al: Extracorporeal membrane oxygenator support in case of severe status asthmaticus. Ann Thorac Surg 31:171–175, 1981

Matthay RA, Berger HJ, Loke J, et al: Effects of aminophylline upon right and left ventricular performance in chronic obstructive pulmonary disease. Noninvasive assessment by radionuclide angiocardiography. Am J Med 65:903–910, 1978

McFadden ER, Jr, Kiser R, DeGroot WJ: Acute bronchial asthma: Relations between clinical and physiologic manifestations. New Engl J Med 288:211–225, 1973

Peress L, Sybrecht G, Macklem PT: The mechanism of increase in total lung capacity during acute asthma. Am J Med 61:165–169, 1976

Pierce RJ, Payne CR, Williams SJ, et al: Comparison of intravenous and inhaled terbutaline in the treatment of asthma. Chest 79:506–511, 1981

Powell JR, Vozeh S, Hopewell P, et al: Theophylline disposition in acutely ill hospitalized patients. The effect of smoking, heart failure, severe airway obstruction, and pneumonia. Am Rev Respir Dis 118:229–238, 1978

Qvist J, Andersen JB, Pemberton M, et al: High-level PEEP in severe asthma. New Engl J Med 307:1347–1348, 1982

Rebuck AS, Read J: Assessment and management of severe asthma. Am J Med 51:783–798, 1971

Roth MJ, Wilson AF, Novey HS: A comparative study of the aerosolized bronchodilators isoproterenol, metaproterenol and terbutaline in asthma. Ann Allergy 38:16–21, 1977

Simons FER, Pierson WE, Bierman CW: Respiratory failure in childhood status asthmaticus. Am J Dis Child 131:1097–1101, 1977

Stalcup SA, Mellins RB: Mechanical forces producing pulmonary edema in acute asthma. New Engl J Med 297:592–596, 1977

Webb-Johnson DC, Andrew JL, Jr: I. Bronchodilator therapy. New Engl J Med 297:476–482, 1977
Webb-Johnson DC, Andrews JL, Jr: II. Bronchodilator therapy. New Engl J Med 297:758–764, 1977
Westerman DE, Benatar SR, Potgieter PD, et al: Identification of the high-risk asthmatic patient. Experience with 39 patients undergoing ventilation for status asthmaticus. Am J Med 66:565–572, 1979

Otto G. Raabe
Robert S. Howard
Carroll E. Cross

22

Aerosol Considerations in Asthma

Understanding of aerosol generation, deposition, and removal processes has become increasingly important to environmental scientists, inhalation toxicologists, physiologists, allergists, pulmonologists, and occupational medicine personnel. Although inhaled aerosols have been used since the time of Hippocrates to treat asthmatic disorders, recent widespread uses of inhaled newer, longer-acting, and more specific β_2-adrenergic agents, muscarinic agents, steroids, and other compounds effecting mediator release, emphasize the importance of understanding the principles of aerosol interactions with the respiratory tract to clinicians caring for patients with asthma and related diseases.

Aerosols have many important advantages over other routes for administration of therapeutic agents to individuals with airway diseases. The diagnostic, prophylactic or therapeutic aerosol is delivered directly to the epithelial surfaces that give rise to bronchospastic reactions. Diagnostic studies such as studies of aerosol deposition, mucociliary clearance, respiratory epithelial permeability and allergic, pharmacologic and irritant "challenge" can only be accomplished via inhalation delivery systems. Prophylactic effects are more complete than from oral or systemic administration, i.e., numerous studies have shown that aerosol therapy is clearly more efficacious in the prevention of bronchospastic reactions provoked by various stimuli (allergens, inhaled irritants, pharmacologic agents, exercise) than are oral and systemic therapies. Finally, therapeutic effects of aerosol treatment are more rapid in onset, generally more effective, and, since smaller doses are

BRONCHIAL ASTHMA, Second Edition
ISBN 0-8089-1814-1

used, are lower in the incidence of systemic side effects. For example, administration of an effective dose of an aerosolized β_2-adrenergic produces a blood level of approximately 1/100th the blood level of a comparably effective dose of an orally or systemically administered β_2-adrenergic agent. Analogous approximate efficacy/blood level interrelationships probably apply for aerosol versus systemic administrations of both muscarinic antagonists and corticosteroids. Aerosol drug administration in asthma allows for an improved separation of local (airway) effects and systemic effects (including side effects), providing the clinician with the opportunity to use a more effective and safer therapeutic option.

Aerosols are defined as relatively stable suspensions of finely-divided liquid droplets or solid particles in a gaseous medium, usually in air. If inhaled, aerosol particles may be deposited by contact upon respiratory epithelial surfaces leading to desirable therapeutic actions, potential injury, or planned diagnostic behavior depending on the particular physical and chemical properties of the particles and the biological characteristics of the respiratory tract. As pharmacologic agents deposited in the respiratory tract can directly influence the wide variety of cells constituting the respiratory epithelium, properly formulated, generated, delivered, and deposited aerosols are important considerations in aerosol pharmacotherapeutics. As tracers of airflow or indicators of lung epithelial anatomy and function, aerosols deposited in the lung can be utilized for various diagnostic studies. Aerosols are used for ventilation scans, for assessing respiratory epithelial permeability and rates of mucociliary clearance, and also for determining the perturbating effects of infections, drugs and environmental toxicants on both permeability and clearance.

This chapter will consider applied principles of aerosol generation and deposition in the airways, methods for characterizing aerosols, the different types of equipment and techniques used for aerosol delivery systems and briefly other applications of aerosol technology to the clinician. The apparent increasing importance of aerosol sciences to the field of environmental inhalation toxicology, which has significant implications to the asthmatic patient, will not be specifically addressed.

AEROSOL PROPERTIES

The Aerodynamic Diameter

The aerodynamic performance of aerosol particles depends upon such physical characteristics as the particle size, shape, and density. It is a combination of these properties that determines the inertial character of a particle. For any particle of a given size, shape, and density, we can, at least mathematically, construct a spherical particle of unit density (1 g/cm^3) that will have exactly the same aerodynamic properties as any given particle. The diameter of this artificial sphere is called the "aerodynamic diameter" (AD). The usefulness of this concept of an equivalent aerodynamic diameter is that aerosol particles having varying sizes, shapes, and densities, are often described in terms of their relative aerodynamic diameters. Should two different aerosols consist of particles having the same distribution of aerodynamic diameters, the inertial behavior of the two aerosols will be identical.

For aerosols of extremely small particles, (diameters less than 0.5 μm), the concepts of aerodynamic diameter and inertial behavior are not very useful because Brownian diffusion is then the predominant mechanism of particle motion. But the inhalable aerosol particles to be used in asthma therapeutics should have aerodynamic diameters larger than this, typically from 1 to 10 μm. Hence, in this discussion, we shall neglect particle diffusion and concern ourselves with the inhalation properties of particles for which the concept of aerodynamic diameter is applicable.

Particle Size Distributions

Medical aerosols are comprised of particles or droplets having a range of physical or aerodynamic sizes, so they must be described in terms of distribution parameters. Referring to aerosols as if they consist of one size of particle is wrong and misleading when, in fact, a range of sizes is mixed together. The lognormal distribution is a natural distribution of sizes that has been observed to apply to size distributions of various types. It has thus become customary to assume that medical aerosols are lognormally distributed with respect to size. With this assumption, it is then possible to completely describe a distribution in terms of only two values, e.g., the median size, and the associated geometric standard deviation. Figure 22-1 shows a representative lognormal distribution (probability density or frequency function) in terms of the count (or number) of particles of various sizes; the characteristic parameters in this case are the count median diameter (CMD) and associated geometric standard deviation (σ_g).

If the particle aerodynamic diameter had been calculated and plotted rather than the physical diameter, the median would have been the count median aerodynamic diameter (CMAD). Numerically half of the particles are smaller than the CMD (or CMAD) and half are larger. Of course, the amount of aerosolized drug deposited is usually more important than the number of individual particles. With that amount usually proportional to the mass, the parameter most often chosen for discussion is the Mass Median Aerodynamic Diameter (MMAD), rather than the CMAD. Half the mass of an aerosol is associated with particles smaller than the mass median, and half with larger particles.

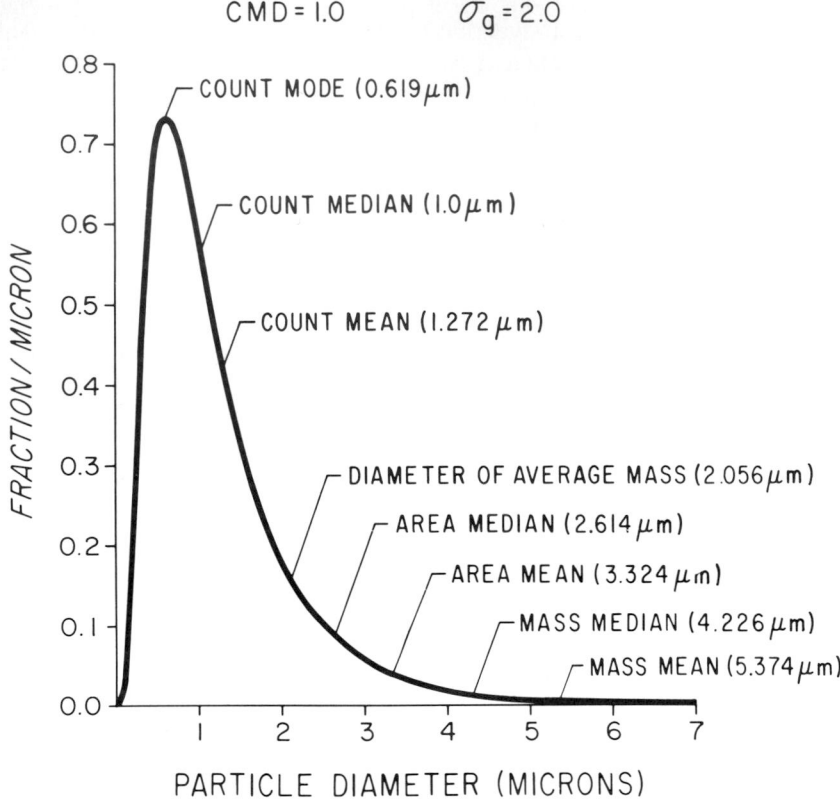

Fig. 22-1. Example of the lognormal particle size distribution describing the particle number distribution with count median diameter (CMD) equal to 1 μm and geometric standard deviation (σ_g) equal to 2.

The geometric standard deviation (σ_g) is quite different from the normal standard deviation. The σ_g is the ratio of the particle size with a cumulative value of 84.1 percent to that of the median size (50 percent cumulative value) rather than the difference between these sizes as in the normal standard deviation. As such, the geometric standard deviation has no units, and must always be greater than 1. But if it is less than about 1.2, we consider the particle size distribution to be sufficiently narrow so that the particle sizes are effectively uniform, equal or "monodisperse." With a larger σ_g, the aerosol would be called "polydisperse," or "heterodisperse" if a mixture of constituents.

The output of an aerosol generator can be assessed by measuring the size distribution of the resulting aerosolized particles. There is a wide diversity of engineering techniques to do this, ranging from simple instruments for the measurement of light scattering or a series of air-jets impinging onto disc inserts ("cascade impactors"), to very sophisticated sensors or collectors that characterize the particle size distribution and chemistry. For most purposes, it is usually enough to report the MMAD and σ_g of an aerosol.

Inhalation Deposition of Particles

The collection in the respiratory tract of inhaled airborne particles, and the initial regional pattern of these collected particles, is called deposition. All particles that ever come in contact with the moist walls of the airways are deposited. Figure 22-2 illustrates the five principal physical mechanisms that may lead to the deposition of inhaled particles in the respiratory tract. Most medical aerosols are electrostatically charged by the aerosol generation processes, and these charged particles may be attracted to the wall of the airway by the image-charge effect. However, the overall influence of charge on the deposition of most medical aerosols is probably small. Likewise, the noninertial incidental contact of a particle with the wall of the airways leads to deposition by interception, but this process is most important only for elongated particle shapes such as fibrous aerosols. Brownian diffusion is significant only for particles less than 0.5 μm, i.e., only for particles much smaller than those used in medical therapeutics. So the two most important physical processes associated with inhalation deposition of medical aerosol are gravitational settling and impaction.

Deposition by gravitational settling occurs throughout the respiratory tract due to the influence of the earth's gravity on small particles suspended in

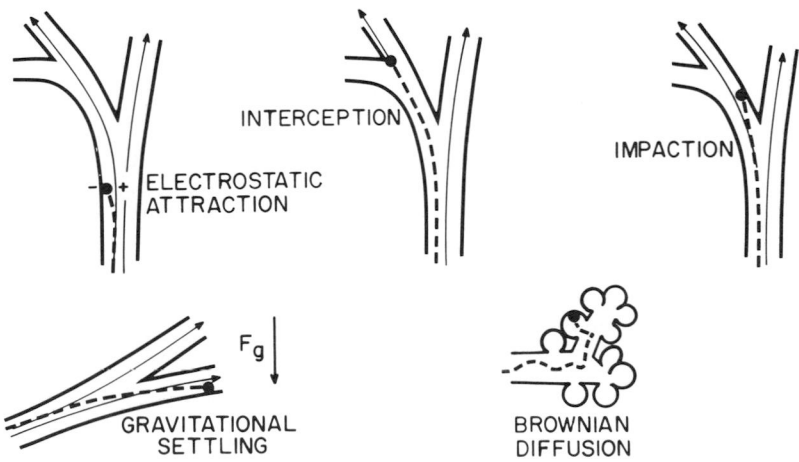

Fig. 22-2. Illustration of five major physical mechanisms of deposition of inhaled airborne particles in the human respiratory tract.

air. The settling speed of small particles increases proportionally with the square of the aerodynamic diameter, and for a 5-μm aerodynamic diameter particle, the gravitational settling speed is about 0.7mm/second. Gravitational deposition is especially important in the distal regions of the bronchial airways and is enhanced by breath-holding, or low frequency breathing, since both these conditions lead to longer residence times for particles in the respiratory tract.

Inertial impaction is the dominant mechanism of deposition of particles larger than 3 μm in aerodynamic diameter and occurs primarily in the nasopharyngeal airways, oropharynx, larynx, and proximal tracheobronchial regions. In this process the airborne particles, because of their inertia, do not follow changes in direction or speed of air streamlines and as a result they may collide with the wall of the airway. For example, if air velocity is suddenly reduced or turned because of the change in flow direction caused by the obstruction of a surface, inertial momentum may carry larger particles across the air streamlines and into the moist surface of the tract where they are deposited.

Even with carefully developed theoretical models and with the support of reliable deposition data, it is not possible to predict exactly in a particular person the quantitative regional deposition of particles of a given inhaled aerosol. Biological variability in airway geometry and tone between individuals, differences in health, confounding factors such as cigarette smoking and differences that relate to age, sex, size, and ventilatory pattern can cause differences in the fraction of an inhaled aerosol that may deposit in the airways and in the site of deposited aerosol within the airway. However, for the purposes of medical aerosol planning, reasonable predictions are made using the available models and data employing certain simplifying assumptions concerning biological factors.

The most widely used model of regional deposition versus particle size was developed by International Commission on Radiological Protection (ICRP) Task Group on Lung Dynamics in 1966. Assuming "typical" anatomical values for normal respiratory parameters for a 70-kg person, the ICRP Task Group then mathematically predicted the deposition throughout the respiratory system of aerosol particles *inhaled and exhaled through the nose* at a rate of 15 breaths per minute at various tidal volumes. The result for a TV=750 ml is shown in Figure 22-3. Deposition occurs both during inspiration and exhalation. At least three cautions, however, must be taken when attempting to apply this model to predict aerosol deposition in asthma therapy:

1. The aerosol particle may change in size as it moves from the generator into the lungs. Usually, the pharmacologically active drug is being carried by liquid droplets. These can undergo relatively rapid evaporation

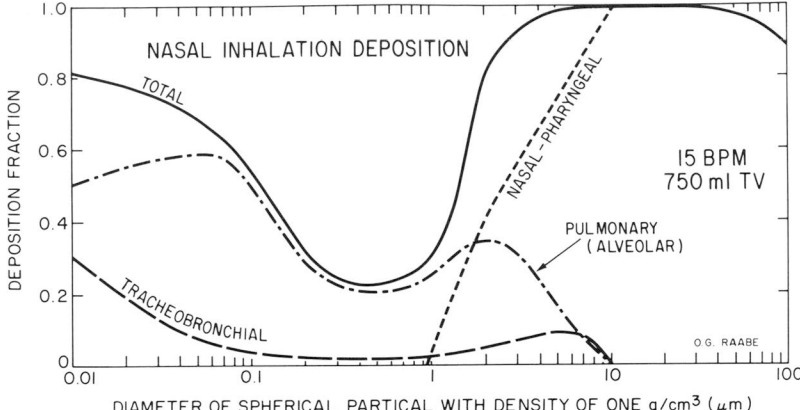

Fig. 22-3. Nasal Inhalation Deposition: Total and regional deposition fractions for aerosols entering the nose for various sizes of inhaled airborne spherical particles with physical density of one gram per cubic centimeter in the human respiratory tract as calculated by the International Commission on Radiological Protection (ICRP) Task Group on Lung Dynamics (1966) for nasal breathing at a rate of 15 breaths per minute (BPM) and tidal volume (TV) of 750 ml.

during their transit, and can thereby result in more than a four-fold reduction in particle size between generation and deposition. On the other hand, a hygroscopic aerosol particle may grow in size during the sojourn through the lung's humidified airways.

2. Therapeutic aerosols are commonly not breathed continuously, but rather are introduced under pressure as a bolus with a very high initial velocity which quickly changes at a poorly defined rate.

3. The ICRP Task Group Model did not consider oral asthmatic aerosol therapy.

Experimental data with human volunteers can be integrated with the ICRP model to provide information on the regional deposition during oral breathing. The site of deposition for oral breathing changes markedly from nasal breathing due to the loss of the filtering action of the nasal airways. Figure 22-4 shows typical deposition patterns versus particle size during steady oral breathing. Again, these results may not apply exactly to a specific patient but show the general trends. Some studies have shown an enhanced deposition in patients with chronic obstructive pulmonary disease (COPD) as well as nonuniform distribution in lung for the deposited particles. Changes in airway caliber and nonuniform ventilation in diseased lungs are implicated.

Tracheobronchial deposition for particles larger than 5 μm as shown in

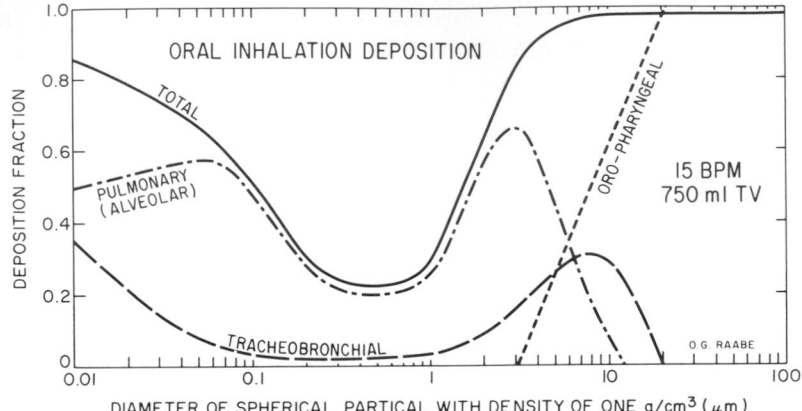

Fig. 22-4. Oral Inhalation Deposition: Total and regional deposition fractions for aerosols entering the mouth for various sizes of inhaled airborne particles with physical density of one gram per cubic centimeter in the human respiratory tract for breathing via the mouth at 15 breaths per minute (BPM) and tidal volume (TV) of 750 ml.

Figure 22-4 is primarily associated with deposition in the trachea and major bronchi. From both theoretical considerations and experimental observations, it is reasonable to set 5 μm as the maximum desirable aerodynamic diameter for inhalable particles that will deposit beyond the proximal tracheobronchial airways.

Clearance, Retention, and Other Medical Applications of Aerosols

After initial deposition, particles associated with inhaled aerosols are subjected to various physical, chemical, and biological processes including dissolution into body fluids with absorption by the blood, uptake by cells by phagocytosis or pinocytosis, and movement with mucus and body fluids. The term clearance is used to describe the translocation, transformation, and removal of deposited particles from the various regions of the respiratory tract. The temporal distribution of uncleared, deposited particles or their resultant transformation products is called retention.

Most medical aerosols consist of droplets and/or water-soluble components that will readily dissolve in body fluids soon after deposition. Ultimate clearance will be via the systemic circulation with transfer to other organs of the body. Systemic treatment can be effected via the inhalation route of drug administration. Somewhat less soluble aerosols may be used where extended retention is desired in one or more regions of the respiratory tract. Very fine (less than 1-μm aerodynamic diameter) radioaerosols can be used for ventilation scanning and offer some advantages over radioactive gases including lower cost and a lesser degree of patient coordination with the necessary respiratory maneuvers. In the special case of particles of a lipophobic radiotracer-DTPA complex, clearance may be from minutes to hours via respiratory tract epithelia and is dependent on cellular integrity and epithelial permeability. Therefore, this technique provides a useful diagnostic tool for evaluating respiratory tract epithelial injury utilizing external imaging techniques.

Relatively insoluble particles deposited in the ciliated region of the tracheobronchial airways are moved with mucus flow towards the epiglottis where they are swallowed or expectorated. This process is relatively efficient in that most particles deposited there are probably cleared within a few hours and all by one day postexposure.

Insoluble particles deposited in the nonciliated bronchioles or the alveoli are not rapidly cleared from the lung. Most are engulfed by and phagocytized by scavenger pulmonary alveolar macrophage cells, and some of these cells may ultimately enter the tracheobronchial mucus flow, but this does not seem to be a rapid process in human lungs. In some instances it takes up to one year to effectively clear half of alveolarly deposited insoluble particles. Some of the macrophages may enter the pulmonary lymph circulation and be transported to tracheobronchial lymph nodes, but this also is a slow process. Consequently, very insoluble particles are tenaciously retained in the lung parenchyma.

AEROSOL GENERATION

Nebulizers

A nebulizer is an atomizer used to produce aerosols of fine particles by breaking a liquid into fine droplets and dispersing them in a flowing stream of gas or air; generated droplet sizes are typically smaller than 10 μm in physical diameter. Nebulizers must be distinguished from common spray atomizers and from spray cans (Fig. 22-5A), which produce much larger droplets. There are two general types of nebulizers: (a) compressed air, or "jet" nebulizers, and; (b) ultrasonic nebulizers. Compressed air nebulizers are of two specific types, the Rayleigh stream and Babington nebulizers.

Rayleigh stream nebulizers employ a jet of air to entrain and shatter a stream of liquid. The expanding jet of air produces a static pressure that is negative with respect to the ambient atmospheric pressure and is utilized to draw liquid via a feed tube into the jet stream. Prior to 1958, medical nebulizers were essentially baffled spray atomizers. The development then of the Wright nebulizer (Fig. 22-5B) provided the prototype for Rayleigh stream

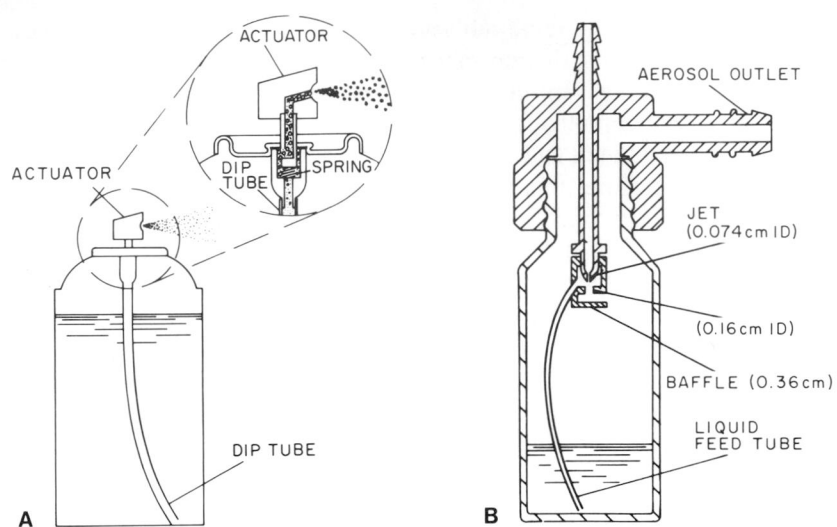

Fig. 22-5. Schematic illustration of a common spray can atomizer (A). This is contrasted with an illustration of the Wright nebulizer (B).

disruption utilizing a proximal jet disrupter baffle that has influenced the subsequent design of modern nebulizers. Wright showed that placement of a baffle obstruction close to the outlet of a Rayleigh jet stream of liquid and air caused a violent disruption of the stream yielding up to a tenfold greater output of inhalable droplets. Some modern nebulizers such as the Lovelace nebulizer and Retec nebulizer use a hemispherical primary baffle in place of the flat baffle used by Wright.

The Babington nebulizer principle (Fig. 22-6) was developed in 1969 as a means of nebulizing viscous liquids. Liquid is allowed to flow over an orifice (usually a rectangular slot) through which compressed air is forced. The surface tension of the flowing liquid over the orifice prevents the formation of a liquid stream, but small droplets are efficiently generated at the surface of the untorn film of liquid as the small parcels of compressed air rapidly traverse the film. A baffle is usually utilized to increase small droplet production by air stream disruption. Babington nebulizers are usually high-output devices suitable for humidification and croup-tent applications.

Ultrasonic nebulizers utilize a standing wave of high frequency ultrasound to produce a small geyser at the surface of a liquid reservoir. Droplets are produced by the high frequency ultrasound vibrations at the geyser's apex. A stream of air is used to carry off the aerosol, but compressed air is not involved in the droplet formation process. A sectional view of a typical ultrasonic nebulizer is shown in Figure 22-7. A high frequency electrical signal (up to 1 megahertz) is transmitted to a piezoelectric transducer that produces mechanical vibrations at the applied frequency. These vibrations

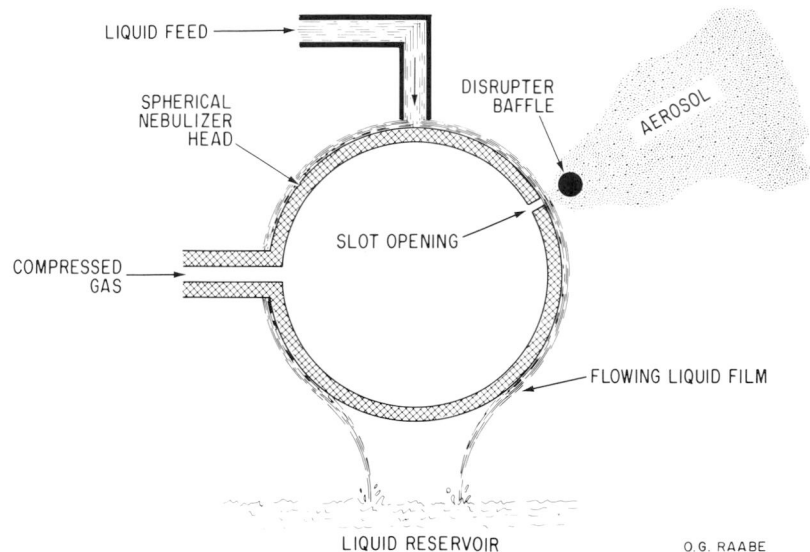

LIQUID FEED

SPHERICAL
NEBULIZER
HEAD

DISRUPTER
BAFFLE

AEROSOL

SLOT OPENING

COMPRESSED
GAS

FLOWING LIQUID FILM

LIQUID RESERVOIR   O.G. RAABE

Fig. 22-6.   Schematic illustration of a Babington nebulizer.

are highly directional and are transmitted via a conductive liquid (water) to the container of liquid to be nebulized as an intense acoustical field that produces adiabatic compressions and rarefactions. The actual magnitude of the vibrations is about 0.2 μm. This turbulence creates a pressure gradient along the axis of the transducer that results in a water geyser from which drops of about 0.3 μm are violently shaken. These small droplets rapidly coagulate to form aerosol droplets up to 10 μm in diameter. Ultrasonic nebulizers are also used for humidification and croup-tent applications.

Nebulizer performance is characterized in terms of the output concentration of inhalable aerosol delivered (microliters of liquid in droplets per liter of carrier air); evaporation losses separate from usable aerosol as a concentration (microliters of water vapor per liter of carrier air); volumetric flow rate of delivered aerosol (liters per minute of carrier air); mass or volume median diameter and geometric standard deviation of the released droplets at time of initial formation; volume of liquid required for proper operation; and operating time with typical reservoir filling. A summary of the operating characteristics of some selected nebulizers is given in Table 22-1.

The most desirable nebulizers for asthma therapy are those with droplet distributions that are initially below 5 μm in volume median diameter, have high aerosol concentrations (above 20 μl per liter), have low evaporation (below 20 μl per liter), yield more than 5 liters/min of aerosol, and operate for more than 15 minutes without refilling. Ultrasonic nebulizers are usually

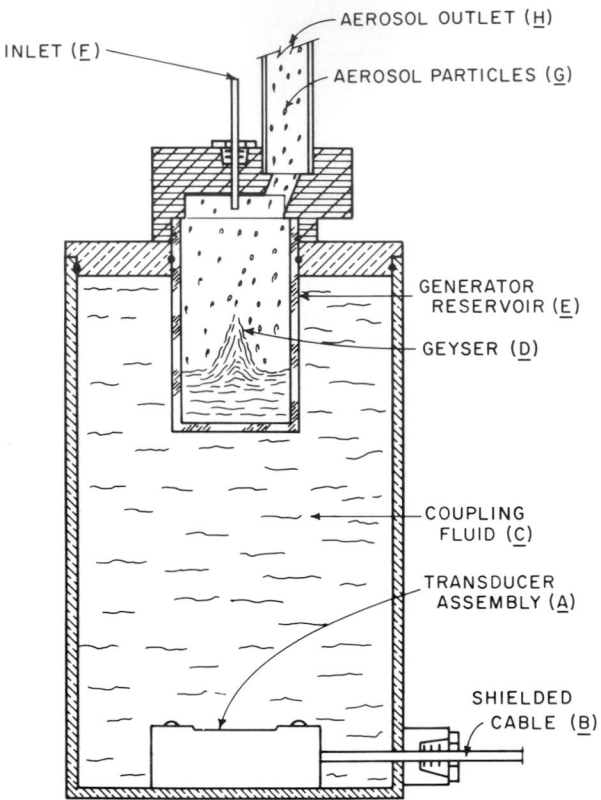

AIR INLET (F)

AEROSOL OUTLET (H)

AEROSOL PARTICLES (G)

GENERATOR
RESERVOIR (E)

GEYSER (D)

COUPLING
FLUID (C)

TRANSDUCER
ASSEMBLY (A)

SHIELDED
CABLE (B)

Fig. 22-7. Schematic illustration of an ultrasonic nebulizer showing the piezoelectric transducer assembly (A), receiving power via the shielded cable (B) generating an acoustical field in the coupling fluid (C) creating an ultrasonic geyser (D) in the generator reservoir (E) with air entering at (F) carrying away aerosol via the aerosol outlet (H).

best used for humidification applications because they heat the liquid being aerosolized (high evaporation losses) and concentrate enough energy in the liquid geyser to denature some chemicals.

Nebulizers can be used to produce aerosols of solid particles since the solvent (usually water) rapidly evaporates from droplets and dissolved or suspended materials yield an aerosol of the residue after the solvent has completely evaporated. Such residue aerosols are much smaller than the droplets from which they are formed. The mass median diameter (MMD_p) of the resultant aerosol can be calculated from the volume median diameter (VMD_d) of the original aqueous droplets using:

$$(MMD_p)^3 \times \rho = (VMD_d)^3 \times c$$

Table 22-1
Representative Operating Characteristics of Selected Nebulizers

Nebulizer Type	ΔP* (psig)	Q† (l/min)	A‡ (µl/l)	W§ (µl/l)	VMD‖ (µm)	σ_g¶	Vol# (ml)	Time** (min)
Dautrebande D-30	10	17.9	1.6	9.6	1.7	1.7	30	100
	20	25.4	2.3	8.6	1.4	1.7	30	70
	30	32.7	2.4	8.2	1.3	1.7	30	55
DeVilbiss No. 40	10	10.8	16	9.9	4.2	1.8	10	30
	15	13.5	15.5	8.6	3.5	1.8	10	28
	20	15.8	14	7.0	3.2	1.8	10	27
	30	20.5	12	7.2	2.8	1.8	10	23
Collison 3-jet	20	7.1	7.7	12.7			100	500
	25	8.2	6.7	12.6	2.0	2.0	100	470
	30	9.4	5.9	12.6			100	430
	40	11.4	5.0	12.6			100	370
Retec X-70N	20	5.2	55	16	5.4	1.9	10	24
	30	7.4	54	11	3.6	2.0	10	19
	40	8.6	53	7	3.7	2.1	10	18
	50	10.1	49	9	3.2	2.2	10	17
Lovelace	20	1.5	40	10	5.8	1.8	4	40
	30	1.6	31	11	4.7	1.9	4	45
Solosphere (Babington)	20	7.1	70	18	6.5	2.4	450	560
With auxiliary air	20	57	26	20	10	2.1	450	130
Mist-O₂-Gen Ultrasonic (Model EN145)	—	28	57	36	4.7	2.3	50	15
DeVilbiss Ultrasonic (Set #4)	—	41	150	33	6.9	1.6	500	60

* ΔP = Applied Gage Pressure
† Q = Volumetric Flow Rate
‡ A = Output Concentration
§ W = Evaporation Output

‖ VMD = Droplet Size Distribution
      Volume Median Diameter
¶ σ_g = Geometric Standard Deviation

Vol = Reservoir Volume
** Time = Approximate Operating
         Time Before Refilling.

where ρ is the physical density (g/cm^3) of the final solid particles and c is the concentration (grams per milliliter) of the solute or suspension in the nebulized liquid droplets.

Metered-Dose Inhaler

Metered-dose inhalers (MDI) release a spray consisting of large droplets of propellant within which the therapeutic agent is carried either as a suspension of fine particles or a solution. The MDI (Fig. 22-8) is essentially a miniaturized modification of commercial pressurized aerosol spray cans used to dispense paint, deodorants, and insecticides (Fig. 22-5A). The formulation to be aerosolized is mixed to approximately 10 ml with a suitable highly volatile liquid propellant, usually a fluorinated hydrocarbon such as dichloro-difluoro-methane (freon) and maintained at the liquification pressure (approximate 3 atm) in a sealed container. Surfactants, various cosolvents, antioxidants, flavorants, and perservatives are often included in the mixture. The pressure in the sealed container forces the mixture through a feed tube into a small metering chamber near the actuator orifice. When the actuator is depressed, it releases the measured volume of the formulation. Although the effective MMAD may exceed 40 μm at the actuator orifice, evaporation of the propellant yields particles or droplets that have MMADs of between 1 and

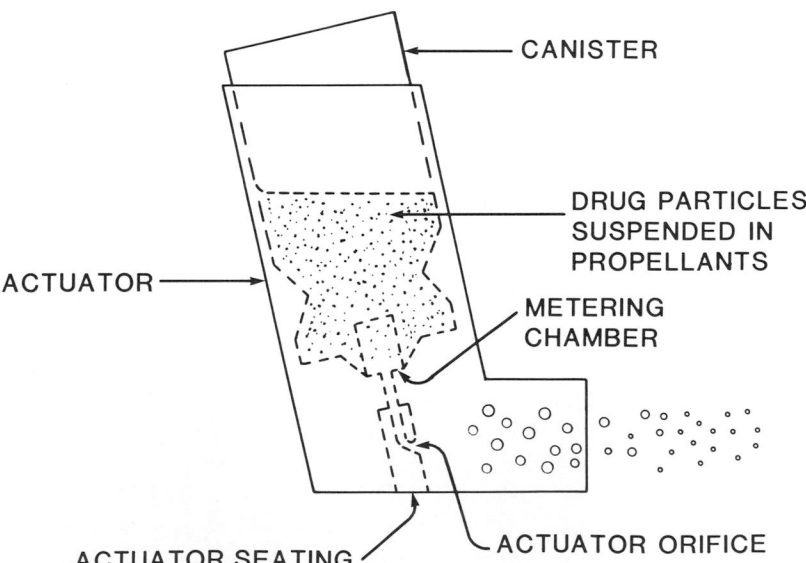

Fig. 22-8. Schematic illustration of the Metered Dose Inhaler used to generate measured pulses of aerosol utilizing a formulation mixed under pressure with a volatile liquid such as a fluorocarbon.

25 μm by the time they reach the oropharynx. The initial velocity of the propellant droplets often exceeds 30 m/sec. Because of the relatively large aerodynamic size and high inertia of the aerosol, most of the particles (approximately 80 percent of the dose) impacts on the oropharynx. Using optimal inhaler technique, approximately 10 percent of the metered dose reaches the lung and 10 percent remains on the delivery device. Unfortunately, many studies have documented that up to 50 percent of patients use a suboptimal inhalation technique; 15 percent of patients are unable to learn even after careful education.

Clinical Considerations

Most asthmatic patients will use commercially available heterodisperse aerosols released from MDIs or from jet nebulizers. The most critical factors in the efficient delivery of the aerosol to respiratory surfaces will be the aerosol size and the inhalation mode. Deposition from an MDI is maximized by activation of the MDI during the course of a slow deep inhalation followed by a 7–10 second breathhold; under these circumstances a maximum of 10–15 percent of the dosage deposits in airways. Because of the high oropharyngeal impaction of particles generated with simple MDIs, and the fact that many patients have difficulty using proper inhalation techniques, a variety of flow smoothing and drying chamber attachments have been developed. For the most part these may not markedly improve overall drug delivery to the bronchial airways because of particle losses in these devices. The droplets formed by MDIs consist of extremely volatile propellant mixed with various other liquid, solid, and dissolved components. Although the propellant may dry quickly, the associated cooling of the droplets delays the evaporation of other liquid constituents. The result is that droplets bigger than 10 μm in diameter may require several seconds to dry. Clearly, it is more important for improvement of the performance of MDIs to design better orifice nozzles that form the initial spray of propellant/medication mixture; if the initial droplet size distribution is reduced in size, the need for drying delays and special spacers can be eliminated.

The aerosol size distribution generated by MDIs depends upon a combination of factors including: (a) propellant properties including container pressure; (b) chemical formulation; (c) physicochemical properties of the constituent mixture including physical density, vapor pressure, viscosity, surface tension, heat of vaporization; and (d) engineering design of the nozzle orifice, actuator, and delivery system. Current MDIs yield dry particles with mass median aerodynamic diameters about 5 μm and geometric standard deviations of about 2. This means that 16 percent of the dosage is associated with particles bigger than 10 μm and 50 percent with particles bigger than 5 μm in aerodynamic diameter.

It is clear from Figure 22-4 that both tracheobronchial and oropharyngeal deposition decrease with decreasing particle size, but what is also important is that the sites of deposition tend to move into the smaller bronchial airways with decreasing size, just as it tends to result in increased pulmonary (alveolar) deposition. Hence, the most desirable range of particles for bronchial airway deposition and asthma therapy is in the range above 1 μm but below 5 μm in aerodynamic diameter. Particles larger than 5 μm will result in 50 to 100 percent deposition in the oropharynx, larynx, and proximal tracheobronchial airways.

Modern compressed air and ultrasonic nebulizers produce droplets size distributions that have medians below 5 μm. Since these water droplets begin to dry rapidly even under saturated conditions, the delivered droplet distributions can be expected to have mass median aerodynamic diameters under 2 μm. Nebulizers therefore tend to yield droplets in the proper size range for asthma therapy. However, nebulizers operate continuously while patients inhale intermittently. If only 40 percent of the breathing cycle involves inspiration, then only 40 percent of a nebulized aerosol can be inhaled. The remainder is usually released into the surroundings or exhaust duct. Also, some liquid is not generated from the reservoir and some aerosol is lost in the hoses and apparatus. Because of the preferential evaporation of solvents, the residual liquid volume retained by the apparatus is more concentrated in solute than that of the original solution. Of the 40 percent that is inhaled, about 40 percent is deposited in the lung, assuming the delivery droplet distribution mass median is less than 2 μm. With considerable individual variation due to factors such as operational technique, anthropomorphic effects and state of airways resistance, fractional deposition in the airways from clinical jet nebulizers, somewhat surprisingly, does not differ much from deposition from MDIs (Fig. 22-9). In the jet nebulizer the majority of the aerosol is retained in the apparatus and the tubing or passes out of the system during exhalation and a much smaller fraction is deposited in the oropharynx compared with MDIs. Only 10 to 15 percent of the medication is deposited in the lung with either device.

Although deposition in the lungs from nebulizers may be increased by changing the inhalation mode, such as by slow deep breathing followed by a breathhold, aerosol deposition from nebulizers is far less dependent on respiratory maneuvers than is deposition from MDIs. Increasing compressed gas flow rates or driving pressures (or operating frequencies in the case of ultrasonic nebulizers), by increasing the percentage of the aerosol mass in the desirable size range (MMAD < 5 μm), can modestly increase lung deposition. It seems that it is far less important to improve the fraction of the dosage reaching the airways from a nebulizer than it is to optimize MDI administration techniques. It appears that some patients, including those most severely ill with severe airways obstruction, benefit from the higher doses of broncho-

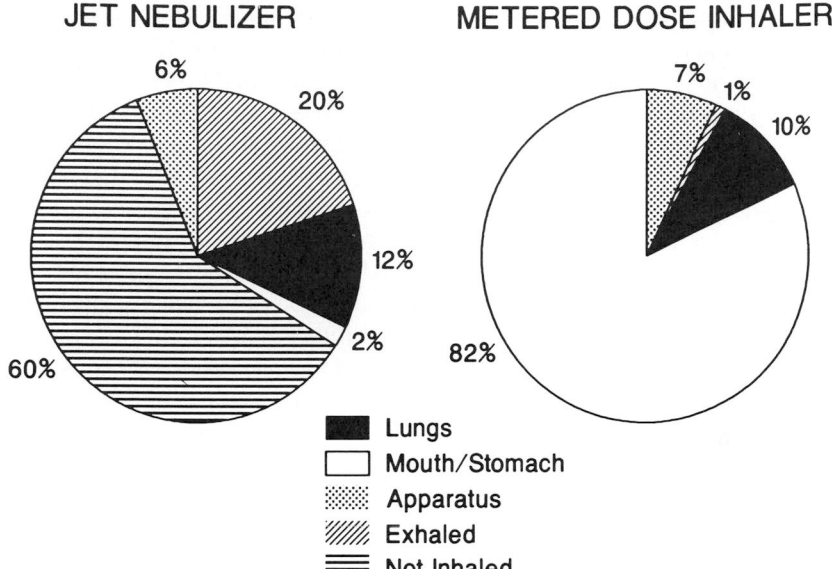

JET NEBULIZER   METERED DOSE INHALER

Lungs
Mouth/Stomach
Apparatus
Exhaled
Not Inhaled

Fig. 22-9.   Deposition patterns for therapeutic aerosols released from an MDI and from a jet nebulizer. Only about 10 to 15 percent of the dose reaches the lungs from each device, but the division of the remainder of the dose between oropharynx, inhalation apparatus and exhaled air is totally different.

dilators available via nebulizers. Other advantages of nebulizers are that they are versatile in dispensing therapeutic solutions or mixtures, need not contain additives such as propellants, surfactants and, in some cases, preservatives, and that output of the therapeutic agent can be varied over a wide range according to the choice of nebulizer and its operating conditions.

Although there is considerable research activity which would permit manufacture and delivery of therapeutic aerosols which would "target" more specific sites within the conducting airways, these currently involve relatively complex technologies that have not as yet found a wide application to asthmatic patients. In addition, specialized aerosols are under development, including the use of aerosols of liposomes that could be expected to significantly prolong, and in some cases, facilitate respiratory tract drug delivery.

SUMMARY

Current strategies in the management of asthmatic and related airway hyperreactivity states focus upon deposition of topically active therapeutic agents upon airway surfaces. To achieve an optimal therapeutic effect, the main considerations of aerosol therapy should be to utilize an aerosol-producing apparatus that generates an inhalable aerosol (<5 μm MMAD) and utilizes an appropriate delivery and inhalation system that will allow the generated aerosol to be deposited efficiently on tracheobronchial airway surfaces. Clinicians should have some understanding of the conditions which potentially modulate airway aerosol deposition and thereby may compromise the effectiveness of aerosol therapeutics. There is presently an increasing use of aerosols for the diagnosis of airway hyperreactivity, the determination of drug efficacy in modulating inhalation challenge responses, in evaluation of the distribution of ventilation, and in determination of bronchotracheal clearance rates and respiratory epithelial permeability.

An understanding of the principles related to aerosol science prepares the clinician to optimally utilize those aerosol therapies that are most efficacious and least toxic for patients with bronchospastic disorders. Problems of suboptimal aerosol deposition can be overcome with proper knowledge and use of aerosol delivery systems. Aerosol therapies can be expected to provide a satisfactory asthma treatment for the majority of patients, provide for a wide safety margin, and should be the cornerstone in the therapeutic armamentarium for all forms of asthma.

ACKNOWLEDGMENT

A portion of this chapter was supported by the United States Department of Energy under contract DE-AC03-76SF00472 with the University of California, Davis.

REFERENCES

Agnew JE, Pavia D, Clarke SW: Airways penetration of inhaled radioaerosol: An index to small airways function. Eur J Respir Dis 62:239–255, 1981

Ahrens RC, Bonham AC, Maxwell GA, et al: A method for comparing the peak intensity and duration of action of aerosolized bronchodilators using bronchoprovocation with methacholine. Am Rev Respir Dis 129:903–906, 1984

Alderson PO, Biello DR, Gottschalk A, et al: Tc-99m-DTPA aerosol and radioactive gases compared as adjuncts to perfusion scintigraphy in patients with suspected pulmonary embolism. Radiology 153:515–521, 1984

Aviado DM: Toxicity of aerosols. J Clin Pharm 15:86–104, 1975

Chan TL, Lippmann M: Experimental measurements and empirical modeling of the regional deposition of inhaled particles in humans. Am Ind Hyg Assoc J 41:399–409, 1980

Clark SW, Pavia D (Eds): Lung Mucociliary Clearance and the Deposition of Therapeutic Aerosols. Chest 80 (Suppl.):789–924, 1981

Clarke SW, Newman SP: Therapeutic aerosols 2: Drugs available by the inhaled route. Thorax 39:1–7, 1984

Clarke SW, Pavia D (Eds): Aerosols and the Lung: Clinical and Experimental Aspects. London, England, Butterworth & Co Ltd, 1984, pp. 275

Cushley MJ, Lewis RA, Tattersfield AE: Comparison of three techniques of inhalation on the airway response to terbutaline. Thorax 38:908–913, 1983

Effros RM, Mason GR: measurements of pulmonary epithelial permeability in vivo. Am Rev Respir Dis 127:559–565, 1983

Giacomelli-Maltoni G, Melandri C, Prodi V, et al: Deposition efficiency of monodisperse particles in the human respiratory tract. Am Ind Hyg Assoc J 33:603–610, 1972

Hatch TE, Gross P: Pulmonary Deposition and Retention of Inhaled Aerosols. New York, Academic Press, 1964

Heyder J, Armbruster L, Gebhart J, et al: Total deposition of aerosol particles in the human respiratory tract for nose and mouth breathing. J Aerosol Sci 6:311–328, 1975

Hidy GM: Aerosols: An Industrial and Environmental Science. New York, Academic Press, 1984, pp. 774

Hinds WC: Aerosol Technology: Properties, Behavior and Measurement of Airborne Particles. New York, John Wiley and Sons, 1982, pp. 424

Itoh H, Smaldone GC, Swift DL et al: Quantitative measurement of aerosol deposition: Evaluation of different techniques. J Aerosol Sci, in press, 1986

Kim CS, Trujillo D, Sackner MA: Size aspects of metered-dose inhaler aerosols. Am Rev Respir Dis 132:137–142, 1985

Konig P: Review: Spacer devices used with metered-dose inhalers: Breakthrough or gimmick. Chest 88:276–284, 1985

Kradjan WA, Lakshminarayan S: Efficiency and air compressor-driven nebulizers. Chest 87:512–516, 1985

Lewis RA, Fleming JS: Fractional deposition from a jet nebulizer: How it differs from a metered-dose inhaler. Br J Dis Chest 79:361–367, 1985

Lippmann M: Regional deposition of particles in the human respiratory tract, in Lee DHK, Falk HL, Murphy SD, (eds): Handbook of Physiology, Section 9: Reactions to Environmental Agents. Bethesda, Maryland, American Physiological Society, 1977, pp. 213–232

Liu BYH (Ed): Fine Particles: Aerosol Generation Measurement, Sampling and Analysis. New York, Academic Press, Inc., 1976, pp. 837

Lourenco RV: Clinical aerosols: II Therapeutic aerosols. Arch Intern Med 142:2299–2308, 1982

Messina MS, Smaldone GC: Evaluation of quantitative aerosol techniques for use in bronchoprovocation studies. J Allergy Clin Immunol 75:252–257, 1985

McFadden ER (Ed): New Concepts in the Topical Treatment of Asthma and Related Diseases. Greenwich, Connecticut, Cliggott Publishing Co., 1982, pp. 80

Miller WF, Geumei AM: Respiratory and pharmacological therapy in COPD, in Petty TL (ed): Chronic Obstructive Pulmonary Disease, (2nd Ed), New York, Marcel Dekker, Inc, 1985, pp. 205–261

Morgan WKC, Ahmad D, Chamberlain MJ, et al: The effect of exercise on the deposition of an inhaled aerosol. Respir Physiol 56:327–338, 1984

Morrow PE, Bates DV, Fish BR, et al: Deposition and retention models for internal dosimetry of the human respiratory tract (Report of the International Commission on Radiological Protection: ICRP: Task Group on Lung Dynamics). Health Phys 12:173–207, 1966

Newman SP: Deposition and Effects of Inhalation Aerosols. Sweden, Rahms i Lund Tryckeri AB, 1983, pp. 113

Newman SP: Aerosol deposition considerations in inhalation therapy. Chest 88:152s–160s, 1985

Newman SP, Clarke SW: Therapeutic Aerosols 1: Physical and practical considerations. Thorax 38:881–886, 1983

Newman SP, Miller AB, Lennard-Jones TR, et al: Improvement of pressurized aerosol deposition with Nebuhaler spacer device. Thorax 39:935–941, 1984

Newman SP, Pellow PGD, Clay MM, et al: Evaluation of jet nebulizers for use with gentamicin solution. Thorax 40:671–676, 1985

O'Brodovich HM, Coates G: Quantitative ventilation-perfusion lung scans in infants and children: Utility of submicronic radiolabeled aerosol to assess ventilation. J Pediatr 105:377–383, 1984

O'Byrne PM, Dolovich M, Dirks R, et al: Lung epithelial permeability: Relation to nonspecific airway responsiveness. J Appl Physiol 57:77–84, 1984

Pratter MR, Irwin RS: The clinical value of pharmacologic bronchoprovocation challenge. Chest 85:260-265, 1984

Raabe OG: Deposition and clearance of inhaled aerosols, in Witschi HR, Nettesheim, P (eds): Mechanisms in Respiratory Toxicology. Boca Raton, Florida, CRC Press, Inc, 1982, pp. 27–76

Raabe OG: Deposition and clearance of inhaled particles, in (Gee JBL, Morgan WKC, Brooks SM eds): Occupational Lung Diseases. New York, Raven Press, 1984, pp. 1–37

Sanders CL, Cross FT, Dagle GE, et al: Pulmonary Toxicology of Respirable Particles. Springfield, Virginia, Tech Inform Center, USDOE, 1980, pp. 676

Shim CS, Williams HM: Effect of bronchodilator therapy administered by canister versus jet nebulizer. J Allergy Clin Immunol 73:387–390, 1984

Smaldone GC, Itoh H, Swift DL, et al: Production of pharmacologic monodisperse aerosols. J Appl Physiol 54:393–399, 1983

Smaldone GC, Messina MS: Enhancement of particle deposition by flow-limiting segment in humans. J Appl Physiol 59:509–514, 1985

Smaldone GC, Messina MS: Flow limitation, cough and patterns of aerosol deposition in humans. J Appl Physiol 59:515–520, 1985

Stahlhofen W, Gebhart J, and Heyder J: Experimental determination of the regional deposition of aerosol particles in the human respiratory tract. Am Ind Hyg Assoc J 41:385–398, 1980

Stuart BO: Deposition and clearance of inhaled particles. Environ Health Perspect 55:369–390, 1984

Tobin MJ: Use of bronchodilator aerosols. Arch Intern Med 145:1659–1663, 1985

Frederick W. Hanson

23

Management of the Pregnant Asthmatic

The obstetrician faced with caring for the pregnant asthmatic must have a thorough understanding of the unique changes in maternal respiratory physiology occurring to meet the increased oxygen needs of pregnancy. Equally important is an awareness of the potential adverse effects of asthma on the increased needs for oxygen by the fetus, as well as any potentially adverse effects of treatment modalities upon the fetus. The physiologic changes and clinical manifestations of asthma appear to be well understood, although the factors that precipitate and aggravate asthmatic attacks are complex. The influences of pregnancy upon this disease are best described as variable. Indeed, as is typical of many medical diseases complicated by pregnancy, predictability of the course of asthma is often difficult. A review of past as well as current obstetric literature reveals a paucity of information relating to pregnancy and asthma.

INCIDENCE

The incidence rate for asthma in the general population has been variously reported to range from 2.6 to 3.1 percent, and asthma in association with pregnancy has been reported to occur at frequency ranges varying from 0.4 to 1.3 percent. The obstetrician is frequently faced, therefore, with counseling and management decisions regarding pregnancy and asthma.

The maternal respiratory system undergoes anatomic, hormonal, and acid-base balance alterations to meet the increased oxygen demands of the pregnant mother and growing fetus. The pregnant uterus and placenta represent a low-pressure arteriovenous shunt, partially compensated by increased cardiac output. The fetus survives and matures in a relatively hypoxic environment with a pO_2 approximating 28.5 mm Hg. Fetal adaptation occurs through several mechanisms, including a more efficient hemoglobin than adult, vascular shunts in the fetal circulatory system, and increased fetal placental flow rates.

Anatomically, the enlarging uterus results in a gradual displacement of abdominal contents and a decrease in the vertical dimension of the thorax. Compensatory mechanisms include an increase in circumference of the thoracic cage, and increase in the substernal angle, diaphragmatic breathing, and increased diaphragmatic excursion.

One of the earliest respiratory changes to occur during pregnancy is an increased minute ventilation due primarily to a rise in tidal volume of up to 40 percent. While tidal volume rises significantly, it does so by decreasing expiratory reserve volume. Vital capacity remains unchanged or is only slightly elevated, and respiratory capacity undergoes a significant increase. Functional residual capacity and residual volume decrease secondary to diaphragm elevation and increased pulmonary ventilation (see Fig. 23-1).

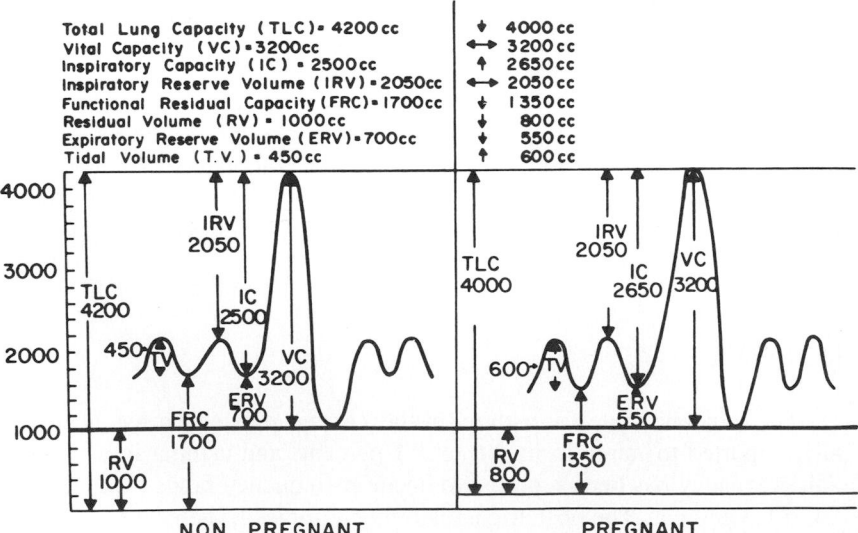

Fig. 23-1. Schematic representation of changes of pulmonary volumes during pregnancy. (From Fishburne JI: Physiology and disease of the respiratory system in pregnancy, A review. J Rep Med 22(4):177, 1979. Used with permission.)

Pulmonary function during pregnancy and the immediate postpartum period has been well studied. With the exception of an increase in ventilation of approximately 42 percent, pulmonary function parameters such as maximum breathing capacity, timed vital capacity, forced expiratory volume in the first second, maximal expiratory flow volume, and forced vital capacity remain unchanged. Respiratory rates rise only slightly, and alveolar ventilation is reported to rise as much as 70 percent. Lung compliance decreases by 50 percent, and specific airway conductance increases. Oxygen consumption increases by approximately 20 percent. The increased minute volume results in increased carbon dioxide expiration, and therefore decreased carbon dioxide. An increased urinary loss of bicarbonate, however, maintains a normal plasma pH.

The precise etiology for the hyperventilation of pregnancy is unknown. Current evidence supports a theory of central stimulation plus respiratory center threshold alteration. Progesterone lowers that threshold and stimulates respiration, which results in hyperpnea and decreased carbon dioxide tension.

PATHOPHYSIOLOGY OF ASTHMA

An excellent detailed discussion of the pathophysiology of asthma occurs earlier in this book (Chapter 3). Briefly, asthma is a disease characterized by hyperreactivity of the lung airways. This hyperreactivity is episodic and chronic in frequency and varies from mild to severe in intensity. Bronchoconstriction, bronchial edema, and bronchial mucus plugs combine to produce a decreased arterial pO_2. Severely affected patients who are unable to compensate have carbon dioxide retention and respiratory acidosis.

EFFECTS OF PREGNANCY ON ASTHMA

As seen in Figure 23-2 most reported series of pregnant asthmatics are divided equally between improvement, aggravation, or unchanged status with regard to the influence of pregnancy on the severity and frequency of asthmatic episodes. Most reported series of pregnant asthmatics are divided equally between improvement, aggravation, or unchanged status with regard to the influence of pregnancy on the severity and frequency of asthmatic episodes. These results may seem paradoxic because one might have anticipated general disease improvement due to increases in free cortisol, prednisolone, and histaminase during pregnancy. Nonetheless, some studies have pointed out that those patients who experienced aggravation of asthma with pregnancy tended to have more severe disease prior to pregnancy. Others have pointed out that those asthmatics who experience improvement of their

EFFECT OF PREGNANCY ON ASTHMA

	IMPROVED %	SAME %	WORSE %
JENSEN	41	15	44
GANDEVIA	48	28	24
TURIAF	50	26	24
SCHAEFER	3	93	4
GAMMAL	35	25	40
HIDDLESTONE	39	35	27
WILLIAMS	42	34	24
WILLAMSON	20	36	54
FEIN	10	67	23
AVERAGE	36	41	23
GLUCK & GLUCK	14	43	43

Fig. 23-2. Effect of asthma on pregnancy outcome. (From Gluck JC, Gluck PA: The effects of pregnancy on asthma: A prospective study. Ann Allergy 37:164–168, 1976. Used with permission.)

disease during pregnancy do so in the first trimester, and that those who deteriorate tend to do so in the second and third trimesters. It must also be noted that the first attack of asthma may occur during pregnancy. Asthma is rarely an indication for therapeutic abortion or cesarean section, however. Finally, pregnant asthmatic patients tend to react similarly in subsequent pregnancies.

The immunology of pregnancy is a fascinating but poorly understood subject. In general, cell-mediated immunity is suppressed in pregnancy. Furthermore, elevated levels of corticosteroids have been shown to decrease the number of circulating monocytes and the absolute number of T cells. Similarly, a variety of factors found in maternal serum, starting at 11–12 weeks of pregnancy, have been shown to decrease T-cell function. Finally, IgE antibodies decrease during pregnancy, and a recent small prospective study demonstrates a potentially useful predictive correlation between levels of IgE and the response of asthma to pregnancy.

EFFECTS OF ASTHMA ON PREGNANCY

Most reported studies as to effects of asthma on pregnancy have indicated little if any increased maternal mortality. Gordon et al. reported on 277 pregnant asthmatics in 30,861 pregnancies, and showed that 5.7 percent of the patients were severe asthmatics and two-thirds of the maternal mortalities (a total of 5) occurred in this group. This latter group also had an incidence of 35 percent low-birth-weight infants, 28 percent perinatal deaths, and even more importantly 12.5 percent neurologically abnormal infants at 1 year. The perinatal death rate was highest for black infants, suggesting that factors other than asthma are also involved. Long-term Collaborative Project data also indicate that at 1 year 5.7 percent of the infants of asthmatic mothers were diagnosed as asthmatic, a seven-fold increase over controls. Such Collaborative Project data also demonstrates a two-fold increase as compared to controls in other respiratory diseases such as bronchopneumonia, acute tracheobronchitis and bronchiolitis.

Bhana and Bejerkedal evaluated 381 pregnancies and demonstrated a two-fold higher incidence of maternal complications such as hyperemesis gravidarum, vaginal hemorrhage, and toxemia in pregnant asthmatics. Likewise, in comparison to controls, pregnant asthmatics experienced a higher percentage of induced labor (14.2 versus 9.1 percent), complicated labor (14.4 versus 9.6 percent), and labor interventions (9.9 versus 7.7 percent). Stillbirths, perinatal and infant mortalities, prematurity, and hypoxia were all increased, but only neonatal deaths were statistically elevated when compared with control populations. Finally, other studies have demonstrated a slight but insignificant increase in spontaneous abortion, unchanged gestational lengths but lower birth weights, and no increased incidence of congenital malformations.

MEDICAL MANAGEMENT OF PREGNANCY

The medical management of asthma is extensively detailed elsewhere in this book (Chapters 20 and 21). the principles of management for the pregnant asthmatic should differ little from that of her nonpregnant counterpart. Thus, the primary concern in management for the obstetrician is the avoidance of hypoxia and its potential deleterious effects upon the fetus. Of secondary concern but near equal importance is the avoidance of unnecessary drugs. Virtually all medications employed in the management of acute and chronic asthma freely cross the placenta. The risks of hypoxia must be balanced against potential drug side effects for the mother and fetus.

The current concensus indicates that patients should avoid specific allergens. Unfortunately, the majority of asthmatic individuals are atopic and therefore sensitive to multiple allergens. Current reports recommend against desensitization procedures during pregnancy. However, other individuals, such as Metzger et al., advise cautious administration of immunotherapy for IgE-mediated disease. These authors compared 121 immunotherapy-treated pregnancies with 147 matched untreated controls. With the exception of a slight increase in abortions, there was no increased incidence of complications in immunotherapy-treated pregnant patients. It is recommended, however, by most authors that antigen concentrations be kept stable during pregnancy to avoid the potential risks of maternal anaphylaxis. It also appears that children from treated pregnancies develop allergic disease with the same frequency as children born to nontreated mothers.

Certain drugs commonly employed in the management of asthma are, however, to be avoided during pregnancy. Patients who have a history of bronchospasm being aggravated by respiratory infections should be aggressively treated when respiratory infections are suspected. Antibiotics are generally safe with the exception of tetracyclines and chloramphenicol. Chloramphenicol has been associated with cardiovascular collapse (gray syndrome) in newborns. Tetracyclines are to be avoided, because of their effects on the developing teeth of the fetus. Efforts should also be directed at improving pulmonary toilet and preventing atelectasis and mucus plugging. Iodine-containing compounds should be avoided since they freely cross the placenta and also will appear in the milk of the breast feeding mother. Many combination drugs used for the treatment of asthma contain iodine. Congenital goiter with airway obstruction can result from the elevated thyroid-stimulating hormone levels that follow the blocking of fetal thyroid binding of organic iodine by iodine.

Briggs et al. have written an excellent reference guide for drugs used in pregnancy and lactation. The majority of drugs used in the treatment of asthma in pregnancy fall into risk categories designated by the authors as B and C. Category B drugs are those for which animal reproduction studies have not demonstrated a risk and there are no controlled studies in pregnant women or animal-reproduction studies have shown an adverse effect (other than decreased fertility) that was not confirmed in controlled studies in women in the first trimester (and there is no evidence of risk in later trimesters). Such category B drugs are phenobarbital; terbutaline; ritodrine; metaproterenol; salbutamol; and prednisone. Category C drugs are those for which either studies in animals have revealed adverse effects on the fetus (teratogenic, embryocidal, or other) and there are no controlled studies in women or studies in women and animals are not available. These drugs should be given only if the potential benefit justifies the potential risk to the fetus. Such category C drugs are: theophylline; aminophylline; ephedrine; epinephrine; betamethasone; dexamethasone; and isoproterenol. Category D drugs are those for which there is a positive evidence of human fetal risk, but the benefits from use in pregnant women may be acceptable despite the risk. Amobarbital is an example of the latter category.

In most cases there is scant data with regard to breast feeding. Theophylline is excreted into breast milk and less rapidly absorbed preparations are advised. Less than one percent of the maternal dose is excreted in breast milk. Similar precautions apply to aminophylline. Phenobarbital is excreted into breast milk but infant sedation has been rarely reported. No breast feeding data is available for the other compounds mentioned.

If asthmatic patients are to undergo abortion, the prostaglandin-containing abortifacients are to be used with extreme caution. These compounds are potent bronchoconstrictors. Finally, idiosyncratic reactions to aspirin and tartrazine dyes have been reported.

It is generally agreed by most authors that should anesthesia be required for obstetric procedures local or conduction anesthesia is preferable to general anesthesia. Halothane, despite its idiosyncratic reactions, would probably be the anesthetic of choice if general anesthesia is required because of its bronchodilating properties. It is also less irritating to the respiratory mucosa. Sedatives should be used with extreme caution because of their depressant effects on the respiratory center and suppression of the cough reflex. Hydroxyzine hydrochloride or hydroxyzine pamoate have been noted to possess teratogenic properties in animal studies. These drugs are considered to have a category C risk factor with no data available with regard to breast feeding.

Disodium cromoglycolate, which inhibits mast cell degranulation, has been used effectively as prophylactic therapy in some asthmatics. No particular pattern of birth defects has been noted for this drug; however, it is not approved for use in pregnancy

In the past, the chronic use of adrenal steroids in pregnant asthmatics has been avoided. Early animal studies indicated that cortisone and adrenocorticotropic hormone were dangerous to the fetus. Moreover, isolated case reports in humans attribute congenital defects, particularly cleft palate, to the use of these compounds. Current literature does not support such suggested associations. Indeed, corticosteroids may be required as life-saving drugs for pregnant patients with asthma. Furthermore, the obstetrician should be alert to signs of adrenal insufficiency in the neonate and is responsible for notifying the anesthesiologist and pediatrician when chronic steroid therapy has been employed.

Bronchodilators for the acute and chronic relief of bronchospasm are absolutely necessary therapeutic modalities. Virtually all of these compounds freely cross the placenta. Theophylline has not been associated with fetal complications. β-adrenergic stimulators such as ephedrine, epinephrine, and isoproterenol hydrochloride are useful and potent bronchodilators. Epinephrine is also an β-adrenergic stimulator and can cause peripheral vasoconstriction in both mother and fetus and temporarily reduce placental perfusion with resultant fetal distress. No long-term fetal effects have been reported. Newer β-adrenergic agents such as metaproterenol sulfate and terbutaline sulfate appear to have better bronchodilating properties with fewer cardiac effects. Unfortunately, they have not been approved for use in pregnancy, although the latter is used extensively to stop premature labor.

Atropine crosses the placenta and can cause fetal tachycardia. It is also drying to mucous membranes and leads to inspissation of mucus plugs. Scopolamine has a marked central sedative effect.

Pulmonary infection, hypoxemia, and dehydration are the major problems to be managed in the hospitalized asthmatic. Oxygen by mask, aggressive antibiotic therapy with proven infection, and intravenous fluids are required. With the few exceptions listed above, management of the pregnant asthmatic is similar to that of her nonpregnant counterpart, and fortunately, the prognosis for both the mother and fetus is good.

REFERENCES

Bhana SL, Bjerkedal F: The course and outcome of pregnancy in women with bronchial asthma. Acta Alergol 27:397–406, 1972

Briggs GG, Bodendorfer TW, Freeman RK, et al: Drugs in pregnancy and lactation— A reference guide to Fetal and Neonatal Risk, Williams & Wilkins, Baltimore/ London, 1983

Burrow GN, Ferris TF: Medical Complications During Pregnancy. W.B. Saunders Company, 1975, pp 602–608

Depp R, Sciarra JJ: Gynecology and Obstetrics. New York, Harper and Row, 1979, 3:8–11

Fishburne JI: Physiology and disease of the respiratory system in pregnancy. J Reprod Med 22(4):177–189, 1979

Gluck JC, Gluck PA: The effects of pregnancy on asthma: A prospective study. Ann Allergy 37:164–168, 1976

Gordon M, Niswander KR, Berendes H, et al: Fetal morbidity following potentially anoxigenic obstetric conditions. VII. Bronchial asthma. Am J Obstet Gynecol 106(3): 421–429, 1970

Greenberg F: The potential teratogenicity of allergy and asthma treatment in pregnancy. Immunol and Allergy Practice 7:15–20, 1985

Hernandez E, Angell CS, Johnson JWC: Asthma in pregnancy: current concepts. Obstet Gynecol 55:739–743, 1980

Huff RW, Hayashi RH: Emergency care in pregnancy, in Queenan JT (ed): Management of High Risk Pregnancy. Oradell, NJ, Medical Economics Company, 1980, Chap. 47, pp 411–413

Lavery JP, Kochenour NK: Asthma, in Queenan JT (ed): Management of High Risk Pregnancy. Oradell, NJ, Medical Economics Company, 1980, Chap. 42, pp 361–368

Leontic EA: Respiratory disease in pregnancy. Med Clin North Am 61(1):111–128, 1977

Metzger WJ, Turner E, Patterson R: The safety of immunotherapy during pregnancy. J Allergy Clin Immunol 61(4):268–272, 1978

Schaefer G, Silverman F: Pregnancy comnplicated by asthma. Am J Obstet Gynecol 82(1):182–189, 1961

Schatz M, Patterson R, Zeitz S, et al: Corticosteroid therapy for the pregnant asthmatic patient. JAMA 233(7):804–806, 1975

Turner ES, Greenberger PA, Patterson R: Management of the pregnant asthmatic patient. Ann Intern Med 6:905–918, 1980

Weinstein AM, Dubin BD, Podleski WK, et al: Asthma and pregnancy. JAMA 24(11):1161–1165, 1979

Williams DA: Asthma and pregnancy. Acta Allergol 22:311–323, 1967

Dennis Fung
N. Ty Smith

24

Anesthetic Considerations in Asthmatic Patients

The perioperative mortality from asthma is low, but "bronchospasm" continues to be a cause of intraoperative death in recent statistics. Although severe, poorly controlled asthmatic patients may present for emergency or urgent surgery, it is uncommon to encounter a situation in which an operation cannot be delayed to gain better control of a patient's asthma. Of frequent concern, however, are the possibility of morbidity from treatment and the task of deciding whether a patient has been adequately prepared preoperatively.

There is currently no "best" method of managing anesthesia in patients with asthma. Instead, the anesthetist has a number of reasonable anesthetic agents and techniques from which to choose. Indeed, the agents and techniques that are ultimately selected for a particular patient will usually reflect the degree of concern that is attached to the special problems that asthmatic patients present and the degree of confidence in an agent's or a technique's ability to control the problem.

The asthmatic patient who is to undergo anesthesia and surgery presents the following special concerns:

1. The emotional stress of the operative experience may trigger an acute asthmatic attack.

2. The asthmatic patient's medications may interact adversely with anesthetic agents.
3. The anesthetic agents may exacerbate or provoke an asthmatic attack.
4. Airway stimulation may result in reflex bronchospasm.
5. Increased production and impaired elimination of secretions may increase the likelihood of postoperative pulmonary infection.
6. The patient may have insufficient respiratory reserve to compensate for the effects of anesthesia and surgery.
7. Artificial ventilation may be inadequate for the patient who is in severe bronchospasm.
8. Other intraoperative catastrophes can mimic asthma and be difficult to diagnose during the course of an operation.

Recommendations for the anesthetic management of asthmatic patients come from a variety of sources. Unfortunately, many of the recommendations are based solely upon clinical experience and case reports. However, some guidance is provided by clinical studies on unanesthetized asthmatics or on anesthetized, nonasthmatic patients. Extrapolations have also been made from animal experiments. Moreover, the development of an animal asthma model (Basenji, greyhound, sensitized to Ascaris) may provide additional insights for recommendations about anesthesia and asthma in the future. Nevertheless, the clinician may be justifiably skeptical of recommendations arrived at by extrapolation. The paucity of specific clinical recommendations can be attributed to the difficulty and hazard of performing controlled clinical studies on asthmatic patients who must have anesthesia and surgery.

In spite of the ignorance and controversy that attend many of the clinical decisions that must be made, advice of a general nature can be derived from the objectives of safe anesthetic practice. For elective surgery, the preoperative management should provide optimal control of the patient's disease and maximize physiologic reserves. The anesthetic agents and techniques that are selected should maintain control of the disease process and make minimal demands on physiologic reserves. Problems related to the anesthetic, the operation, and the patient's disease should be anticipated; suitable monitoring for problems should be applied; and measures for successful management of problems should be immediately available. These objectives and special concerns in managing asthmatic patients lead naturally to the clinical decisions that must be made. These decisions can be grouped according to their relevance to the preoperative, intraoperative, and postoperative periods.

PREOPERATIVE DECISIONS

How severe is the patient's asthmatic condition? Severity can be assessed by history and physical examination. Pulmonary function testing can be used to measure the degree of impairment. An attempt has been made to classify asthmatic patients, the implication being that a course of management can be prescribed once the patient has been placed in the appropriate class. Without an intelligent classification, there is a tendency to arrive at arbitrary and inconsistent preoperative management decisions. Table 24-1 illustrates a classification and the matching of each class with an appropriate preoperative management.

Is the patient's asthma optimally controlled? Although the asthmatic process is, by definition, reversible, not every asthmatic patient can be made "normal." Associated irreversible pulmonary disorders and the urgency of the surgical procedure may prevent attaining a normal state. If reversible airway obstruction is present and if bronchial secretions can be reduced, however, delay of elective surgery is warranted. The following considerations suggest that the patient's condition can be improved:

1.   Onset of symptoms in a previously asymptomatic patient or worsening of symptoms. Exacerbation may be related to preoperative anxiety, failure to continue medication, recent respiratory infection, and/or exposure to inhaled irritants, such as seasonal pollen, cigarette smoke, or atmospheric pollutants. Anxiety regarding the operation can usually be controlled without delaying surgery and is discussed under the question of preanesthetic medication. The other exacerbating factors may indicate that delay would benefit the patient. Since some patients are unable to accurately assess their asthma status and others will deny worsening symptoms when they exist, objective evidence concerning reversibility is desirable.

Table 24-1
Preoperative Classification and Management of Asthmatic Patients

Class	Criteria for Classification	Management
I	Asymptomatic. No recent episodes of asthma. Not on bronchodilator therapy.	None specific.
II	Asymptomatic. Recurrent asthma but presently without bronchospasm. Currently on bronchodilator therapy.	Pulmonary function testing and measurement of theophylline levels to determine adequacy of therapy.
III	Symptomatic. Currently experiencing bronchospasm.	Delay surgery until theophylline therapy is optimal. Corticosteroids. Examination for causes of refractoriness to therapy and for complications of asthma.

2. New physical findings of asthma or more pronounced findings in a patient who is usually clear of such signs. The anesthetist is usually unable to determine this phenomenon from a single preoperative visit unless the patient has been examined on previous occasions. Reexamination by the patient's primary physician and communication of the findings and impressions to the anesthetist would be helpful.

3. Demonstration of reversible obstruction during pulmonary function testing. Between attacks, the asthmatic patient may be asymptomatic and exhibit normal physical findings. Spirometry may nevertheless show obstruction. Although the efficacy of preoperative pulmonary function tests in asymptomatic asthmatics has not been systematically examined, measurement of FEV_1 has been recommended as part of the assessment in all asthmatics, and treatment with bronchodilators and bronchial drainage is advised if the FEV_1 is less than 70 to 80 percent. Since the pulmonary laboratory may be unable to schedule testing on short notice, and since adjustment of bronchodilator therapy may be required, arrangement for testing should be made in advance of surgery. Although bedside tests to detect diminished expiratory flow have been described (e.g., match test, flow-dependent incentive spirometer), their sensitivity is arguable and reversibility by bronchodilators is difficult to demonstrate.

In the adult who has not been under close medical supervision, nonasthmatic causes of dyspnea, productive cough, and wheezing should be considered. In addition, dehydration, anemia, pulmonary infection, and obesity should be recognized and corrected preoperatively, as much as practical. Preoperative respiratory therapy, including bronchial drainage with instruction in effective removal of airway secretions and chest expansion, is indicated in patients with severe asthma. It is believed that the primary benefit will be improved respiratory reserves postoperatively, particularly in those patients who will require extensive postoperative recovery. Prophylactic initiation or augmentation of bronchodilators to therapeutic blood levels has been recommended. A course of perioperative corticosteroid has also been suggested. Neither recommendation has been subjected to controlled evaluation.

What intraoperative problems can be anticipated preoperatively?

1. Bronchospasm. In patients with a history of asthma, the incidence of intraoperative wheezing is 6.5 percent. Patients over the age of 20 years are more likely to develop wheezing than are young patients. However, the older asthmatic patients probably include those with nonallergic bronchospastic conditions. The patient's response to previous anesthetics is difficult to evaluate unless details of previous care are known, and,

even then, the patient's potential for developing bronchospasm may have changed. The likelihood of intraoperative bronchospasm in any given patient cannot be predicted; it should be therefore anticipated that every asthmatic patient has the potential for developing severe bronchospasm. Substances and circumstances that are known to trigger asthma should be noted and avoided. Since airway secretions may be a significant factor in the onset of bronchospasm, the airway should be cleared just before induction.

2. Hypoxemia. It is generally recognized that the patient with labored breathing will become hypercapnic and hypoxemic when given respiratory-depressant drugs, and that pharmacologic sedation is hazardous. Even in less severe asthma, however, abnormal ventilation-perfusion ratios can result in an increased $AaDO_2$. A further increase in $AaDO_2$ associated with induction of anesthesia may cause serious hypoxemia unless the inspired oxygen concentration is increased. Administration of isoproterenol intravenously during anesthesia will also cause an increase in $AaDO_2$ by increasing pulmonary shunt. Preoperative arterial blood gas analysis will identify patients with hypoxemia. However, routine preoperative arterial sampling in patients with an asthmatic history is not indicated except in the poorly controlled asthmatic or in the patient who will be exposed to significant respiratory hazards such as thoracotomy and upper abdominal surgery. Additional intraoperative monitoring, including arterial catheterization for arterial blood sampling, pulse oximetry, and end-tidal CO_2 analysis, should be considered.

3. Problems related to the treatment of asthma. Drugs such as theophylline, may interact with inhalational agents, particularly halothane and to some extent, enflurane, that sensitize the myocardium to the effects of catecholamines. Whether this potential interaction is significant at therapeutic blood levels of theophylline is not known. Intraoperative ventricular dysrhythmias have been reported with theophylline concentrations above therapeutic range. Nevertheless, there seems to be no indication for discontinuing theophylline preoperatively. Patients who have received an adrenal-suppressing course of corticosteroids within 6 months should receive hydrocortisone preoperatively and intraoperatively to prevent stress-induced adrenal insufficiency. The need for steroid coverage has been questioned by some authors, but since hypotension is not an infrequent perioperative event, corticosteroid coverage can usually be justified to eliminate adrenal crisis as a possible etiology. During the 1960s, bilateral carotid body resection (glomectomy) was performed on selected, severe asthmatics. These patients may manifest depressed ventilatory responses to hypercapnia and an absent response to hypoxia. Accordingly, particular care is required in the use of sedatives and in weaning these patients from ventilatory support.

Can asthmatic patients have outpatient surgery? In many instances the decision of suitability is based on the ASA (American Society of Anesthesiologists) classification of physical status. ASA I, and II, and selected III patients may be suitable for outpatient procedures. Asymptomatic and well-controlled asthmatics are usually in classes I and II. Inclusion of marginally or poorly controlled asthmatics may be feasible, depending on the procedure, the anticipated duration, and the presence or absence of additional disease, particularly that involve the cardiovascular system. Additional risks to asthmatic patients may preclude outpatient anesthesia from consideration. For example, since preanesthetic medication is frequently not given to outpatients, anxiety may be a problem; additional monitoring may not be available; finally, the efficiency required of outpatient facilities is incompatible with the delay required to carefully assess and treat a symptomatic patient.

A dilemma arises when a previously well-controlled, asymptomatic patient arrives on the morning of surgery with acute asthma. Investigation into the cause for the exacerbation is warranted. A course of action that has been suggested is to give an inhaled bronchodilator and observe the patient for improvement; if improvement follows, the procedure is undertaken. While such a remedy may be expedient, if the patient develops a serious dysrhythmia from the bronchodilator or develops severe intraoperative bronchospasm, it may be difficult defending the decision to proceed with an elective operation.

What preanesthetic medication is recommended? Control of anxiety is given special attention, although the relationship between asthmatic exacerbation and acute emotional stress is not always clear. Much of the anxiety associated with the operation and anesthetic can be reduced by simple explanation and positive previews of the anticipated events. In patients who do not show signs of impending respiratory failure (rising PCO_2 or labored breathing), there are no contraindications to any of the usual premedications. A narcotic in combination with a minor tranquilizer and parasympatholytic can be safely used. Histamine release and increased airway resistance are well-documented effects of intravenous morphine administration; yet narcotics are used without apparent adverse effect. Unlike morphine, fentanyl does not release histamine and would cause less concern if preoperative analgesia is required. Hydroxyzine and the neuroleptic agent, droperidol, lower airway resistance. Diazepam has no effect on airway resistance. The significance of these airway effects has been questioned because the measurements used may have been insensitive to changes in small airway resistance. On the other hand, anesthetic problems have not been reported with these agents. In patients who have excessive secretions, the antisialogogic effect of atropine may be detrimental; although the volume of secretions is reduced, their increased viscosity impairs elimination. Phenothiazines, such as diphenhydramine, also have a drying effect. Barbiturates, such as pentobarbital and secobarbital, have been used with satisfactory results. Theoretically, histamine-2 receptor antagonists should be avoided but in a study involving postoperative nonasthmatics, no decrease in airway conductance was seen following intravenous cimetidine.

Bronchodilator therapy should be continued. Patients who continue to use hand-operated inhalers of β-agonists, such as epinephrine and isoproterenol, present a special concern. Such patients may be emotionally, as well as pharmacologically, dependent upon the ready availability of their device. Preoperative access to self-administered β-agonists poses the danger of overtreatment and myocardial irritability. On the other hand, such patients may experience emotionally induced exacerbation if denied the security of their device. Substitution of a bronchodilator, such as metaproterenol, with low β-adrenergic activity, is a partial solution to this dilemma. If the patient is allowed to retain the device, regardless of the bronchodilating agent, electrocardiogram (EKG) evidence of excessive cardiac β-adrenergic effects should be a warning to delay the induction of anesthesia.

A short perioperative course of corticosteroids has been recommended for patients who are poorly or marginally controlled. Cromolyn sodium has also been suggested. While these are reasonable suggestions, their usefulness and the absence of significant hazards has yet to be documented in surgical patients.

INTRAOPERATIVE DECISIONS

Decisions concerning intraoperative management are usually made preoperatively. Although improvisation and flexibility are often necessary, a last-minute change in anesthetic plan without good indications carries with it the risk of unexamined or hastily considered consequences of the new course of action.

Either local or regional anesthesia is preferred over general anesthesia if the operation and patient are appropriate. The primary advantages of this approach are that endotracheal intubation is not performed and spontaneous ventilation is preserved. In addition, analgesia can often be continued postoperatively by using long-acting agents or continuous techniques. Special consideration must be given to minimizing the emotional stress that can accompany a difficult block and awareness during the operation, as well as to the unique properties of local anesthetics. For example, epinephrine in local anesthetic solutions might augment the β-adrenergic effects of bronchodilators. The antidysrhythmic property of the local anesthetic should counter the increased myocardial automaticity, however. The use of epinephrine-containing solutions of lidocaine is not contraindicated in the presence of bronchodilators, but the EKG should be monitored.

Isolated cases have been reported of bronchospasm following regional anesthesia to the arm when a sympathetic ganglion block has been inadvertently obtained. There is no apparent anatomic explanation for this phenomenon since sympathetic innervation to the airways is scarce or lacking. Other reports describe bronchospasm after induction of spinal or epidural anesthesia. A systematic study of the effects of regional anesthesia or sympathetic block has not been reported, and clinical experience does not suggest a significant problem. However, in a recent review of 27 anesthetic deaths, the only patient who died of severe bronchospasm developed problems after the induction of epidural anesthesia (Kennen and Boyan, 1985).

What induction agents should be used?   Asthma is not a contraindication to intravenous induction using thiopental, methohexital, diazepam, or ketamine. Several anesthetic agents, however, are known to cause histamine release. Administration of morphine, meperidine, d-tubocurarine, and occasionally thiopental result in significant elevation of plasma histamine. It has been customary to recommend against the use of these drugs in asthmatic patients in spite of evidence that histamine may not be the culprit in asthmatic episodes. There remains concern that the release of histamine is accompanied by release of an asthma-inducing peptide or that asthmatics may be more sensitive to histamine than are nonasthmatics. The ultra short-acting barbiturates may increase the incidence of coughing and possibly of reflex bronchoconstriction. Diazepam, which has no effect on airway resistance, may be a reasonable substitute for the drugs listed above. Ketamine decreases airway resistance in nonasthmatic patients and, to a greater degree, in symptomatic asthma patients, but the patient must be able to tolerate the cardiovascular effects of ketamine. This agent offers the advantages of bronchodilatation, high inspired oxygen concentration, and rapid induction. Its bronchodilating action may depend upon the release of endogenous catecholamines. Consequently, its usefulness and safety in catecholamine-depleted patients and in the presence of halothane needs to be determined. Seizures have occurred following ketamine induction in patients who were taking aminophylline; therefore, ketamine should be avoided or given with diazepam when a patient has been on aminophylline. In the wheezing patient with a full stomach and in asthmatics who cannot tolerate the circulatory effects of intravenous thiopental, intravenous ketamine may be the induction agent of choice. An alternative to intravenous induction is a calm inhalation induction with halothane in the well-premedicated patient. This is the common practice for managing a cooperative asthmatic child. In an uncooperative child intramuscular or intravenous ketamine may be the induction technique of choice.

What anesthetic agents can be used?   There are no absolute contraindications to use of any of the general anesthetic agents. However, the patient must be able to withstand the effects of an anesthetic concentration that is sufficient to obtund the response to surgical stimulation and the endotracheal tube. Halothane, because of its bronchodilating property, is the most widely recommended choice. In fact, halothane is frequently used to eliminate intraoperative wheezing. Enflurane and isoflurane have also been shown to act as bronchodilators in experimental asthma, but they are more disagreeable to inhale than halothane and possibly present a greater risk for stimulating coughing especially isoflurane. Diethyl ether was recommended at one time because it is also a bronchodilator, but it increases airway secretions, prolongs induction, and is flammable. The effects of nitrous oxide have not been studied in asthmatic patients. Nitrous oxide can diffuse rapidly into a poorly ventilated air-filled space resulting in expansion of the space and dilution of the oxygen concentration. Theoretically, these effects could be of concern in asthmatics with pulmonary air trapping or severe ventilation-perfusion mismatch. Whether a significant problem exists is unknown; nevertheless, caution is advised in the use of high nitrous oxide concentrations in severe asthmatics.

It might be anticipated that nitrous oxide in combination with a narcotic (balanced anesthesia) would predispose to intraoperative bronchospasm, since balanced anesthesia is considered "light," and narcotics can cause bronchoconstriction. Narcotics have been used to facilitate controlled ventilation during status asthmaticus, and the addition of nitrous oxide to provide anesthesia would seem reasonable. Experience with patients suffering from status asthmaticus cannot necessarily be extrapolated to asthmatic patients during surgery, however. The risk of bronchospasm during balanced anesthesia as compared with halothane anesthesia is not known, nor it is known whether balanced anesthesia will make wheezing worse. When inhaled agents are a special hazard because of other conditions, e.g., congestive heart failure, intracranial tumor, or malignant hyperthermia, the relative risks of anesthesia with narcotic nitrous oxide versus that with a potent inhalation agent must be carefully considered. In a patient who is susceptible to malignant hyperthermia the potent inhaled anesthetics are contraindicated, and balanced anesthesia will be required.

High-dose narcotic anesthesia without nitrous oxide has become popular as a technique for patients who have limited myocardial reserve. High-dose fentanyl suppresses the cardiovascular response to endotracheal intubation. Its effectiveness in suppressing reflex bronchoconstriction has not been documented, but bronchospasm does not appear to be a problem. Postoperative ventilatory support will usually be required.

Which neuromuscular blocking agents should be used?   In the asthmatic patient the primary hazard of neuromuscular blocking agents is that their use tempts one to insert an endotracheal tube before the patient is adequately anesthetized: paralysis prevents skeletal muscle-mediated cough but not reflex bronchospasm. Many of the commonly used neuromuscular blocking agents have been implicated in the production of bronchospasm. Histamine release following the administration of d-tubocurarine, metocurine, atracurium or succinylcholine has been demonstrated. To date the only relaxants that have escaped blame are pancuronium and vecuronium. There is one case reported of tachycardia (210 beats per minute) in a 7-year-old child who received pancuronium while being ventilated for status asthmaticus. Although pancuronium usually causes only a modest (10 percent or less) increase in heart rate, it can interact with drugs used to treat asthma, resulting in exaggerated tachycardia. Animal experiments and clinical reports suggest that neuromuscular block by competitive drugs is antagonized by aminophylline and also by hydrocortisone. Whether a clinically noticeable dose increase is required in the presence of these drugs has not been determined.

What is the best method for accomplishing tracheal intubation? Because airway stimulation is a leading cause of bronchospasm during anesthesia (Shnider and Popper, 1961), tracheal intubation should be avoided if the airway can be managed satisfactorily without an endotracheal tube. When intubation is required, anesthesia with isoflurane, enflurane or halothane will usually prevent reflex bronchospasm. The addition of local anesthetic topical spray or aerosol before intubation is controversial, and many anesthetists will not include it. An occasional patient will develop bronchospasm following topical spray. In healthy, awake volunteers, topical anesthesia with lidocaine aerosol fails to prevent an increase in distal airway resistance after insertion of the endotracheal tube (Gal and Suratt, 1980). In surgical patients the application of tracheal spray before intubation does not reduce the incidence of subsequent wheezing. Thus, topical spray may be ineffective and occasionally harmful. Intravenous lidocaine (1 mg/kg) or atropine are effective in blocking reflex bronchoconstriction (Hirshman, 1983). If halothane or enflurane must be avoided, induction and intubation with ketamine anesthesia and muscle relaxation may produce satisfactory results.

INTRAOPERATIVE BRONCHOSPASM

Asthmatic patients should be monitored continuously during operation and in the immediate postoperative period for the onset of bronchospasm. The following observations are suggestive of bronchospasm:

1.   Wheezing or bilateral wheezing audible on chest auscultation. If access

to the patient's chest is limited by drapes and equipment, the anesthetic circuit hoses can be auscultated.

2. Prolonged expiratory time and slow, prolonged filling of the reservoir bag.
3. Increased peak airway pressure during volume-limited ventilation, or decreased tidal volume during pressure-limited ventilation.
4. Overexpansion of the chest and minimal excursion during the ventilation cycle.

Although the most likely cause of wheezing and difficult ventilation in an asthmatic patient is bronchospasm, these findings are nonspecific. Wheezing sounds can be produced by airway secretions, a foreign body, pneumothorax, pulmonary edema, straining during light anesthesia, and partial obstruction of the endotracheal tube. Difficult ventilation can be produced by straining during light anesthesia, tension pneumothorax, and obstruction of the endotracheal tube. The greatest threats to life are endotracheal tube obstruction and tension pneumothorax; immediate diagnosis and treatment are required. Inspection of the endotracheal tube, deflation of the cuff, passage of a suction catheter, and, if necessary, replacement of the endotracheal tube are the steps in management of tube obstruction. Inspection of the chest and sternal notch, auscultation, and if necessary, insertion of pleural needles are the steps in management of tension pneumothorax. Surgical stimulation of the carina or contact of the endotracheal tube against the carina can trigger bronchospasm. Local anesthetic infiltration of the carina or retraction of the endotracheal tube will relieve these problems.

The management of intraoperative bronchospasm consists of preventing provocation, removing provoking factors, maintaining oxygenation and ventilation, and reversal of bronchoconstriction.

Prevention.   Preoperative control of airway secretion is considered a major step in the prevention of intraoperative bronchospasm. Anesthetic agents that may initiate bronchospasm should be avoided (see Table 24-2). Anesthetic concentrations should be sufficient to obtund the response to tracheal intubation, airway stimulation, e.g., suctioning and surgical stimulation. Unnecessary airway stimulation, such as movement of the endotracheal tube or the patient's head, should be minimized. Prophylactic intravenous lidocaine should be considered when a potentially provoking maneuver is required.

Removal of provoking factors. Intraoperative removal of secretions requires attention to the following details: continuous auscultation of breath sounds; warming and humidification of inhaled gases; access to the endotra-

Table 24-2
Drugs That May Produce Adverse Effects in Asthma Patients

A. Drugs that have provoked bronchospasm

Agent	*Evidence*
Bupivacaine, aerosol	Reported in two asthmatic subjects
d-tubocurarine	Two case reports
Enflurane	One case report of a delayed exacerbation of asthma after recovery from an uncomplicated anesthetic
Gallamine	One case report
Pancuronium	Two case reports
Pentazocine	A case report in an asthmatic who was also sensitive to aspirin
Propranolol	Provoked wheezing in awake asthmatics
Succinylcholine	Three case reports
Thiopental	Case report of anaphylaxis with bronchospasm

B. Drugs that may increase bronchial tone

Agent	*Evidence*
Barbiturates	Studies on excised lung tissue
Cyclopropane	Studies on excised lung tissue; dog studies
d-tubocurarine	Controlled studies in patients with airway disease
Fentanyl	Controlled study in intubated nonasthmatics during anesthesia
Lidocaine, aerosol	Initial decrease in expiratory flow rates in awake asthmatics
Meperidine	Dog study
Morphine	Controlled study in intubated nonasthmatics during anesthesia
Neostigmine	Increased airway resistance in awake, nonasthmatic subjects
Propranolol	Increased airway resistance in awake, nonasthmatic and asthmatic subjects

cheal tube; and an adequate supply of catheters, sterile gloves and sterile saline.

Oxygenation and ventilation. The inspired oxygen concentration should be increased to compensate for ventilation-perfusion mismatch. A volume-limited mechanical ventilator should be available and should have the ability to control inspired flow rate and expiratory time. Peak airway pressures up to 70 cm H_2O may be needed. Uncontrollable deterioration of gas exchange requires expeditious completion of the operation. If the patient's bronchospasm continues past the end of surgery, some means of delivering oxygen and high pressure ventilation, such as the Jackson-Rees modified T-piece, will be necessary during transport to the recovery area; an ordinary resuscitation bag or demand valve may not be suitable if peak airway pressure is over 45 cm H_2O. A volume-limited ventilator and respiratory therapist should be in the recovery room or critical care unit when the patient arrives.

Reversal of bronchoconstriction. An increase in anesthetic concentration is usually the first measure taken if it is appropriate and can be done safely. The addition of halothane, enflurane, or isoflurane to augment the anesthetic and provide bronchodilation should be considered if balanced anesthesia is being given. An aerosolized bronchodilator with predominant beta-adrenergic action, such as metoproterenol, can be administered via the endotracheal tube using the side arm of a T-adaptor or an in-line adaptor. If the patient has not been receiving aminophylline, intravenous administration should be started. Although the pharmacokinetics of aminophylline in anesthetized surgical patients have not been studied, the guidelines for treatment of awake patients are usually recommended. Since there is possible interaction with halothane or enflurane, a conservative approach might be to give half the usual loading dose and half the maintenance infusion rate with determination of blood theophylline concentrations during longer operations. Theophylline toxicity is a major risk for asthmatic patients; consequently these preparations should be given by controlled infusion. Intravenous isoproterenol (0.1 to 0.3 mcg/kg/min) may be required in patients who cannot be adequately ventilated. If the patient did not receive preoperative corticosteroid, 100 mg of hydrocortisone intravenously has been recommended. The effects of therapy can be monitored by observing the electrocardiogram for evidence of β_1-adrenergic effect and the blood pressure, breath sounds, and peak airway pressure for β_2-adrenergic effects.

POSTOPERATIVE DECISIONS

What is the safest way to extubate? There is good reason to favor extubation of the asthma patient while the responses to airway stimulation are still obtunded by deep anesthesia. This course is feasible if spontaneous ventilation is satisfactory, if the airway can be safely managed without an endotracheal tube, and if a full stomach is not suspected. Satisfactory ventilation and airway safety require recovery from neuromuscular blockade. Reversal using atropine and neostigmine has not been evaluated in asthmatics. Rare cases have been reported in nonasthmatics of bronchial hypersecretion following neostigmine and requiring 2–3 mg of atropine. Neostigmine and other cholinesterase inhibitors can cause parasympathetic bronchoconstriction, but this effect is also prevented by atropine. The safest alternative in severe asthmatics may be postoperative sedation and ventilation until neuromuscular function recovers spontaneously and completely. When the patient must be awake before extubation, the possibility of bronchospasm should be anticipated. If bronchospasm develops during recovery from the anesthetic, extubation in the operating room has at least two advantages. First, the anesthetist is present when the patient is extubated and can observe his response prior to transport to the recovery room. Second, reintubation can be readily performed. If the patient is to be extubated outside the operating room, a physician should be in attendance to evaluate the patient before and after extubation and to reintubate the trachea if necessary. Bronchospasm that is caused by the presence of the endotracheal tube will frequently subside following extubation. When it persists and other causes of wheezing have been eliminated, continuing pharmacologic management with either inhaled or intravenous bronchodilators may be required. Impending respiratory failure is an indication for reintubation and mechanical ventilation.

How should postoperative analgesia be managed?   The need for analgesia must be assessed on an individual basis. This is especially the case in asthmatics because of the significant respiratory hazards. In patients who have good postoperative ventilatory reserves (effective cough, lung expansion, and gas exchange) narcotic analgesia can be used. There is no evidence supporting the use of one narcotic over another, although limited respiratory depression is claimed for mixed agonist/antagonist opioids. Again, histamine release by morphine is of concern, but fentanyl is too short acting for this purpose unless it can be given by continuous infusion or patient-controlled analgesia.

In patients who have questionable or inadequate postoperative ventilatory reserves, continuous epidural or brachial plexus block can be used. Hypotension is more likely following epidural analgesia if epinephrine is included in the local anesthetic that is injected. This occurs because of the combined sympathetic block and β-adrenergic vasodilation. A similar interaction between epidural analgesia and systemically administered adrenergic bronchodilators may occur; therefore the patient's blood pressure should be monitored closely following local anesthetic or bronchodilator administration. Recent interest in epidural narcotic analgesia may lead to improved management of postoperative pain in asthmatics. However, the frequent occurrence of pruritus after epidural morphine suggests that there may be problems due to histamine release. In addition, there is a small risk that patients who are receiving epidural opioids will experience delayed respiratory depression, and consequently they must usually be observed in a critical care unit. There has not been a clinical evaluation of epidural narcotic analgesia in asthmatics.

EMERGENCY ANESTHESIA

One of the most difficult challenges in anesthesia is the asthmatic patient who presents for emergency surgery. Many of the triggering and exacerbating factors are present and occasionally uncontrollable in these patients: fever, sepsis, pneumonitis, dehydration, ventilatory embarrassment, pain, and anxiety. Anesthetic induction poses a particular problem. Since these patients often have a full stomach, the anesthetist must use either an awake intubation or a "rapid-sequence" induction. The former carries with it the risk of bronchospasm in a frightened patient with inadequate topical anesthesia. With a rapid sequence induction, the anesthetist is in a dilemma. The entire anesthetic dose must be given at once. If it is too small, bronchospasm is very probable. If it is too large, hypotension (thiopental) or hypertension (ketamine) may ensue. Nevertheless, ketamine is probably the agent of choice in a rapid sequence induction. Finally, there is the problem of extubation, mainly because of a potentially full stomach. Extubation during light anesthesia could result in bronchospasm. We feel, nevertheless, that the full stomach takes precedent; hence we will lighten anesthetic depth before extubation in the hope that bronchospasm will not occur. If it does, one can quickly deepen anesthetic depth and proceed again, this time taking active measures, such as that of administering aminophylline and steroids to prevent bronchospasm.

REFERENCES

Aldrete JA: Asthma and the anesthesiology. Postgrad Med 44:93–96, 1968; 45:210–213, 1969

Aviado D: Regulation of bronchomotor tone during anesthesia. Anesthesiology 42:68–80, 1975

Barrett JP: Clinical epilog on bronchomotor tone. Anesthesiology 42:1–3, 1975

Barton MD: Anesthetic problems with aspirin-intolerant patients. Anesth Analg 54:376–380, 1975

Converse JG, Smotrilla MM: Anesthesia and the asthmatic. Anesth Analg 40:336–342, 1961.

Cottrell JE, Wolfson B, Siker ES: Changes in airway resistance following droperidol, hydroxyzine, and diazepam in normal volunteers. Anesth Analg 55:18–21, 1976

Crago RR, Bryan AC, Laws, AK, et al: Respiratory flow resistance after curare and pancuronium, measured by forced oscillations. Can Anesth Soc J 19:607–614, 1972

Don HF, Koopman W, Mathieu A: Asthma and other allergic disorders: Current immunologic concepts and anesthetic considerations. In Mathieu A, Kahan BD (eds): Immunologic aspects of anesthetic and surgical practice. Grune & Stratton, Orlando, FL, 1975, pp. 289–313

Gal TJ, Suratt PM: Resistance to breathing in healthy subjects following endotracheal intubation under topical anesthesia. Anesth Analg 59:270–274, 1980

Gold MI: Anesthesia for the asthmatic patient. Anesth Analg 49:881–888, 1970

Gold MI, Helrich M: A study of the complications related to anesthesia in asthmatic patients. Anesth Analg 42:283–293, 1963

Heinonen J, Muittari A: The effect of diazepam on airway resistance in asthmatics. Anaesthesia 27:37–40, 1972

Hirshman CA: Airway reactivity in humans. Anesthesiology 58:170–177, 1983

Huber FC, Guiterrez J, Corrsen G: Ketamine: its effects on airway resistance in man. South Med J 65:1176–1180, 1972

Keenan RL, Boyan CP: Cardiac arrest due to anesthesia. A study of incidence and causes: JAMA 253:2373–2377, 1985

Kingston HGG, Hirshman CA: Perioperative management of the patient with asthma. Anesth Analg 63:844–855, 1984

Sealy WC, Young WG, Jr, Houck WS, Jr, et al: The use of steroids for the control and prevention of serious respiratory embarrassment during and after intrathoracic operations. J Thoracic Cardiovasc Surg 39:109–116, 1960

Shnider SM, Papper EM: Anesthesia for the asthmatic patient. Anesthesiology 22:886–892, 1961

Tarhan S, Moffitt EA, Sessler AD, et al: Risk of anesthesia and surgery in patients with chronic bronchitis and chronic obstructive pulmonary disease. Surgery 74:720–726, 1973

Unger L, Johnson JH: Surgery in asthmatic patients. South Med J 53:633–637, 1960

Vaughn J, Casson H, Hirshman CA: Anesthetic management of a child with asthma and presumed susceptibility to malignant hyperthermia. Anesthesiology 59:283–285, 1983

Theodore A. Goodman
Joe P. Tupin

25

The Psychobiology of Asthma: Implications for Treatment

Bronchial asthma has been a focus of the psychosomatic medicine literature since the pioneering work of French and Alexander, who viewed the symptoms produced by asthma as an attempted resolution of a psychologic conflict arising from the mother-child interaction. Since this theory was based on psychoanalytic theory, the necessary treatment for asthma would be pschoanalysis, in an attempt to resolve the psychologic conflict, and thus, its somatic manifestation, asthma. Both etiology and treatment were handled with facility, although no attention was paid to the intervening mechanisms whereby an unconscious conflict could elicit specific pathophysiologic alterations in the bronchus.

In the intervening years, theories of psychopathology have undergone significant development and change, and have been augmented by increasing knowledge of neuroendocrinology and neuroimmunomodulation. We are now in a position to have a far more sophisticated understanding of how emotions, perceptions, and thoughts can, for example, effect the pulmonary mast cell and bronchial smooth muscle, and produce asthmatic symptoms.

The intent of this chapter is threefold. First, we present preclinical and clinical evidence of the impact of emotion and personality factors in producing a predisposition to asthma, and in precipitating an asthmatic attack in both children and adults. Second, we examine the evidence that central nervous system (CNS) events such as thought, perception, and emotion can

BRONCHIAL ASTHMA, Second Edition
ISBN 0-8089-1814-1

541

produce specific effects upon the immune system in general, and in particular, upon both immune and autonomic function in the lung. Third, we discuss the psychiatric management of the child and adult asthmatic in clinical practice, including special considerations in the treatment of psychiatric disorders in patients with asthma.

EMOTION AND PERSONALITY IN ASTHMA

A study of 487 asthmatic patients of all ages in 1958 showed that the predominant precipitating factor of an asthmatic attack was extrinsic allergic factors in 29 percent, respiratory infections in 40 percent and psychological factors in 30 percent (although in one-half of these patients, allergic factors were also present but felt to be of secondary significance). More than one etiologic factor was present in about three-fourths of the entire group, and psychologic factors were present in 70 percent, although it was the sole precipitant in only 1.2 percent. This early study points out not only the significance of psychologic factors, but also the degree to which they are interrelated to other factors, whether infectious, allergic, or irritant. Not surprisingly, teasing apart and separately evaluating this psychologic component has been difficult to do in carefully controlled studies, although the literature abounds with phenomenologic studies of individual patients or small groups of patients.

Preclinical Data

Suggestion is the induction in a patient of a mental state that is contrary to reality or to the patient's past experiences. In this state of suggestibility, the patient responds compliantly and readily. While elegant suggestions may be utilized to effect change in psychotherapy, suggestion is frequently and unwittingly used for example, when a patient is told that an injection "won't hurt a bit."

In addition to its use as a psychotherapeutic tool, suggestion has also been used in experimental settings as one means of demonstrating and further defining the role of mental phenomena in the production of asthmatic symptoms. Particularly noted for this work is Luparello and his colleagues who, over a period of ten years, have systematically explored the effects of suggestion upon asthma. In their earlier studies, they were able to produce bronchoconstriction in asthmatic patients given nebulized saline when they were led to believe that they were inhaling an allergen. This phenomena was observed in 19 of 40 asthmatic subjects (but not in control subjects), and 12 developed asthmatic symptoms. These symptoms were reversed when the subjects were given further nebulized saline, although now they were led to believe they were being administered a bronchodilator! Subsequently, the same group demonstrated that carbachol produced less of an increase in airway resistance when given to asthmatic patients if they were led to believe that they were being given a bronchodilator. Both bronchoconstriction and bronchodilatation thus could be produced through suggestion, which was also able to modify the effects of medication. Not all studies have supported these findings, but in general, positive findings have been found in those studies where airway resistance or specific airway conductance were measured, rather than peak flow or spirometric variables. This is consistent with the hypothesis that the effects of suggestion are ultimately mediated via the parasympathetic nerve fibers of the proximal airways.

Stein, in 1982, cited two interesting vignettes that occurred during an experiment on emotion and asthma. He was attempting to make a systematic study of the effects of specific emotional stimuli upon pulmonary resistance using a whole body plethysmograph, the description of which sounds similar to being locked in a bank vault. When a 32-year-old man with asthma was placed in the device, he became markedly anxious and claustrophobic. This precipitated a severe asthmatic attack. Although this man was in psychotherapy, he did not discuss this experience until several years later, when he spontaneously associated the feelings he experienced during the experiment with issues concerning separation from significant individuals in his life. His anxiety was thus produced by the body plethysmograph because it apparently evoked memories and feelings associated with an important conflict in his life. The patient's elaboration of this unconscious connection as revealed over the course of therapy helps us to understand why his reaction was of such intensity.

Stein's second subject, a 43-year-old housewife with a 25-year history of asthma, also experienced a spontaneous asthma attack during the experiment. Although the first subject was markedly dysphoric prior to his attack, however, the second subject repeatedly remarked upon how helpful her doctors were, how the experiment was going to benefit her, how "wonderful" the experiment was, and, immediately prior to her attack, how "this is the best I've felt in weeks." As you might suspect, this subject was as anxious as the first, but used different defense mechanisms to cope with her anxiety. These vignettes illustrate two principles. First, that asthma can be precipitated by emotion, and second that emotional responses to a particular stimuli can appear, at least on a superficial level, to be so variable and idiosyncratic, that links to concomitant physiologic responses can be confusing and difficult to appreciate without careful study.

To more rigorously evaluate the effects of emotion upon asthmatic symptoms, Levenson conducted an interesting experiment where asthmatic and nonasthmatic children were shown three movies, all of which were intended to elicit an emotional response in the viewer. The first film was of asthmatic children in the hospital, the second of three severe industrial accidents, and the third of a mother giving her child away for adoption. All three movies produced a significantly greater increase in pulmonary resistance in the asthmatic children than in the normal controls. The intent of the study was to demonstrate that thematically relevant stressors would produce more of an effect upon asthmatic subjects than thematically neutral stressors. However, a more parsimonious interpretation of the results is that the intensity of an emotional response, regardless of the type of stressor eliciting it, is related to the degree of bronchoconstriction or asthmatic symptoms produced. This might suggest that asthmatic patients would show a high degree of emotional reactivity to a given stressor. However, as will be described below, a clear picture has emerged of significantly decreased expression in asthmatic children of anger, pleasure, or surprise to given stimuli when compared to nonasthmatic children.

The question arises, then, whether this decreased expression of emotion is an adaptive conditioned response in the asthmatic individual, arising to protect against the onset of an asthmatic attack, or, whether the phenomenon is a contributory factor in the etiology of the disease process, as predicted by psychoanalytic theory and described by French and Alexander. While this question cannot be answered at present, hopefully light can be shed upon the issue by an examination of personality factors that have been associated with asthma.

The Clinical Data

CHILDREN

A broad range of personality traits and of psychopathology has been described in children with asthma. Weiner, in an extensive review of the subject in 1977, summarized a series of studies that attributed all of the following traits to asthmatic children: immaturity, lack of self-confidence, insecurity, overanxiousness, restlessness, potential aggressiveness, bossiness, timidity, politeness, and imaginativeness. Clearly, this approach to an understanding of the personality of the asthmatic child is so broad and overinclusive that it is of little utility, and suffer from small sample sizes, inadequate or no control groups, and lack of attention to the issue of cause and effect.

One of the first studies to begin to address these problems was by Fine in 1963 and compared hospitalized asthmatic children to their nonasthmatic siblings, and found that the subjects were both more dependent and introverted, and explosive and uncontrolled than their siblings. Also noted was the finding that asthmatic children inhibited themselves from crying, especially during times of conflict, although they also had a low frustration tolerance, which led to the observed explosive behavior. Unfortunately, this study employed a questionable control group, making it impossible to address the issue of cause and effect with respect to asthma and psychopathology. As subsequent research began to use other chronically ill, hospitalized children as controls, it began to appear that many of the traits previously described as peculiar to asthma were in fact the result of chronic disease, and that the asthmatic children did not differ psychologically from other children with chronic disease.

However, before we adopt this "physiogenic" notion of asthma, that is, that particular personality traits result from asthma, and dismiss the "psychogenic" theory, that particular pesonality traits are associated with the development of asthma, it is necessary to examine the fascinating work of Chess, based upon the theory of temperament developed by Chess and Thomas over the past twenty years. This theory assumes that development of personality occurs as the result of an interaction between temperament, which is a constellation of traits *present at birth,* and environment. In applying this theory to a study of asthmatic children 3 to 7 years of age, they found that this group differed significantly in temperament from both normal controls, and a control group matched for age with chronic eczema or allergic rhinitis. Of the nine categories of temperament they have been studying, the asthmatic children in the present study were characterized by lower regularity, lower adaptability, lower intensity of reaction, lower mood value, and lower persistence than the group of controls. Since temperament has been shown by this group, through careful longitudinal study of a large cohort, to be a set of traits present at birth and persisting into adulthood, we are faced with a persuasive argument that there are indeed particular traits, defined by Chess and Thomas as nine dimensions of temperament, which are associated with the development of asthma. This does not however, imply that this specific profile of temperament in asthmatic children is not further modified by life experience and by the disease itself as, for example, through conditioning of muted emotional responses to stress.

ADULTS

As is the case with children, a multiplicity of personality traits have been identified in adult asthmatics, and it has become clear that no personality type or types characterize the asthmatic patient. However, personality, from an analytic perspective, consists, at least in part, of a group of defense mechanisms that arise to diminish the anxiety elicited by a psychological conflict. While different people may develop differing defense mechanisms, and thus different personalities, Alexander felt that all asthmatic patients experienced the same or similar core psychological conflicts or traits. This theory is of historical significance, and arises from his theory of psychosomatic specificity; that specific conflicts produced specific psychosomatic diseases. According to this theory, the conflict central to asthma is separation anxiety. This connection is supported by the multitude of studies demonstrating precipitation of asthma by separation of the patient from an important figure in his or her life. Furthermore, exploration of the families of these patients has revealed an overcontrolling, engulfing mother, a relationship that frequently leads to conflicts around separation and issues of independence versus dependence.

Unfortunately, this theory has not stood the test of time. Of particular note are the studies by Knapp and his co-workers that have demonstrated that conflict surrounding separation is not invariably present in asthmatic subjects, but that many other conflicts are recognizable. Perhaps most interestingly, they showed that in 83 percent of their patients with asthma, there were prominent feelings of helplessness, and that this same percentage (but not necessarily the same patients) suffered from depression of varying, but often significant severity. Feelings of helplessness in animal models, and depression in human subjects, have been shown to alter immune responsiveness, and may be of central importance in understanding the psychologic components of asthma, as will be discussed below.

ALEXITHYMIA

Alexithymia is a term coined by Sifneos, taken from the Greek (a = lack, lexis = work, thymos = emotion or mood), to describe a constellation of findings he noted to be particularly prominant in patients with psychosomatic illnesses. The patients he described as alexithymic seemed to have an impoverished fantasy life resulting in a rigid, uncreative way of thinking. They tended to avoid the stress of conflict through taking action instead of using words, and were markedly constricted in their expression of emotion. Most dramatically, they had extreme difficulty in recognizing feelings and describing those feelings with words.

In comparing control patients with various psychiatric disorders to patients with *psychosomatic* illnesses, he found a twofold increase in alexithymic characteristics in the latter group. Sifneos hypothesized that alexithymic traits result from deficits in neural pathways associated with emotional responses, and therefore are of etiologic significance with respect to psychosomatic disease. This theory is an attempt to provide a biologic model to support the psychogenic theories of Alexander. Other investigators feel they can identify two types of alexithymia. Primary alexithymia, analogous to Sifneos' conceptualization, and secondary alexithymia, resulting from, and as a psychological defense against the discomfort and dysphoria of a chronic physical illness.

Several questionnaires are now available that can identify alexithymic patients, and that have high intertest reliability. Use of these scales has demonstrated the stability of alexithymic traits over time. Subgroups of alexithymics have also been identified. One group is overly tense and communicates affective distress by focusing on physical symptoms. The second, and much more common subgroup denies equally intense affective distress through counterdependent, self-assured behavior. The observation of these traits in adults is interesting in light of the study by Fine, where analogous characteristics were seen in children with asthma, but not in their unaffected siblings. Further, the description of primary and secondary alexithymia helps to understand why Chess found alexithymic-like characteristics as a precursor to asthma, while other investigators found lessened emotional responsiveness as a response to the disease. The traits described in asthmatic children of inhibition of crying, dependency, and low frustration tolerance with subsequent loss of control and explosive behavior thus might be the progenitor of the adult manifestations of alexithymia, and demonstrate the potential significance of alexithymia as an etiologic factor in asthma. Of even greater significance than etiologic considerations are the implications of alexithymia with respect to treatment of asthma, which will be considered.

THE CNS AND IMMUNE MECHANISMS —
THE RELEVANCE TO ASTHMA

The concept that the CNS could have modulatory effects upon the immune system was first proposed by Russian scientists at the turn of the century, but only recently have these effects begun to be systematically explored.

Cunningham emphasizes the multiple levels at which a stimulus perceived by the mind is processed and altered before a somatic effect, such as immunosuppression occurs. The most proximal level in this schema is the perception of emotion. Personality variables, in this context, can then alter the experience of that emotion, perhaps enhancing or diminishing its impact upon the limbic system and hypothalamus. Transduction of the electrical impulses reaching the hypothalamus to neurohormonal signals then trigger the endocrine response of the anterior pituitary. It is the complex hormonal response of the pituitary in addition to direct autonomic innervation of elements of the immune system, which can modulate immune responses, and thus effect asthmatic symptoms.

The effects of stress upon multiple aspects of immune function have been convincingly documented both in animal experiments and in humans. In building upon this base, others have begun to examine the ability of personality variables to modify these stress effects. For example, a study of academic stress in dental students demonstrated that those students who had a constellation of personality traits the investigators termed an "inhibited power syndrome" had significantly lower levels of salivary IgA during high stress periods than did the group of students characterized as "relaxed affilitative." Another study looked at the same two groups of personality characteristics in undergraduate students and showed that the "inhibited power" group had high levels of sympathetic activation (measured as adrenergic and noradrenergic metabolites in 24-hour urine collections), and also reported higher levels of illness.

The role of the hypothalamus in these immunomodulatory effects have been demonstrated through two different approaches. In the first approach, selective lesions were made in the anterior hypothalamus of rats. These lesions decreased multiple measures of immune response, including circulating antibody levels. The second approach was to measure single neuron firing rates in the ventromedial nucleus of the rat hypothalamus. The firing rate of these neurons doubled at the time of antigen challenge, although there was no change in firing rate in control rats injected with inert vehicle only.

The pituitary response to hypothalamic input during stress involves the pro-opiomelanocortin (POMC) system, and elevations of all of the end products of this prohormone have been shown to be elevated under situations of stress, including ACTH (and thus cortisol), β-endorphin, β-lipotropin and α-MSH.

In addition to stress, various psychopatholgic states, and depression in particular, have also been shown to cause similar release of POMC peptides in a manner quite analogous to that seen in situations of experimental and naturally occurring stress. In fact, depressive episodes have not infrequently been misdiagnosed as Cushing's Disease due to the observed dysregulation of the hypothalamic-pituitary-adrenal axis. Furthermore, individuals subject to depression, and many individuals when depressed can be shown to have an "external locus of control." This is a concept used to differentiate individuals who feel they have control over their lives (an internal locus of control) from those who feel they are controlled by external events (an external locus of control). In an elegant series of experiments by Shavits and his co-workers, it was shown that learned helplessness, an animal model of external locus of control and depression is associated with elevated circulating levels of β-endorphin, and produce defects in several subpopulations of lymphocytes. These findings may be directly relevant to asthma due to the high incidence of depression and helplessness which was found by Knapp et al. in their group of asthmatic patients described earlier. Demonstration of alterations in the levels of prostaglandin E_1 and E_2 in depression may also be relevant to the impact of psychopathology upon asthma.

The mechanism through which neurotransmitters, neuromodulators, and neurohormones present in the peripheral circulation exert their effects upon the immune system has been well delineated. Lymphocytes, neutrophils, and

mast cells have been shown to possess receptors for many of these substances. Binding to a receptor either activates (e.g., β-adrenergic agonists) or
inhibits (α-adrenergic agonists) adenyl cyclase, or activates guanyl cyclase
(cholinergic agonists). It is the ratio of cGMP/cAMP that determines the
functional status of the immune cell. Recently receptors on lymphocytes have
been found for many of the burgeoning number of putative peptide neuromodulators, and these too effect the cGMP/cAMP ratio in the effector cells of
the immune system.

In addition to the potential neurohormonal effects on the immune system, many anatomic connections between the autonomic nervous system and
the immune system have been described. Sympathetic nerve endings have
been histologically demonstrated to be in close proximity to lymphocytes in
both thymus and spleen. If these splenic nerves are cut, up-regulation of β-
receptors on splenic lymphocytes occurs, demonstrating the functional nature
of this anatomic relationship. Furthermore, chemical sympathectomy of an
animal produces a decrease in both T-and B-cell response to antigen challenge.

In addition to the afferent and efferent connections of elements of the
immune system, a cholingergic reflex arc has been demonstrated to produce
bronchoconstriction in the dog, and anterior hypothalamic lesions may
decrease bronchoconstriction. Therefore, input from higher CNS centers may
affect not only the immune mediated aspects of asthma, but the vagally
mediated bronchoconstrictive component as well. This is not surprising in
view of the ability of suggestion to decrease carbachol-mediated bronchoconstriction.

A final series of experiments dramatically demonstrates that purely
"mental" events can modulate immune responsiveness. Robert Ader was
studying taste aversion conditioning. This is a particularly powerful conditioning paradigm where a single pairing of a novel drinking solution
(saccharin-flavored water) with a noxious stimulus (cyclophosphamide,
which was injected in doses producing gastrointestinal distress), produced an
aversion to saccharin in the mice for up to three months. Unexpectedly, some
of the mice so treated died well after the immunosuppressive effects of the
cyclophosphamide had resolved. In studying this phenomena, Ader found
that re-exposure to saccharin water consistently and reproducibly depressed
both cellular and humoral immunity in mice conditioned by the saccharin
water/cyclophosphamide pairing. Such a result, and the heretic hypothesis
that immune responses could be conditioned to be suppressed by a neutral
stimulus like saccharin water led to many independent attempts to replicate
these observations. These efforts supported Ader's original observation, and
have almost uniformly demonstrated that immune responses can be conditioned.

While Ader's experiments demonstrated conditioned immunosuppression, of perhaps greater relevance to asthma is conditioned immunoenhancement. This phenomenon has also been demonstrated in rats who were given allogenic skin grafts. These grafts were protected by a plaster cast applied to the rats' abdomens, and these casts became the conditioned stimulus. After the rats had rejected their grafts, they were then anesthetized and placed in plaster casts again without receiving a second graft. Nonetheless, they showed a rise in cytotoxic T lymphocytes alloantigen specific for the previously grafted tissue! Thus, both immunosuppression and immunoenhancement have been shown to occur in response to the mind's interpretation of perceived stimuli.

The conceptual similarity of these conditioning experiments to suggestion, hypnosis, and the placebo effect is striking. Recent studies demonstrating that elevations in plasma of both sympathetic neurotransmitters and the stress- and depression-related POMC peptides can occur in conditioned animals in anticipation of the occurrence of previously experienced stressful events opens an avenue to begin examination of the neurohormonal mediators of the modulation of asthmatic symptoms by psychologic factors.

It has been observed that the incidence of atopic disorders, and in particular asthma, is increased in patients with affective disorders, that is, both major depression and manic-depressive illness. There are also case reports of dramatic improvements in asthmatic symptoms with treatment of mania with lithium carbonate. These observations support the contention that neuroimmunomodulation is of relevance in asthma. Recently, histamine sensitive suppressor T-cell function was measured in patients with asthma before and following an imagery procedure similar to self hypnosis. Improvement in suppressor T-cell function was observed in those patients who subjectively felt that their asthmatic symptoms had improved as a result of the procedure. This is the first study to examine conditioned immunomodulation in asthmatic patients, and again demonstrates the relevance of these concepts to asthma.

PSYCHIATRIC CONSIDERATIONS IN THE TREATMENT OF ASTHMA

Up to this point, we have examined personality factors that are associated with the presence of asthma, psychologic factors related to the perception or amelioration of an asthmatic attack, and have drawn upon work in the area of neuroimmunomodulation to see through which neurohormonal systems these effects might be mediated.

In considering psychosocial treatment of the asthmatic patient, however, we need to consider in addition the psychologic complications of the illness itself, and the role of these complications in perpetuation or exacerbation of asthmatic symptoms. These factors should be assessed in the initial evaluation of the patient with asthma in order to determine what psychosocial interventions, if any, are needed to minimize asthma related morbidity.

Assessment

All too often, such an assessment is not made in the absence of more florid psychopathology, which demands recognition and referral for psychiatric treatment. This may occur in part because the physician is uncomfortable performing a role for which he or she has had little formal training. One means of overcoming this difficulty, especially in larger asthma clinics, is the multidisciplinary treatment team approach, where a psychiatrist with experience in evaluation of the asthma patient is available for both patient evaluation and treatment, as well as for consultation with staff. However, even in the absence of such a consultant, a fairly brief and straightforward interview directed toward obtaining information in several specific areas will provide the physician with the data necessary to reach a decision regarding treatment of psychiatric or psychosocial issues. The areas of interest are: precipitants of asthmatic symptoms, social and family support, accuracy of self assessment of disease severity, including the severity of the impact of the disease upon daily living, and psychopathology.

PRECIPITANTS

The precipitants of an asthmatic attack effect not only medical treatment decisions, but psychiatric treatment decisions as well. Earlier we discussed the impact of emotion and suggestion upon precipitation of an asthmatic attack. One should question patients in both of these areas. Do emotional outbursts such as crying, laughing, anxiety, or anger trigger an attack? Are attacks precipitated in settings where previous attacks have occurred, or by thinking about or seeing objects associated with prior attacks? Such psychophysiologic precipitants, when identified in a patient, have been shown to correlate with more positive outcomes to specific psychiatric interventions. In particular, in those individuals where emotion is a prominent factor in the initiation of bronchospasm, relaxation training, usually in combination with other behavioral techniques can be an effective treatment. On the other hand, in patients demonstrating a prominent degree of suggestibility with respect to asthmatic symptoms, suggestion and hypnosis have proven to be useful adjuncts to treatment.

SOCIAL SUPPORT AND PSYCHOSOCIAL ASSETS

The response of asthma to treatment has been shown to correlate closely with a patient's psychosocial assets. In fact, it can be anticipated that individuals who have low social status, poor interpersonal relationships, lack of positive family support, and poor work history will respond less well to treatment and require higher doses of medication to control symptoms. By questioning patients in these areas, one can determine whether psychosocial intervention is needed to avoid a poor treatment outcome. Especially in the case of children, structural change within the family may be possible, although draconian changes such as removing the child from the home are now used only as a last resort.

ACCURACY OF DISEASE ASSESSMENT

One should spend some time with the patient to gain an understanding of how the patient views the illness. How much of an impact does asthma have on the patient's life? How frightening are attacks? What is the effect of the illness upon the family or friends? Of course these attitudes are a reflection of one's personality, and thus of the defense mechanisms used to cope with the anxiety produced by a chronic illness. Patients (or families of child patients) who are at either extreme on the continuum of minimizing versus exaggerating symptoms and the effects of those symptoms are at greater risk for inappropriate self-treatment and have been shown to require more frequent and longer hospitalizations. This continuum can be measured using the panic-fear subscale of the MMPI, a highly standardized self administered psychological testing instrument. This subscale is correlated with the degree to which patients exaggerate or minimize their symptoms. Patients scoring either high or low on this subscale averaged rehospitalization rates three to four times greater than patients with an intermediate score on the test over a one- and two-year followup period. In the individuals judged at risk, short-term psychotherapy geared to discussion of reality issues related to the disease process could be of benefit.

PSYCHOPATHOLOGY

We have earlier come to the conclusion that although no particular personality type is associated with asthma, that certain "temperaments," as defined by Chess et al., are. However, evaluation of these traits is time consuming, and would prove to be of little benefit in the management of the asthmatic. These traits are an enduring aspect of one's personality, and despite the fact that they are associated with asthma, there is no evidence that modification of these traits would have any effect upon the course of disease. However, psychopathology of all degrees of severity may coexist with asthma, and have effects upon disease severity, compliance with treatment, and the degree to which the disease interferes with normal functioning. Consequently, it is necessary to make an assessment concerning the degree, if any, of psychopathology in a given patient, and the degree to which it does impact upon the disease and its treatment.

While a thorough assessment of psychopathology and personality is not practicable in a busy clinical practice, the physician should be alert to the more obvious signs of psychopathology that impact upon the disease and its management. In particular, patients showing signs of depression should be questioned about its severity and for the presence of vegetative signs such as anergia, early morning awakening, anhedonia, or weight loss. Anxiety itself may directly affect the severity of asthma symptoms, or be a symptom of an atypical depression. These individuals should be referred to a psychiatrist for treatment. Likewise, where a question of psychotic symptoms arise, a psychiatrist will need to diagnose and stabilize the patient in order to maximize patient compliance.

In the case of possible personality disorders, again a consultation with a psychiatrist could prove useful. While psychotherapy would be indicated only if the patient desires such treatment, the consultant would be able to provide the primary physician with specific recommendations that could improve patient cooperation and compliance, and thus decrease morbidity or inappropriate utilization of increasingly costly and scarce medical resources. Such a beneficial effect of even brief periods of psychotherapy (and even single evaluative sessions) have been demonstrated in studies conducted in Health Maintenance Organizations. In these studies, rates of medical utilization over a five-year followup period decreased substantially (in one study up to 60 percent) following brief psychotherapeutic intervention.

In patients with personality disorders in particular, but in any patient, the physician should also remain cognizant of the possibility that a patient's symptoms are being exaggerated, or perpetuated and maintained for secondary gain. The child with school phobia is allowed to stay home from school. The child with a distant, aloof mother gets more attention when his asthmatic symptoms worsen, or the husband gets more nurturance from his wife. Even more obvious are cases concerning disability insurance, especially if there is pending litigation. Particularly in this latter situation, a successful treatment outcome is impossible until the legal situation is resolved. However, in any of these or similar situations of secondary gain, following an assessment, a psychiatrist may help to devise a strategy to eliminate the need or desire to achieve secondary gain, and thus the need to remain ill. Such a strategy may be in the form of suggestions to the treating physician, or might be effected through brief therapy of several session duration with the psychiatrist.

Earlier we discussed the concept of alexithymia and its significance in asthma. The assessment of alexithymia is important for several reasons. The alexithymic individual minimizes his emotional symptomatology, in part because of his own lack of awareness of these symptoms, and an inability to verbalize accurately their intensity. The treating physician thus might not achieve an accurate appraisal of the severity of the illness or the response to treatment unless he recognizes and takes into consideration whether or not a patient is alexithymic.

The alexithymnic has also been shown to require more frequent and longer hospitalization for asthma. Therefore, recognition might lead to more intensive treatment and followup of these patients, decreasing their increased risk of morbidity. Another derived subscale of the MMPI is available that identifies alexithymic patients. This test has a sensitivity of 82 percent. While it has been used predominantly in research settings, it could easily be utilized for particular patients when clinically indicated.

PSYCHOMAINTENANCE OF PHYSICAL SYMPTOMS

In evaluating these various psychological parameters, we have attempted to look at those factors that will have an impact upon the course of illness in patients with asthma. Dirks has coined the term psychomaintenance for this concept: the psychologic, behavioral, and social perpetuation and exacerbation of physical illness. In extensive studies of psychomaintenance in asthma, he has developed a Battery of Asthma Illness Behavior, which employs the MMPI and the subscales already described, as well as a Respiratory Illness Opinion Survey, and an Asthma Symptom Checklist. Using this battery of tests, he was able to predict rehospitalization within six months with from 72 percent to 84 percent accuracy based upon psychological factors alone! This indicates how important assessment and treatment of these psychologic and social factors are in management of the asthmatic patient.

Treatment

Following the assessment procedures outlined, the need for intervention at a psychobiologic or social level will have been clarified, and of course treatment recommendations are an integral part of that assessment. In the past, when the assessment and treatment of psychosomatic illnesses was guided by psychoanalytic theory as formulated by Alexander, there were no alternatives to individual psychotherapy (despite the fact that in only a limited number of cases was this the appropriate treatment modality). Today, however, multiple treatment techniques, many of which are short term and cost effective are available for treatment of specifically targeted symptoms. In a given case, one or more of these techniques may be employed in a multisystems approach to care of the asthmatic patient.

HYPNOSIS AND SUGGESTION

Hypnosis and suggestion are considered together because in many respects, these techniques are indistinguishable from each other. The major difference between them is that while both employ suggestion, in hypnosis, the patient is in a relaxed, "hypnotized" state where he is more receptive to the suggestion.

Suggestion is appropriately used in an acute setting by the primary care giver, often to augment the effectiveness of administered medication. In such settings, as well as in experimental settings, suggestion alone is about half as effective as medication alone in alleviating bronchoconstriction, and the effects of medication and suggestion are additive.

In a chronic setting, use of suggestion during an hypnotic interview or series of interviews is the treatment of choice in patients who have been found during the assessment to be suggestible. Typically, when hypnosis is used alone, the patient will be treated over a course of four to eight sessions. The sessions consist of trance induction followed by either direct or indirect suggestion tailored to the particular asthma precipitants experienced by the patient. Usually, the patient will be taught self hypnosis, and instructed to hypnotize himself or herself perhaps several times a day, employing autosuggestion while in the trance state.

Large numbers of case reports showing dramatic results from hypnosis are to be found in the literature. However, only two studies were fairly well controlled and had large numbers of subjects. In both studies, patients in the hypnosis group fared better than patients in the control group. Differences were not large, but were statistically significant. However, patients in the hypnosis group were randomly selected from the pool of asthmatic patients without regard to their suggestibility, hypnotizability, or the precipitants of their attacks. In appropriately selected patients, hypnosis should do even better than was evident in these studies, and is clearly a valuable adjunctive treatment.

BEHAVIOR THERAPY: RELAXATION, SYSTEMATIC DESENSITIZATION, AND BIOFEEDBACK

Again, there are some similarities between relaxation training and hypnosis since hypnosis requires relaxation before a trance state can be achieved. However, in relaxation training, any suggestions are directed specifically toward the goal of achieving relaxation. Combinations of relaxation training with systematic desensitization or with biofeedback have also been studied. Earlier, the ability of emotional arousal to precipitate asthmatic symptoms was discussed, and studies linking autonomic (sympathetic) activation with alterations in immune response were presented. The theoretical rationale for relaxation training is that it will lessen autonomic arousal, thus decreasing direct autonomic effects on the bronchial smooth muscle, and indirectly alter immune responsiveness. The addition of systematic desensitization to relaxation training involves exposing the patient, either through imagination or in vivo, to a hierarchy of increasingly close, and thus increasingly anxiety provoking, approximations of the stimuli that have in the past provoked attacks. However, this is accomplished at a rate where anxiety to a given level of stimulus has resolved before the next higher level of stimulus is introduced. Theoretical justification of this technique has previously centered around the emotional arousal theory of asthma precipitation. The conditioning experiments of Ader and others now provide an additional avenue for exploration of the effects of systematic desensitization: perhaps patients are not only conditioned to have lesser emotional responses to anxiety provoking stimuli, thus decreasing autonomic arousal, but are also undergoing conditioning of immune responsiveness, accounting for the intermediate and long-term benefits seen in patients undergoing systematic desensitization.

Several biofeedback techniques have been used to treat asthma. Electromyographic techniques have been used as an adjunct in relaxation. Respiratory biofeedback has been used to directly train patients in increasing pulmonary efficiency. Case reports of thermal biofeedback, where patients are taught to increase skin temperature have also shown positive and sometimes dramatic outcomes, probably again by serving as an adjunct to relaxation techniques. Finally, electroencephalogram (EEG) sensorimotor biofeedback has been reported in a single case report to have had a dramatic effect on asthma symptoms in a 6-year-old boy. In this technique, the patient is trained to produce a so-called sensorimotor rhythm of 12–14 Hz from regions overlying the Rolandic cortex. The technique was applied to asthma with the hope it would decrease bronchial hyper-reactivity since it has been shown to be efficacious in increasing voluntary motor inhibition and in decreasing motor activity in patients with psychomotor seizures.

Because of poor study design, studies attempting to evaluate relaxation training alone or in combination with systematic desensitization or biofeedback are difficult to interpret. However, despite the methodologic and statistical shortcomings of many studies, critical reviews of behavior therapy in general agree that while the benefits of relaxation therapy alone have not been demonstrated, the combination of relaxation with another behavioral technique does produce both subjective and objective improvement of asthma symptoms.

PSYCHOTHERAPY

Two psychotherapeutic modalities have been employed in the treatment of asthmatics: individual and group psychotherapy. Given the appropriate set of circumstances, one of these techniques might constitute an appropriate adjunct to treatment. However, meta-analyses of studies of asthmatic patients in individual psychotherapy have been unable to document the efficacy of the procedure. This may be in part due to the fact that no studies to date have satisfied the criteria for adequate research design. This does not imply that individual psychotherapy is of no benefit. In appropriately selected patients, there have been clear improvements in patient-physician interaction/compliance with treatment and subsequent improved adjustment to chronic disease. However, what the studies have shown is that individual psychotherapy has not yet been shown to affect the disease process itself.

With respect to group psychotherapy, while research findings have been more variable, with some reports of dramatic improvements in group members, again, poor experimental design precludes drawing definitive conclusions.

Before leaving the topic of psychotherapy, a brief comment about the alexithymic patient is necessary. Since these individuals are unable to express feelings and emotions, they are not good candidates for this form of treatment. Rather, one of the behavioral therapies is usually better suited as means of treatment.

EDUCATION

Since much of the morbidity of asthma occurs as a result of a lack of understanding, misunderstanding, or poor compliance, patients can frequently benefit from formal educational sessions where the physiology of the disease process and principals of pharmacologic management are elucidated for the patient. This has been used in particular with children, often in the setting of asthma self-help groups. If such a program is available, it is a very cost effective first line treatment and may obviate the need for more intensive and costly psychosocial intervention.

PSYCHOPHARMACOTHERAPY OF THE PATIENT
WITH ASTHMA

It was noted earlier that depressed patients have a higher incidence of a history of atopic disorders. Conversely, many asthmatic patients become depressed, both as a response to their chronic disease, or as an untoward side effect of corticosteroid treatment.

The physician treating depression in the asthmatic patient should be cognizant of several issues pertinent to this group of patients. Approximately one to six persons per thousand are allergic to the dye Tartrazine (ED&C yellow #5). However, the incidence of this allergy in asthmatics is higher, and 10 percent–40 percent of aspirin-sensitive asthmatics respond adversely to Tartrazine. This dye is contained in several antidepressant medications, and these should be avoided in asthmatics, especially those with aspirin sensitivity. Antidepressants containing tartrazine include doxepin (Adaptin, Pennwalt, Rochester, New York 14623), desipramine (Norpramin, Merrill-Dow, Cincinnati, Ohio 45215), imipramine (Tofranil, Geigy Pharmaceuticals, Ardsley, New York 10502), and trazodone (Desyrel, Mead Johnson, Evansville, Indiana 47721). Should a reaction occur, its recognition is important to avoid a vicious cycle of increasing steroid use to control allergic symptoms, leading to increasing depressive symptoms which is then treated with further increase in the offending antidepressant.

The use of MAO inhibitors should also be avoided in patients who require treatment with sympathomimetic drugs. Despite the fact that epinephrine is metabolized by catechol-o-methyl transferase and not monoamine oxidase, a hypertensive reaction has been pointed out to be a possible result of the combination.

Finally, despite the absence of any studies of this question, the use of tricyclic antidepressants with high anticholinergic properties has been suggested as a possible means of reducing bronchospasm in the asthmatic patient while at the same time treating their depression.

REFERENCES

Ader R, Cohen R, Bojerg D: Conditioned suppression of humoral immunity in the rat. J Comparative Physiological Psychology 96:517–521, 1982
Alexander F, French TM, Pollock GH: Psychosomatic Specificity. University of Chicago Press, Chicago, 1968
Alquist J: Hormonal influences on immunologic and related phenomena, in Ader R (ed): Psychoneuroimmunology. Academic Press, New York, 355–425, 1981
Besedovsky H, Sorkin E, Felix D, et al: Hypothalamic changes during the immune response. Eur J Immunol 7:323–325, 1977
Brown EL, Fukuhara JT, Feiguine RJ: Alexithymic asthmatics: the miscommunication of affective and somatic states. Psychother Psychosom 36:116–121, 1981
Connors CK: Psychological management of the asthmatic child. Clin Rev Allerg 1:163–177, 1983
Cunningham AJ: Mind, body & immune response. In Ader R (ed): Psychoneuroimmunology, Academic Press, New York, 609–616, 1981

Dirks JF, Schraa JC, Brown EL, et al: Psychomaintenance in asthma: Hospitalization rates and financial impact. Br J Med Psych 53:349–354, 1980

Dirks JF, Robinson SK, Dirks DL: Alexithymia and the psychomaintenance of bronchial asthma. Psychother Psychosom 36:63–71, 1981

Dirks JF: Bayesian prediction of psychomaintenance related to rehospitalization in asthma. J Pers Assess 46:2, 1982

Erskine-Milliss J, Schonell M: Relaxation therapy in asthma: a critical review. Psychosom Med 43:365–372, 1981

Fritz FK: Childhood asthma. Psychosomatics 24:959–967, 1983

Gorczynski RM, MacRae S, Kennedy M: Conditioned immune response associated with allogenic skin grafts in mice. J Immunol 129:704–709, 1982

Hollaender J, Florin I: Expressed emotion and airway conductance in children with bronchial asthma. J Psychosom Res 27:307–311, 1983

Horton DJ, Suda WL, Kinsman RA, et al: Bronchoconstrictive suggestion in asthma: a role for airways hyperreactivity and emotions. Am Rev Respir Dis 117:1029–1038, 1978

Jemmott JB, Borysenko M, McClelland DC, et al: Academic stress, power motivation and decrease in secretion rate of salivary secretory immunoglobulin A. Lancet 21:1400–1402, 1983

Kim SP, Ferrara A, Chess S: Temperature of asthmatic children. J Pediatr 97:483–486, 1980

Knapp PH, Nemetz SJ: Personality variations in bronchial asthma. Psychosom Med 19:443, 1957

Knapp PH, Nemetz SJ, et al: The context of reported asthma during psychoanalysis, Psychosom Med 32:167, 1970

Lerro FA, Hurnyak MM, Patterson C: Successful use of thermal biofeedback in severe adult asthma. Am J Psychiatry 137:735–736, 1980

Levenson RW: Effects on thematically relevant and general stressors on specificity of responding in asthmatic and nonasthmatic subjects. Psychosom Med 41:28–39, 1979

Liebman D, Minuchin S, Baker L: The use of structural family therapy in the treatment of intractable asthma. Am J Psychiatry 131:535–539, 1974

McClelland DC, Floor E, Davidson RJ, et al: Stressed power motivation, sympathetic activation, immune function and illness. J Hum Stress 6:11–19, 1980

Polonsky WH, Knapp PH, Brown EL, et al: Psychological factors, immunological function and bronchial asthma. Psychosom Med 47:77, 1985

Richter R, Dahme B: Bronchial asthma in adults: there is little evidence for the effectiveness of behavioral therapy and relaxation. J Psychosom Res 26:533–540, 1982

Shavit Y, Lewis JW, Terman GW, et al: Opioid peptides mediate the suppressive effect of stress on natural killer cell cytotoxicity. Science 223:188–190, 1984

Sifneos PE: The prevalance of 'alexithymic' characteristics in psychosomatic patients. Psychother Psychosom 22:255–262, 1973

Spector S, Luparello T, Kopetzky MT, et al: Response of asthmatics to methacholine and suggestion. Am Rev Respir Dis 113:43–50, 1976

Stein M: Biopsychosocial factors in asthma. In West LF, Stein M (eds): Critical Issues in Behavioral Medicine 12:159–182, 1982

Tansey MA: EEG sensorimotor biofeedback training and the treatment of a six-year-old asthmatic child. Am J Clin Biofeedback 5:145–149, 1982

Thompson WL, Thompson TL: Treating depression in asthmatic patients. Psychosomatics 25:809–812, 1984

Weiner H (ed): Bronchial asthma. In Psychobiology and Human Disease, Elsevier, New York, 1977, pp. 223–317.

Williams DA, Lewis-Faning E, Rees L, et al: Assessment of the relative importance of the allergic, infective and psychological factors in asthma. Acta Allergol (Kbh) 12:376, 1958

Edwin L. Klingelhofer
M. Eric Gershwin

26

Preventive Medicine and Patient Education

Prevention or control of asthma depends on patients acquiring and using information about their disease effectively, and developing the skills to behave and then behaving in a manner consistent with this information.

The majority of asthma sufferers experiences mild, intermittent, and transitory systems. They do not perceive that working out an elaborate preventive strategy is worth the time and effort involved. These individuals arrive at adequate coping procedures largely through a process of trial and error. Usually these will consist of the use, when needed, of an over-the-counter medication or a prescription drug in a dusty container exhumed from the back of the medicine chest. For more stubborn cases this haphazard approach often does not work out so well.

A CAUTIONARY TALE OF FAILURE

Roger and Emmy are in their mid-thirties and have been living together for the last six years. Both developed asthma and allergic rhinitis in childhood, with symptoms linked initially to the pollen season. Emmy's attacks are still mainly seasonal but Roger's have become year round and their onset is associated with exposure to a variety of substances; pollens, dust, viral infections, aspirin, and wine are the ones he knows about.

BRONCHIAL ASTHMA, Second Edition
ISBN 0-8089-1814-1

Their medical histories are surprisingly similar. When their symptoms first appeared they were each taken to their family doctors who, after a perfunctory examination, prescribed an oral antihistamine and theophylline. This tactic worked well enough but the side effects of the medication were so distressing that they went on to consult allergists who conducted skin tests, found positive reactions to a number of different pollens, and started a course of immunization shots. The shots helped some, they report, but were not continued long enough to desensitize them to the antigens. They disliked the process immensely, the injections, the necessity to appear at the allergist's office regularly, and to wait around there with nothing happening after the shot had been given.

After high school they both left home, Roger to attend college on the West Coast and Emmy to pursue a musical career. They stopped the shots—but not the hay fever and asthma.

During college Roger's asthma became much more persistent and severe and he had to seek emergency treatment on three occasions, all at the time of the year when grass was pollenating. The college health service referred Roger to an allergist who, after reviewing his situation, put him on a regular schedule of theophylline—he doesn't remember the dosage—with an aerosol beta-agonist backup for more acute episodes. Roger took the medication faithfully. He was graduated from college, moved to Los Angeles, married his college sweetheart, and had the marriage fail under conditions of considerable stress and tension after three years. During this period Roger's asthma worsened. He broke with the opinion of his doctor and concluded that his asthma was psychogenic in origin and that he was nothing more than a slave to his medications. He abruptly stopped using them and (with the demise of his marriage) moved to Northern California.

During this same period Emmy noticed that her asthma was getting worse. She blamed that on constant travel, contending it brought her in contact with pollens to which she was sensitive. She too consulted an allergist who put her on antihistamines and aerosols. She had to have something because she played in and was lead singer in a bluegrass band and without medication she simply could not perform.

Emmy, too, wound up in Northern California, became tired of her medication and its side effects and gave up on it. Besides it was costing her a lot of money she didn't have. She and Roger first met in the waiting room of an herbalist they had gone to for what they both believed would be more "organic" and less drastic and harmful treatment.

Now, six years later, Roger is still considerably troubled by asthma. He observes the regimen prescribed by the herbalist which, he believes, has been somewhat helpful but, as he puts it, "sometimes I do things that aren't too smart. Like, if there's a bottle of good red wine around, I may take a few hits of it. I know what'll happen but I just can't resist."

Emmy, too, is still asthmatic. She now finds that she will sometimes lapse into asthma when she has a viral infection but she is less bothered with pollens, in large measure because the area of Northern California where she lives does not grow the plants to which she formerly reacted. That fact may also explain Roger's marginal improvement.

Last winter Emmy was in bed with a severe cold and fever and moderate asthma symptoms. A friend who visited her during this episode asked if she was doing anything for it.

"Rest and teas," Emmy wheezed.

"Don't you want some Contac or something?" the friend asked. "I'd be glad to go out and get it for you just to help you breathe better."

"I'd die before I took any of that stuff," Emmy gasped.

This cautionary tale of failure in treatment probably typifies the experiences of many asthmatics. It owes much to the breakdown of preventive strategies (either through ignorance of or neglect of them) combined with nonexistent or failed efforts to educate the patients about the nature and care of their disease.

SELF-MANAGEMENT PROGRAMS

Unfortunately, a reactive, symptom-centered approach is also quite apt to characterize treatment of moderate to severely troubled patients. Here the results are likely to be unsatisfactory. It is only recently that systematic programs for the management and control of asthma have begun to be formulated—most of them aimed at children. These programs, which have been tagged as "self-management" or "self-care," all aim to bring moderately to severely asthmatic children to the point where they can, with a minimum of medical intervention, prevent or minimize the severity of asthmatic episodes and live as normal a life as possible. The principles and procedures that have been developed for them are equally valid for adults although there seems to have been little effort to formulate programs aimed at helping adults manage their asthma more aggressively and with greater degrees of self-involvement and responsibility for decision-making. (The State University of New York at Buffalo's Adult Asthma Self-Management Program is a notable exception to this statement. So, too, is the ALA's self-instruction booklet, *Help Yourself to Better Breathing*, which is aimed at adult audiences.)

The various asthma self-management programs which are enumerated a bit farther on have been faulted because they are, in the main, too brief and conceptually too narrow to mediate the substantial and durable changes necessary if the complex, intractable, and uniquely individual mix of attitudes and behaviors that govern asthma treatment are to be altered. Thoresen and

Kermil-Gray have offered the framework for a four-dimensional social learning model that enumerates some of the welter of interactive cognitive, physiological, behavioral, and social and environmental factors that must be addressed if a program of training in self care is to be effective. The extant training programs do not attain anything approaching this level of complexity. Indeed, most of them only concentrate on one or two of the behavior change skills which Thoreson and Kermil-Gray identify as being effective in managing asthma. The skills they identify are:

1. relaxation and breathing exercises
2. self-monitoring
3. problem solving
4. decision-making
5. behavior analysis
6. stimulus control
7. rearranging consequences
8. positive self-statements
9. contracting and use of token economies
10. positive reinforcement.

The elements in this list add up to mishmash; some of them identify helpful behavior, while others consist of general strategies or contingencies for bringing about the changes sought that are applicable to any training or learning situation at all.

The three training programs most readily available to patients are *ACT for Kids*, which was developed by the University of California at Los Angeles Health Services Research Center and is offered by the Asthma and Allergy Foundation of America (AAFA), *Superstuff*, which has been prepared by and is available through the American Lung Association (ALA), and *Winning Over Wheezing*, which was originally developed at National Jewish Hospital in Denver, tried out extensively in Hawaii, and is now available from William H. Rorer, Inc., the pharmaceutical firm. These three programs are described and discussed in some detail below.

Four other programs have been developed under sponsorship of the National Heart, Lung, and Blood Institute's Division of Lung Diseases and are just now being made available for general use under American Lung Association sponsorship. They are *Open Airways*, which grew out of a program originally developed at Columbia University College of Physicians, the American Institute for Research's individual and group education programs, *Air Wise* and *Air Power*, which were tested at Kaiser-Permanente Medical Group clinics in Santa Clara and San Jose, California, and *Living With Asthma*, which was put together and assessed at Denver's National Asthma Center.

At least five additional programs have been tried but they are purely local in nature and, for that reason, are not accessible to most physicians or their patients.

ACT (Asthma Care Training) consists of five 1-hour sessions aimed at asthmatic children aged 6–12 years and their parents. The program which, ideally, is given to 5–8 person groups, can be conducted in clinics, physicians' offices, hospitals, or classrooms by elementary school teachers, health educators, or nurses with teaching experience. The existence and venue of ACT sessions would be known to hospitals or the local allergy society. The sessions which require active participation in a variety of individual and group activities are organized around a common theme—"You're in the Driver's Seat"—and uses highway symbols and analogies to achieve their goals, which are to:

1. identify personal symptoms ("Warning Signals")
2. identify aggravators ("Roadblocks")
3. explain preventive and treatment strategies ("Tune-ups")
4. facilitate decision-making and promote problem-solving ("Road Maps")
5. teach general health habits ("Maintenance and Service")

For the child the program aims to develop mastery skills over the disease and to give experience in decision-making; parents are taught how to nurture the child and create an environment conducive to decision making.

The approach strikes one as being somewhat cluttered and superficial although evaluations indicate that it is effective in reducing emergency room visits and parental panic. However, when ACT graduates and controls were compared the program did not affect frequency of office visits or number of hospitalizations, although the number of days in hospital for the ACT group was fewer. The limited amount of time devoted to each element in the program and to practicing its target skills may help explain its slight success.

Superstuff is a self-teaching approach designed to give parents and elementary school children more self-confidence, self-control, and know-how in dealing with their asthma. It does this by having children work through a series of games, puzzles, and other exercises aimed to train them to react appropriately to various aspects of the disease. Parents are supplied with a news magazine that offers the salient facts in control of asthma. The kit may be purchased from physicians or the local ALA office.

Superstuff is attractively designed and inviting. It is doubtless fun for the child but it blurs the importance of its message and purpose by making them incidental to the process of working through the exercises. To be maximally useful the child's progress through the workbook, the heart of the program, needs to be monitored and reviewed, and the message frequently reinforced and driven home by parents—and this function is played down in the instructions that accompany the package.

Superstuff has been cursorily evaluated. The materials have been judged as understandable, appealing, and useful by their consumers and use of them has been associated with "improvement." In essence, though, it slights a serious and stubborn problem by placing its emphasis on fun and games rather than on its serious purpose and the significant gains to be achieved from using the information to be had from and the skills to be learned in the materials. As it is the learnings sometimes seem to be incidental to the context in which they are imbedded.

Winning Over Wheezing is an asthma self-help program offered to children from 5 to 16 years and their parents. Like the other programs discussed it aims to improve knowledge about the disease, provide training in breathing and relaxation, and foster self-management. It also stresses physical fitness; exercise (swimming is favored) forms an integral part of every training session.

The program consists of 11 weekly sessions for the children. These sessions are divided into two parts, 45 minutes devoted to classroom work followed by 45 minutes of supervised exercise.

Parents attend three separate 90-minute meetings that inform them about the disease and encourage them to let their children take responsibility for the management and care of their asthma.

The program has been evaluated by having parents respond to a questionnaire upon completion of the program. They testify overwhelmingly that the program was helpful in general and in moving the child to accept more responsibility for asthma care. However, half of the children showed no improvement in their willingness to participate in physical activities even though their skills had improved. Knowledge about asthma on the part of the children was judged to have increased, and participation in the program was associated with a decline in the frequency of asthmatic attacks, their severity, and in the amount of medication used.

This testimony is impressive and the program is sufficiently long at least to offer the possibility of bringing about some useful and durable changes. However, these evaluative statistics apply to families in which both child and parent completed the program and no information is supplied about the incidence of fallout or dropout which is, or can be an evaluative statement.

This program, (manual, slide show, cassette tape, posters, and training booklets) has been made available to pediatricians by William H. Rorer, Inc., Fort Washington, PA, 19034. Pediatricians or the local pediatric society should know of the existence of local courses.

While any one of these three self-help programs is not likely, in and of itself, to effect the radical change in entrenched habits and attitudes which will result in an aggressive and competent preventive posture, they all contain elements that are essential to such an outcome. If they are reinforced by physician and parents and if the strategies taught are checked and monitored they can make an enormous difference in the outlook and in the general health and well being of asthmatic children. The problem here (as with any other program of long-term care) is to secure consistent and unfailing adherence to its elements. This means that some altogether human attributes like slacking off because the regimen is boring or not immediately or intrinsically rewarding, or giving up on or cutting back on medication, or succumbing to the temptation to do things which it is known will exacerbate the asthma symptoms need to be anticipated and countered. To have the strength and the resoluteness to do this, parents and children must have consistent support and explicit encouragement from their physician.

In practice, most patient education gets done and the specification of preventive measures, which is an irreducible part of that activity, is carried out in the doctor's office. The quality of the results of that process are extremely variable and, it is safe to say, rarely approach the goal of having asthmatics maximize their ability to prevent or be more assertive in looking after their symptoms. For that reason this chapter devotes itself to steps physicians can take and strategies they can follow to help their asthmatic patients know more about and achieve better control of their symptoms.

The variable results of physician-mediated attempts to educate asthmatic patients owe much to the inability of physician and patient to cope effectively with the inherent complexity of the task. To take a common example, asthma symptoms often reappear or fail of control because the patient gives up on taking necessary medication. This can be a deliberate act ("I wanted to see if I could get along without the stuff") or an inadvertent one ("It just slipped my mind"); it can result from properties of the medication itself (disagreeable taste; untoward side-effects); cost can play a role ("I couldn't afford to get the prescription refilled"). It can happen because there are a number of medications that have to be taken in a fixed order on a hard and fast schedule which the patient has difficulty remembering and following because of personal limitations or inadequate instructions. The medication may suddenly lose its effectiveness because other blocking drugs are being taken for other conditions or (sometimes) the new drugs may actually mobilize the asthma symptoms. Whatever the reason, nonadherence to medication regimens may result from any of a large number of causes. In the case of asthmatics, the evidence suggests that nonadherence is more often the rule than the exception. To have patients stick to their medication schedules more firmly requires that physicians recognize the welter of causes for this failure and to take time to provide this information and a rationale that will motivate and enable their patients to stay the course.

From this example it will be seen that preventing or minimizing the severity of asthma attacks is a skill as arcane and many-faceted as the disease itself. The information and the attitudes inherent in a competent program of prevention are not transmitted in a brief, one-directional session in which a set of instructions and admonitions are given in a rush.

Asking physicians to assume this patient education burden may seem excessive or outside their proper sphere of responsibility. Yet, there is much that can be done and the physician is in the best spot to do it.

One can think of prevention (and education for prevention) of asthma as occurring at the end of a rational, time-ordered sequence or chain of steps. Each of the steps (which are loosely adapted from and build on Hindi-Alexander's steps to asthma self-management) are spelled out in Figure 26-1 along with a suggested list of physician and patient behaviors at each point. The steps and the physician's role in each one are elaborated in the sections that follow the figure.

STEPS TO PREVENTION

As noted, we regard effective prevention and control of asthma symptoms to be primarily an educational matter. There are several mass asthma prevention programs for children readily available and the physician may choose to remand patients to one or another of them if they are available in the locality. The trouble with some such programs is that they are not always ongoing and, more important, people tend to resist attending them unless they are in a crisis situation. Consequently, most patient education on this subject is still carried out in the physician's office and the indications are that it is not particularly effective in bringing patients to the point where they are able to manage their symptoms competently. The reasons for this reside in both parties concerned. Patients may not understand or accept the diagnosis; they often do not comprehend, neglect, or refuse to follow treatments specified; they will not or cannot cooperate in various strategies aimed at ameliorating the disease; they are less than zealous in carrying out avoidance procedures; they acquire and act on misinformation or myth, or develop attitudes about the disease which interfere with treatment; and they fail to heed and take appropriate action at the appearance of prodromal symptoms. These failures occur because information or advice is not transmitted or comprehended or, worse, is interpreted incorrectly; they are compounded because of inability or unwillingness of patients to push for clarification, because of diffidence, the fear of appearing stupid, or because of explanations that are simply beyond them. They are further aggravated by personal, social, and economic factors which may find them getting important secondary gains from having the disease or running the risk of precipitating an asthma attack or suspending a treatment or preventive stratagem because of

STEPS TO PREVENTION OF ASTHMA

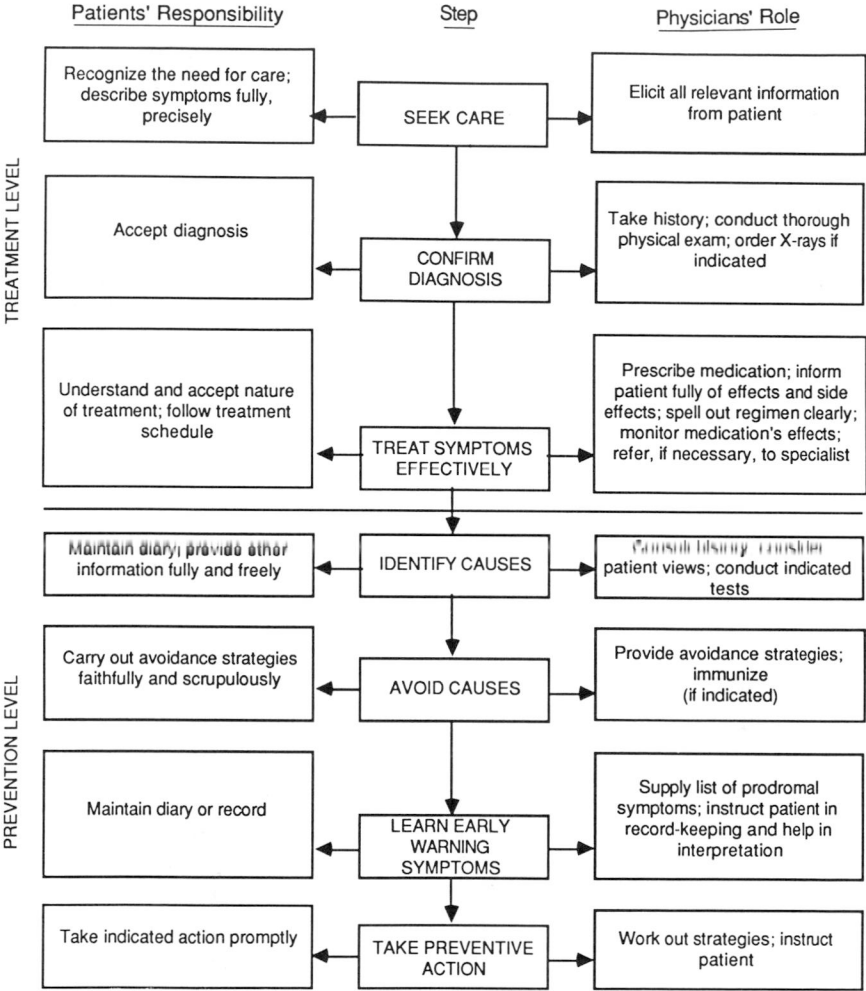

Patients' Responsibility	Step	Physicians' Role
Recognize the need for care; describe symptoms fully, precisely	SEEK CARE	Elicit all relevant information from patient
Accept diagnosis	CONFIRM DIAGNOSIS	Take history; conduct thorough physical exam; order X-rays if indicated
Understand and accept nature of treatment; follow treatment schedule	TREAT SYMPTOMS EFFECTIVELY	Prescribe medication; inform patient fully of effects and side effects; spell out regimen clearly; monitor medication's effects; refer, if necessary, to specialist
Maintain diary, provide other information fully and freely	IDENTIFY CAUSES	Consult history, consider patient views; conduct indicated tests
Carry out avoidance strategies faithfully and scrupulously	AVOID CAUSES	Provide avoidance strategies; immunize (if indicated)
Maintain diary or record	LEARN EARLY WARNING SYMPTOMS	Supply list of prodromal symptoms; instruct patient in record-keeping and help in interpretation
Take indicated action promptly	TAKE PREVENTIVE ACTION	Work out strategies; instruct patient

(TREATMENT LEVEL covers SEEK CARE through TREAT SYMPTOMS EFFECTIVELY; PREVENTION LEVEL covers IDENTIFY CAUSES through TAKE PREVENTIVE ACTION.)

Fig. 26-1. Patient and physician responsibilities at each step to prevention of asthmatic symptoms.

social (peer) or economic pressure—eating wrong foods at a party, cutting out or reducing medication to save money, etc.

Physicians, for their part, may be guilty of any of the standard sins of omission or commission which most often include failure to listen to the patient, failure to explain the causes and treatment adequately and in language the patient can understand, not talking to or talking down to the patient, failure to cover effects (including side effects) of medication. To these add misdiagnosis, wrong or inappropriate treatment, palpable distrust of the patient's capacity to progress toward an effective self-care or preventive posture, or (in some instance) making the patient unnecessarily dependent on the physician out of psychological or economic considerations.

Educating a patient in prevention and self-care is a complicated, frustrating, unrewarding business. Given all of the elements that can and do go wrong the wonder is (to paraphrase Dr. Johnson) not that it is not done well but that it is done at all. Nevertheless it is possible (if the time is taken and the energy invested) for physicians to carry out this important aspect of comprehensive health care much more effectively. The sections which follow name the steps toward and suggest ways the physician can help patients develop proficiency and confidence in controlling and preventing the onset of asthmatic disease.

Step 1—Seek Care

The decision to seek care is a significant step because it denotes recognition of a condition beyond the capacity of the individual to manage and implies the motivation to do something about it. However, the decision is complicated by the variety of medical (and nonmedical) treatment facilities available, some of which like the mushrooming network of walk-in care clinics offer little or nothing in the way of continuity or follow-up and others of which are probably inappropriate for the condition.

Once the patient has appeared for treatment, the physician's role is to secure and weigh all pertinent information. What transpires, of course, will depend on prior experience with the patient and the completeness of information appearing in the chart. The physician will certainly want and will attempt to create an atmosphere in which there is a complete recital of the factors that have prompted the visit.

This process of acquiring information will be facilitated if the initial interview is conducted comfortably and informally; for example in office (instead of examining room where the patient is perched insecurely on the edge of a hard, backless, examining table). The patient should be encouraged and helped to provide all information relevant to the decision to seek treatment. At this stage open-ended questions or requests "Tell me what is troubling you" "How do you feel right now?" are more likely to elicit fuller, more informative replies. If this sort of question, as it sometimes does, opens a floodgate of information the patient can be interrupted and put on track by interjecting something like "Tell me more about so-and-so," where the so-and-so represents disclosures specific to the present visit.

Step 2—Confirm the Diagnosis

The symptoms of asthma are commonly seen and so well-known as to be almost unmistakable. However, the interim diagnosis should be affirmed by taking a good history which explores the patient's background thoroughly. The history should be supplemented by a physical examination which includes a careful listen to the chest, evaluation of other organs, an X-ray (if this is a first visit) and any necessary laboratory work that can be ordered to nail down the preliminary diagnosis of asthma or to rule out other asthma-mimicking possibilities like cystic fibrosis. (Chapters 7 and 8, Part I, above, deal comprehensively with the differential diagnosis of asthma). At all points in this confirmatory process the patient should know exactly what is being done, why it is being done, and what bearing it has on the process.

Once there is a confident diagnosis of asthma the patient (or parent) will need information about the nature of the disease and its care. This information is effectively presented in the AAFA's *Handbook for the Asthmatic,* or ALA's *The Asthma Handbook.* They can be given to the patient with the explanation that it will be useful in understanding the disease and dispelling some of the myths that surround it. If a child is involved, AAFA's *Allergy in Children* is also valuable.*

The patient should be encouraged to read these short and well-designed booklets carefully and to bring questions about any points not understood. To prompt questioning (and more active participation in the learning process) encourage the patient to mark any unclear or confusing parts of the booklet and to write questions or comments in its margins. Request that they be brought along to the next visit, or phoned in if no consultation is planned soon.

Step 3—Treat the Symptoms

The treatment devised for an asthmatic will depend on the age of the patient and the cause, severity, and obstinacy of the symptoms. In prescribing treatment it has been found that less than full adherence to the regimen occurs in something like one-half of all cases. Adherence is associated with belief that the disease is a threat to health, that the action being proposed will be efficacious, and knowing (understanding) what is being recommended and its purpose. Social support and stability of the patient's primary group are also important correlates to following treatment as is the continuity, supportive-

---

* These and all other publications cited in these sections are available, inexpensively and in quantity, from the organization or agency which produced it.

ness, and personal nature of the care being provided. The attending physician is in a position to capitalize on or make allowances for these factors in devising a treatment plan that will encourage close compliance with it.

In addition, adherence (particularly to courses of medication) is dependent on the complexity of the process and the skill with which it is used. In prescribing a medication, its name, its purpose, its impact on symptoms, and its possible side effects should be spelled out clearly and the patient asked to repeat them. ("Now, please tell me what you are going to do and what will happen.") Asking the patient if she or he "understands" simply invites affirmation. If necessary the instructions should be written out, clearly, in step order. (Not understanding instructions and not having information about medication's side effects are two of the major reasons associated with failing to adhere to treatment; another reason for discontinuing medication is that it does not seem to be exerting any effect on the symptoms. In the case of asthma this is especially prone to happen because some of the medications take time to establish themselves or may be taken improperly. One survey of school-age asthmatic children revealed that a majority of them were using their inhalers improperly so their effect was being lost.)

The physician should also warn the patient about the temptation to and the dangers of playing games with medication—trying to get along without it or overdosing. Abuse, particularly of inhalers, is commonplace; what amounts to overuse should be specified and the number of doses permissible under various conditions clearly stated.

The handbooks named above are helpful in explaining the reasons for complying with treatment procedures and indicate what the patients can do to seek clarification. Winthrop-Brean Laboratories (90 Park Avenue, New York, NY 10016) provide a useful free pamphlet entitled *What you should know about your aerosol bronchodilator.*

If, after a fair trial, the treatment does not work or if the symptoms are outside the experience and competence of the attending physician, it may be necessary to refer the patient to a specialist. This step can offer a bolt-hole to terminate treatment although this possibility can be minimized with careful and open explanations of the reasons for it and its consequences. The AAFA's pamphlet, *The Role of the Trained Allergist and Clinical Immunologist in Cost Effective Patient Care* is useful here.

Once the symptoms are being treated effectively the physician can begin to think about working out preventive strategies with the patient.

Step 4—Identify the Causes

Identifying the cause of asthma is not difficult in itself. In the bulk of asthmatics the trigger is likely to be known to the patient or is readily inferable from the history and physical examination. Where the triggers are obscure (as they are increasingly coming to be as the environment is invaded and degraded by chemicals) nailing them down may be more difficult but a good history and a carefully maintained patient diary should unmask them. If a diary should be required, the physician can help by supplying a format the patient can use conveniently. One such format addressed to the patient appears below.

WHAT ARE ASTHMA'S CAUSAL AGENTS AND HOW CAN I TELL WHICH ONES ARE MAKING ME SICK?

Finding the causal agent is the single most important step you can take toward taking charge of your asthma. Unless you establish what is making you wheeze you will have trouble treating it and you will always be troubled by it.

There are a large number of factors that can precipitate asthma attacks. The most important ones are:

1. colds or upper respiratory infections
2. allergens (dusts, pollen, molds, animal dander, etc.)
3. foods and especially food additives
4. vigorous exercise
5. emotional responses including hyperventilation
6. certain drugs, especially aspirin
7. air pollutants including tobacco smoke, ozone, and sulfur dioxide.

The surest way to pinpoint which of these factors is causing your asthma is to fill out and maintain the ASTHMA FINDER carefully and faithfully. The ASTHMA FINDER and instructions for completing it follow. This may appear to be (and is) an absurdly simply way to go about finding what is making you wheeze. However if it is properly maintained for an adequate period of time it will almost certainly enable you to pick out what is causing your symptoms.

To use the ASTHMA FINDER (Fig. 26-2) you will want to link your or your child's symptoms to the possible causes listed on the form. Here is how to describe your asthma symptoms:

0 = No wheezes at all
1 = Mild wheezing that only you or your doctor can hear or feel
2 = Wheezing that people in your immediate vicinity can hear
3 = Wheezing that can be heard at some distance across a fairly large room (for instance)
4 = Severe wheezing requiring immediate therapy at home, in the doctor's office or at the emergency room.

For _____ Week of _____ to _____ 19 _____
            (Name)   (Month)   (Date)

	Mon	Tue	Wed	Thu	Fri	Sat	Sun	TOTAL
HOW SEVERE WERE YOUR SYMPTOMS?								
No wheezing 0								
Very mild wheezing 1								
Audible wheezing 2								
Loud wheezing 3								
Severe wheezing 4								
WAS THE WEATHER								
Cold?								
Snowy/Rainy?								
Windy?								
DID YOU HAVE ANY INFECTIONS?								
Flu								
Cold								
Sinusitis								
Other*								
WHERE DID YOU GO? WHAT DID YOU DO?								
Work								
School								
Home								
Travel/Recreation/Dine out								
Out-of-doors								
Vigorous exercise								
Other*								
WERE YOU EXPOSED TO								
Smoke, tobacco?								
Dust, pollens, mold, dampness?								
Auto emissions or fumes?								
Detergents, soaps, etc?								
Cosmetics, perfumes?								
Insecticides?								
Animals, pets?								
Chemicals, solvents?								
Other*								
DID YOU WEAR OR COME IN CONTACT WITH								
Wool?								
Fur?								
Feathers or down?								
DID YOU TAKE ANY DRUGS?								
Aspirin								
Other pain/headache remedy								
Cold medicine*								
Nose drops*								
Antibiotics*								
Other*								
DID YOU EXPERIENCE ANY UNUSUAL STRESS, TENSION, ANXIETY, CONFLICT?								
WHAT DID YOU EAT?								
Grains or cereals (breads, breakfast foods, pastries)								
Milk or milk products (Ice cream, cheese, sour cream, cottage cheese, yogurt)								
Eggs or egg products								
Poultry								
Meats (Fresh or processed)								
Fish or shellfish								
Raw fruits or vegetables								
Snacks including candies								
Chocolate								
Nuts or nut butter								
Popcorn								
Chewing gum								
Beverages, including tea								
Coffee								
Cola, soda								
Alcoholic drinks								
WHEN DID THE SYMPTOMS SHOW?								
Morning								
Afternoon								
Evening								
During the night								

*Specify

Fig. 26-2. Weekly record of exposure to common asthma triggers. (From Gershwin ME, Klingelhofer EL: Asthma: Start Living and Stop Suffering! Reading, Massachusetts, Addison-Wesley, 1986, pp 43–44. Used with permission.)

Directions for Using the ASTHMA FINDER

TO COMPLETE THE FORM

Fill out the ASTHMA FINDER each day in the evening just before going to bed. It should take you no more than ten minutes.

For the SYMPTOMS section, if you had no symptoms at all that day, check 0; if your symptoms were mild and did not keep you from your regular activities, check 1; if your symptoms were moderate and prevented you from carrying out some activities, check 2; if your symptoms were severe enough to keep you from work or school, or confined to home or bed, check 3; if your symptoms were so severe as to require hospitalization or emergency treatment, check 4.

For all other sections, check every item for which you have a "yes" answer that day. In the FOODS section make a special effort to record *everything* that you consumed.

TO INTERPRET THE FORM

At the end of the week count the number of check marks you have made for each item and record the number in the "Total" column at the extreme right.

Relate the entries in the SYMPTOMS section to those in all of the other sections: For example, if you checked "0" symptoms all week, what other categories or items had no checks that week? If you did have symptoms, which of the other boxes throughout the form were checked only on days preceding or on which you had symptoms? If you were troubled with symptoms throughout the whole week, which boxes had checks every day? Write any suspected match-up of symptoms and causes below.

Dates	**Symptoms?**	**Possible Causes**
_____	_____	_____
_____	_____	_____
_____	_____	_____
_____	_____	_____
_____	_____	_____

If it should be necessary to order tests—office or laboratory—their form and function should be carefully and fully explained beforehand. The Handbooks cited earlier explain testing procedures simply and clearly.

Step 5—Avoid the Causes

To prevent asthma symptoms from occurring the most important step the patient can take is to avoid contact with the responsible allergen, whatever it is.

Successful avoidance calls for intelligent and unflagging attention to the task of shutting out the cause. Here there are a number of different sources of information that can be supplied to the patient. The National Institute of Allergy and Infectious Diseases has produced a series of pamphlets on drug, dust, food, and pollen allergy which are available from the Superintendent of Documents, U.S. Government Printing Office, Washington, DC 20402. All of these publications contain sections on avoidance of the subject allergen. The AAFA has a similar series covering hay fever, mold, food, drugs, and exercise. The American Academy of Allergy and Immunology, 611 East Wells Street, Milwaukee, WI 53202, has issued a series of short free pamphlets giving tips on control of various allergens including a useful one on exercise-induced asthma, and the ALA has leaflets covering air pollution, dust disease, hay fever, the common cold, and cigarette smoking. The ALA's *Handbook* also deals fairly comprehensively with triggers and what can be done to avoid them and has a valuable section on handling the emotional or stressful factors which often intensify the severity of the asthmatic reaction.

All of the foregoing reveals that there is no dearth of information around to enable patients to avoid or (with help) neutralize their symptoms. How to encourage or motivate patients to use the information and follow the avoidance procedures reflexively is a different kettle of fish. What evidence there is shows that prevention is likely to fall through because the actions called for are complicated, of long duration, and/or interfere with other actions the patient may wish to take. To counter these powerful tendencies (invitations) to get careless about causes, the physician needs to maintain continuity and individuality of care, make it easy for and encourage the patient to keep in close touch, recruit or point the way to social support which will help maintain vigilance, unfailingly stress and monitor beliefs about the seriousness of the disease and the efficacy of the treatment, and verify that patients understand recommendations and their purposes.

Any patient behaviors that show adherence to the regimen—keeping up with medication during asymptomatic periods, doing breathing exercises regularly, being careful about triggers, making sound decisions about self-care, etc.,—should be reinforced. Praise and approval by the physician, especially when delivered as soon as possible after the event are powerful incentives to continue the behavior.

Importantly, the physician has to put aside the temptation to condemn the patient for failing to avoid a trigger and paying the price for the failure with an attack. Such lapses can and ought to be turned into important learning experiences in which the patient confronts the consequences of the lack of vigilance on failure to comply.

Step 6—Learn Early Warning Symptoms

With help, most asthmatics can learn to identify prodromal symptoms well in advance of an attack and take effective counter measures. The ALA and AAFA *Handbooks* devote space to the enumeration, description, and detection of early warning signs which, for asthma, can take a surprisingly wide range of forms.

Picking out the early warning signs can be aided by keeping a systematic record. The Asthma Early Warning Indicator which follows will involve and inform the patient in the process of detecting these conditions. It provides a simple, standardized method of compiling this information and interpreting it so that some sort of conclusion is reached.

The ASTHMA EARLY WARNING INDICATOR (Fig. 26-3) will help you to pick out the signals or triggers of an impending asthmatic reaction if you do not already know them. To complete it, go back over your most recent episode, trying very hard to remember sensations or other bodily signs that *preceded* the full onset of your symptoms. In the appropriate spaces check all of these prodromal (as they are called) symptoms that you can recall. Then,

ASTHMA EARLY WARNING INDICATOR

Check (✓) any sign that preceded each of the last four episodes;
double check (✓✓) any that occurred 24 hours or fewer before the episode.

TYPES OF REACTION	SPECIFIC SIGN OR INDICATOR	NOTICED DURING EPISODE				# ✓s	COMMENTS OR HUNCHES
		1	2	3	4		
Pulmonary	Tightness in chest						Episode 1:
	Shortness of breath						
	Wheezing						
	Cough						
	Mucus in chest						
Ear, Nose, and Throat	Runny nose						Episode 2:
	Nasal congestion						
	Earache/Inflammation						
	Scratchy or sore throat						
Psychological	Irritable						
	Hyperactive/Excitable						Episode 3:
	Anxious/Depressed						
Other	Headache						
	Tiredness/Fatigue						
	Muscle pain/Cramps						
	Low grade fever						Episode 4:
	Restless sleep						
	Other						

Fig. 26-3. Chart recording appearance of prodromol symptoms for asthmatic episodes. (From Gershwin ME, Kingelhofer EL: Asthma: Start Living and Stop Suffering! Reading, Massachusetts, Addison-Wesley, 1986, pp 43–44. Used with permission.)

keep the same record for the next three episodes. After the record is completed, examine it carefully and note any recurring patterns and monitor them regularly; every day.

One useful way to systematize patient self-monitoring is to prescribe, instruct in, and encourage the regular, daily use of a peak-flow meter to take and record readings of respiratory conditions. It is especially useful in pointing to slight, early changes in breathing and lung capacity.

In addition to prodromal symptoms, there are activities or experiences which are likely to put the individual at risk—exposure to cigarette smoke, food additives or dyes, exercise. Where one is likely to be thrust into a situation where exposure to an allergen is unavoidable then the early resort to direct preventive action may be called for.

Step 7—Take Preventive Action

At the appearance of early warning symptoms or exposure to a situation that carries the threat of an asthmatic reaction, preventive tactics which have been worked out and rehearsed in advance with the patient should be invoked. These steps may entail the prophylactic use of medication or resort to other strategies depending on the nature of the trigger. If exercise induces the patient's asthma, for example, the physician should know of and offer suggestions as to appropriate activities or warm-up steps, or advise on pre-medication that can be taken that will foreclose or mitigate the possibility of an attack.

Along with addressing the prodromal symptoms or the situations that are likely to result in an asthmatic attack the physician has a final and crucial responsibility in achieving an acceptable level of prevention in patient care. That is to offer a specific program aimed at improving the patient's inherent ability to resist asthmatic episodes. Such a program has two components, the first of which is aimed at creating conditions which directly ameliorate asthma's symptoms when they occur. This may be accomplished by instructing the patient in breathing improvement and mucus-producing exercises which are spelled out in the Handbooks. In addition, Riker Laboratories, 19901 Nordhoff Street, Northridge, CA 91325 has two useful free booklets on these subjects and the ALA also offers a pamphlet entitled *Breathe Easy Relaxation Exercises.*

On a more general level the physician is concerned with the overall health status of the patient and should do whatever is possible to see to it that the asthmatic patient knows and practices good health habits—that he or she does not smoke cigarettes or dope, is not overweight, gets appropriate exercise regularly, maintains an adequate diet, supplemented if necessary, avoids or knows how to deal with emotional stress, etc. These goals can best be achieved by informing the patient as to how and why they are important in establishing control over asthma and then going on to indicate specifically what needs to be done and what opportunities there are to achieve these goals. Simply admonishing the patient to take off weight or quit smoking or get more exercise is time and words wasted. The patient probably knows these things already and needs information and help in specific things that can be done to achieve them.

CONCLUSION

The cases of Roger and Emmy presented at the outset of this chapter illustrate the myriad of things that can go wrong in the treatment and prevention of asthma—perfunctory and interrupted and episodic care, nonadherence to medication and treatment regimens, acceptance of myths about the cause of asthma, resort to questionable healers, carelessness about avoiding known causes of symptoms, refusal to accept or invoke treatment that would effectively control symptoms during moderate to severe attacks.

Prevention and control of asthma is, at heart, an educational process. While there are useful packaged self-care programs around they are primarily aimed at children and they are inclined to be too brief and lack the rigorousness that would make them effective in helping most patients achieve an effective level of understanding and control of their disease.

The bulk of preventive education about asthma has been and still is being provided by the personal physician. This educational mission, judging from the available evidence, has not been done very effectively, partly because of the stubbornness and durability of the disease itself, partly because physicians do not carry out the educational aspect of their calling as well as they might. This chapter outlines the steps that are involved in achieving the best preventive or control posture possible in the case of the asthmatic patient and sketches some of the specific affirmative actions that physicians can take at each of these way points to aid the patient to attain this goal.

REFERENCES

Bartlett EE: Educational self-help approaches in childhood asthma. J Allergy Clin Immunol 72(5):(Part 2) 545–554, 1983

Blessing-Moore J, Fritz G, Lewiston N: Self-management programs for childhood asthma. Chest 87(1)(Suppl):107S–110S, 1985

Center for Interdisciplinary Research in Immunologic Diseases, UCLA, National Institute of Allergy and Infectious Diseases, Asthma and Allergy Foundation of America: Self management educational programs for childhood asthma, v.1.,

Conference Summary, v. 2., Manuscripts, Conference Report, Los Angeles, June 11–12, 1981

Clark NM, Feldman CH, Freudenberg N, et al: Developing education for children with asthma through study of self-management behavior. Health Educ Q 7:278–297, 1980.

Creer TL, Renne CM, Christian WP, et al: Behavioral contributions to rehabilitation and childhood asthma. Rehab Lit 37(8):226–232, 247, 1976

Fireman P, Friday GA, Gira C, et al: Teaching self-management skills to asthmatic children and their parents in an ambulatory care setting. Pediatrics 68(3):341–348, 1981

Gershwin ME, Klingelhofer EL: Asthma: Start Living and Stop Suffering! Reading, Massachusetts, Addison-Wesley, 1986 (in press).

Goldstein RA: Special presentation: Self-management of asthma programs in the USA. Int Archs Allergy Appl Immun 77:79–80, 1985

Grabenstein JD, Summers RJ, Renard RL: A comprehensive allergen extract monograph with advice for the patient. Ann Allergy 54:185–194, 1985

Hindi-Alexander MC: Decision making in asthma self-management. Chest 87(1) (Suppl):100S–104S, 1985

Hindi-Alexander MC: Response: educational self-help approaches in childhood asthma. J Allergy Clin Immunol 72(5): Part 2, 555–560, 1983

Hindi-Alexander MC, Cropp GJA: Evaluation of a family asthma program. J Allergy Clin Immunol 74(4) Part I: 505–510, 1984

Kinscht JP, Rosenstock IM: Patient's problems in following recommendations of health experts in Stone GC, Cohen F, Health Psychology. San Francisco, California, Jossey-Bass, 1979

Lewis CE: Response: implementing asthma self-management education in medical care settings—issues and strategies. J Allergy Clin Immunol 72(5) Part 2: 622–624, 1983

Maiman LA, Green LW, Gibson G, et al: Education for self-treatment by adult asthmatics. JAMA 241(18), 1919–1922, 1979

McKenney JM: The clinical pharmacy and compliance in Haynes R, Taylor DW, and Sackett DL: Compliance in Health Care. Baltimore, Maryland, The Johns Hopkins University Press, 260–277, 1979

Mullen PD, Mullen LR: Implementing asthma self-management education in medical care settings—issues and strategies. J Allergy Clin Immunol 72(5) Part 2: 611–621, 1983

Rachelefsky GS, Lewis CE, de la Sota A, et al: ACT (Asthma Care Training) for kids: A childhood asthma self-management program. Chest 87(1)(Suppl): 98S–100S, 1985

Robinson LD, Jr: Evaluation of an asthma summer camp program. Chest 87(1) (Suppl): 105S–107S, 1985

Thoresen CE, Kermil-Gray K: Self-management psychology and the treatment of childhood asthma. J Allergy Clin Immunol 72(5) Part 2: 596–606, 1983

Arif Seyal
M. Eric Gershwin

27

Future Directions in Asthma

The historical review of asthma begins with several interesting hypotheses: Aretaeus in the 2nd century speculated that asthma was due to acute paroxysms of foul and viscid humors in lungs. Galen believed that the brain poured secretions into lungs. Van Helmont believed that asthma was the equivalent of epilepsy in lungs. Despite this relatively inauspicious beginning, modern pharmacotherapy and physiology are leading to an unravelling in our understanding of pathophysiology, pathogenesis, and immunology of asthma.

The definition of asthma has remained unchanged for several years and is stated by the American Lung Association to be a disease characterized by increased responsiveness of trachea and bronchi to various stimuli manifested by difficulty in breathing caused by a generalized narrowing of airways. The narrowing is dynamic and changes in degree, either spontaneously or because of therapy. The basic defect appears to be an altered state that leads periodically to increased contraction of smooth muscles and hypersecretion of bronchial mucus. In some instances illness seems to be related to an altered immunologic state, such as atopy, in others underlying cause cannot be determined.

This definition of asthma, even though it is clinically useful, raises several critical questions. What are the mechanisms for airway hyperresponsiveness? What stimuli are significant to set off this reaction? What is the altered state or states of host that predisposes to the development of this clinical picture? In this chapter, the final contribution to this volume, we hope

BRONCHIAL ASTHMA, Second Edition
ISBN 0-8089-1814-1

to delineate critical areas of future study and define newer approaches to the treatment of asthma.

Clearly, asthma is a heterogeneous disease with a wide variety of distinct but overlapping clinical anatomic, functional, and etiologic features. The most important step in the elucidation of the pathoetiology of asthma will be the separation of subgroups of patients. This will allow individualization of management and offer more precise control of symptomatology. It will also lead to the issue of whether asthma is more than one disease. The final issues will be answered by the molecular biologist, not the clinician.

During the past several years it has become apparent that in asthma, although bronchospasm can be triggered by variable stimuli, the underlying process is characterized by a series of interactions. Bronchial hyperreactivity is known to occur in almost all asthmatics and can be demonstrated by inhalation challenge even in asymptomatic asthmatic individuals. What leads to this hyperreactivity? The genesis of this is not well known. However, there is some evidence that part of it may be genetic and part may be acquired. Based on available data it appears that the inflammatory reaction may play a part in this acquired form of hyperreactivity. On the basis of experimental data it is now known that immunologic and nonimmunologic insults to the airways of animals can produce both exudative and proliferative reactions with the formation of airway edema and immunomigration of inflammatory cells into the lumen through the epithelium. Further evidence comes from studies that have demonstrated accumulation of granulocytes and mononuclear cells at the site of allergic reactions for some hours after the antigen challenge and in recent studies by demonstrating increase in serum HMW-NCA (high molecular weight neutrophil chemotactic activity) followed by increased C3b receptors on neutrophils and monocytes during antigen-induced bronchospasm.

The pathology of asthma, with increased mucus production, mucosal edema, desquamated ciliated epithelium, thickened basement membrane, hypertrophied smooth muscles, and accumulation of lymphocytes and eosinophils all underscore the role of inflammation. The mechanism by which these inflammatory cells lead to bronchial hyperactivity needs to be elucidated. These components may be interrelated and play a variable role in different groups of asthmatics. Yet several questions must be raised: Are steroid-dependent asthmatics those in whom cellular inflammation plays a major role? Are there patients with autoantibodies directed at beta receptors? Is hyperirritability reversible? Can the new concepts of gene cloning be used to modify high IgE responsiveness? Can the action of IgE be modified at the level of the target cell? What is the role of soluble factors in amplifying/suppressing these effects?

Further studies are needed not only to answer these questions but also to delineate the exact role of glucocorticoids in modifying responses. Newer agents that would inhibit inflammation without any significant side effect are needed to achieve good control of the disease in subsets of asthmatic. Also new formulation of aerosolized steroids are needed that will deliver more medication per puff without causing hypophyseal-pituitary adrenal axis suppression.

Cromolyn sodium and aerosol steroid preparations have been used during the past several years although their exact mode of action is not yet clear. Cromolyn can, however, be considered among the anti-inflammatory drugs for asthma because it inhibits the late inflammatory phase of IgE-mediated allergic reaction. Additional studies will need to better identify the exact site(s) of action of these available agents, their role in altering hyperactivity, and develop more effective forms for their administration.

Therapeutic efficacy of currently available agents (beta-adrenergic agonists and methyl xanthine) for the treatment of bronchial asthma may be in part due to their ability to prevent generation of inflammatory mediators from mast cells or other inflammatory cells. Efforts now should be directed for possible developments of drugs that will be capable of preventing the interaction of inflammatory mediators with target cell receptors. Much more information regarding the structure and function of these mediators and target cells will be needed before receptor blocking or specific inhibitors of the mediators can be developed. Finally, much work needs to be done on inhibition of mucus formation.

There is a significant relationship between neurologic and humoral regulation of airway reactivity. The presence of imbalance of the autonomic nervous system has been well documented in allergic patients. This autonomic imbalance is manifested by alpha-adrenergic and cholinergic hyperresponsiveness and beta-adrenergic hyposensitivity. In a small subgroup of atopic individuals antibodies to beta receptors have been demonstrated but their exact significance is not known. Possible area of investigation in this avenue could include genetically determined differences in adrenergic reactivity and possible role of infections (particularly those of viral infections, respiratory syncytial virus) in childhood leading to autonomic imbalance later in life. In this regard it will be interesting to follow the efficacy of new classes of drugs, especially atropinelike agents such as Atrovent (Boehringer Ingelheim Ltd., Ridgefield, Connecticut) in reducing mucus production, decreasing cough, and perhaps improving hyperirritability.

Bronchial allergy contributes to asthma in more than 80 percent of children and in 30–50 percent of adults, but prevention of exposure to allergens may be limited except in some circumstances. Avoiding antigen is still the simplest, and when applicable the most useful treatment the allergist has to offer. Diagnostic reliability and treatment efficacy, however, requires more specific indentification and purification of allergens for use in skin, bronchial challenge or Radioallergosorben testing (RAST) and, of course, immunotherapy. Efforts have been directed towards modification and refinement of antigens. The selection of responsive patients and the monitoring of immunologic response to treatment requires using refined techniques to suppress antibody and mediator response to therapy. The availability of monoclonal IgE, generated by hybridomas, may allow more scientific appraisals of antibody-antigen mast cell interaction. The recent successful cloning of epsilon genes will be even more valuable. Similarly, current work on regulation of IgE production by T cells indicates that a unique set of regulatory factors exists to enhance or inhibit the synthesis of IgE. Further understanding of the nature and mode of action of these suppressive and enhancing factors may provide us a basis for reversing the allergic disease, including allergic asthma.

Epidemiological studies have shown that the incidence of asthma and the rate of hospitalization for acute asthma has increased significantly during the last 15–20 years. This has happened in spite of our increased understanding of pathophysiology, pathology, and immunology and the availability of newer therapeutic agents. Is this due to increased urbanization and industrialization leading to multitude of occupational exposures and air pollution in our cities? Nutritional factors may also play a role. Food additives and preservatives have been found to produce bronchospastic response in asthmatic patients. Restaurant foods that have been treated with vegetable fresheners containing sulfites have been found to be the likely cause of exacerbation of asthma in up to five percent of asthmatics. Ironically, sulfites have also been used as preservatives in certain aerosolized bronchodilators. We do not know the exact mechanism of this action. What other food additives and preservatives may trigger similar response in asthmatics and nonasthmatic individuals? Sadly the exact magnitude of this problem is not known. Studies are needed to refine the methods of diagnosis of food allergies and their relationship with asthma.

Our understanding of asthma has advanced significantly in pace with the historical landmarks of medicine. Studies of specific genetically determined altered state of bronchial reactivity, evaluation of a multitude of allergic and nonallergic stimuli that can trigger the asthmatic state in the predisposed individual and identification and refinement of various pharmacologic and/or immunologic modalities for interrupting this bronchial response, are major avenues for our further understanding of the disease. The final pathway of such approaches will definitely lead to improved quality of life for the millions of children and adults who suffer from the chronicity of asthma.

REFERENCES

American Lung Association: Chronic Obstructive Lung Disease, 5th Ed., New York, American Lung Association, 1977, p 15
Carroll MP, Durham SR, Walsh Y, et al: Activation of neutrophils and monocytes

after allergen and histamine-induced bronchoconstriction. J Allergy Clin Immunol 75:290, 1985

Davis A, Vickerson F, Worsley Y, et al: Determination of dose-response relationship for nebulized ipratropium in asthmatic children. J Pediatr 105:10002, 1984

Hiroshima M, Yodoi J, Ishizaka K: Regulatory role of IgE binding factors from rat T lymphocytes. J Immunol 125:1442, 1980

Holgate ST, Church MK, Cushley MJ, et al: Pharmacologic modulation of airway calibre and mediator release in human models of bronchial asthma, in Kay AB, Austin KF, Lichenstein, LM (eds): Asthma: Physiology, immunopharmacology and treatment. 3rd International Symposium. London, England, Academic Press, Inc. 1984, pp. 391–415

Kaliner M, Shelhamer JH, Davis PB, et al: Anatonomic nervous system abnormalities and allergy. NIH Conference. Ann Intern Med 96:349, 1982

Kenton J, Helm B, Ishizaka P: Properties of a human immunoglobulin epsilon chain fragment synthesized in E. coli. Proc Natl Acad Sci 81:2955, 1955

Leung D, Brozek C, Frankel R, et al: IgE specific suppressor factors in normal human serums: In vitro and in vivo effects. Clin Res 31:164A, 1983

Liu FT, Albrandp KA, Bry CG: Expression of a biologically active fragment of human IgE epsilon chain in E. coli. Proc Natl Acad Sci 81:5369, 1984

Nagy L, Lee TH, Kay AB: Neutrophil chemotactic activity in antigen induced late asthmatic reactions. N Engl J Med 306:497, 1982

Ricci M, Maggi E, Del Prati Y, et al: IgE synthesis in vitro induced by T cell factors from patient with elevated serum IgE levels. J Allergy Clin Immunol 71:913, 1983

Stevenson DD, Simon RA: Sensitivity to ingested metabisulfite in asthmatic subjects. J Allergy Clin Immunol 68:26, 1981

Ventor JE, Fraser CM, Harrison LE: Antibodies to β_2-adrenergic receptors: a possible cause of adrenergic hyporesponsiveness in allergic rhinitis and asthma. Science 207:1361–1363, 1980

Arif Seyal

M. Eric Gershwin

Self-Assessment Examination

ANSWER THE FOLLOWING MULTIPLE CHOICE AND TRUE OR FALSE QUESTIONS

True or False Questions 1–4
(A = True, B = False)

Stimuli that can provoke an acute episode of asthma may include the following:

1. Infection

2. Physical exertion

3. Immunodeficiency

4. Metabisulfite

Select the best answer

5. Stimulation of the vagus nerve produces bronchospasm by the following mechanism:

    a. Direct effect on small airways
    b. By release of acetylcholine that constricts large airways
    c. By reduction in glandular and goblet cell secretions
    d. All of the above

587

6. Vagally mediated reflex bronchospasm can result from stimulation of receptors located in:

    a. Lower airways
    b. Larynx
    c. Irritant and cough receptors
    d. Chemoreceptors
    e. All of the above

7. All of the following drugs and chemicals except one can produce bronchospasm in susceptible individuals:

    a. Aspirin
    b. Indomethacin
    c. Clonidine
    d. Inderal (Propranolal)
    e. Tartrazine

8. Which of the following statements regarding leukotrienes are true?

    a. Leukotrienes are derivatives of arachidonic acids
    b. Leukotrienes are probably the most potent naturally occurring bronchoconstrictors hereto identified
    c. Leukotrienes produce arteriolar vasoconstriction
    d. Indomethacin pretreatment may enhance the airway response to inhaled leukotrienes

9. Which of the following are preformed in mast cells and released immediately?

    a. $PGE_{2\alpha}$
    b. SRS-A
    c. Histamine
    d. All of the above
    e. None of the above

10. Mast cells have receptors for the:

    a. Fc portion of IgM
    b. Fc portion of IgE
    c. Fab portion of IgG
    d. Fab portion of IgE

11. An increased number of mast cells may be seen in bronchoalveolar lavage in which of the following respiratory ailments.

    a. Sarcoidosis
    b. Extrinsic allergic alveolitis

c. Cryptogenic fibrosing alveolitis
d. Allergic bronchial asthma
e. All of the above
f. None of the above

12. Mast cells may be degranulated nonimmunologically by all of the following except:

a. Allergen-IgE
b. Polycationic amines
c. Radiocontrast media
d. Opiates
e. Enzymes

13. Clumps of bronchial epithelial cells in sputum called Creola bodies:

a. Are seen in bronchogenic carcinoma
b. Are characteristic of bronchial asthma
c. Also contain clumps of eosinophils and mast cells
d. All of the above
e. None of the above

14. Significantly increased blood eosinophilia may be seen in the following disorders except:

a. Trichinosis
b. Malaria
c. Churg-Strauss syndrome
d. Ascariasis
e. Hyper-IgE syndrome

15. The predominant 5-lipoxygenase pathway metabolite of arachidonic acid produced by human eosinophils is:

a. LTD_4
b. LTE_4
c. LTC_4
d. Prostaglandin E_2
e. All of the above

16. The rate of hospitalization for acute asthma during the last 10 years has:

a. Significantly decreased in children
b. Increased in adults and children
c. Remained almost constant
d. Significantly decreased in adults only
e. None of the above

17. The highest incidence of asthma both for males and females is between the ages of:

    a. 0–9 years
    b. 10–19 years
    c. 20–40 years
    d. 45 years and above

18. The majority of the patients with childhood asthma:

    a. Will have severe asthma at age 35
    b. Will be disease free at age 30
    c. Do not respond to oral theophylline therapy
    d. All of the above
    e. None of the above

19. Histological examination of the airways of an asthmatic subject would be expected to reveal the following:

    a. Degranulated mast cells
    b. Extensive inflammation of submucosal glands
    c. Denuded epithelium
    d. All of the above

A 4-year-old female has had asthma since age 2 and has been followed by her family physician. She is being referred to you for further evaluation treatment of asthma. Her vital signs include blood pressure 100/58; pulse 110; respiratory rate 28 without intercostal retractions, temperature 37°C (oral); weight 20 kg. Examination of lungs reveal scattered expiratory wheezes bilaterally. Her current medications include anydrous theophylline (S.R.) 50 mg bid.

20. The differential diagnosis of wheezing at this age includes:

    a. Bronchialitis
    b. Asthma
    c. Congenital malformation
    d. Foreign body inhalation
    e. Cystic fibrosis
    f. All of the above

21. At age 2 her asthma was most likely due to:

    a. Viral infections
    b. Allergens
    c. Mycoplasma infection
    d. Exercise
    e. All of the above

22. Other important points of the history to more clearly delineate the patients clinical state include:

    a. Exercise tolerance
    b. Sleep interruption due to cough and wheezing
    c. Growth pattern
    d. School attendance
    e. Frequency of acute attacks of wheezing
    f. All of the above

23. What therapeutic measures will you take after evaluation in your office?

    a. Start oral Prednisone immediately
    b. Institute cromolyn sodium therapy
    c. Adjust her theophylline dose
    d. Add albuteral and beclomethasone
    e. Order skin testing

24. A child with severe asthma often has the following characteristics:

    a. Virtually daily wheezing
    b. Tendency to become tight suddenly with cyanosis
    c. Sleep interruption due to cough and wheezing
    d. Poor exercise tolerance
    e. All of the above

25. Major risk factors for respiratory difficulty at age 2 include:

    a. Smoking parents
    b. Recurrent bronchiolitis
    c. Croup
    d. Family history of asthma
    e. All of the above

26. Theophylline clearance in children is _____ than in adults.

    a. Greater
    b. Less
    c. About the same

27. In planning a comprehensive treatment program of severe asthma, an evaluation of the role that psychogenic factors play in the disease is always indicated.

    a. True
    b. False

28–32. House dust mite is known to be an important cause of asthma in childhood. Which of the following historically derived observations are characteristic of asthmatic children sensitive to house dust mites?

A = True, B = False

28. Perennial symptoms

29. Symptoms exacerbate in bed at night

30. Symptoms are worse in winters

31. Symptoms are worse in early morning hours

32. Symptoms are aggravated on exposure to dusting and domestic cleaning

33–36. Match the following with the correct response

    a. Responds to diethylcarbamazine
    b. Chronic eosinophilic pneumonia
    c. Nitrofurantoin toxicity
    d. Positive serum precipitating antibodies against Aspergillus

33. A 32-year-old male present to your office with episodes of cough, wheezing, low grade fever and purulent sputum containing brown plugs. The patient's laboratory findings includes a total eosinophil count of 2400/mm³. Chest x-ray film shows right lower lobe atelectasis. Serum IgE is 2500 ng/ml.

34. A 28-year-old male Pakistani student with cough and wheezing worse at night. Chest x-ray finds miliary markings. Markedly elevated serum IgE.

35. 56-year-old female who is being treated for recurrent urinary tract infection presents cough, dyspnea, and fever. Chest x-ray shows bibasilar infiltrates. The total blood eosinophil count is 6500/mm³.

36. A 27-year-old female with cough, dyspnea, malaise, and night sweats. Chest x-ray shows nonsegmental infiltrates described by radiologist as photographic negative of pulmonary edema.

A 41-year-old farmer was hospitalized in mid-February with sudden onset of fever, chills, malaise, dry cough, and dyspnea. Physical examination showed temperature 103.4°F, respiratory rate was 26/min, pulse 110, slight cyanosis and bilateral crepitant rales. Chest x-ray showed bilateral patchy infiltrate. Total white blood cell count was 13500/mm³. Diff. polys. 72% Bands. 8% Lymphs. 15% Eos. 4% Monos 1%. gram stain of sputum shows oral flora.

37. On the basis of above data the differential diagnosis of this condition would include the following:

    a. Acute viral illness
    b. Acute bacterial pneumonia
    c. Hypersensitivity pneumonitis
    d. Sarcoidosis
    e. a–c are correct
    f. All of the above statements are correct

38. Soon after hospitalization blood cultures were drawn and the patient was started on I.V. ampicillin. Within 18 hours he felt much improved. His temperature was normal. There was no cyanosis. He complained of slight cough but no shortness of breath. Improvement in his symptomatology was most probably due to:

    a. Antibiotic therapy
    b. Natural course of viral illness
    c. Removal of patient from his environment
    d. All of the above

39. All of the following will help establish the diagnosis of hypersensitivity pneumonitis except:

    a. Increased serum IgE level
    b. Increased serum IgG and IgA
    c. Positive dual skin test to appropriate antigen
    d. Bronchoalveolar lavage showing elevated IgA and IgG level
    e. Precipitating antibodies

40. Appropriate therapy for hypersensitivity pneumonitis includes the following:

    a. Avoidance of exposure
    b. Use of corticosteroids in acute and subacute cases
    c. Bronchodilator therapy
    d. A and B
    e. All of the above are correct

41. The basic pathologic process seen in hypersensitivity pneumonitis includes:

    a. Eosinophilic infiltrates in the interstitial spaces
    b. Neutrophilic infiltrate of alveolar septa and interstitium
    c. Eosinophilic pneumonia
    d. Lymphocyte interstitial infiltrates and granuloma formation

42–46. Match the following precipitating agents with appropriate occupation:

42. Hair dresser   A. T.D.I. (Toluene Diisocyanate)

43. Polyurethane worker   B. Persulfate

44. Silofillers   C. Nitrogen Dioxide

45. Printers   D. Ethylenediamine

46. Rubber Industry Workers   E. Vegetable Gum

A 16-year-old male presented in the Allergy Clinic with a history of shortness of breath and chest tightness after playing tennis. Maximum chest tightness was felt 10 minutes after finishing the game and lasted about 30 to 45 minutes. He was otherwise healthy and had no history of atopy. He had no pets. Use of tobacco and drugs were denied. On examination, there is no manifestation of allergic diathesis. Cardiopulmonary exam is normal. Routine office spirometry shows no signs of obstruction.

47. At this you should:

   a. Tell the mother the patient is normal
   b. Immediately order skin test for grass and weeds allergy
   c. Start long acting theophylline
   d. Obtain comprehensive pulmonary function studies

48. Your initial impression will be:

   a. Grass pollen allergy
   b. Psychophysiologic shortness of breath
   c. Exercise-induced asthma (EIA)
   d. None of the above

49. In exercise-induced asthma (EIA) pulmonary function tests, performed by utilizing the cycloergometer, would show:

   a. No change in FEV_1 during exercise but marked fall of FEV_1 soon after the exercise
   b. Improved FEV_1 during first 2 minutes after exercise followed by a fall of FEV_1
   c. Steady fall of FEV_1 soon after starting exercise
   d. None of the above

50. Pulmonary function studies in the above patient confirms the diagnosis of exercise induced asthma (EIA). You would now:

   a. Advise mother the patient should stop any kind of exercise
   b. Advise albuteral inhaler prior to exercise

    c.   Start cromolyn sodium 20 mg with spinhaler q6 hour

    d.   Start long-acting theophylline immediately

51.   In most asthmatics vigorous exercise of 12–15 minutes is associated with:

    a.   Bronchospasm

    b.   Hyperinflation

    c.   Hypoxemia

    d.   Fall of FEV_1

    e.   All of the above

52.   What type of exercise would be most suitable for this patient with EIA:

    a.   Biking

    b.   Running

    c.   Swimming

    d.   Tennis

53.   All have been found in association with exercise induced asthma except:

    a.   Decreased bronchoconstriction with repeated exertion

    b.   Importance of environmental conditions (eg, ambient air temperature and humidity)

    c.   Found more commonly in boys

    d.   Seen frequently in normal people

54.   All except one of the following drugs are effective in preventing EIA:

    a.   Cromolyn sodium

    b.   Albuteral inhaler

    c.   Theophylline

    d.   Corticosteroids

55.   Which of the following statements are true about pregnant women with asthma:

    a.   No significant change is noted in FEV_1

    b.   There is an increase in minute ventilation as noted in non-asthmatic pregnant patients

    c.   Approximately 50% of the asthmatics show no change in the severity of asthma during pregnancy

    d.   All of the above

    e.   None of the above

56. While treating a pregnant asthmatic your primary concern is the avoidance of hypoxemia and its potential deleterious effects upon fetus. Decreased fetal oxygen tension could result from:

    a. Reduced uterine blood flow from vasoconstriction of uterine arteries associated with hypocarbia

    b. Mechanical effect of hyperventilation leading to decreased maternal venous return

    c. Shift in oxyhemoglobin dissociation curve to the left

    d. All of the above

57–61. Answer A if true and B if false.

The following drugs are considered "safe" for the treatment of asthma during pregnancy:

57. Theophylline

58. Cromolyn sodium

59. Atropine

60. Beclomethasone

61. Terbutaline

You are called to the emergency room to see a 32-year-old male with 15 years history of asthma, admitted in acute respiratory distress. On examination he is using his accessory muscles for respiration and has intercostal retractions. His vital signs show blood pressure 142/84; pulse 108; respiratory rate 28/min, temperature 99°. Examination of the lungs reveal bilateral inspiratory and expiratory wheezes. Arterial blood gases shows: PO_2 68, PCO_2 35, pH 7.48. Chest x-ray is clear. The patient has been treated with epinephrine subcutaneously two times without any significant improvement.

Based on the above information, answer the following questions.

62. You would now undertake the following steps:

    a. Start 100% oxygen mask

    b. Mechanical ventilation

    c. Oxygen by 28% venturi mask

    d. No supplemental oxygen

63. Further history reveals the patient had symptoms of an upper respiratory tract infection 2 days prior to this visit in the emergency room. Now he is afebrile and has a nonproductive cough. You would now procede with the following therapy:

    a.   Start intravenous antibiotics   c.   Aerosolized B-agonist
    b.   Oral theophylline   d.   Peroral antibiotics

64. After several minutes of appropriate management, the patient feels better and is able to confirm that he had taken oral theophylline approximately 8 hours prior to being seen in the emergency room. Review of his outpatient chart notes a theophylline blood level taken 2 hours after the theophylline administration orally at 14 μg/ml. While patient's serum theophylline blood level is being analyzed what would be the estimated serum theophylline level at this point assuming T1/2 of 6 hours.

    a.   2 μg/ml   c.   0 μg/ml
    b.   7 μg/ml   d.   14 μg/ml

65. All except one of the following measures will not be helpful in the treatment of asthma in acute exacerbation

    a.   Beta agonists
    b.   Intravenous aminophylline
    c.   Cromolyn sodium by spinhaler
    d.   Large doses of intravenous steroids

66. The lab reports a serum theophylline blood level of 7.5 μg/ml. Now to achieve a therapeutic serum theophylline level of 15 μg/ml you would administer a loading dose of aminophylline as follows:

    a.   No loading dose needed
    b.   2 mg/kg over 20–30 minutes
    c.   3.5 mg/kg over 20–30 minutes
    d.   6.5 mg/kg over 20–30 minutes

Match the following:

The following may affect theophylline clearance:

67. Smoking

68. Erythromycin

69. Liver disease   A.   Decrease

70. Phenobarbital therapy   B.   Increase

71. Acute viral infection   C.   No effect

72. Cimetidine

73. Indocin

74. Acidemia

75. What would you expect 4 hours after administration of intravenous solumedral to a patient with severe asthma:

    a. Improved FEV_1
    b. Reduction in ventilation-perfusion mismatch
    c. Reduction in hypoxemia
    d. All of the above
    e. None of the above

76. Prolonged corticosteroid therapy has the following effect on bronchial response to inhalation allergen challenge:

    a. Inhibit the late response only
    b. Inhibit the immediate response only
    c. Inhibit both immediate and late responses
    d. None of the above

True and False: Answer questions 77–81
(A = True, B = False)

77. Beclomethasone is not absorbed into systemic circulation at commonly prescribed dosages.

78. Corticosteroids may prevent the release of mediators from human lung mast cells.

79. Rapid clearance of inhaled steroids from bronchi may account for low incidence of local adverse effects.

80. Corticosteroids may enhance the effects of beta-adrenergic agents.

81. Glucocorticoids may suppress the bronchospastic response to methacholine inhalation challenge.

82. When is the peak serum theophylline level achieved after an intravenous bolus of aminophylline?

    a. Immediately
    b. 30–60 minutes
    c. 2–3 hours
    d. 4–6 hours

83. Indications for endotracheal intubation in status asthmaticus include:

    a. Deterioration of mental status
    b. Increasing PCO_2
    c. Respiratory rate of 30/min
    d. Persistent wheezing
    e. All of the above

84. Which of the following is considered true of the bronchopulmonary inhalation challenge with occupational agents?

    a. A positive response is reflected by a decrement of at least 20–25% in FEV_1

    b. Testing is contraindicated when the patient's FEV_1 is less than 50% of level predicted

    c. Challenge test should begin with doses well below the threshold level

    d. All of the above

    e. None of the above

85. Asthmatics are known to have airways that are exquisitely sensitive to a variety of inhaled substances. Which of the following is true about airway reactivity in asthmatics?

    a. Airway reactivity of asthmatics to histamine occurs at doses that are generally 1/100 that required to produce similar response in normals

    b. Airway reactivity to leukotriene D in asthmatics is slightly delayed in onset and somewhat prolonged in duration

    c. Bronchoconstriction in response to leukotriene D occurs at one-third the dose required to produce a similar response in normals

    d. A and B are true

    e. A–C are true

86. Acute asthma and anaphylactoid phenomenon following the oral intake of the usual dosage of aspirin have been attributed to:

    a. Products of the lipoxygenase pathway of arachidonic acid metabolism

    b. Products of the cyclooxygenase pathway of arachidonic acid metabolism

    c. Direction action on sympathetic nervous system

    d. IgE antibodies

    e. All of the above

    f. None of the above

87. Sulfiting agents have recently been identified as potentially causing acute bronchospasm in asthmatics. Which of the following foods and drinks contain sodium metabisulfite?

    a. Salad dressing made with vinegar

    b. Cheez Whiz

    c. Tang

    d. Wine and beer

    e. All of the above

88. Immunotherapy has been found to be reliably more effective than placebo in the treatment of extrinsic asthma with which of the following agent/agents:

 a. Ragweed pollens
 b. House dust mite
 c. Cat pelt allergens
 d. All of the above
 e. None of the above

89. The best results of immunotherapy can be achieved by using which one of the following techniques:

 a. Coseasonal
 b. Preseasonal
 c. Perennial
 d. All of the above
 e. None of the above

90. Which one of the following statements are true about sensitivity to sulfiting agents?

 a. Approximately 5% of the asthmatics may be sulfite sensitive
 b. Positive response to a provocative sulfite challenge in a nonasthmatic may be manifested by urticaria
 c. Fatal anaphylactoid reactions have been reported
 d. A and B are true
 e. All of the above statements are true

91. Cromolyn sodium has been shown to block provocation of asthma by sulfiting agents.

 a. True
 b. False

92. Epidemiologic risk factors of allergic bronchopulmonary aspergillosis include all except:

 a. Diagnosis in all ages
 b. Highest incidence between ages 20 and 40
 c. Male sex predominence
 d. Almost all patients have preexisting asthma
 e. All of the above

93. Radiographic changes in ABPA are most frequently seen in which area(s)?

 a. Lower lobes
 b. Upper lobes

c. Periphery
d. Hilar
e. (a) and (c)
f. (b) and (d)
g. All of the above
h. None of the above

94. Which of the following may cause a false negative serologic test in ABPA?

a. Theophylline
b. Steroids
c. Beta agonists
d. Cromolyn

95. Bronchospasm occurring during anesthesia induction would most likely be due to:

a. Hydroxyzine
b. Pentobarbital
c. D-Tubocurare
d. Nitrous oxide

96. In an aspirin-intolerant patient with arthritis, which of the following medications might be expected to aggravate the asthma?

a. Indomethacin
b. Motrin
c. Naprosyn
d. Clinoril
e. All of the above

97. Immunotherapy causes:

a. Production of IgG-blocking antibodies
b. Decreased responsiveness of basophils to antigen challenge
c. Decrease in specific IgE levels
d. All of the above
e. None of the above

98. Complications of asthma in children include:

a. Atelectasis
b. Pneumothorax and pneumomediastinum
c. Chest wall deformities
d. Acute respiratory failure
e. All of the above

99. Bitoterol (a new B adrenergic bronchodilator) is different from other beta adrenergic agonists in that it:

    a. Is not itself active but must be hydrolized in the lung to an active compound
    b. Is not absorbed systemically when given by aerosol
    c. Has a half life of 2.5 hours
    d. Works immediately

100. Several clinical studies have demonstrated that ketotifen may have the following properties:

    a. Effective as prophylactic drug for both extrinsic and intrinsic asthmatics
    b. Moderately effective in the treatment of allergic rhinitis
    c. May cause drowsiness
    d. All of the above

ANSWERS

1. a	26. a	51. e	76. c
2. a	27. a	52. c	77. a
3. b	28. a	53. d	78. b
4. a	29. b	54. d	79. a
5. b	30. b	55. d	80. a
6. e	31. b	56. d	81. a
7. c	32. a	57. a	82. b
8. all true	33. d	58. a	83. b
9. c	34. a	59. b	84. d
10. b	35. c	60. a	85. e
11. e	36. b	61. b	86. f
12. a	37. e	62. c	87. e
13. b	38. c	63. c	88. e
14. b	39. a	64. b	89. c
15. c	40. d	65. c	90. e
16. b	41. d	66. c	91. a
17. a	42. b	67. b	92. e
18. b	43. a	68. a	93. f
19. d	44. c	69. a	94. b
20. f	45. e	70. b	95. c
21. a	46. d	71. a	96. e
22. f	47. d	72. a	97. d
23. c	48. c	73. c	98. e
24. e	49. b	74. b	99. a
25. e	50. b	75. d	100. d

Index